Handbook of
Health Behavior Research IV
Relevance for Professionals and
Issues for the Future

Handbook of
Health Behavior Research IV
Relevance for Professionals and Issues for the Future

Edited by

David S. Gochman

University of Louisville
Louisville, Kentucky

Plenum Press • New York and London

Library of Congress Cataloging-in-Publication Data

Handbook of health behavior research / edited by David S. Gochman.
       p.   cm.
     Includes bibliographical references and indexes.
     Contents: I. Personal and social determinants   II. Provider
determinants -- III. Demography, development, and diversity --
IV. Relevance for professionals and issues for the future.
     ISBN 0-306-45443-2 (I). -- ISBN 0-306-45444-0 (II). -- ISBN
0-306-45445-9 (III). -- ISBN 0-306-45446-7 (IV)
     1. Health behavior. 2. Health behavior--Research.   I. Gochman,
David S.
     [DNLM: 1. Health Behavior--handbooks. 2. Research--handbooks.   W
49 H236 1997]
     RA776.9.H363   1997
     613--dc21
     DNLM/DLC
     for Library of Congress   97-14565
                                                                   CIP

ISBN 0-306-45446-7

© 1997 Plenum Press, New York
A Division of Plenum Publishing Corporation
233 Spring Street, New York, N. Y. 10013

http://www.plenum.com

Printed in the United States of America

DEDICATION

Throughout my career I have been helped and encouraged by many persons. There are a few whose help was so special that my debt to them is enormous. It is in recognition of what I owe them that this *Handbook* is dedicated to Zelda S. Ackerman, O. J. Harvey, and D. Eldridge McBride, and to the memories of John H. Russel, William A. Scott, and John P. Kirscht. Mrs. Ackerman, my advisor in New York City's High School of Music and Art (now LaGuardia High School), facilitated my early entrance into academia. "Mac" McBride and John Russel, inspired and committed teachers, advisors, and counselors during my formative years at Shimer College, served as role models and continued as my friends over the decades. Bill Scott and O. J. Harvey were encouraging and supportive advisors during my graduate training at the University of Colorado. Bill taught me methodological rigor and innovation, and O. J. encouraged me to think in new and divergent ways. Both of them maintained high standards for their own performance, and demanded no less from me and others.

Jack Kirscht was a pioneer in health behavior research, a community activist, and a person of great wit, humor, and charm. In 1967 he convinced me to come to the University of Michigan's School of Public Health and to bring my research interests in cognitive development and structure to the area of health behavior. He was also a contributor to my 1988 book. Health behavior research lost a giant with his untimely death. He is very much missed by many as a friend and colleague and as a teacher and scholar.

Contributors

Tom Baranowski, Department of Behavioral Science, M. D. Anderson Cancer Center, University of Texas at Houston, Houston, Texas 77030

Carolyn L. Blue, Helen R. Johnson School of Nursing, Purdue University, West Lafayette, Indiana 47907-1337

Jo A. Brooks, Helen R. Johnson School of Nursing, Purdue University, West Lafayette, Indiana 47907-1337

John G. Bruhn, Provost and Dean, Pennsylvania State University at Harrisburg, Middletown, Pennsylvania 17057-4898

David R. Buchanan, School of Public Health and Health Sciences, University of Massachusetts, Amherst, Massachusetts 01003

Henry P. Cole, Behavioral Research Aspects of Safety and Health (BRASH) Working Group, University of Kentucky, Lexington, Kentucky 40506-0350

K. Michael Cummings, Department of Cancer Control and Epidemiology, Roswell Park Cancer Institute, Buffalo, New York 14263

Robert H. Daugherty, 4403 Lynnbrook Drive, Louisville, Kentucky 40220

Elizabeth W. Edmundson, Department of Kinesiology and Health Education, University of Texas at Austin, Austin, Texas 78712

Ann Randolph Flipse, Clinical Skills Program, University of Miami School of Medicine, Miami, Florida 33101

June A. Flora, Stanford Center for Research in Disease Prevention, Stanford University School of Medicine, Palo Alto, California 93404-1825

Eugene B. Gallagher, Department of Behavioral Science, University of Kentucky College of Medicine, Lexington, Kentucky 40536-0086

Helen C. Gift, National Institute of Dental Research, National Institutes of Health, Bethesda, Maryland 20892-6401

Karen Glanz, Cancer Research Center of Hawaii, University of Hawaii, Honolulu, Hawaii 96813

David S. Gochman, Kent School of Social Work, University of Louisville, Louisville, Kentucky 40292

Marsha Davis Hearn, Department of Nutrition and Dietetics, Georgia State University, Atlanta, Georgia 30303

G. Christian Jernstedt, Department of Psychology and C. Everett Koop Institute, Dartmouth College, Hanover, New Hampshire 03755

Steven H. Kelder, School of Public Health, University of Texas Health Science Center at Houston, Houston, Texas 77225

Rona L. Levy, School of Social Work, University of Washington, Seattle, Washington 98105-6299

Leslie A. Lytle, Division of Epidemiology, School of Public Health, University of Minnesota, Minneapolis, Minnesota 55454-1015

Maggie L. Moore-West, Department of Family and Community Medicine, Dartmouth Medical School, Hanover, New Hampshire 03755

Tore Nilstun, Department of Medical Ethics, University of Lund, S-222 22 Lund, Sweden

Joseph F. O'Donnell, Department of Medicine, Dartmouth Medical School, Hanover, New Hampshire 03755

Brian Oldenburg, School of Public Health, Queensland University of Technology, Red Hill, Queensland 4059, Australia

Virginia A. Reed, Department of Psychology, Dartmouth College, Hanover, New Hampshire 03755

Leon S. Robertson, Yale University and Nanlee Research, Branford, Connecticut 06405-5115

Caroline Schooler, Stanford Center for Research in Disease Prevention, Stanford University School of Medicine, Palo Alto, California 93404-1825

James W. Swinehart, Public Communication Resources, 1310 Bolton Road, Pelham Manor, New York 10803-3602

B. Alexander White, Kaiser Permanente, Portland, Oregon 97227-1098

H. Jean C. Wiese, Department of Behavioral Science, University of Kentucky College of Medicine, Lexington, Kentucky 40536-0086

Preface to All Volumes

THE STATE OF THE ART

The *primary* objective of this *Handbook* is to provide statements about health behavior research as a basic body of knowledge moving into the 21st century. It is expected that the *Handbook* will remain in use and current through 2005, at least. The *Handbook* presents a broad and representative selection of mid-1990s health behavior findings and concepts in a single work. While texts and books of readings are available in related areas, such as health psychology (e.g., DiMatteo, 1991; Stone et al., 1987), medical anthropology (e.g., McElroy & Townsend, 1989; Nichter, 1992), medical sociology (e.g., Cockerham, 1995; Helman, 1990; Wolinsky, 1988), behavioral health (e.g., Matarazzo, Weiss, Herd, Miller, & Weiss, 1984), behavioral risk factors (e.g., Hamburg, Elliott, & Parron, 1982), and changing health behaviors (Shumaker et al., 1990), none of these works was intended to address basic research-generated knowledge of health behavior, and none was intended to transcend individual disciplines. Accordingly, none of these works presents a broad and representative spectrum of basic health behavior research reflecting multidisciplinary activities. One work with a title identical to this one but for one word, the *Handbook of Health Behavior Change* (Shumaker et al., 1990), deals almost exclusively with applications. This *Handbook* thus presents the reader with the "state of the art" in health behavior research, something not found elsewhere.

In the context of this primary objective, it was not intended that the chapters be journal articles. Authors were encouraged to provide extensive coverage of their topics and to provide original findings to the degree that such findings were relevant. They were not encouraged to write research reports, and the reader should not expect the chapters to read as though they were journal articles.

HEALTH BEHAVIOR AS BASIC RESEARCH

Health behavior is not a long-established, traditional area of inquiry, comparable to chemistry or psychology, but a newly emerging interdisciplinary and multidisciplinary one. Health behavior is still establishing its identity as a domain of scientific research.

Although the earlier work (Gochman, 1988) that helped define it is now nearly a decade old, there are still relatively few institutional or organizational structures, i.e., departments and programs, that reflect the field, and few books and no journals are directed at it.

A *second* objective of the *Handbook* is to reaffirm the identity of health behavior and help secure its position as an important area of basic research, worthy of being studied in its own right. In the context of their discussion of the emergence of medical anthropology, Foster and Anderson (1978, pp. 2–3) stated: "When a sufficient number of researchers focus on the same, or related, topics, and as significant new data begin to appear, the stage is set for the emergence of a new discipline or subdiscipline. But some spark is essential to coalesce these emerging interests around a common focus; usually, it seems, an appropriate name supplies this spark." It is hoped that this *Handbook* will provide such a spark.

LEVELS OF ANALYSIS

Personal, Social, and Provider Determinants

A *third* objective, very much related to the first two, is to view health behavior research as transcending particular behaviors, specific illnesses or health problems or strategies for intervention, or single sets of determinants. One major way of achieving this objective is to look at health behavior in transaction with a range of personal, social systems: as an outcome or product, as well as a factor that affects these systems (in this context, the term *system* is often used interchangeably with *unit* or *entity*), rather than primarily as a set of risk factors or as targets for interventions directed at behavioral change. Volumes I and II of this *Handbook* thus deal largely with characteristics of the system of concern, and focus on specific health behaviors, or specific health problems or conditions, as ways of demonstrating the impact of these systems.

Volume I begins with conceptualizations of health and health behavior and then moves from smaller to larger systems, demonstrating how health behavior is determined by—and often in transaction with—personal, family, social, institutional and community, and cultural factors. These levels of analysis cannot be neatly differentiated, and at times the distinctions between them are arbitrary: Families, organizations, and institutions are all social systems. Moreover, although all individuals differ in their responses to and interpretations of family, social, and cultural norms, personalities and cognitive structures nonetheless reflect family, social, and cultural factors; additionally, families, social groupings, and organizations all reflect elements of the culture in which they exist. Furthermore, the categorizing and sequencing of sections and chapters in no way reflect an attempt to exclude material that deals with other levels of determinants; they serve primarily to facilitate focusing more on one of these determinants than on others. Volume I concludes with an integration that relates categories of health behaviors to characteristics of personal and social systems, identifies common themes, and suggests future research directions.

Since so much of health behavior is determined by providers—the health professionals and institutions that comprise the care delivery system—Volume II examines the way encounters with health providers determine health behaviors, and how health behaviors and the providers reciprocally affect one another. Volume II begins with an overview section on communication, continues with a section on interactional and structural determinants, i.e., professional characteristics, perceptions, power, and role relations, and organizational, locational, and environmental factors; and then presents major sections on the impact of provider characteristics on adherence to and acceptance of both disease-focused and lifestyle regimens.

Populations and Professional Applications

Volume III begins with an overview section on the demography of health behavior and continues with an examination of health behaviors in a range of populations selected on the basis either of the life-span continuum; of a health status risk due to an existing condition, a socially constructed label, or restrictive economic and environmental conditions; or of membership in defined communities. Volume IV examines the relevance of knowledge generated by health behavior research for the training and clinical (and other) practice activities of health professionals; for health services management and health policy; and for planned applications in school, family, community and workplace settings, and the media. Volume IV aims to position health behavior research in the 21st century through a discussion of the four major disciplines that inform health behavior research: health psychology, medical anthropology, medical geography, and medical sociology. Volume IV also presents a working draft of a taxonomy of health behavior and of a matrix framework for organizing health behavior knowledge.

Glossary and Index

Each of the volumes concludes with a glossary of health behavior concepts and definitions, and an index. Both of these reflect the contents of the entire *Handbook*.

A FRAMEWORK FOR ORGANIZING HEALTH BEHAVIOR KNOWLEDGE: A WORK IN PROGRESS

A Taxonomy for Health Behavior

Reviewing the contributed chapters in a volume with the editorial objective of integration led to the development of a "work in progress" taxonomy of health behaviors that became a primary organizing principle for the final chapter of each of the first three volumes. The taxonomy continued to evolve from Volume I to Volume III. The integration of Volume I would have been modified and organized slightly differently had it been written *after* those for Volumes II and III, but the fundamentals remained the same. Virtually all of the health behavior findings reported could be subsumed under one of six categories: health cognitions; care seeking; risk behaviors; lifestyle; responses to illness, including adherence; and preventive, protective, and safety behaviors.

A Matrix Framework

The working taxonomy appears in a different way in Volume IV. With one minor modification—the distinction between nonaddictive and addictive risk behaviors—it combines with the range of personal and social systems used as organizing principles in Volumes I and II, and in the integration chapters for Volumes I through III, to become part of a matrix framework for organizing health behavior knowledge. This framework is presented in Chapter 20 of Volume IV, entitled "Health Behavior Research, Cognate Disciplines, Future Identity, and an Organizing Matrix: An Integration of Perspectives."

DIVERSITY OF PERSPECTIVES

A *fourth* objective is to assure that the reader is exposed to varied perspectives in conceptual models, disciplines, populations, and methods, as well as to nonmedical frames of reference. The *Handbook* exposes the reader to a range of theories and models. The contributors bring expertise from their training or professional involvements in varied disciplines, including (in alphabetical order) anthropology, biology, communications, dentistry, education, engineering, ethics, geography, health management and policy, health promotion and health education, medicine, nursing, psychiatry, psychology, public health, social work, and sociology.

DIVERSITY OF READERS

A *fifth* objective is to assure the relevance of the *Handbook* for persons in a number of fields who are interested in issues related to research in health behavior. The potential readership includes researchers in the social and behavioral sciences who want to know more about health behavior in general, or particular aspects of it, or who want to develop their own health behavior research; students in courses that integrate social and behavioral science and health, in disciplines such as anthropology, psychology, and sociology, and in professional programs in dentistry, medicine (including psychiatry), nursing, public health, and social work; professionals who provide, plan, implement, and evaluate health services and programs: fitness and exercise physiologists; family planners; health educators and promoters; health managers; health planners; hospital administrators; nutritionists; pharmacists; physicians in community and family practice; physiatrists; public health dentists, nurses, physicians; rehabilitation therapists; social workers; and so forth.

THE PRACTICAL RELEVANCE OF HEALTH BEHAVIOR RESEARCH

The practical value of increasing knowledge and understanding of health behavior through rigorous, systematic research is implicit in the grave concern with health status in many contemporary societies. Solutions to an appreciable number of health problems require large-scale efforts at local, regional, and national levels to develop and enforce policies to control, minimize, and ultimately reduce air, land, and water pollution; the hazards of transportation; and the risks of the workplace environment. Many of these solutions transcend individual health behaviors. Solutions to other health problems, however, involve policies, programs, and processes that interact with the personal health behavior of individuals and the population at large, in their family, social, workplace, institutional, and community milieus.

As material in Volume IV demonstrates, attempts to change individual health behaviors, either through individual therapeutic interventions or through larger-scale health promotion or health education programs, have been less than impressive. Many attempts are purely programmatic, hastily conceived, and lacking in theoretical rationale or empirical foundation. A major reason for this is the lack of *basic* knowledge about the target behaviors, about the contexts in which they occur, and about the factors that determine and stabilize them. Basic research in health behavior, aside from being worthy of study in its own right, may very well increase the effectiveness of interventions and programs designed to bring about behavioral change.

DELIBERATE OMISSIONS

Notably absent from the *Handbook* are chapters devoted to topics such as "Type A" personality, psychosomatics, and stress. While these considerations may be linked to health status, and sometimes to health behavior, they have been omitted because they are more generally models for understanding the etiology of disease and illnesses. Furthermore, while "holism" has become a catchword among many who disavow the traditional medical model, the term has come to include charlatanism and cultism, as well as some impressive approaches to treatment. At present, it remains more a statement of faith suggesting future research alternatives than a body of well-thought-through, rigorously conducted research. Moreover, caution against a reverse "ethno-centrism" and overly romanticized views of non-high-technological medicine is cogently provided by Eisenberg and Kleinman (1981). In their words (Eisenberg & Kleinman, 1981, p. 10): "Healing ceremonies can be efficacious, but hardly substitute for antibiotics or surgery." Accordingly, there is no section on "holism" or "holistic medicine" or "holistic health" in the *Handbook*.

REFERENCES

Cockerham, W. C. (1995). *Medical sociology* (6th ed.). Englewood Cliffs, NJ: Simon & Schuster.

DiMatteo, M. R. (1991). *The psychology of health, illness, and medical care: An individual perspective.* Belmont, CA: Brooks/Cole.

Eisenberg, L., & Kleinman, A. (Eds.). (1981). *The relevance of social science for medicine.* Dordrecht, Netherlands: Reidel.

Foster, G. M., & Anderson, B. G. (1978). *Medical anthropology.* New York: Wiley.

Gochman, D. S. (Ed.). (1988). *Health behavior: Emerging research perspectives.* New York: Plenum Press.

Hamburg, D. A., Elliott, G. R., & Parron, D. L. (Eds.). (1982). *Health and behavior: Frontiers of research in the biobehavioral sciences.* Washington, DC: National Academy Press.

Helman, C. G. (1990). *Culture, health and illness* (2nd ed.). London: Wright/Butterworth.

Matarazzo, J. D., Weiss, S. M., Herd, J. A., Miller, N. E., & Weiss, S. M. (Eds.). (1984). *Behavioral health: A handbook of health enhancement and disease prevention.* New York: Wiley.

McElroy, A., & Townsend, P. K. (1989). *Medical anthropology in ecological perspective* (2nd ed.). Boulder, CO: Westview.

Nichter, M. (Ed.). (1992). *Anthropological approaches to the study of ethnomedicine.* Amsterdam, Netherlands: Gordon and Breach Science Publishers.

Shumaker, S.A., Schron, E. B., Ockene, J. K., Parker, C. T., Probstfield, J. L., & Wolle, J. M. (Eds.). (1990). *The handbook of health behavior change.* New York: Springer.

Stone, G. C., Weiss, S. M., Matarazzo, J. D., Miller, N. E., Rodin, J., Belar, C. D., Follick, M. J., & Singer, J. E. (Eds.). (1987). *Health psychology: A discipline and a profession.* Chicago: University of Chicago Press.

Wolinsky, F. D. (1988). *The sociology of health: Principles, practitioners, and issues* (2nd ed.). Belmont, CA: Wadsworth.

Preface to Volume IV

Volume IV deals explicitly (and almost exclusively) with ways in which knowledge generated by health behavior research is relevant to health professionals. A number of chapters in Volumes I through III mention the application of basic health behavior knowledge with implications for professional practice. Chapters in Volume II, dealing with communication (Chapter 1), interactional and structural determinants (Chapters 2 through 5), and adherence to disease-focused and lifestyle regimens (Chapters 6 through 20), consider many linkages between health behavior knowledge and clinical issues such as patient satisfaction, care seeking, and increasing acceptance of, and participation in, disease-reducing and health-advancing programs. Chapters in Volume III dealing with development (especially Chapters 3 and 4) and with groups "at risk" (especially Chapters 6 through 13) consider linkages between health behavior knowledge and behavioral changes that result from planned interventions. The relevance of such knowledge, however, was not itself the major thrust of these discussions.

In contrast, Part I of Volume IV deals explicitly with the relevance of health behavior knowledge for the education, training, and clinical practice of health professionals; Part II with its relevance for health managers and policy makers; and Part III with its relevance for health promotion and health education interventions in a range of settings.

In Part IV, Chapter 19 provides an integration of the contributed material on applications and relevance. Chapter 20 provides an integrative analysis of the major disciplines that generate health behavior research, including a matrix framework for organizing health behavior knowledge and a view toward the future.

The glossary integrates concepts and definitions used throughout all four volumes of this *Handbook*.

Acknowledgments

Many persons provided greatly valued assistance during the nearly four years from the time the *Handbook of Health Behavior Research* was conceptualized until its publication, and I owe all of them my thanks. The substantial help I received from some of them merits special recognition. Among the support staff at the Raymond A. Kent School, I especially wish to thank Shannon R. Daniels and Kelley E. Davis for their expeditious and careful photocopying of what must have seemed like tons of manuscripts, Jane Isert for her dedication in assuring that calls and mail from contributors and from the publisher reached me in a timely way, and Sally Montreuil-Palmarini for expediting mailings of material to contributors.

Among the highly professional and committed staff at the University of Louisville's Ekstrom Library, special thanks go to all of the reference librarians, and particularly to Carmen Embry (now at Barrier Islands Art Center) for some insightful content suggestions; Sharon Edge for her expediting access to materials; and S. Kay Womack (now at the University of Oklahoma) for her astute and knowledgeable guidance through computer and other literature searches, particularly in areas in which little had been written that was adequately indexed.

Thomas R. Lawson, Director of the Kent School, deserves recognition for his continued encouragement of my scholarly activities, his efforts in securing a sabbatical leave for me to assure the *Handbook*'s timely completion, and his generosity in providing necessary supplies and personnel resources.

A great debt is owed to all of the authors whose scholarly chapters grace the *Handbook*, and add immeasurably to its value, for the care they devoted to their work, and for their receptivity and constructive responses to the high density of editorial suggestions made throughout the *Handbook*'s progress. A number of authors and others also provided suggestions about potential contributors for several topics. Among those whose help in this quest was exceptional were M. Robin DiMatteo, Eugene B. Gallagher, Russell E. Glasgow, Michael R. Kauth, Jeffrey Kelley, James E. Maddux, Lillian C. Milanof, R. Prasaad Steiner, and David P. Willis.

Gene Gallagher, along with Zeev Ben-Sira (whose untimely death occurred prior to the final revision of his chapter), John G. Bruhn, Patricia J. Bush, Henry P. Cole, Reed Geertsen, Marie R. Haug, Richard R. Lau, Alexander Segall, and Ingrid Waldron had all contributed to the 1988 book. Their willingness to contribute anew to this one is most appreciated.

Finally, Richard Millikan merits special recognition for the excellence of his copyediting work, his ability to perceive issues that cross-cut the four volumes, and for his skill in helping me clarify my own thinking; and Eliot Werner, Executive Editor at Plenum Publishing Corporation, deserves special thanks for his vision and encouragement in the area of health behavior research, for his faith in the value of the *Handbook*, and for being laid back and calming in the face of my "overfunctioning" and obsessive-compulsivity.

Contents

Chapter 3.   Health Behavior Research: What Physicians Must Know   43

Ann Randolph Flipse

**Chapter 4.   Health Behavior Research and Medical Training and
                Practice: A Social Context** **53**

H. Jean C. Wiese and Eugene B. Gallagher

Chapter 8. **Relevance of Health Behavior Research to Health Promotion and Health Education** 143

Karen Glanz and Brian Oldenburg

Chapter 9. **Relevance of Health Behavior Research to Public Health Professionals** 163

David R. Buchanan

I
PROFESSIONAL TRAINING AND PRACTICE

The need for increasing health behavior content in the training of health professionals, particularly in medicine and dentistry but not in these areas alone, has long been documented. (Although health behavior is often generically referred to as social and behavioral science content, it is a distinct subset of this broader domain and should not be confounded with it.) Health professionals' perceptions of their patients (e.g., Tannenbaum, Weschler, & Massarik, 1961/1975); communication with patients (e.g., Elder, 1963/1975), including the relationship between social factors and communication (e.g., Schatzman & Strauss, 1975); and different models of professional–patient interaction (e.g., Szasz & Hollender, 1956/1975) were all identified in the 1950s and 1960s as critically relevant to professional practice and thus appropriate targets for training.

In advocating a new practice paradigm and new competencies for the future, Bruhn's overview (Chapter 1) discusses a number of ways in which knowledge generated by health behavior research is relevant to the training and practice of a range of health professions. The specific relevance of health behavior research for training and practice in medicine, nursing, social work, dentistry, health promotion and health education, and public health is the major focus of Part I.

MEDICINE

The narrow scientism of the medical curriculum, which was indicted years ago for its failure to include a broad spectrum of social and behavioral science knowledge (e.g., Millon, 1975), continues to typify the training and professional socialization of physicians. Paradoxically, despite numerous "reforms," medical education has changed very little; its focus on technology and the "hard" sciences marginalizes any efforts to introduce humanistic or social content (Bloom, 1988; Conrad, 1988). While there remains "concern for teaching physicians the humanistic, psychosocial, and cultural aspects of patient care" (Light, 1988, p. 312), little has been changed to accomplish this objective. Moreover, students apparently acquire methods of "academic triage" to figure out what their instructors really want them to know and thus discard material related to the social context of medicine (Conrad, 1988, pp. 324–325). By the time they complete their training, they have been well socialized into the medical model. British data, for example, indicate that as they advance through their training, medical students increasingly use the disease concept to embrace a larger range of conditions, showing the impact of the "scientific" disease

1

model in their programs (Stefan & McManus, 1989).

In their cogent overview of medical practice, Eisenberg and Kleinman (1981) noted the historical concern about physicians who demonstrate an overly narrow disease focus, rather than a broader, more person-oriented one. They argued, however, that this divergence in perspectives reflected community and societal factors more than flaws in medical education. They noted, though, that the emphasis in contemporary medical education on increased specialization and increased technology has exacerbated this divergence, and they expressed concern that medical interventions may be less effective because of it. They advocate increased social and behavioral science content in medical training as a way of countering this narrowness and thereby assuring that medicine can deliver its technological skills with increasing effectiveness.

While a late 1980s survey showed that over 80% of American and Canadian medical programs include some content in social or behavioral sciences, medical humanities, or behavioral medicine, the hours of instruction in these areas comprised less than 5% of total teaching time in any program (Baumgart & Costello, 1988). Moreover, no program listed content labeled as "health behavior." Departments of preventive medicine, the programs of which would presumably be based to a far greater degree than others on health behavior content, have historically played only minor or marginal roles in medical curricula (Baumgart & Costello, 1988).

Insights about how "feeling" components are "socialized out" of medical training are provided by Hafferty's (1988) analyses of cadaver humor. Hafferty notes that the tradition of cadaver humor fosters emotional toughness; it serves to eliminate unacceptable expressions of anxiety and fear. Noting the increasing number of women enrolled in medical schools, Hafferty observes that cadaver humor decreasingly depicts women as passive, pliant victims. Hornig-Rohan (1986) wrote as a medical student that medical training glosses over problems that professionals

will eventually face in dealing with patients' personalities, problems, life events, and deaths.

Grinker (1975) argues for a "systems theory" approach to medical thinking and attacks the historical "atomistic" perspective of medicine and medical training that results in patients being thought of as specific disorders or organs. He urges that patients' emotions and thoughts, their frustrations, disappointments, hopelessness, and other behavioral manifestations be considered along with their somatic complaint or symptom. Knowles (1968/1975) stated as far back as 1968 that "... medicine is a social as well as a physical and biological science ... and that it needs the humanities and social sciences and the effects of their study as never before in ... history ..." (p. 7). Such content, he urged, should be part of the premedical program, and the medical curriculum as well. Knowles identified historical barriers that have prevented this from happening, but encouraged medical education to incorporate this content nonetheless.

Asserting that "never has the time been more opportune for reexamination of the social science curiculum in medical education," MacLeod and McCullough (1994, p. 1368) identified a range of relevant health behavior knowledge from health psychology, medical anthropology, medical geography, and medical sociology, including the social determinants of health, such as its linkages to socioeconomic status, and "the means by which we may achieve greater user involvement in health decision making" (p. 1370).

The social and organizational environments of medical education impede the changes that are necessary to introduce health behavior content. These environmental constraints include the external pressures on medical schools, such as sources of funds, and linkages with pharmaceutical houses that serve as barriers to curricular change, as well as internal issues such as the lack of a consensus about such content on the part of medical school faculties (Bloom, 1988). Medical students tend to strengthen their identification with other physicians rather than to maintain any prior inclination to identify with their patients (Conrad, 1988). MacLeod and Mc-Cullough (1994), arguing that medical schools do not provide attractive environments for behavioral and social scientists, suggest that universities offering health professional training have a responsibility to maintain an environment that encourages collaboration, cross-fertilization, and integration of multidisciplinary interests relevant to health.

Specific Content.   More specific to health behavior, Mechanic and Newton (1965/1975) urge, for example, that physicians need to understand dimensions of illness behavior, the significance to the patient of the presenting symptoms, the dynamics of the process of eliciting relevant information from patients, and the social and institutional context in which medicine is practiced and further urge that medical education should incorporate such content. Medical training runs counter to generating "caring" behaviors. Very little in the curriculum focuses on physician–patient interaction; technical incompetence is systematically criticized, but inadequate bedside manner is not (Conrad, 1988).

Petersdorf and Feinstein (1981) documented the inclusion of medical sociology content in medical curricula, defining medical sociology to include a broad range of health behavior topics, including personal, familial, societal, institutional, and community effects on health and illness, as well as the interpersonal aspects of medical practice. Although this content was included in some way in a number of curricula, it was absent from a far larger portion. Petersdorf and Feinstein further noted that the enthusiastic supporters of medical sociology content "were not nearly as eloquent in expounding their positive views, as the detractors were in relieving themselves of their negative biases" (p. 40).

Kendall and Reader (1988) provided concise analyses of some of the innovations undertaken by a select group of medical schools between the 1950s and 1980s, as well as evaluations of their impact and endurance. Evidence suggests that reforms tend to be less than widespread or permanent. While some social science content either was included or helped frame the innovations, health behavior content did not appear to have had any prominent role in the reforms.

Segall (1984), addressing the importance of educating physicians for clinical prevention, identified physician–patient interactions—including communication and decision processes—support of family and friends, and patient motivation as areas in which physicians require increased knowledge and sensitivity and as areas that should be targets of medical school curricula.

The three chapters by Reed, Moore-West, Jernstedt, and O'Donnell (Chapter 2), Flipse (Chapter 3), and Wiese and Gallagher (Chapter 4) amplify at length the relevance of health behavior research for medical training and practice and the impediments to reforming medical education and training. The three chapters are highly consistent and convergent; each discusses selected health behavior theoretical models as well as the importance of health behavior knowledge for understanding the social, ethnic, and cultural context of medicine.

Each chapter identifies an innovative curriculum model that incorporates health behavior research, yet each chapter highlights some special area. Reed and her colleagues emphasize how health behavior research points to the importance of physician communication skills and how these skills, in turn, facilitate the imparting of health behavior information to patients. Flipse highlights the ethnic and social context in which patient care occurs, and Wiese and Gallagher point to increasing consumerism and external market influences on medicine.

NURSING

Nursing as a profession has been far more hospitable than medicine to social and behavioral science content and to knowledge generated by health behavior research. In the late 1980s, Baumgart and Costello (1988) observed that health behavior content was becoming a reality, despite lack of consensus about ensuring minimum guidelines. Drawing upon a critical examination of the health belief model as well as on application of the Triandis model to health and illness, Facione (1993) demonstrated the utility of health behavior content for culturally sensitive nursing. Health behavior knowledge about patients' needs for information, gathered through the Patient Learning Need Scale (Bubela et al., 1990), was used to assist nurses in discharge planning for hospitalized patients. Concepts from health behavior models were integrated with nursing models to develop the health-promoting self-care system model to advance patients' self-care behaviors (Simmons, 1990). Drawing upon health behavior data, Butterfield (1990) challenged nurses to focus on changes in the larger social, political, and economic systems as well as in the individual patient.

In Chapter 5, Blue and Brooks provide additional documentation of the degree to which health behavior content has increasingly become part of professional socialization in nursing, and how nursing has integrated health behavior concepts and models in the development of its own theories for both clinical and community practice.

SOCIAL WORK

Social work has historically been responsible for the "social component" in illness, i.e., for understanding the personal, family, social, institutional, and cultural contexts in which health actions occur (e.g., Bartlett, 1961). Social work borrows concepts from a number of disciplines, and in the health field it borrows broadly from anthropology, medicine (including psychiatry), public health, psychology, and sociology. It has especially been concerned with the meaning of illness for patients and their families, recognizing that the impact of illness can have "as many different meanings as there are possible combinations of such factors as personality development, social conditions, environmental pressures, ways

of becoming ill or handicapped, methods of treatment, and possible end results" (Elledge, 1953, p. 49, cited in Bartlett, 1961, p. 140). Social work has also had major responsibility for assuring adequate communication between professionals and patients and among professionals themselves (Bartlett, 1961; Dinerman, 1979). Moreover, social work has a major responsibility for teaching physicians about the total social experience of the patient, particularly the patient's cultural, social, familial, and vocational background, and about the linkage between these influences and the patient's problem (e.g., Thomson, 1973).

Traditionally, however, social work has been reluctant to use empirical knowledge to bolster its practice, preferring instead to use concepts broadly without thinking critically about their validity. Social work has changed since the mid-1980s and, as a result of the continually changing curricular standards of the Council on Social Work Education, is becoming increasingly committed to research and empiricism. This increasing commitment should make social work more receptive to health behavior knowledge.

In Chapter 6, Levy identifies critical areas of social work practice that can be served by health behavior research. At the same time, she notes that there is little specific attention given to health behavior in professional training. (The editor of this *Handbook* offers one of the few courses in health behavior research as a foundation for direct, family, agency, and community-level social work interventions.)

DENTISTRY

Some years ago, Kegeles and Cohen (1971) concluded that social science research had been a "humanizing force for the profession" of dentistry and anticipated that incremental research findings would ultimately have an impact upon dental curricula. They noted then, however, that social science research findings had not had any appreciable impact upon dental education, nor had social scientists teaching within dental schools, although the number of social scientists employed in dental contexts had increased. In the years since Kegeles and Cohen's report, there has been little appreciable change in the degree to which health behavior knowledge has been incorporated in the training of dental professionals. In Chapter 7, Gift and White demonstrate the relevance of health behavior content for a broad range of professional oral health activities and note, as well, the degree to which dentistry's commitment to technology impedes the incorporation of nontechnological material in professional training and clinical and community dentistry.

HEALTH PROMOTION AND HEALTH EDUCATION

Professional training programs in health promotion and health education (HP/HE) would seem to be based systematically on health behavior knowledge. While such content is assuredly part of these programs, its formalization and institutionalization varies with the level of the program. In Chapter 8, Glanz and Oldenburg note the increase in coverage of health behavior knowledge in HP/HE since the early 1980s, discuss its role in training, and demonstrate its relevance for professional activities. In Part III, Kelder, Edmundson, and Lytle (Chapter 14), Schooler and Flora (Chapter 15), Baranowski and Hearn (Chapter 16), Cole (Chapter 17), and Swinehart (Chapter 18) address specific planned HP/HE applications.

PUBLIC HEALTH

In the controversy about whether public health training should be narrowly defined and relocated within medical schools or whether it should remain more broadly defined and located in schools of public health that are autonomous of medical training (Kahn & Tollman, 1992), proponents of the latter position stress the impor-

tance of promoting public health as a multidisciplinary professional calling that would be considerably limited in the patient/illness-centered contexts of medical schools. For these purposes, professional training must emphasize not only the "hard" science and technology base that underlies public health interventions, but also the social and behavioral science knowledge relevant to target populations. Kahn and Tollman (1992) reported survey data showing that students and alumni both endorse increased behavioral science content. In Chapter 9, Buchanan discusses the role of health behavior knowledge in public health training and practice in epidemiology and biostatistics, environmental health, nutrition, exercise, occupational health, maternal and child health, and international health.

REFERENCES

Bartlett, H. M. (1961). *Social work practice in the health field*. New York: National Association of Social Workers.

Baumgart, A. J., & Costello, E. A. (1988). Health behavior research and the training of health professionals. In D. S. Gochman (Ed.), *Health behavior: Emerging research perspectives* (pp. 363–379). New York: Plenum Press.

Bloom, S. W. (1988). Stucture and ideology in medical education: An analysis of resistance to change. *Journal of Health and Social Behavior, 29*, 294–306.

Bubela, N., Galloway, S., McCay, E., McKibbon, A., Nagle, L., Pringle, D., Ross, E., & Shamian, J. (1990). Factors influencing patients' informational needs at time of hospital discharge. *Patient Education and Counseling, 16*, 21–28.

Butterfield, P. G. (1990). Thinking upstream: Nurturing a conceptual understanding of the societal context of health behavior. *Advances in Nursing Science, 12*(2), 1–8.

Conrad, P. (1988). Learning to doctor: Reflections on recent accounts of the medical school years. *Journal of Health and Social Behavior, 29*, 323–332.

Dinerman, M. (1979). In sickness and in health: Future social work roles. *Health and Social Work, 4*(2), 6–22.

Eisenberg, L., & Kleinman, A. (Eds.). (1981). *The relevance of social science for medicine*. Dordrecht, Holland: Reidel.

Elder, R. G. (1963/1975). What is the patient saying? In T. Millon (Ed.), *Medical behavioral science* (pp. 411–417). Philadelphia: W. B. Saunders. [Reprinted from *Nursing Forum*, 1963, *2*, 25–37.]

Elledge, C. H. (1953). The meaning of illness. *Medical Social Work, 2*(2), 49.

Facione, N. C. (1993). The Triandis model for the study of health and illness behavior: A social behavior theory with sensitivity to diversity. *Advances in Nursing Science*, *15*(3), 49–58.

Grinker, R. R., Sr. (1975). Biomedical education as a system. In T. Millon (Ed.), *Medical behavioral science* (pp. 10–18). Philadelphia: W. B. Saunders.

Hafferty, F. W. (1988). Cadaver stories and the emotional socialization of medical students. *Journal of Health and Social Behavior, 29*, 344–356.

Hornig-Rohan, M. (1986). Developing physicians for the 21st century: The future of medicine/36th Annual Convention of the American Medical Student Association. *Advances, Institute for the Advancement of Health, 3*(2), 62–67.

Kahn, K., & Tollman, S. M. (1992). Planning professional education at schools of public health. *American Journal of Public Health, 82*, 1653–1657.

Kegeles, S. S., & Cohen, L. K. (1971). *Role of social sciences in dentistry*. In N. D. Richards & L. K. Cohen (Eds.), *Social sciences and dentistry: A critical bibliography* (pp. 365–377). The Hague: A. Sijthoff.

Kendall, P. L., & Reader, G. G. (1988). Innovations in medical education of the 1950s contrasted with those of the 1970s and 1980s. *Journal of Health and Social Behavior, 29*, 279–293.

Knowles, J. H. (1968/1975). Medical education and the rationalization of health services. In T. Millon (Ed.), *Medical behavioral science* (pp. 5–10). Philadelphia: W. B. Saunders. [Reprinted from J. H. Knowles (Ed.), *Views of medical education and medical care*, 1968, Cambridge: Harvard University Press.]

Light, D. W. (1988). Toward a new sociology of medical education. *Journal of Health and Social Behavior, 29*, 307–322.

MacLeod, S. M., & McCullough, H. N. (1994). Social science education as a component of medical training. *Social Science and Medicine, 39*, 1367–1373.

Mechanic, D., & Newton, M. (1965/1975). Social considerations in medical education: Points of convergence between medicine and behavioral science. In T. Millon (Ed.), *Medical behavioral science* (pp. 19–28). Philadelphia: W. B. Saunders. [Reprinted from *Journal of Chronic Diseases, 18*, 291–301.]

Millon, T. (1975). Behavioral perspectives in medicine. In T. Millon (Ed.), *Medical behavioral science* (pp. 3–5). Philadelphia: W. B. Saunders.

Petersdorf, R. G., & Feinstein, A. R. (1981). An informal appraisal of the current status of "medical sociology." In L. Eisenberg & A. Kleinman (Eds.), *The relevance of social science for medicine* (pp. 27–48). Dordrecht: Holland.

Schatzman, L., & Strauss, A. (1975). Social class and modes of communication. In T. Millon (Ed.), *Medical behavioral science* (pp. 402–411). Philadelphia: W. B. Saunders.

Segall, A. (1984). Physician education in clinical prevention. In J. D. Matarazzo, S. M. Weiss, J. A. Herd, N. E. Miller, & S. M. Weiss (Eds.), *Behavioral health: A handbook of health enhancement and disease prevention* (pp. 1204–1213). New York: Wiley.

Simmons, S. J. (1990). The health-promoting self-care system model: Directions for nursing research and practice. *Journal of Advanced Nursing, 15*, 1162–1166.

Stefan, M. D., & McManus, I. C. (1989). The concept of disease: Its evolution in medical students. *Social Science and Medicine, 29*, 791–792.

Szasz, T. S., & Hollender, M. H. (1956/1975). A contribution to the philosophy of medicine: The basic models of the doctor–patient relationship. In T. Millon (Ed.), *Medical behavioral science* (pp. 432–440). Philadelphia: W. B. Saunders. [Reprinted from *Archives of Internal Medicine*, 1956, *97*, 585–592.]

Tannenbaum, R., Weschler, I. R., & Massarik, F. (1961/1975). The process of understanding people. In T. Millon (Ed.), *Medical behavioral science* (pp. 393–402). Philadelphia: W. B. Saunders. [Reprinted from R. Tannenbaum et al., *Leadership and organization: A behavioral science approach*, 1961, New York: McGraw-Hill.]

Thomson, R. (1973). Can the social worker teach the physician? *Journal of Medical Education, 48*, 585–587.

1

Relevance of Health Behavior Research to Training and Practice in the Health Professions

An Overview

John G. Bruhn

HEALTH BEHAVIOR: THE BASIS FOR A PRACTICE PARADIGM

A Philosophy of Practice: Some Tenets

Beginning in the middle of the 20th century, the health professions—particularly medicine—acquired vast new scientific and technological knowledge. This new body of information enabled these professions to become more effective in the diagnosis and treatment of disease. While the science of the health professions has advanced, however, the art of healing has been neglected (Miller et al., 1975). Practice in the health professions has been focused on treating, curing, and returning patients to their former

John G. Bruhn • Provost and Dean, Pennsylvania State University at Harrisburg, Middletown, Pennsylvania 17057-4898.

Handbook of Health Behavior Research IV: Relevance for Professionals and Issues for the Future, edited by David S. Gochman. Plenum Press, New York, 1997.

conditions. It is necessary to resynthesize the art of healing with the scientific aspects of patient care and to reestablish a philosophy of practice that acknowledges patients to be more than their diseases.

This chapter suggests a philosophy of practice for today's health professionals that is comprised of three major tenets:

1. *Understand that the body is in a constant state of change, continually responding to internal and external stimuli or challenges to its equilibrium*. How individuals cope with challenges is linked with and affects the physiological mechanisms of the body. When individuals cope, they react emotionally and make behavioral choices. When their daily reactions to challenge and behavioral choices become ineffective, unsatisfying, or inappropriate, they may become sick. Staying healthy is a process; how healthy a person feels at any given time is tied to how well that person copes with challenge. Health behavior research has shown that people's perceptions

are important predictors of their health actions (e.g., Becker, 1974). There are exceptions, however, to these personal assessments. Hypochondriacs, for instance, never feel that they are coping well; at the other extreme, persons may be sick by clinical standards, but deny even significant indications that they are not coping adequately. Research on the health belief model has shown that the personality characteristic of "perceived vulnerability" consistently predicts persons' expectations of their general vulnerability to illness (Gochman, 1988).

Health behavior research has also shown that people's health-seeking behaviors are based, to a great extent, on their perceptions of their bodily state, rather than on their bodies' actual physical conditions (e.g., Bibace & Walsh, 1981). People make assumptions that, along with their expectations, help to shape their attributions of health and illness. How people attribute cause is important in understanding health behavior. People are especially motivated to seek causal attributions during periods of high uncertainty; unfamiliar symptoms lead to speculative inferences, which make for erroneous attributions (Janis & Rodin, 1979). Since most illnesses produce some degree of fear and distress, a high level of emotionality surrounding perceived changes in health is likely to result in inaccurate inferences about what is wrong and to lead in turn to inappropriate action or inaction. People also may put off getting proper medical attention and seek out other types of advice and help while trying to attribute cause.

How healthy people remain depends on how well they cope with the changing and diverse challenges or risks in their environments and lifestyles. Indeed, part of remaining healthy and coping satisfactorily depends upon people's ability to be flexible, on how they view changes and new challenges, and how willing they are to modify the ways in which they cope with them. Illness requires temporary or permanent changes in people's lifestyles. People usually have no choice regarding these changes, unless they refuse to accommodate to illness. Changing lifestyles to enhance health is difficult, especially when there is no imminent threat of illness.

Individual health care, however, is perpetual. Health behavior research has shown that people choose how healthy they want to be according to how they perceive their vulnerability (e.g., Dielman, Leech, Becker, Rosenstock, & Horvath, 1980). People who rationalize that they are not at risk may take little or no action to enhance their health (e.g., Gochman, 1985). People are reluctant to alter behavior patterns that represent powerful, predictable, and immediate sources of gratification; that are deeply ingrained in their values and beliefs; and that are reinforced by those with whom they associate (Bruhn, 1988).

Health is part of an individual's philosophy of life. Change in a person's philosophy of life usually requires change in that person's values as well as a significant modification of the person's social network and social support system. Major community-based cardiovascular disease prevention programs have attempted to reduce cardiovascular disease by reducing risk factors in entire communities (Shea & Basch, 1990). The most important finding from these studies is that health behavior change occurs at multiple social levels, including those of the individual, the group, the organization, and the community. Health behavior and lifestyle change is not only a matter of changing individual behaviors, especially if any change is to be sustained. Individual behaviors must be meaningfully related to each other and tied to an individual's values, beliefs, and priorities.

2. *Health has special meaning for each individual; this meaning must be changed if the individual's behavior is to be changed.* The definition people give health often relates to the degree of control they believe they have over their health. Some people who have learned that they are helpless to change a situation for the better do not try. Others may feel that they are helpless to affect the course of events in certain situations. Health behavior research has shown that individuals' beliefs about the degree of con-

trol they have over changing situations are good predictors of their behavior (e.g., Kirscht, 1972). Beliefs, however, are linked with values; believing that one has control over, for example, one's health status will produce healthful behavior only if health is highly valued. It has been found, for example, that women who believe in self-control of their health and who place a high value on health are more likely to engage in breast self-examination than those who do not (Lau, 1988). Health professionals with knowledge of their patients' health locus of control beliefs can design therapies or regimens that are consistent with those beliefs and that maximize compliance. Communications about proper preventive health behaviors and the proper utilization of health professionals can be targeted to audiences with different types of beliefs about control.

A health professional's practice is a process of influencing patients' health behavior. The health care literature often talks about "managing patients" and difficulties in getting patients to "comply" with advice or regimens. Such phraseology indicates that the professional–patient relationship is construed, not as a process, but as a praxis. Roter (1988) noted that compliance was associated with patterns of provider behavior during the physician–patient encounter that included more information giving, less question asking, more positive talk, and more partnership building. This association seems to apply to all types of interactions between health professionals and clients, well or sick.

Perhaps one of the more important but less frequently discussed aspects of health behavior change involves the kind of health behavior modeled by health professionals. For example, patients cannot be expected to take dietary and exercise advice from an overweight health professional who does not exercise. Health professionals model their health values (Holcomb et al., 1985; Wells, Lewis, Leake, & Ware, 1984; Young, 1988). The iatrogenic consequences of medical intervention can be prevented by modeling procedures, such as cardiac catherization, endoscopy exams, or preparing children to undergo

anesthesia. Little is mentioned, however, about the impact of the physical appearance, health behavior, and informal comments made by health professionals on their patients' beliefs and values regarding health (Janis & Rodin, 1979; Shapiro & Shapiro, 1984).

3. *The health professional is only an instrument in the promotion of health and treatment of disease.* Individuals are responsible for self-management of their bodies, minds, and spirits. When something goes awry so that people can no longer manage their health or need confirmation of the state of their health, they consult a health professional. Health professionals are not healers, but they are one aspect of the process of healing or restoring health. They should also be advocates for keeping people healthy. The promotion of health and treatment of disease is a dialogue or partnership. Health professionals are providers of technical knowledge and resources, but individuals must have the motivation to retain or regain their health and cooperate in the process. Clinical contact alone does not ensure that individuals will continue to be good self-managers of their health, but contact with a health professional is an important source of social support for individuals who do not have such support.

Health professionals often regard themselves to be successful when their patients "comply" with their advice or regimen, yet compliance does not mean that a disease has been cured or that a problem has been solved. Neither does noncompliance mean that a patient has failed. Health behavior research has shown consistently that there may be many reasons a patient does not "comply" (e.g., Kirscht & Rosenstock, 1979). Effective dialogue between the health practitioner and the patient helps ensure that the health professional will gain information to fashion advice or a regimen that is acceptable to the patient and compatible with the patient's life situation. The patient, on the other hand, learns the responsibility of self-care and self-management. Past conceptions of the active, dominant health professional and the passive, submissive patient do not fit with responsibility for one's own health and its maintenance. Patients need to seek second or third opinions, to ask questions, to obtain information, and to inquire about the competencies and costs of health professionals and health facilities. Future health professionals need to learn that patient advocacy is not a challenge to them and their profession, but a welcome change on the part of the lay public, indicating that patients are the ultimate gatekeepers of the quality of their health.

Education Reform for Health Professionals

A report issued by the Pew Health Professions Commission (O'Neil, 1993) stated that the education and training of health professionals in the United States is not adequate to meet the health care needs of the American people. The commission noted that the curricula of schools in a number of health professions (medicine, dentistry, nursing, allied health, pharmacy, public health, health care administration, and veterinary medicine) need to be rebalanced to include prevention, community health, the behavioral sciences, and patient outcomes management.

Medicine

The call for such reform, particularly in medical education, is not new. Enarson and Burg (1992) reviewed the results of 15 reform initiatives in medicine from 1906 through 1992. They noted that while these initiatives have contributed to changes in accreditation, licensing exams, and an institutional voice in policies on medical education, most reform initiatives have not yielded significant changes in medical education. Concern about reform in medical education has been heightened in the mid-1990s by the federal government's proposal to reform health care. While a survey of medical educators indicates a perception of the need for reform, the issues of the redistribution of power and finances make reform more appealing to deans than to most faculty (Cantor, Cohen, Barker, Shuster, &

Reynolds, 1991). Much of the dialogue about reform in medical education has therefore focused on the curriculum, which provides a semblance of reform, but ensures no substantial change (Bloom, 1988). The aggregate effect of successive waves of self-examination by medical schools essentially has been to bring about no change in how physicians are prepared to practice medicine (Swanson, 1989). Preparing medical students to practice medicine more effectively involves more than rearranging disciplines (Ginzberg, 1993). Blumenthal and Meyer (1993) warn that if no substantial changes are made in the structure and attitudes of academic medical centers, other health care organizations may take over some of their functions. Community-based institutions could well qualify for training programs now conducted in university health science centers.

The basic challenge for reform in medical education, therefore, is a call for a new type of physician who is prepared to make fundamental changes in the provision of health care. Boelen (1992) noted that future physicians should be able to (1) address and improve the quality of care by responding to the patient's total health needs with integrated preventive, curative, and rehabilitative services; (2) make optimal use of technology, bearing in mind ethical and financial considerations; (3) promote healthful lifestyles and empower individuals and groups to take responsibility for their own health protection; (4) strike a balance between patients' expectations and those of society at large; and (5) work effectively in teams within the health sector and between the health sector and the community. Medical practitioners of the future must help to create and empower competent consumers of health care (Todd, 1992).

Allied Health Sciences

Reform of education in the health professions is not limited to medical education. Allied health education is relatively isolated from other health professions and even from disciplines within its own field. Modes of teaching have remained traditional and approaches to care have become specialized, following the medical model. In many instances, allied health still is attempting to define itself and find its place within the health care team. Concerns about gaining independence from physician referrals and defining areas of knowledge and skills of specific allied health disciplines have prevented allied health practitioners from teaching, learning, and practicing in teams (Rettie, 1993; Robinson, 1993).

Dentistry

The traditional model for dental education is for every graduate to enter private practice. Clinical education continues to occur predominately in dental school clinics. Students receive limited experience in community settings and have few opportunities to work as members of health care teams. Dentistry needs to develop a more integrated curriculum and provide experience in delivering care to diverse segments of the population in community-based settings. Dental care must become recognized as an integral part of health care (O'Neil, 1993).

Nursing

Nursing has gained attention in recent years as members of the profession have moved out of generic staff roles in hospitals and gained new competencies in the delivery and management of care, especially in primary care settings. There is need, however, for more interdisciplinary teaching and practice involving allied health, medicine, pharmacy, and other professions. Nursing has developed, and should continue to develop, teaching programs in the school, home, and other community settings (O'Neil, 1993).

Pharmacy

Pharmacy education is in the process of further professionalization. The Pharm.D. degree is accepted as the terminal degree in the profession. Pharmaceutical care in the future will require the pharmacist to work toward definite

drug therapy outcomes, to collect more information and apply more judgment, and to work more closely with patients, physicians, and other health care professionals (Hepler, 1990). New, expanded roles for pharmacists include counseling and direct participation in patient care. The focus of pharmacy is changing from product to patient, requiring changes in the pharmacy curriculum. Curricular reform must include the design of techniques to help students develop competencies in critical thinking, problem solving, communication, ethical behavior, leadership, teamwork, and lifelong learning. A variety of ambulatory clinical training models need to be developed to provide opportunities for students in pharmacy and in other health professions to learn together (O'Neil, 1993).

New Competencies

The Pew Health Professions Commission (Shugars, O'Neil, & Bader, 1991) outlined an agenda for action in the preparation of health practitioners for the year 2005. Several new competencies established by this agenda for the future will depend on findings from health behavior research. These competencies include emphasizing prevention strategies; helping individuals, families, and communities to maintain and promote healthful lifestyles; providing counseling for patients in situations that involve ethical issues; understanding health through different cultural values; and understanding determinants of health such as environment, behavior, socioeconomic conditions, and genetics.

Health Behavior as a Relevant Vehicle for Teaching

As Stellar (1992) points out, chronic diseases consume a major portion of health care. Control of these diseases is dependent on lifestyles, behavior modification, and coping strategies. Health-promoting and disease-preventing behaviors are therefore of great importance to health practitioners, not only for their role in cost containment, but also for the general welfare of society.

Curricula in the health professions could be framed within the theme of prevention. Prevention provides a context for viewing all factors that impinge on a person's health; behavior provides a mechanism or vehicle for understanding how health can be lost or maintained through one's actions or inactions. Blumenthal (1993) points out that prevention receives little attention during the clinical years of medical school, and little has been written about new approaches to teach it. The University of Pennsylvania, for example, has made a beginning with a single "integrative neuroscience" course that integrates behavioral science into the teaching of neurology, neuroscience, neuropathology, and psychiatry. This approach not only teaches the basic neuroendocrine mechanisms involved, but also teaches them in a clinical context wherein the realities of the lives of patients can be addressed (Stellar, 1992). Similarly, health behavior research provides students with examples as well as a context for understanding how behavior can be an etiological factor in disease causation and a necessary factor to bring about or maintain good health.

Medicine

Applications of health behavior research to medicine have been effective in the areas of smoking, alcohol, and diabetes management (Duryea, Ransom, & English, 1990). If medicine can produce biological immunity in susceptible hosts, it is reasoned, then psychology can produce psychological immunity in susceptible targets.

Inoculation Theory. Inoculation theory was formulated to provide subjects with enhanced resistance to the verbal appeals of persuaders. Immunization interventions are efficient when used in situations in which susceptibility to pressure and persuasion is significant. Several researchers have reported that emphasizing methods for resisting peer pressure to begin smoking results in a substantial reduction in reported smoking behavior among students. Inoc-

ulation theory used in preventive alcohol education programs has been shown to be effective in decreasing the frequency of riding with drunk drivers and helping students resist pressures to engage in health-risking behaviors. More current applications of inoculation theory have involved efforts to teach teenage diabetics to improve compliance with their self-care protocols by resisting the persuasive appeals of peers. In numerous other possible applications of inoculation theory, the promotion of health-enhancing behavior brings together the concepts of personal autonomy and choice.

Nursing

Health behavior research and a commitment to prevention provide a useful framework for answering questions that arise in nursing practice (Nemcek, 1990).

Health Belief Model

The health belief model, a major health behavior research formulation, was developed to explain why and under what conditions people take preventive actions (e.g., Rosenstock, 1966). Perceptions directly affect the likelihood of taking preventive actions. These perceptions are affected by various demographic, social, psychological, and structural factors. For example, individuals who perceived themselves to be susceptible to swine flu, believed an inoculation would be beneficial, and perceived the vaccine to be safe were likely to obtain the inoculation (Aho, 1979; Cummings, Jette, Brock, & Haefner, 1979; Rundall & Wheeler, 1979a). Perceived vulnerability, benefits, and barriers have been found to correlate, for example, with vaccination behavior (Larsen, Olsen, Cole, & Shortell, 1979), participation in Tay-Sachs disease screening (Becker, Kaback, Rosenstock, & Ruth, 1975), obtaining preventive checkups (Rundall & Wheeler, 1979b), complying with exercise programs (Tirrell & Hart, 1980), and mothers' obtaining frequent pediatric services for their children (Becker, 1974).

Social Linkages

A lack of preventive care has been associated with powerlessness, hopelessness, and social isolation. These factors relate closely to the presence or absence of social networks and social support (e.g., Mitchell, Billings, & Moos, 1983). It is important for health practitioners not only to understand the barriers to patient compliance with preventive regimens, but also to utilize the patient's family, friends, and other supportive ties in enhancing compliance. Health behavior research has provided practical insights into clinical approaches to modify health behavior.

Social and Cultural Contexts

Dressler (1989) made a strong appeal for considering disease and risk factors for disease in a social and cultural context. He pointed out that the Type A behavior pattern, given its variable predictive efficacy, should not be considered a serious predictor of cardiovascular disease. Yet, when considered in a social and cultural context, it may be a serious predictor. Dressler believes that current teaching and research in cardiovascular disease are too narrowly focused on individuals and that much clinical decision making fails to consider the framework in which patients live out their lives. Health behavior research provides a framework or model that takes into account how disease is produced in varying social contexts and discourages simplistic causal notions of risk.

Problem-Based and Value-Based Learning

Problem-based learning provides a practical and useful framework for learning by health professionals. The basic philosophy behind problem-based learning is that students learn best when the context of their learning closely resembles that of the problems they will face as professionals and when they actively assume responsibility for their learning. Problem-based learning

in medicine has existed since the 1960s. For the most part, it has been adopted within a traditional curriculum or a parallel track for a small number of students. Only a few medical, nursing, and allied health schools have adopted problem-based learning as the framework for their entire curricula (Des Marchais, Bureau, Dumais, & Pigeon, 1992). Problem-based learning is not a panacea, but it is an alternative to the traditional Socratic method of teaching in the health professions.

The problem-based approach has strengths and weaknesses (Albanese & Mitchell, 1993; Norman & Schmidt, 1992), and its effectiveness has yet to be shown through rigorous evaluation (Friedman et al., 1990). There is evidence, for example, that problem-based learning does not enhance performance on the national board exams in medicine (Mennin, Friedman, Skipper, Kalishman, & Snyder, 1993). The advantages seem to be in the qualitative aspects of learning medicine. A multidisciplinary course taught at Dartmouth Medical School, in which humanistic and social science principles are formally integrated into the clinical curriculum, has been especially effective. Almy et al. (1992) noted that in many medical schools, human values are emphasized wherever possible during clinical clerkships; they pointed out, however, that students need to incorporate principles from several different disciplines into complex clinical decisions. At Dartmouth, as a result of a problem-based course in the fourth year, students develop a deep interest in and understanding of patients and society and of priority setting for health care expenditures. Problem-based learning has not yet appeared, to any significant extent, in the curricula of the schools of other health professions (Bruhn, 1992).

McKenna, Ledbetter, and Ramaeker (1989a,b) emphasized the importance of teaching students in the health professions about values and the process of valuing. In the health professions, values are usually taught informally through role modeling. Macklin (1993) noted that the values learned are only as good as the role models who do the teaching. She stressed that the major aim in teaching ethics to future health professionals is to get them to think about what they are doing. Such thinking requires the ability to identify morally relevant considerations, to recognize the different and perhaps competing rights or interests at stake, and to question how a proposed course of action complies with or violates accepted, time-honored ethical principles.

There is no empirical evidence that students who have progressed through a problem-based or value-based curriculum provide better health care to their clients. There is anecdotal evidence, however, that students from problem-based programs are more concerned with the holistic aspects (the person as a functioning whole) of patient care, are more effective in communicating with patients, and have better organizational skills (Bruhn, 1992). Thus, teaching principles of health behavior helps to broaden the perspectives of students to become holistic practitioners. Health behavior research from cultural anthropology has provided sources of data on different cultural conceptions of health and illness, which provides a broader perspective of health and illness (Segall, 1988).

Thomas (1992) said that the dilemma of modern medicine and the central flaw in medical education is the irresistible drive to *do something*. Value judgments that underlie actions and the consequences of actions often are not examined. Lock and Lella (1986) pointed out that medical education in its usual form perpetuates value-laden attitudes that are reinforced with percentages, absolutes, stereotypes, and statistical averages. There is little exposure to the differing ideas of other cultures concerning health and illness. The goal of education in the health professions should be for students to arrive at informed value commitments to develop the ability to assess their own values in the light of each patient's situation, so that the clinical encounter becomes a partnership of appreciation. Students need to be made aware of their own biases and value judgments through self-reflection and a tolerance of ambiguity (Lock & Lella, 1986).

HEALTH BEHAVIOR COMPETENCIES FOR FUTURE HEALTH PRACTITIONERS

Several conferences and commissions have examined the competencies of health professionals, especially medical graduates, to meet the current and future health needs of the public (Gastel & Rogers, 1989; Marston & Jones, 1992; O'Neil, 1993; Shugars et al., 1991). One of the key questions asked was: "What should be the outcomes of undergraduate clinical education, and where and how should clinical education be taught to achieve these outcomes?" These conferences and commissions emphasized that schools of the health professions must increase their emphasis on the health of society so that health professionals can assess the impact of their actions on communities as well as on individual patients. Special attention must be given to the development in future health professionals of specific skills, especially in communication, critical appraisal (clinical judgment), and population analysis, as well as professional attitudes that include empathy, integrity, and professional responsibility.

Many of these competencies and skills require knowledge of the principles of health behavior and an application of findings from health behavior research. In particular, the five areas of competencies discussed below appear to be essential for health care professionals to effectively practice in expanded and proactive roles.

Understanding Psychological and Social Mediators of Health and Illness

The first essential health behavior competency is an understanding of the general psychological and social mediators of health and illness. Lifestyle factors are disproportionately identified as causal links to risk factors associated with public health morbidity and mortality. Accidents among the young and aged, cancer and heart disease associated with dietary practices and cigarette smoking, and AIDS associated with drug abuse and sexual behaviors are examples of the clear implication of behavior in the etiology of disease. As behavioral scientists collaborate with biomedical colleagues, sophisticated biological and behavioral techniques are being used to study brain–behavior relationships, how genetics influences behavior, and how hormonal factors affect brain–behavior development.

The relationship of behavioral factors to the immune system is a promising area of research that could expand understanding of disease onset (Kiecolt-Glaser & Glaser, 1992). Data on marital disruption provide evidence that chronic psychological distress may have significant negative effects on both the qualitative and the quantitative aspects of immune function (Kennedy, Kiecolt-Glaser, & Glaser, 1990). Although many of the physiological pathways are unclear, one longitudinal study showed greater autonomic arousal in interacting married couples to be a very strong predictor of subsequent decline in marital quality. Poorer health ratings at a 3-year follow-up also were correlated strongly with greater declines in marital satisfaction (Levenson & Gottman, 1985).

Another study examined the immunological correlates of chronic distress associated with caring for a relative afflicted with Alzheimer's disease (Kiecolt-Glaser et al., 1987). Alzheimer's caregivers were found to have significantly poorer immune function than their matched comparison subjects. Specifically, caregivers had lower percentages of helper T-lymphocytes, lower helper/suppressor ratios, and higher antibody titers, and were more distressed, than their comparison counterparts.

Assessing Individual and Family Health Risks

A second essential health behavior competency is the ability of health professionals to assess the health risks of individuals and families. Much of what is understood about risk factors derives from epidemiological studies. The epidemiological approach differentiates factors that contribute to illness from those that affect the course of an illness. In preventing disease, it is useful to proceed on the basis of specific understanding of disease mechanisms, but sometimes the mechanisms are unknown. There is substantial evidence that some factors are risks for certain diseases, even though researchers do not understand the workings of the mechanisms that link psychosocial factors and biological systems. For example, education is one of the best predictors of good health, longevity, and the use of preventive and other health services. Education is associated with life changes and many attributes associated with health, such as habits, coping abilities, and self-esteem (Mechanic, 1989).

Marital status is another important predictor of health. While marriage favors men more than women, both gain more than the unmarried. Marriage is thought to provide more stability in lifestyle; it involves strong expectations and personal commitments and goals that go beyond oneself.

Religious participation is another predictor of health. Churchgoing also is related to more regularity in lifestyle and conventionality. Religious participation also may be associated with health behaviors with respect to smoking, drinking, and sex.

Social support and social networks are other predictors of health. Large social networks provide tangible and emotional assistance when needed, and group association may serve as a basis for self-esteem and satisfaction.

How well individuals adapt to abrupt and involuntary change in their lives, such as losing a spouse, being placed in a nursing home, unemployment, or forced retirement, is another predictor of health. These changes may profoundly affect lifestyle, accelerate aging effects, and hasten mortality.

The Centers for Disease Control found, after reviewing the leading causes of mortality and morbidity among persons in all age groups, that nearly all contributing behaviors can be categorized into six areas: (1) behaviors that result in unintentional and intentional injuries; (2) tobacco use; (3) alcohol and other drug use; (4) sexual behaviors that contribute to unintended pregnancy and sexually transmitted diseases, including HIV infection; (5) dietary behaviors that result in disease; and (6) physical inactivity (Kolbe, Kann, & Collins, 1993).

There is some evidence that risk factor education works. Frank, Winkleby, Fortmann, and Farquhar (1993) documented knowledge and behavior change in two California communities that were used as control cities in the Stanford Five-City Project. Over a decade, residents of two communities became better informed about the advantageous effects of cholesterol-specific diets, weight loss, exercise, and reduced smoking.

The perception of risk for becoming ill is considered critical to individuals' decisions to engage or not engage in healthy behaviors. Perception of risk is a key factor in the success of efforts to educate people about health risks. Prohaska, Albrecht, Levy, Sugrue, and Kim (1990) examined self-perceptions of risk for AIDS in a survey of 18- to 60-year-old adults in Chicago. They found that increased exposure to the media and greater belief in the accuracy of the media as a source of information about AIDS did not affect people's perceptions of risk, either positively or negatively. Similarly, knowing someone with AIDS did not increase the likelihood that individuals would consider themselves at risk. These researchers found that increased perceptions of risk for AIDS were related to worry about one's health and fear of the threat of AIDS. They noted the perception of personal risk depends upon multiple perceptual, behavioral, and situational factors, and prevention efforts must focus on changing people's perceptions rather than giving people facts.

People's perceptions of risk are closely related to their personality attributes. There is some evidence that there are disease-prone personalities (Carmody, Crossen, & Wiens, 1989). A genetic disease-prone personality, characterized by depression, anger/hostility, and anxiety, is associated with at least five different diseases (coronary heart disease, asthma, ulcers, rheumatoid arthritis, and headaches). Generalized emotional distress and interpersonal alienation appear to be features of the disease-prone personality. The disease-prone personality and self-perceptions of risk are interrelated and are affected by other factors, such as life situation, lifestyle, beliefs, and values, as is demonstrated by the difficulty in promoting voluntary behavioral changes in seropositive individuals and the relative ineffectiveness of HIV screening programs (Cleary et al., 1991). Clearly, future health practitioners are challenged not only to understand the complexity of variables involved in assessing health risk, but also to consider the uniqueness of patients and their families in planning risk interventions.

Intervening to Modify Health Risks

Health professionals, by virtue of their positions as helpers and healers, have always had permission to intervene in people's lives to eliminate disease and distress. It is a relatively new role, however, for them to suggest what individuals should do to live healthier lives and reduce risks for disease—a third essential health behavior competency. Efforts to induce voluntary behavior change in relatively healthy individuals have had some success, as evidenced by the reduction in tobacco smoking, the increase in wearing of seat belts, and the alteration of diet and exercise patterns. Efforts to reduce drug and alcohol consumption seem to meet with episodic results. These interventions have applied health behavior principles to populations, but the mass media, the major option available for influencing large-scale behavior change, usually influence only a small proportion of the audience. McAlister (1991) suggested that health behavior change in a population can best be achieved by combining and reinforcing the media efforts with interpersonal contact. When local residents select the messages to be conveyed and establish the goals and policies for the educational effort, health behavior change becomes a two-way process between the population and the health professionals.

Skidmore and Roberts (1991) stated several principles of community education for health professionals to consider when planning health interventions:

- All aspects of an intervention should be congruent with community values and culture.
- An intervention should be developmentally appropriate to the target group.
- An intervention should have a "connection" with the life situation and lifestyle of the targeted group.
- An intervention should be directed at the major decision-making group in the community.

That these principles often are not applied to intervention at the individual level probably is the reason that patient non-compliance is poorly understood. Too often, health professionals focus on simple, objective factors in an attempt to embrace patient compliance; e.g., "the physician should speak in easy to understand language" or "have the patient reiterate the provider's directives" (Masur, 1981).

The reasons patients do not comply with provider advice, follow a prescribed regimen, or return for care are far more complex than those embodied in the patient–health professional interaction. Improving compliance is a matter not only of educating the patient, but also of educating the health professional to consider the many factors that contribute to the uniqueness of each patient.

Promoting Healthful Behaviors

Promoting healthful behaviors—a fourth essential health behavior competency—has not been a high priority in the training of health professionals for the several reasons that health professionals do not generate income by keeping people healthy, gain more satisfaction from curing than from preventing illness, see education and prevention as strategies that compete or conflict with the specialist model, do not feel competent in the knowledge or skills of disease prevention, view health promotion as time-consuming, and gain no respect or support from their peers for promoting health (Relman, 1982).

If health professionals are to do more than restore function to the sick, society at large and schools of the health professions will have to balance the quality and quantity of life. Health professionals have come to value the length of life, not its quality, which reinforces a mechanistic, specialized approach to remedying bodily ills. The mind and spirit are excluded from diagnosis and treatment as confounding factors. Health professionals can promote better health only if body, mind, and spirit are considered equal partners in health and disease.

Partnering Health Care

Interdisciplinary teams now are common in many health care settings. The purpose of teaming is the sharing of knowledge and skills to provide better, more convenient care for the patient. Despite a lot of rhetoric about health care teams, they have usually consisted of other health professionals assembled by the physician to deal with the specifics of a given patient. Health care teams have not been an integral part of the traditional delivery of health services, and health professionals other than physicians have not assumed (or been permitted to assume) the leadership of teams. Health problems are too complex, however, to support the assumption that any one health discipline has all the answers (e.g., Stahelski & Tsukuda, 1990). Health care teams should therefore be the usual mode of delivering care.

Thus, students preparing for the health professions need to gain an understanding of what other health professionals do and how their services can be used—a fifth essential health behavior competency. In addition, they need to learn how to share their knowledge and skills for the benefit of the patient. One of the greatest barriers to the formation of teams is the fear that health professionals will invade each other's turf (Bruhn, Levine, & Levine, 1993). The best way to increase trust, cooperation, cohesiveness, and effective decision making is for health professionals to learn together. Such joint learning will not occur in the face of the separateness that currently characterizes the curricula in the schools of the health professions. Health behavior research has shown that common values and shared communication can enhance patient–provider communication. Health providers must also share values and communication if their primary focus is indeed to be the patient, not power and status (Kirscht & Rosenstock, 1979).

Substantial changes in educating health professionals are needed if the delivery of health services is to be made more effective, efficient, and humane. Values that stress the importance of credentials and the differential power, prestige, status, and autonomy they give a profession are instilled during the educational preparation of health professionals. Elitism detracts from collaboration and teamwork. Instead of focusing on combining their expertise to provide optimum care, professionals are devoting energy to protecting their turf and identity. As professionals defend their own interests, patients became victims. More time and energy are expended in making sure professionals win than in making sure patients win (Bruhn et al., 1993).

Much has been said and written about health care teams. The instances in which they work are uncommon throughout much of health care today. As Hirschhorn (1991) pointed out, empowerment in a team environment is balanced with collaboration. Team members focus on the task at hand, and the team manager manages boundaries. Team teaching and team-administered care are based on the premise that a variety of resources can be brought to bear to accomplish a task. Not only bringing resources together, but also successfully orchestrating the resources, is what makes a combined effort effective. Simply getting a physician, a nurse, a social worker, and an occupational therapist together does not necessarily mean they will make a team, even if they have a common operating philosophy and task. *How* they work together determines whether there will be a win/win outcome. *How* to collaborate can best be learned from modeling, trial and error, and experience.

A behavioral shift is needed in the health professions—a shift from preserving the status quo to behaving in an innovative, cooperative, and aggressive manner. Behavior changes must be preceded, however, by changes in perceptions and attitudes. The concerned parties—health professionals, their students, and their patients—must feel that it is important for all to win, whether with respect to quality health education or to quality services. A win/lose philosophy has not led to a system of education of health professionals, or a system of health services delivery, that meets the changing needs of society. Territoriality has effectively preserved professional interests and benefits. Boundaries between health professionals and patient care have been idealized and protected from all change except that initiated by health professionals. Only recently have patients been granted "rights" and permitted to be advocates for their own care.

Shortell (1982) noted that while health care professionals increasingly are trained to take a holistic view of patients, many fail to take a holistic view of themselves as health care professionals. Health professionals tend to view each other in a segmented and instrumental manner; each represents to the others a means of doing a job. Given this perception of other professionals in conjunction with differences in professional culture, it is far easier to understand patients than to understand coworkers.

Values give people's personal and professional lives structure, direction, and meaning. Health care professionals, in particular, practice in clinical and programmatic settings in which value conflicts and dilemmas are daily occurrences. Often when conflicts between health professionals occur, the patient is blamed (Butterill, O'Hanlon, & Book, 1992). Health behavior research has shown that organizational structure, power within the organization, communication within the organization, and boundaries within the organization are potential sources of conflict that affect the quality of patient care. The need for a common value base will help health professionals see themselves as members of a team rather than as representatives of their respective disciplines (Aaronson, 1991; Clark, 1994; Keliher, 1992; Sands, Stafford, & McClelland, 1990).

Proposals for change include joint nurse–physician management of patient care units, nurses as voting members of hospital governing boards, and the development of voluntary nursing staff organizations paralleling those of the voluntary medical staff. When a hospital's demand for nurses exceeds its supply, nurses can be in a favorable economic position to press for change. Some attributes of Theory Z management, particularly consensual decision making and developing holistic views of people, could facilitate changes in the roles of nurses and other health personnel with respect to sharing power and decision making. For these changes to occur, however, physicians and administrators will have to give up some of their autonomy and professional elitism (Shortell, 1982).

The key question is whether health care managers are willing to place their careers in the service of values and risk the possibility of new values, such as quality care. As Shortell points out, concern for quality involves more than managerial preference. It involves the development of a distinctive organizational philosophy and culture that is shared by all participants. Such a development will require major shifts in professional boundaries.

NEW SATISFACTIONS AND PRIORITIES OF FUTURE HEALTH PRACTITIONERS

Reasons for Choosing a Health Profession

Individuals choose to enter helping professions for numerous reasons that are more complex than the desire to help people. Oken (1978) has described some psychological themes common to physicians, among them the denial and undoing of anxiety about death, perfectionism, a push toward active mastery, the use of cognitive mastery for dealing with unpleasant feelings, and

authoritarianism. Oken points out that many of these traits are functionally helpful in the job of a physician, which involves uncertainty, high expectations on the part of patients, and the effects and end results of chronic and incurable disease. Current criticisms of physicians, however, focus more on their interpersonal behavior (or quality of care) than on their technical competence. Carson (1977) asked, "How do physicians achieve personability in a professional relationship?" His answer is: by listening empathetically and questioning imaginatively. It is obvious that patients expect physicians to become part of their treatment. Rogers (1974) noted the need for physicians who, in addition to having a deep personal commitment to the skilled technology of medicine, understand medicine's broad humanistic caring function and are not afraid to expand their roles to improve the quality of life and the health care of patients.

While physicians are not the only health professionals with these responsibilities, their predominance, power, and prestige in the health care area make them the most common targets of criticism. The reasons for choosing to enter other health professions could equally be scrutinized by patients and the public. Criticism of the quality of care applies to all health professionals. Students need to examine their willingness to accept broad social responsibilities before considering a health profession as a career choice. To prepare health professionals who will accept these responsibilities, it will be necessary to broaden the education of health professionals and to select the best candidates to enter professional schools.

Congruency between Personal and Professional Goals

Schroeder (1992) noted serious dissatisfaction among practicing physicians—discontent that seems especially great among internists. Interest in generalist careers has plummeted. A Lewis Harris survey commissioned by the national Alpha Omega Alpha honorary medical society in the early 1990s indicated that medical school applicants are altruistic, agree that helping others is an important career consideration, and value the opportunity to be useful socially. The survey also found that college students as a whole tended to have a positive image of physicians (Schroeder, 1992). Applications to medical school peaked at the end of the Vietnam war in 1974–1975. A steady decline in applicants followed, with the low figure of 26,721 occurring in 1988–1989. The 1990–1991 cycle saw a major upsurge in applications to 33,600. Factors that discouraged students from pursuing medicine as a career included concerns about preserving enough time for self and family, indebtedness, the hard work of medicine, the attractiveness of other careers, and discouragement by practicing physicians.

A survey of older physicians conducted by the American Medical Association in 1987 indicated that the believe medicine to be in worse shape than when they entered medical school (Schroeder, 1992). Yet there has been substantial progress in medicine as a field, and the financial rewards are considerable. Schroeder points out, however, that there is still a need to improve both the "field" and the "factory." Health professionals in general lead demanding lives, yet some health professions, such as nursing, occupational therapy, and physical therapy, continue to have a strong appeal to young people. The current generation seems to value greater congruency between personal and professional goals.

Broader Ethic of Responsibility

A study of patients' perceptions of the role of the family practice physician in providing health promotion services indicated that 70% of the 450 patients questioned believed that physicians should counsel all patients concerning yearly Pap smears, breast self-examinations, and smoking cessation. A sizable majority believed that physicians should provide sex education to teens and discuss social support systems and home safety issues with patients. Patients also

thought that physicians should refer them to other professionals for dental care, marital problems, and financial problems (Price, Desmond, & Lash, 1991). Godin and Shephard (1990) stated that the potential preventive role of the physician is not yet being exploited effectively. Only about 25% of people who regularly exercise reported that they had been advised to do so by their physicians. These authors suggested that other types of health professionals such as physician assistants and physical therapists might be better able to promote exercise than physicians.

Evidence suggests that an intensive, multidisciplinary curriculum introduced into a community hospital family medicine residency program can increase physicians' use of preventive strategies with their patients and of easy-to-follow protocols for managing common problems (Patterson, Fried, & Nagle, 1989). The residency years, however, come too late in the process of medical education to influence attitudes and behavior about prevention. More than half of the seniors graduating from United States medical schools rate their curricula inadequate in regard to health promotion and disease prevention, and data suggest that current medical school curricula turn students away from career choices that foster prevention (Wheat, Killian, & Melnick, 1991).

Health professionals must also address themselves to new responsibilities to humanity. The personal values and ethics involved in transactions between health professionals and their patients are but one part of the total human situation and cannot be divorced from the values held by society. Increasingly, the health professions are being asked to assume a position of leadership in the reexamination of societal values.

In designing better ways to make quality health care available, affordable, and accessible, there is no doubt that prevention and holistic care should be the underpennings of a "system" of care. There is a need for a new professional ethic for all health professionals—an ethic of accountability to patients as well as peers (Bruhn & Smith, 1972).

Obviously, there is a significant challenge to

the health professions to make training and practice better meet the needs of a changing and complex society. Health behavior theory, principles, and research can contribute enormously to the curricula of schools of the health professions. The role of the social and behavioral sciences in the education of health professionals has often been belittled as "common sense" or "something that could be learned after the essentials of a curriculum." A sophisticated public is requiring, however, that all health professionals take a second look at themselves and how they practice. As Thomas (1992) said, what was expected from shamans, millennia ago, is still required of contemporary masters of the professions—to *do* something. As Thomas further notes, however, shamans employed a lot of nontechnology that was immensely effective. They skillfully used the principles of health behavior!

REFERENCES

Aaronson, W. E. (1991). Interdisciplinary health team role taking as a function of health professional education. *Gerontology and Geriatrics Education, 12*, 97–110.

Aho, W. P. (1979). Participation of senior citizens in the swine flu inoculation program: An analysis of health belief model variables in preventive health behaior. *Journal of Gerontology, 34*, 201–208.

Albanese, M. A., & Mitchell, S. (1993). Problem-based learning: A review of literature on its outcomes and implementation issues. *Academic Medicine, 68*, 52–81.

Almy, T. P., Colby, K. K., Zubkoff, M., Gephart, D. S., Moore-West, M., & Lundquist, L. L. (1992). Health, society, and the physician: Problem-based learning of the social sciences and humanities—Eight years of experience. *Annals of Internal Medicine, 116*, 569–574.

Becker, M. H. (1974). The health belief model and personal health behavior. *Health Education Monographs, 2*(4) [entire issue].

Becker, M. H., Kaback, M. M., Rosenstock, I. M., & Ruth, M. V. (1975). Some influences on public participation in a genetic screening program. *Journal of Community Health, 1*(1), 3–14.

Bibace, R., & Walsh, M. E. (Eds.). (1981). *Children's conceptions of health, illness, and bodily functions.* San Francisco: Jossey-Bass.

Bloom, S. W. (1988). Structure and ideology in medical educa-
tion: An analysis of resistance to change. *Journal of Health and Social Behavior, 29*, 294–306.

Blumenthal, D. S. (1993). Prevention in the medical curriculum: Reform and opportunity. *American Journal of Preventive Medicine, 9*, 122–123.

Blumenthal, D. S., & Meyer, G. S. (1993). The future of the academic medical center under health care reform. *New England Journal of Medicine, 329*, 1812–1814.

Boelen, C. (1992). Medical education reform: The need for global action. *Academic Medicine, 67*, 745–749.

Bruhn, J. G. (1988). Lifestyle and health behavior. In D. S. Gochman (Ed.), *Health behavior: Emerging research perspectives* (pp. 71–86). New York: Plenum Press.

Bruhn, J. G. (1992). Problem-based learning: An approach toward reforming allied health education. *Journal of Allied Health, 21*, 161–173.

Bruhn, J. G., Levine, H. G., & Levine, P. L. (1993). *Managing boundaries in the health professions.* Springfield, IL: Charles C. Thomas.

Bruhn, J. G., & Smith, D. C. (1972). Social ethics for medical educators. In M. B. Visscher (Ed.), *Humanistic perspectives in medical ethics* (pp. 288–297). Buffalo, NY: Prometheus Books.

Butterill, D., O'Hanlon, J. O., & Book, H. (1992). When the system is the problem, don't blame the patient: Problems inherent in the interdisciplinary inpatient team. *Canadian Journal of Psychiatry, 37*, 168–172.

Cantor, J. C., Cohen, A. B., Barker, D. C., Shuster, A. L., & Reynolds, R. C. (1991). Medical educators' views on medical education reform. *Journal of the American Medical Association, 265*, 1002–1006.

Carmody, T. P., Crossen, J. R., & Wiens, A. N. (1989). Hostility as a health risk factor: Relationships with neuroticism, Type A behavior, attentional focus, and interpersonal style. *Journal of Clinical Psychology, 45*, 754–762.

Carson, R. A. (1977). What are physicians for? *Journal of the American Medical Association, 238*, 1029–1031.

Clark, P. G. (1994). Social, professional, and educational values on the interdisciplinary team: Implications for gerontological and geriatric education. *Educational Gerontology, 20*, 35–51.

Cleary, P. D., Van Devanter, N., Rogers, T. F., Singer, E., Shipton-Levy, R., Steilen, M., Stuart, A., Avorn, J., & Pindyck, J. (1991). Behavior changes after notification of HIV infection. *American Journal of Public Health, 81*, 1586–1590.

Cummings, K. M., Jette, A. M., Brock, B. M., & Haefner, D. (1979). Psychosocial determinants of immunization behavior in a swine influenza campaign. *Medical Care, 17*, 639–649.

Dielman, T. E., Leech, S. L., Becker, M. H., Rosenstock, I. M., & Horvath, W. J. (1980). Dimensions of children's health beliefs. *Health Education Quarterly, 7*, 219–238.

Des Marchais, J. E., Bureau, M. A., Dumais, B., & Pigeon, G. (1992). From traditional to problem-based learning: A case report of complete curriculum reform. *Medical Education, 26*, 190-199.

Dressler, W. W. (1989). Type A behavior and the social production of cardiovascular disease. *Journal of Nervous and Mental Disease, 177*, 181-190.

Duryea, E. J., Ransom, M. V., & English, G. (1990). Psychological immunization: Theory, research, and current health behavior applications. *Health Education Quarterly, 17*, 169-178.

Enarson, C., & Burg, F. D. (1992). An overview of reform initiatives in medical education. *Journal of the American Medical Association, 268*, 1141-1143.

Frank, E., Winkleby, M., Fortmann, S. P., & Farquhar, J. W. (1993). Cardiovascular disease risk factors: Improvements in knowledge and behavior in the 1980's. *American Journal of Public Health, 83*, 590-593.

Friedman, C. P., de Bliek, R., Greer, D. S., Mennin, S. P., Norman, G. R., Sheps, C. G., Swanson, D. B., & Woodward, C. A. (1990). Charting the winds of change: Evaluating innovative medical curricula. *Academic Medicine, 65*, 8-14.

Gastel, B., & Rogers, D. E. (Eds.). (1989). *Clinical education and the doctor of tomorrow*. New York: New York Academy of Medicine.

Ginzberg, E. (1993). The reform of medical education: An outsider's reflections. *Academic Medicine, 68*, 518-521.

Gochman, D. S. (1985). Family determinants of children's concepts of health and disease. In D. C. Turk & R. D. Kerns (Eds.), *Health, illness, and families: A life-span perspective* (pp. 23-50). New York: Wiley.

Gochman, D. S. (1988). Health behavior research: Present and future. In D. S. Gochman (Ed.), *Health behavior: Emerging research perspectives* (pp. 409-424). New York: Plenum Press.

Godin, G., & Shephard, R. J. (1990). An evaluation of the potential role of the physician in influencing community exercise behavior. *American Journal of Health Promotion, 4*, 255-259.

Hepler, C. D. (1990). The future of pharmacy: Pharmaceutical care. *American Pharmacy, NS30*(10), 23-29.

Hirschhorn, L. (1991). *Managing in the new team environment: Skills, tools, and methods*. Reading, MA: Addison-Wesley.

Holcomb, J. D., Mullen, P. D., Fasser, C. E., Smith, Q., Martin, J. B., Parks, L. A., & Wente, S. M. (1985). Health behaviors and beliefs of four allied health professions regarding health promotion and disease prevention. *Journal of Allied Health, 14*, 373-385.

Janis, I. L., & Rodin, J. (1979). Attribution, control and decision making: Social psychology and health care. In G. C. Stone, F. Cohen, & N. E. Adler (Eds.), *Health psychology* (pp. 487-521). San Francisco: Jossey-Bass.

Keliher, M. N. (1992). In defense of the interdisciplinary team and the role of the child and youth care worker. *Journal of Child and Youth Care, 7*, 25-33.

Kennedy, S., Kiecolt-Glaser, J. K., & Glaser, R. (1990). Social support, stress, and the immune system. In B. R. Sarason, I. G. Sarason, & G. R. Pierce (Eds.), *Social support: An interactional view* (pp. 253-266). New York: Wiley.

Kiecolt-Glaser, J. K., & Glaser, R. (1992). Psychoneuroimmunology: Can psychological interventions modulate immunity? *Journal of Consulting and Clinical Psychology, 60*, 569-575.

Kiecolt-Glaser, J. K., Glaser, R., Shuttleworh, E. C., Dyer, C. S., Ogrochi, P., & Speicher, C. E. (1987). Chronic stress and immunity in family caregivers of Alzheimer's disease victims. *Psychosomatic Medicine, 49*, 523-535.

Kirscht, J. P. (1972). Perceptions of control and health beliefs. *Canadian Journal of Behavioral Science, 4*, 225-237.

Kirscht, J. P., & Rosenstock, I. M. (1979). Patients' problems in following recommendations of health experts. In G. C. Stone, F. Cohen, & N. E. Adler (Eds.), *Health psychology* (pp. 189-215). San Francisco: Jossey-Bass.

Kolbe, L. J., Kann, L., & Collins, J. L. (1993). Overview of the Youth Risk Behavior Surveillance System. *Public Health Reports, 108*, 2-10.

Larsen, E. B., Olsen, E., Cole, W., & Shortell, S. (1979). The relationship of health beliefs and a postcard reminder to influenza vaccination. *Journal of Family Practice, 8*, 1207-1211.

Lau, R. R. (1988). Beliefs about control and health behavior. In D. S. Gochman (Ed.), *Health behavior: Emerging research perspectives* (pp. 43-63). New York: Plenum Press.

Levenson, R. W., & Gottman, J. M. (1985). Physiological and affective predictors of change in relationship satisfaction. *Journal of Personality and Social Psychology, 49*, 85-94.

Lock, M., & Lella, J. (1986). Reforming medical education: Towards a broadening of attitudes. In S. McHugh & T. M. Vallis (Eds.), *Illness behavior: A multidisciplinary model* (pp. 47-58). New York: Plenum Press.

Macklin, R. (1993). Teaching bioethics to future health professionals: A case-based clinical model. *Bioethics, 7*, 200-206.

Marston, R. Q., & Jones, R. M. (Eds.). (1992). *Medical education in transition*. Princeton, NJ: Robert Wood Johnson Foundation.

Masur, F. T. (1981). Adherence to health care regimens. In C. K. Prokop & L. A. Bradley (Eds.), *Medical psychology: Contributions to behavioral medicine* (pp. 442-470). New York: Academic Press.

McAlister, A. L. (1991). Population behavior change: A theory-based approach. *Journal of Public Health Policy, 12*, 345-361.

McKenna, A., Ledbetter, M., & Ramaeker, L. (1989a). Integrating values education into an allied health curriculum. Part I. *Radiologic Technology, 60*, 499-502.

McKenna, A., Ledbetter, M., & Ramaeker, L. (1989b). Integrating values education into an allied health curriculum. Part II. *Radiologic Technology, 61*, 41-46.

Mechanic, D. (1989). *Painful choices: Research and essays on health care*. New Brunswick, NJ: Transaction Publishers.

Mennin, S. P., Friedman, M., Skipper, B., Kalishman, S., & Snyder, J. (1993). Performances on the NBME I, II, and III by medical students in the problem-based learning and conventional tracks at the University of New Mexico. *Academic Medicine, 68*, 616-624.

Miller, S., Remen, N., Barbour, A., Nakles, M. A., Miller, S., & Garell, D. (1975). *Dimensions of humanistic medicine*. San Francisco: Institute for the Study of Humanistic Medicine, Mt. Zion Hospital and Medical Center.

Mitchell, R. E., Billings, A. G., & Moos, R. H. (1983). Social support and well-being: Implications for prevention programs. *Journal of Primary Prevention, 3*, 77-98.

Nemcek, M. (1990). Health beliefs and preventive behavior: A review of research literature. *AAOHN Journal: Official Journal of the American Association of Occupational Health Nurses, 38*, 127-137.

Norman, G. R., & Schmidt, H. G. (1992). The psychological basis of problem-based learning: A review of the evidence. *Academic Medicine, 67*, 557-565.

Oken, D. (1978). The doctor's job—an update. *Psychosomatic Medicine, 40*, 449-461.

O'Neil, E. H. (1993). *Health professions education for the future: Schools in service to the nation*. San Francisco: Pew Health Professions Commission.

Patterson, J., Fried, R. A., & Nagle, J. P. (1989). Impact of a comprehensive health promotion curriculum on physician behavior and attitudes. *American Journal of Preventive Medicine, 5*, 44-49.

Price, J. H., Desmond, S. M., & Losh, D. P. (1991). Patients' expectations of the family physician in health promotion. *American Journal of Preventive Medicine, 7*, 33-39.

Prohaska, T. R., Albrecht, G., Levy, J. A., Sugrue, N., & Kim, J. (1990). Determinants of self-perceived risk for AIDS. *Journal of Health and Social Behavior, 31*, 384-394.

Relman, A. S. (1982). Encouraging the practice of preventive medicine and health promotion. *Public Health Reports, 97*, 216-219.

Rettie, L. (1993). The future of allied health in higher education: Where does it belong? *Journal of Dental Education, 57*, 623-625.

Robinson, T. C. (1993). Overview of allied health issues in contemporary health care. *Journal of Dental Education, 57*, 616-618.

Rogers, D. E. (1974). The doctor himself must become the treatment. *Pharos of Alpha Omega Alpha, 37*, 124-129.

Rosenstock, J. M. (1966). Why people use health services. *Milbank Memorial Fund Quarterly, 44*, 94-127.

Roter, D. L. (1988). Reciprocity in the medical encounter. In D. S. Gochman (Ed.), *Health behavior: Emerging research perspectives* (pp. 293-303). New York: Plenum Press.

Rundall, T. G., & Wheeler, J. R. (1979a). Factors associated with utilization of the swine flu vaccination program among senior citizens. *Medical Care, 17*, 191-200.

Rundall, T. G., & Wheeler, J. R. (1979b). The effect of income on use of preventive care: An evaluation of alternative explanations. *Journal of Health and Social Behavior, 20*, 397-406.

Sands, R. G., Stafford, J., & McClelland, M. (1990). "I beg to differ": Conflict in the interdisciplinary team. *Social Work in Health Care, 14*, 55-72.

Schroeder, S. A. (1992). The troubled profession: Is medicine's glass half full or half empty? *Annals of Internal Medicine, 116*, 583-592.

Segall, A. (1988). Cultural factors in sick-role expectations. In D. S. Gochman (Ed.), *Health behavior: Emerging research perspectives* (pp. 249-260). New York: Plenum Press.

Shapiro, A. K., & Shapiro, E. (1984). Patient-provider relationships and the placebo effect. In J. D. Matarazzo, S. M. Weiss, J. A. Herd, N. E. Miller, & S. M. Weiss (Eds.), *Behavioral health: A handbook of health enhancement and disease prevention* (pp. 371-383). New York: Wiley.

Shea, S., & Basch, C. E. (1990). A review of five major community-based cardiovascular disease prevention programs. Part II. Intervention strategies, evaluation methods, and results. *American Journal of Health Promotion, 4*, 279-287.

Shortell, S. M. (1982). Theory Z: Implications and relevance for health care management. *Health Care Management Review, 7*, 7-21.

Shugars, D. A., O'Neil, E. H., & Bader, J. D. (Eds.). (1991). *Healthy America: Practitioners for 2005, an agenda for action for U.S. health professional schools*. Durham, NC: Pew Health Professions Commission.

Skidmore, J. R., & Roberts, R. N. (1991). Rural Navajo early intervention health promotion: Community principles and behavioral applications. *Behavior Therapist, 14*, 29-30.

Stahelski, A. J., & Tsukuda, R. (1990). Predictors of cooperation in health teams. *Small Group Research, 21*, 220-233.

Stellar, E. (1992). The significance of the behavioral sciences. In R. Q. Marston & R. M. Jones (Eds.), *Medical education in transition* (p. 73). Princeton, NJ: Robert Wood Johnson Foundation.

Swanson, A. G. (1989). Medical education reform without change. *Mayo Clinic Proceedings, 44*, 1173-1174.

Thomas, L. (1992). *The fragile species*. New York: Scribner.

Tirrell, B. E., & Hart, L. K. (1980). The relationship of health beliefs and knowledge to exercise compliance in patients after coronary bypass. *Heart and Lung, 9*, 487-493.

Todd, J. S. (1992). Health care reform and the medical education imperative. *Journal of the American Medical Association, 268*, 1133-1134.

Wells, K. B., Lewis, C. E., Leake, B., & Ware, J. E., Jr. (1984). Do physicians preach what they practice? *Journal of the American Medical Association, 252*, 2846-2848.

Wheat, J. R., Killian, C. D., & Melnick, D. E. (1991). Reevaluation of medical education: A behavioral model to assess health promotion/disease prevention instruction. *Evaluation and the Health Professions, 14*, 305-318.

Young, E. H. (1988). Health promoting behaviors of family practice residents: Do they compare with the general public? *Family Medicine, 20*, 437-442.

2

Health Behavior Research and Medical Training

A New Paradigm

Virginia A. Reed, Maggie L. Moore-West, G. Christian Jernstedt, and Joseph F. O'Donnell

INTRODUCTION

Despite rapid advances in the technology of the health sciences and in understanding of the basic biology of diseases at the molecular level, most of the disease processes that in the postantibiotic age cause disability and death have behavioral roots. The statistics concerning behavioral risk factors noted in youth are particularly alarming. For example, among American high school students, 73.9% indicated that they had tried smoking by their senior year, while 24.7% admitted to

smoking daily over the past month. Furthermore, 48% indicated that they had had at least one alcoholic drink within the past month. With regard to sex, 70% responded that they had had sexual intercourse by their senior year, with 18.5% reporting having had four or more sexual partners. As for suicide, 24% indicated that they had given serious consideration to the thought of suicide over the past year. Finally, 22% indicated that they had carried a weapon in the past month (Kann et al., 1995).

Health behavior research can and should provide a significant contribution to the goal of achieving optimal understanding and control of the many behaviorally related disease processes. Additionally, incorporation of health behavior research into the process of medical education should provide physicians with awareness, knowledge, and tools that can assist them in helping individual patients. Despite the significance of the role that health behavior research could play in medical education, however, the actualization of that role was, at the mid-1990s, relatively minor.

Virginia A. Reed • Department of Psychology, Dartmouth College, Hanover, New Hampshire 03755. **Maggie L. Moore-West** • Department of Community and Family Medicine, Dartmouth Medical School, Hanover, New Hampshire 03755. **G. Christian Jernstedt** • Department of Psychology and C. Everett Koop Institute, Dartmouth College, Hanover, New Hampshire 03755. **Joseph F. O'Donnell** • Department of Medicine, Dartmouth Medical School, Hanover, New Hampshire 03755.

Handbook of Health Behavior Research IV: Relevance for Professionals and Issues for the Future, edited by David S. Gochman. Plenum Press, New York, 1997.

The first section of this chapter provides a historical context for the current relative lack of inclusion of health behavior research in medical education. This section also provides examples of promising new trends. The second section focuses on research on communication skills and the impact these skills can have on medical training. The final section of the chapter focuses on meta-analysis as a most useful tool for interpreting studies in the field of health behavior research.

A NEED FOR A NEW PARADIGM OF HEALTH IN MEDICAL EDUCATION

In the late 1980s, Baumgart and Costello (1988) noted that the topic of health behavior, despite its prominence in the arenas of popular culture and social policy, remained underrepresented in the training of North American health professionals. The authors felt, however, that socioeconomic trends would lead to significant changes in the content and structure of health sciences education and would spark increased interest in health behavior research. Their cautiously optimistic assessment was based on the apparent harkening of the health professions of nursing, social work, and health education to the call of social policy experts, although the interface between policy and medical education remained a tenuous one.

The shift in health care policy toward both managed health care and outcomes-based research is reminiscent of earlier times when social and health policy changes were predicted to dictate reform in our educational institutions (Funkenstein, 1968). The pattern of response by medical schools in the United States has historically been to develop a variety of reforms—often embedded within the strengths and philosophies of individual departments and institutions—that assume various roles in courses, electives, or teaching style. Vicissitudes of these reforms often become the individual school's barriers to the next generation of reforms.

Increasing health care costs and the subsequent development of managed care institutions (Rivo, Mays, Katzoff, & King, 1995) should have a decisive effect on medical education. One might have predicted, as did Baumgart and Costello (1988), that through the mid- to late 1990s, perhaps more than at any other time, the opportunity existed for programs and research endeavors to be informed by the increasingly sophisticated results of health behavior research. Gochman (1988) defined health behavior research as research on the determinants of health behavior, as well as on health behavior itself—research, in other words, that relates to the improvement or restoration of health and to the maintenance of health. There is a powerful rationale for the use of health behavior research in developing content and programs in medical education; therefore, health behavior research will be the point of departure in the following discussion of barriers to reform in United States medical schools. Emphasizing medical practice, not treatment, as a critical determinant in health behavior makes it critically important to focus on medical education as the primary socializing agency for medical deportment in order to understand the entire breadth of health behaviors.

Proposed Reform in Medical Education

Two mid-1990s documents (Christakis, 1995; Swanson & Anderson, 1993) examined the historical process of reform in medical education. Christakis (1995) identified 19 reports concerning undergraduate medical education reform published between 1910 and 1993. His goal was to identify the values and agendas that created a need for reform and to describe patterns, if they existed, throughout the decades. The choice of reports was based on their focus in undergraduate medical education and on their breadth of recommendations. Christakis (1995) indicated that the major themes of these reports consistently affirmed society's expectation that medical schools would serve society. He also found that the core objectives were consistent among the 19 reports: serving the public interest, addressing the physician workforce, coping with an increasingly complex medical knowledge base, and supporting rising interest in generalism. In the examination of the specifics of the proposed reforms, the themes that emerged were manner of teaching, content of teaching, faculty development, and organizational factors. While Christakis (1995) posited that the similarity in proposed reforms over an 83-year period suggested a consistency of social vision for the profession, another interpretation may be that there has been such a weak responsiveness to these visions on the part of the institution of medical education that the visions must constantly be resuggested.

The second document, "Educating Medical Students: Assessing Change in Medical Education—The Road to Implementation" (ACME-TRI) (Swanson & Anderson, 1993), identified recurrent problems in medical education from the 1930s to the mid 1980s, documented that most medical schools had not solved these problems, and summarized the barriers to problem solution. The second phase of the report provided information for the implementation of reform.

ACME-TRI summarized findings of a project surveying North American medical school deans. The dimensions of the survey were based on 18 recommendations from three major documents on medical education published by the Association of American Medical Colleges in the 1980s (Swanson & Anderson, 1993) that reconfirmed findings from the 1932 Commission on Medical Education (Rappeleye, 1932). Some of the findings of ACME-TRI that relate specifically to the subject of innovation and health behavior models lay in the areas of curriculum structure and content. Authors of the report found that the majority of preclinical teaching continued to be conducted by basic science departments, with most of the teaching done by lecture. The length of time scheduled for required instruction ranged from a low of 799 hours to a high of 2389 hours at the responding institutions. The time available

for elective courses in the preclinical disciplines was minimal. There had been very few changes made within the preclinical curriculum to respond to the request for relevancy of content or to reforming teaching techniques to include more individualized instruction.

The clinical years continued to consist primarily of experiential learning in tertiary settings, with some supplementary instruction provided in seminars and lectures. Over the past decade, there has been more of a move into the outpatient ambulatory care setting, a move with specific implications for student understanding of the patient within a socioeconomic and behavioral context (Swanson & Anderson, 1993).

When students were queried as to the adequacy of different content areas in their curriculum, they consistently responded that the content areas dealing with the more behavioral aspects of health care were inadequate. These aspects included nutrition; medical care cost control; management of the patient's socioeconomic, educational, and emotional problems; care of the ambulatory patient; public health and community medicine; and the role of medicine in the community. In contrast, more traditional content areas, such as biochemistry, anatomy, and interview skills, were all considered to be adequately or excessively represented (Swanson & Anderson, 1993).

The results of both Christakis (1995) and the ACME-TRI Report (Swanson & Anderson, 1993) point to the continued need for change in medical education as well as to a reassertion of the professional value of a social vision. Health policy experts and social theorists have long advocated approaches like that of health behavior research in order to integrate a certain social consciousness into medical education (Forman, 1994). Despite consistent assertion of the need and rationale for change, change has not come about. Certain elements have mitigated against implementation of innovations in the United States, with the result that academic research and teaching endeavors have maintained a fairly traditional approach. A review of the literature suggests a number of elements that have served as impediments to implementation of innovation.

External Forces

Cultural Impact on Medical Education. Perhaps the single most important dimension in education is the process of acquiring and disseminating knowledge. Drawing from Kuhn's (1970) theory of paradigms, knowledge base is critical when it is interpreted as that which defines not only events, but also the types of research used to explain events, the manner of teaching to emphasize such explanations, and the process of implementing programs to reinforce understanding. Schon (1984, 1987) described the professional's way of knowing as one of technical rationality and positivism. The model stems from a belief in rational and linear thinking as well as in the ultimate ability of technology to solve any and all problems. Technology's legacy to medicine has taken several trajectories.

With medicine's metaphorical view of the body as something akin to the machine, more and sicker people are being hospitalized for shorter periods of time. Students' contacts with patients are becoming briefer and more narrowly focused. Procedures yield higher payments than do visits with the physician, reinforcing briefer and far more limited relationships.

Many proponents of educational reform have depicted the disease model of medical knowledge as critical in framing health care in the United States. Gunderman (1995) termed this approach "reductive isolation." This dominant model of disease emphasizes quantification, objectivity, and measurement. Such an orientation has led some physicians to view the patient in a snapshot fashion, as a disease, and to pay little attention to the impact of disease in the context of the patient's life. In most ways, the medical understanding of disease stands in opposition to the health behavior model. As one student stated (Gunderman, 1995, p. 677):

> Disease begins to seem inevitable in medical school. We forget that most people are healthy, and we forget to ask why. We understand the roots of disease well, but the roots of health almost not at all.

Gunderman (1995) contrasted the prevailing model of disease with that of the ascendant interrelation. This model involves understanding interrelationships as well as the etiology of health and illness. In the words of Gunderman (1995, p. 680):

> We cannot understand the eye, despite its many likenesses to a lens or a photoreceptor, without reference to seeing. We cannot understand the structures of living organisms without reference to their activities of living. In the human case, we cannot understand human biology without reference to human life.

Tresolini, Shugars, and Lee (1995), in a report funded by the Pew Foundation, emphasized that biomedical science and technology have been the orientation of medical education over the past 50 years. They credit this focus to the remarkable progress in biomedical research and technological developments for diagnosis and treatment of diseases. Yet they warn that such a focus is limited and cannot address the current health care problems, which embody etiology and management so complex as to require examining multifactorial influences on health and illness. Questioning how curriculum might function within such a paradigm, they developed case studies of five medical schools that reported offering an integrated approach to teaching. They found that the most important institutional characteristic was the strong presence of an explicitly stated mission, philosophy, or theoretical model that embraced an integrated approach as a base for the curriculum. Within the mission statements, there were themes of community service and a school orientation that focused outward to the community. Tresolini et al. (1995) identified, within the approaches to teaching the integration of psychological, social, and biological factors in health care, four themes that were based on several levels of relationships: the physician–patient relationship, the physician–community relationship, the physician–other practitioners relationship, and the faculty–student relationship.

Tarlov (1992) suggested that the most important effect on medical education would be the reconceptualization of health. He redefined health as a capacity, a relative ability to perform, and a continuous variable to measure. Health is also the use of that capacity to achieve expectations and to negotiate the demands of the social and physical environment toward optimal functioning (Tarlov, 1992).

Boelen (1995) asked faculty and administrators for an examination of the social accountability of medical education. Hamilton (1995) called for reexamining the model of the social origins of health and disease. Lomas (1994) suggested the need to distinguish between the content of medicine and the context for medical practice.

Social Factor of Financial Support. The manner in which medical education is primarily financed places a burden on innovations and supports the traditional disease paradigm. Historically, much of medical education has been financed by the services provided by the faculty, either in research support or in clinical services (Ganem, Beran, & Krakower, 1995). As a result, educational endeavors tend to be held hostage to the economic demands of institutional maintenance. Faculty whose time is consumed by direct services may not have the time either to devote to teaching or to offering new and innovative ideas that could contribute to the understanding of health behaviors. Expediency has become valued, encouraging the continuance of the impersonal lecture, the tertiary care team teaching, and, ultimately, the "see one, do one, teach one" approach. The marriage of medical education to large medical centers has resulted in medical educators' following an ideology of institutional maintenance rather than one of freedom of ideas, resulting in what Bloom (1988) termed "innovation without reform." The aforementioned rise in health care costs and the subsequent development of managed care institutions and their economic dominance over centers of medical education (Rivo et al., 1955) only strengthen the assumption that an ideology of institutional maintenance will continue to be a dominant factor in medical education.

It is difficult to consider how medical education can move toward incorporating an entirely new approach to understanding disease or health. Such a knowledge paradigm would have to dominate the majority of medical schools. Thus, it is imperative to consider the pervasive strength of knowledge when calling for significant reform and to examine how new knowledge is diffused within the educational community.

Internal Forces or Structural Impediments

Structure of Medical Education. In examining innovation, it is helpful to understand how processes of reform interface with institutional structure. The basic organization of medical education has changed little since the reforms based on the Flexner Report (Flexner, 1910). Though there have been some structural educational innovations at some institutions such as Case Western Reserve University, the University of New Mexico, and Brown University (Moore-West, Regan-Smith, Dietrich, & Kollisch, 1990), most schools continue to operate within a model of departmental decision making (Swanson & Anderson, 1993). Such a structure has militated against the idea of integration, core knowledge, and competencies and instead has maintained the vestiges of specialized, technology-based knowledge domains. Given physical space and time in the curriculum as signs of power, departments compete for both, allowing little opportunity for integration and generalism.

The University of Pittsburgh recently centralized its governance and found distinct advantages in terms of providing rational and integrative mechanisms for reform, especially dealing with general education focusing on the doctor–patient relationship (Reynolds et al., 1995). The university found that a centralized administration allowed new initiatives to be developed in a coordinated and expedient manner and provided a mechanism for dealing with time issues in the curriculum.

Departments of behavioral sciences emerged in the 1950s and 1960s. Like other departments, they worked to claim space and time. It is perhaps an indication of failure that there are so few departments of behavioral science left in United States medical schools. Although behavioral science is included as one of the basic sciences on the National Board of Medical Examiners Part I Examination (NBME I), it has all but disappeared as an academic domain. Many behavioral scientists work in psychiatry or in departments of family medicine or community medicine. Their roles are often clinical and their teaching supervisory. The departmentalized role of teaching and the decrease in the status of behavioral science departments have lessened opportunities for behavioral science teaching and research to be a resource for innovation in medical schools as they are now structured (Straus, 1994).

The Association for the Behavioral Sciences and Medical Education (ABSAME) is an association of a diverse group of medical educators, crossing all domains of medical specialty as well as the social and behavioral sciences. In 1994, ABSAME produced a document calling for the integration and dissemination of behavioral science domains throughout the process of medical education, with content being framed within the relationship among health, illness, and disease (Association for the Behavioral Sciences and Medical Education, 1994). Although these are positive strides in the direction of new models of behavioral science content, leading to more health behavior research, it is difficult to imagine any significant modification in content organization without a primary focus on reorganizing the structure of medical education.

Admissions. Although interest in the types of students admitted to medical school has risen again due to the increasing attention to primary care, admission policies have traditionally been driven by student academic performance. This focus may be due, in part, to the failure to develop competency measures to supplement or replace the standardized national board scores. Until schools have and use criteria other than knowledge of content by which to measure success, they continue to select students largely on the basis of the science grade point average (GPA) and the scores on the Medical College Admission Test (MCAT), both of which have increased over the past decade (Barzansky, Jonas, & Etzel, 1995). Although there is some association between MCAT scores and GPA, on one hand, and preclinical performance and NBME I performance, on the other, these associations tend to disappear in the clinical years (Moore-West et al., 1990). Much of both this initial association and its subsequent lack may be attributed to the artifact of measurement, whereby ratio variables are more highly correlated than are ordinal or clinical score variables, and where reliability is an issue (Golden, 1994). Performance on basic fact exams has not been predictive of performance on clinical skills exams. Interestingly, research on demographic variables suggests that applicants who are more likely to enter primary care areas may not come from what has been typically described as a pre-med background—young, unmarried, urban university, high achiever, science major—but may tend to be married, older, and have lower entering academic scores (Hojat, Gonnella, Erdmann, Veloski, & Xu, 1995).

Lack of Institutional Goals. Students applying to medical school have little information about the process of medical school selection and the distinguishing characteristics of medical schools, thus making informed choice difficult. A preliminary study (Walsh, Stevens, & Moore-West, 1994) examined perceptions of medical school applicants about the information necessary to making career decisions, specifically decisions concerning medical school. Most students had little specific information on medical education except knowledge of the application process and the particular school's entry requirements.

Each medical school, however, has its own

character, learning climate, and social atmo-sphere and thus creates a unique environment for students. As previously mentioned, Tresolini et al. (1995) found that the institutional charac-teristic most important for success in implement-ing an innovative integrated curriculum was the strong presence of an explicitly stated mission, philosophy, or theoretical model that embraced an integrated approach as a basis for the curricu-lum. With few medical schools having specified exit goals or required competencies for their graduates, applicants have little knowledge of the philosophy, mission, and learning environ-ment of the schools to which they are applying. Schools such as Brown University have devel-oped a series of competencies required of all graduates (Smith, 1994). Attention to such issues provides the potential to move beyond the most basic set of information on applications (GPA/ MCAT and NBME performances) to a more so-phisticated level.

Innovative Programs Influenced by Health Behavior Research

Despite the various elements of medical education that do not readily lend themselves to the integration of health behavior research, this summary does not deny that health behavior re-search is being utilized within areas of teaching and research at some medical schools. Although innovations have been introduced across the country, these reforms are most often course-oriented and remain within the boundaries of the particular institution.

At Dartmouth Medical School, a program called Partners in Health Education was created to support opportunities for medical students to work with public school teachers in teaching health awareness to children (O'Donnell, 1992). A unique element of this program was that it served as one of the early points of contact be-tween Dartmouth Medical School and the area's public schools, combining the medical expertise of a physician, the prevention and education ex-

pertise of a health educator, and the community needs articulated by a school nurse.

Community Service Learning Programs. Across the country, community service programs are springing up at medical schools. Many of these programs are designed to promote health education, disease prevention and wellness, and strategies oriented to community health improve-ment or to meet the needs of the underserved. These programs are an interesting phenomenon for several reasons. Many are student-initiated. Tarallo-Falk (1995) described such programs as creating more of a sense of empowerment and meaning among the students than the traditional curriculum. They are often based in health be-havior research, directed at changes in health behavior at the community level, and focused on prevention or health education as a form of inter-vention. They are also likely to be introduced into the medical student's socialization process at a very early stage (Tarallo-Falk, 1995), providing a potential reframing of the professional role for the entering physician.

The students of Dartmouth Medical School's Community Service Committee—the recipients of the 1995 American Medical Student Associa-tion's Paul Wright Excellence in Medical Educa-tion Award—developed a variety of community services that students may elect. Among them are programs directed at student peer education on smoking, substance abuse, and domestic vio-lence; student-run clinics for smoking cessation; a senior medication awareness program to ex-plain drug effects and side effects to elders to increase their understanding; and a community outreach project designed to help rural college-bound students to matriculate and remain in col-lege (American Medical Student Association, 1995). The content of such programs is largely driven by health behavior research.

It appears that students may be drawn to the opportunity to provide social service out of moral conviction and social vision that deter-mine the students' priorities for health care. Many of these programs have adamantly defended their right to offer service apart from the formal curriculum and apart from administrative control. The students' needs for autonomy in their community service programs may well be a warning to medical educators that institutional inaction is leaving a legacy of distrust among a new generation of students.

At the University of California at Davis School of Medicine, a student-run elective, Health Care to Underserved Populations, provides information on volunteering in communities (American Medical Student Association, 1995). Students present information on underserved groups and invite local experts to discuss their research. Rush University requires each student to complete a first-year experience in community health (Eckenfels, 1992). From this experience, students generated a community service program, the Rush Community Service Initiatives Program (RCSIP), to expand upon their required experiences. As of 1995, the RCSIP had seven community service projects involving about 200 students and 25 physicians on a volunteer basis.

Patient Education and Community Health Promotion

A survey of all United States medical schools was conducted to determine the number of schools that included instruction in the areas of patient education and community health promotion, areas in which health behavior research would play a prominent role (Little, 1992). A total of 77 institutions responded; 65% of those reporting stated that they offered instruction in patient education and 74% that they offered instruction in community health promotion. Those offering such courses indicated that they felt that the material was valuable, but that they had little course time in which to offer an adequate amount of material (Little, 1992). Tufts Medical School, drawing from attempts at other medical schools such as Tulane, George Washington, and Columbia to include resources from their allied schools in public health, developed a unique four-year

combined M.D.–M.P.H. program (J. Evans, 1992). With support from the Health to the Public initiative sponsored by the Pew Charitable Trusts and the Rockefeller Foundation, Tufts also provides forums for other interested medical schools. Utilizing the resources of the public health schools, Tufts offers an undergraduate program to train future physicians within a population-based, community-oriented approach to health care as well as an education in the clinical and research skills that are critical to health promotion and disease prevention (Boyer et al., 1992).

Rational Decision-Making Models

Another set of reforms with a basis in health behavior research and theory is that subset of communication skills known generally as "decision analysis." These approaches are based on the rational decision-making model and are often reliant on population-based data sets. The development of clinical decision making, pioneered by researchers such as Sox (Sox, Blatt, Higgins, Marton, 1988) and Holmes-Rovner (Holmes-Rovner et al., 1994), is a product of the rational model of decision making around clinical and administrative issues. Students are trained to work with patients, helping them make decisions about their health care by providing information trees weighted by specificities and sensitivities. Adding the patients' values, or utilities, places the patients in a far more informed position to make the most appropriate decisions regarding their own health care needs.

An interesting trajectory of health behavior research that focuses on physician practice patterns and how they relate to health-seeking behavior is the use of small-area research. Researchers such as Wennberg (1990) examine physicians' practice patterns within a specific geographic region in order to understand the development and sanctioning of practice norms. This approach places physician practices in a particular area under scrutiny by comparing one geographic area of practice with another. For instance, patterns in elective surgeries (e.g., frequency, types, patient type) are examined in order to understand the nature of physician preference in health care decision making. The resultant model of doctor–patient interaction is called the shared decision-making model (Wennberg, 1990). In this model, patients are presented with all available information in order to be able to make the most informed decision possible regarding their care. Patients are presented with videotapes explaining all options available to them along with the possible benefits and side effects of each option. It is the physician's obligation to provide the patient with all the information possible rather than to offer advice or to filter information.

Moral decision making has evolved into a process of examining the context of a patient's normative, spiritual, and cultural values and attitudes when working toward a decision between the physician's value structure and that of the patient (Smith, Balint, Krause, Moore-West, & Viles, 1994). Negotiation becomes the process of decision making around an outcome that places the physician's belief system and expectations on the same level as those of the patient. Research data are drawn into the relationship in a manner that acknowledges the patient's belief system and values and is combined with the clinical data in a manner that allows the patient to make an informed decision within the context of an understanding and supportive relationship.

Health behavior research has made significant inroads into health care professions other than medicine and has created some movement in undergraduate medical education. The institution of medical education will undergo change over the next decade in response to the various societal demands of health care reform. Whether innovations such as those just described will be successfully disseminated depends not only upon the conceptualized reforms, but also upon the strategies with which these reforms are introduced. A very important element in evaluating innovation diffusion is examining the process of change and identifying the potential barriers within that process (Moore-West & O'Donnell, 1985).

ROLE OF COMMUNICATION SKILLS IN DISSEMINATING HEALTH BEHAVIOR INFORMATION

Over the course of a 40-year career, the average physician providing primary care will conduct at least 200,000 patient interviews (Epstein, Campbell, Cohen-Cole, McWhinney, & Smilkstein, 1993). Each interview provides an opportunity for the physician not only to diagnose and treat the patient, but also to establish and maintain rapport with the patient and to educate the patient by providing health behavior information. These processes, however, are mediated by the physician's ability to communicate. Effective communication skills have been associated with improved patient satisfaction (B. J. Evans, Stanley, & Burrows, 1992) and recall of information (Lewis, Pantell, & Sharp, 1991), both of which can lead to increased patient compliance with medical regimens (Bartlett et al., 1984).

Increased compliance leading to optimal health and functioning is an elusive goal of health behavior messages. Winett (1995) suggests that the efficacy of health behavior information is influenced by the salience of that information and how it is framed and tailored to the individual or the audience for whom it is intended. Prochaska and DiClemente (1983) proposed a model of behavior change, the stages of change model, that describes the occurrence of change as resulting from a series of evolutions for the patient. These evolutions begin with the stage at which behavior change is not yet being considered and continue through stages of planning to change, changing, and, finally, maintaining the change. Physicians who are skilled at communicating health behavior information are most likely skilled at determining where along the readiness continuum individual patients are. The health behavior messages delivered to these patients are likely to be tailored to address not only the patients' need for information, but also their readiness to hear and assimilate the information into health behavior change. High-level communication skills are therefore required to assess and address the subtleties and nuances of patient readiness for health behavior information and change.

Past Research

Since the 1970s, researchers have studied the natural course of communication skill development in medical students and the effect of various programs designed to increase those skills. Helfer (1970) found that medical students' communication skills declined as the students progressed through medical school. He speculated that students enter medical school with certain innate communication skills and abilities that tend to be lost as the students focus their time and energy on organic processes and pathological conditions. As a result of the work of Helfer and others (e.g., see Stillman, Burpeau-DiGregorio, Nicholson, Sabers, & Stillman, 1983), medical schools began to place increasing emphasis on communication skills, and many introduced programs into the curriculum to enhance development of these skills. This emphasis has continued, and today virtually every medical school in the United States teaches interviewing and communication skills (Novack, Volk, Drossman, & Lipkin, 1993).

While many studies have been conducted to examine the effect of various programs for instilling or improving communication skills in medical students, there is enormous variability in the scope, topics, methodology, and quality of the research (Reed & Jernstedt, 1994). Modern experimental research has evolved to a stage at which groups of studies, rather than single studies, must be used to understand important subjects. Meta-analysis (described and discussed in the next section) provides a tool that allows for the quantitative combining, cumulating, and comparing of results of many studies in a coherent and consistent manner.

Anderson and Sharpe (1991) conducted a meta-analysis of 40 experimental interventions designed to improve patient or health care provider communication skills. They reported moderate to large effect sizes for interventions designed to improve interviewing skills in medical students. Reed and Jernstedt (1994) reported preliminary findings of a meta-analysis of 163 studies exploring communication skills in physicians and medical students. They found that studies of interventions designed to enhance communication skills used a variety of outcome measures that could be cast into five domains: communication skills, knowledge, diagnostic abilities, patient satisfaction, and attitude. Reed and Jernstedt's (1994) findings suggest that programs ostensibly designed to enhance communication skills showed positive and significant effect sizes only for the domains of diagnostic abilities and knowledge, not for communication skills.

The two domains in which changes do tend to occur are those upon which medical schools have always been most directly focused. Thus, it appears that even when medical schools target the development of communication skills, efforts to improve these skills may reinforce other skills more than those targeted.

A Theoretical Model

United States medical education and public health recommendations have called for an increased emphasis on preventive medicine (Muller, 1984; U.S. Preventive Services Task Force, 1989). As implementation of these recommendations proceeds, the ability of physicians to communicate effectively on the topic of health behavior becomes increasingly important. Influences on the development of communication skills can be described in terms of a unified theoretical model of adult behavior change, based on the work of Bandura (1978) (illustrated in Figure 1), the basic components of which are the Person, the Environment, Behavior, and Outcome. This model illustrates a theory of personal efficacy and has been previously used to describe learn-

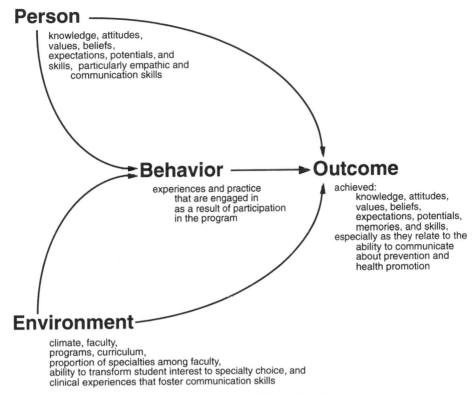

Figure 1. A unified theoretical model of adult behavior change.

ing experiences (Jernstedt & Chow, 1980). Since communication skill development is a learning experience targeted in medical education, this model provides an appropriate way to conceptualize the concomitants of such skill development.

According to this model, each individual brings certain previous experiences and personal characteristics to the medical school learning situation. In the model, this blend of personal characteristics and experiences is represented as the Person. The qualities of the Person vary from student to student, reflecting not only students' inherent abilities and traits, but also the wealth of educational and life experiences to which each student has been previously exposed. In describing the development of communication skills, the Person includes both the skills, abilities, and

potentials relative to communication that each student brings to this point in his or her life, and the actualization of those abilities and potentials.

The climate, faculty, programs, and experiences of the medical school are represented in the model as the Environment. Again, these qualities vary from school to school, and may vary within schools over time as faculty and curricula change and as changes in the health care system are reflected in the clinical experiences and milieu experienced by the students.

The student's actual behavior is represented in the model as Behavior. Behavior would include behavior engaged in as part of the training, and thus would include the practice of skills students undertake as they learn the role of the physician.

The Outcome consists of the medical communication skills and concomitant attributes that the student achieves as a result of the interaction of the Person, the Environment, and the Behavior (Jernstedt & Reed, 1995a,b).

Using this theoretical model as a way to think about the development of communication skills, one concludes that if schools desire to enhance or improve the communication skills that students take with them as one of the outcomes of their medical education, then the range of characteristics of the three contributing elements—the Person, the Environment, and the Behavior—are all candidates for interventions designed to improve such skills.

The Person.   For the purposes of this chapter, the Person includes the innate skills, abilities, and potentials relative to communication that each student brings to the medical school experience in particular, as well as the actualization of those abilities and potentials to this point in his or her life. It also includes the attitudes, values, expectations, and beliefs that the student brings, relative to health behavior as well as to all other aspects of his or her life.

It may well be that different students are more or less predisposed to the development of excellent medical communication skills. For example, it is considered important that medical students develop empathic skills in order to communicate effectively with patients (e.g., Evans, Stanley, & Burrows, 1993). While numerous programs have been designed to help students develop empathic skills, it may be that the students most able to improve and refine their empathic skills have more of those skills upon entering medical school. If that were the case, then one way to improve the communication skills of groups of physicians would be to consider empathic skills as a selection factor in admission to medical school.

Other characteristics, values, and attitudes are also likely predictors of communicative propensity and skill. Theoretically, one way to evaluate the strength of relationship between the two would involve two kinds of assessment tools. One tool would assess broad parameters of student characteristics, attitudes, and values. A second tool would evaluate the communication skills of groups of incoming students, and then would reevaluate the skills of these same groups of students four years later at the conclusion of their medical education. The effect of the medical education process and program on groups of students—those with a predisposition to develop good communication skills and those without—could then be assessed. If a strong relationship were found between certain attributes and communication skill, and if graduating students with excellent medical communication skills were a priority for that school, then the relevant attributes could be assessed and weighted in the admission process. Preferential selection of students has been used successfully to meet other goals of medical education, such as influencing specialty choice (Rabinowitz, 1988, 1990).

The Environment.   In the model, the climate, faculty, programs, and curriculum of the medical school are represented as the Environment. Each medical school has a unique environment, contributed to by the values inherent in the institution as expressed in its written philosophy and its stated or unstated goals and objectives. For example, some schools place more emphasis on research; others place more on practice components. Some schools are known for their dedication to producing primary care physicians; others are known more for graduating students interested in subspecialty areas. It is probable that whatever is most valued at a particular school is most likely to receive the largest share of the attention, resources, and effort. When resources and attention are directed toward a particular outcome or set of outcomes, it is not surprising that those outcomes prevail.

Again, the specialty choice literature provides an example. Schools that are known for producing the largest proportion of family medicine physicians appear to be schools that not only are successful at translating initially expressed interest in primary care into actual selection of a primary care specialty for residency, but also are able to attract students who were not initially interested in family medicine but subsequently developed an interest (Godkin & Quirk, 1991).

Thus, it follows that schools that place more emphasis on incorporating health behavior research into both the curriculum and the experiences available to students may be more likely to produce physicians who will model this emphasis in their practice.

The Behavior. The Behavior that students engage in as part of their medical education provides experience and practice in learning both the skills and the role of the physician. As students participate in preceptorships and clinical rotations, they observe, try out, and refine their skills in many areas, receiving feedback from faculty and mentors. Practice and subsequent feedback are powerful learning tools, but the literature on learning indicates that immediate learning and long-term learning are facilitated in different ways (Druckman & Bjork, 1994). Researchers studying communication skills in medical education have explored both the acquisition of skills and the retention of those skills, with far fewer studies being done on the latter. Individual studies have shown mixed results regarding the retention of skills initially taught (Craig, 1992; Stillman, Sabers & Redfield, 1977).

If one of the goals of a medical school is to improve students' communication skills, then an ideal training program would take into account the differences in optimal learning strategies for short-term and long-term learning. Effective, satisfying medical interviews have many features in common; they also have unique features. A critical need in learning is for the learning to be transferable across situations (Druckman & Bjork, 1994). Thus, the point of teaching medical students communication skills is the hope that the skills acquired will generalize to their performance across time and situations.

The Outcome. As illustrated in Figure 1, the Outcome is the result produced by the interaction of the Person, the Environment, and the Behavior. In the health behavior context, it includes the medical communication skills and

knowledge, the perceptions of the environment, the memories of the learning experience, the new expectations, and the attitudes, values, and beliefs that the student achieves as a result of being a unique Person in the particular educational Environment who underwent the specific learning experiences (Jernstedt & Reed, 1995a,b).

If physicians are to be effective disseminators of health behavior information, they must have factual knowledge of practices and behaviors that enhance health and a high level of communication skills that enable them to assess patient readiness to hear and change actual behavior. As medical schools prepare physicians for the 21st century, increased emphasis on prevention and wellness must be matched by emphasis on the ability to communicate these messages effectively. Each of the three contributing elements of the theoretical model, the Person, the Environment, and the Behavior, should be comprehensively researched in terms of its contributions to and effect on the desired Outcome. One example of such research currently being conducted is the C. Everett Koop Institute at Dartmouth Medical Education Assessment Program (Jernstedt & Reed, 1995a,b; Reed & Jernstedt, 1995). The extensive psychological literature on learning, retention, and performance should be tapped as a resource in designing new programs to enhance the development of communication skills. Evaluation must be seen as a necessary, desirable, and inherent part of the medical education process if the goals of improving communication skills and of improving medical education are to be realized.

RESEARCH AND METHODOLOGICAL ISSUES FOR THE FUTURE: ROLE OF META-ANALYSIS

Foundations of Meta-Analysis

Some excellent evaluation research methods have been used for millennia in conducting forms of health behavior research. For example, the prophet Daniel described the direct empirical comparison of results from experimental and comparison groups fed different diets (cited in Calvin, 1852). Recently, however, a fundamental change in the basic philosophical foundations of research methods has been emerging. This change is characterized by a shift from a focus on the single research study and the description of its outcome by its statistical significance to a focus on the cumulation of research findings across studies and the description of their outcomes by the magnitudes of their effects. Historically, statistical analysis of outcomes from health behavior and other research has been built upon Fisher's (1935) work with agricultural plots. A foundation built on the statistical significance of single studies, whether or not it is still appropriate for manipulating the application of fertilizer to crops, is inappropriate for dealing with modern behavioral research issues, especially in health behavior and other medical areas. One problem is that research is a human process, and a given study can be subject to an array of biases unique to the particular researchers conducting that study (Johnson, 1940). A second problem, and a most serious one for health behavior research, is that reliance on statistical significance can result in ignoring research outcomes that may have important impacts on medical outcomes for patients (Rosnow & Rosenthal, 1989). There are other problems, as well (Schmidt, 1992).

Due in part to this traditional foundation, analyses of experimental results have focused almost exclusively on the probability of statistical significance of the observed outcomes. In particular, researchers, by computing the measure, p, the probability that the null hypothesis is true, have been concerned with whether their results could have been obtained by chance alone. The result of this focus on the statistical significance of the outcome is that the magnitude of the outcome has been all but ignored. The magnitude of an observed outcome, expressed as an effect size, may be even more important than the statistical significance, especially for the type of research conducted in the health behavior field. Effect size indicates how important the observed

outcome may be. Ideally, both statistical significance and effect size should be reported for all outcomes. Fortunately, it is possible to compute effect sizes from many of the standard statistical numbers reported in published research (Rosenthal, 1991).

Meta-analysis is a method of cumulating research across many individual studies, employing effect size as an outcome measure. The use of meta-analytical techniques in psychological and educational research, for example, has transformed the cumulation of research findings since its first full description by Glass, McGaw, and Smith (1981). All future research in health behavior should be conducted and reported in a manner to facilitate the use of meta-analytical summaries of research findings.

Meta-Analytical Methods

There is no single method of conducting meta-analyses. There is, however, an underlying sequence to the general process of meta-analysis:

1. Search for all reports on the particular topic or phenomenon under investigation (e.g., as described earlier in this chapter, find all studies of programs designed to increase communication skills in medical students).
2. Collect all retrievable studies that were located in the search.
3. From the reported results in each study, compute one or more effect sizes for that study. Code each computed effect size for the values of any variables of interest that may be correlated with the effect size. For example, in the communication skill meta-analyses, studies were coded for type of training intervention, study design, and other such variables (Anderson & Sharpe, 1991; Reed & Jernstedt, 1994).
4. Cumulate those effect sizes across published reports, making appropriate statistical adjustments for various sources of error or bias.

5. Average the effect sizes found for the various levels of variables and the various groups that were part of each study.

While these basic steps are present in nearly all meta-analyses, different statisticians and meta-analysts have been concerned about different potential sources of error and bias in this process. Rosenthal (1991) provides an overview of general techniques. Glass et al. (1981) and Hedges and Olkin (1985) provide many formulas for computing effect sizes from the different types of statistical results that can be found in studies. Hunter and Schmidt (1990) provide a unique set of computation tools that are directed particularly at dealing with sampling and measurement error in reported results of research studies. Cooper and Hedges (1994) provide a comprehensive handbook that ranges broadly across most of the important issues in meta-analysis.

Each of these authors introduces important considerations for conducting a modern meta-analysis. Unfortunately, no single source currently combines the best of each writer's recommendations and procedures (though authors Reed and Jernstedt of this chapter are in the process of developing such material). Thus, researchers in health behavior must themselves integrate the methods of these authors. Such an integration of methods results in a recommendation that future meta-analyses must provide four basic sets of measurements: (1) the basic effect size, (2) the corrections in the effect size for standard sources of procedural and statistical bias, (3) the corrections in the effect size for sampling and other measurement errors, and (4) measures of the confidence intervals of the computed effect size.

Recommendations for Future Research on Health Behavior

The style of research reporting currently in use in health behavior publications evolved before the arrival of meta-analytical methods. As a result, many current researchers do not report the statistics that are necessary to calculate effect sizes. Journal editors should require that all individual quantitative research studies include in their published reports the statistical results needed by the meta-analysts who are likely to employ that article in future analyses. These statistics can be as simple as the means and standard deviations, reported separately for each variable and each group that was included in the study.

The goals of research programs should be reconsidered in light of the power of meta-analysis. Researchers must ask themselves whether their research goals would be best served by conducting a meta-analytical cumulation of previous research or by conducting a new individual study. Furthermore, health behavior researchers ought to consider where there are gaps in cumulative knowledge when deciding on research directions to pursue. It may well be true that additional meta-analyses of the vast body of currently existing research are needed more than new individual studies.

Implications of New Research Methods

Meta-analysis, as a research technique, suggests the need for the entire research community to participate in making decisions about necessary and important research topics. Ideally, one can imagine a community of health behavior researchers in which national or regional gatherings guide a division of effort whereby some researchers contribute unique new individual studies while others cumulate existing work. This approach will require a shift in values, since the long-established research tradition values original, single-study research as more exciting, original, and leading edge than the cumulation of others' published work in meta-analysis.

As most researchers who have recently conducted meta-analytical studies have found, however, modern meta-analysis is a complex, creative, and enormously challenging technique. In fact, there is a pressing need for statistical researchers who can make the new methodological discoveries that will be necessary to exploit fully the potential of meta-analysis for health behavior research.

One hopes that a widespread use of meta-analysis in health behavior research would lead to new understandings of how knowledge is best expanded and collated. This modern tool could thus help lead to conclusions about health behavior issues that are more stable and useful, and better understood, than those achieved to date.

CONCLUSION

Changes in the health care system, in the design and focus of medical education, and in the development of new research methodologies all contribute to creating a window of opportunity for health behavior research to be incorporated more fully into the training of health professionals. Understanding the benefits of health behavior research to medical education and the present and historical barriers to its widespread incorporation are first steps in changing the system. A number of creative and innovative programs are already in place. Christakis (1995) indicated that medical schools have historically been expected to serve the society in which they exist. It is time to place renewed emphasis on the fulfillment of this expectation.

AUTHORS' NOTE. For inquiries concerning the need for a new paradigm, contact Maggie L. Moore-West. For inquiries concerning the role of communication skills, contact Virginia A. Reed. For inquiries concerning meta-analysis or the C. Everett Koop Institute—Medical Education Assessment Program, contact G. Christian Jernstedt.

REFERENCES

American Medical Student Association. (1995). The AMSA Paul R. Wright Excellence in Medical Education Award, Washington DC.

Anderson, L. A., & Sharpe, P. A. (1991). Improving patient and provider communication: A synthesis and review of communication interventions. *Patient Education and Counseling, 17,* 99–134.

Association for the Behavioral Sciences and Medical Education. (1994). *Behavioral sciences curriculum guide.* Unpublished. Rochester, NY: ABSME.

Bandura, A. (1978). The self system in reciprocal determinism. *American Psychologist, 33,* 344–358.

Bartlett, E. E., Grayson, M., Barker, R., Levine, D. M., Golden, A., & Libber, S. (1984). The effects of physician communications skills on patient satisfaction, recall, and adherence. *Journal of Chronic Diseases, 37*(9/10), 755–764.

Barzansky, B., Jonas, S., & Etzel, I. (1995). Educational programs in U.S. medical schools. *Journal of the American Medical Association, 274,* 716–722.

Baumgart, A. J., & Costello, E. A. (1988). Health behavior research and the training of health professions. In D. S. Gochman (Ed.), *Health behavior: Emerging research perspectives* (pp. 363–379). New York: Plenum Press.

Bloom, S. W. (1988). Structure and ideology in medical education: An analysis of resistance to change. *Journal of Health and Social Behavior, 29,* 294–306.

Boelen, C. (1995, July). Prospects for change in medical education in the twenty-first century. *Academic Medicine, 70*(Supplement), 21–28.

Boyer, M. H., Madoff, M. A., Bennett, A. J., Dean, D. H., Hyde, J. N., Minihan, P. M., & Barbeau, E. M. (1992). Tuft's four year combined M.D.-M.P.H. program: A training model for population-based medicine. *Academic Medicine, 67*(6), 363–365.

Calvin, J. (1852). *Commentaries on the Book of the Prophet Daniel.* Edinburgh: Calvin Translation Society.

Christakis, N. (1995). The similarity and frequency of proposals to reform U.S. medical education. *Journal of the American Medical Association, 274,* 706–711.

Cooper, H., & Hedges, L. V. (Eds.) (1994). *Handbook of research synthesis.* New York: Russell Sage Foundation.

Craig, J. L. (1992). Retention of interviewing skills learned by first-year medical students: A longitudinal study. *Medical Education, 26,* 276–281.

Druckman, D., & Bjork, R. A. (Eds.). (1994). *Learning, remembering, believing: Enhancing human performance.* Washington, DC: National Academy Press.

Eckenfels, E. (1992). A brief summary of the history and purpose of the Rush Community Service Initiatives Program. Unpublished correspondence with E. Eckenfels, Director, Rush Community Service Initiatives Program, Head, Section of Community and Family Medicine, Rush Medical School.

Epstein, R. M., Campbell, T. L., Cohen-Cole, S. A., McWhinney, I. R., & Smilkstein, G. (1993). Perspectives on patient-doctor communication. *Journal of Family Practice, 37*(4), 377–387.

Evans, B. J., Stanley, R. O., & Burrows, G. D. (1992). Communication skills training and patients' satisfaction. *Health Communication, 4*(2), 155-170.

Evans, B. J., Stanley, R. O., & Burrows, G. D. (1993). Measuring medical students' empathy skills. *British Journal of Medical Psychology, 66,* 121-133.

Evans, J. (1992). The health of the public approach to medical education. *Academic Medicine, 67,* 719-723.

Fisher, R. A. (1935). *The design of experiments.* Edinburgh and London: Oliver and Boyd.

Flexner, A. (1910). *Medical education in the United States and Canada.* New York: Carnegie Foundation for the Advancement of Teaching.

Forman, S. (1994). Social responsibility and the academic medical center: Building community based systems for the nation's health. *Academic Medicine, 69,* 97-101.

Funkenstein, D. H. (1968). The learning and personal development of medical students and the recent changes in universities and medical schools. *Journal of Medical Education, 43,* 883-897.

Ganem, J., Beran, J., & Krakower, J. (1995). Review of U.S. medical school finances, 1993-1994. *Journal of the American Medical Association, 274,* 723-730.

Glass, G. V., McGaw, B., & Smith, M. L. (1981). *Meta-analysis in social research.* Beverly Hills: Sage.

Gochman, D. S. (Ed.). (1988). *Health behavior: Emerging research perspectives.* New York: Plenum Press.

Godkin, M., & Quirk, M. (1991). Why students chose family medicine: State schools graduating the most family physicians. *Family Medicine, 23*(7), 521-526.

Golden, G. (1994). The role of evaluation in behavioral science training. Discussant: M. Moore-West. *Annals of Behavioral Science and Medical Education, 1,* 19-25.

Gunderman, R. (1995). Rethinking our basic concepts of health and disease. *Academic Medicine, 70,* 676-683.

Hamilton, J. (1995, July). Establishing standards and measurement methods for medical education. *Academic Medicine, 70*(Supplement), 51-56.

Hedges, L. V., & Olkin, I. (1985). *Statistical methods for meta-analysis.* New York: Academic Press.

Helfer, R. E. (1970). An objective comparison of the pediatric interviewing skills of freshman and senior medical students. *Pediatrics, 45*(4), 623-627.

Hojat, M., Gonnella, J., Erdmann, J., Veloski, J., & Xu, G. (1995, January). Primary care and non primary care physicians: A longitudinal study of their similarities, differences, and correlates before, during and after medical school. *Academic Medicine, 70*(Supplement), 17-27.

Holmes-Rovner, M., Alexander, E., O'Kelly, B., Rome, W., Wu, S., Lovell, K., & Alfano, M. (1994). Compensation equity between men and women in academic medicine: Methods and implications. *Academic Medicine, 69,* 131-137.

Hunter, J. E., & Schmidt, F. L. (1990). *Methods of meta-analysis: Correcting error and bias in research findings.* Newbury Park, CA: Sage.

Jernstedt, G. C., & Chow, W. K. (1980). Lectures and textual

materials as sources of information for learning. *Psychological Reports, 46,* 1327-1339.

Jernstedt, G. C., & Reed, V. A. (1995a, October). *A model for the longitudinal, comprehensive assessment of medical education.* Paper presented at the Research in Medical Education Conference at the Annual Meeting of the American Association of Medical Colleges, Washington, DC.

Jernstedt, G. C., & Reed, V. A. (1995b). The C. Everett Koop Institute—Medical Education Assessment Program. Hanover, NH: Department of Psychology, Dartmouth College.

Johnson, H. M. (1940). Pre-experimental assumptions as determiners of experimental results. *Psychological Review, 47,* 338-346.

Kann, L., Warren, C. W., Harris, W. A., Collins, J. L., Douglas, K. A., Collins, M. E., Williams, B. I., Ross, J. G., & Kolbe, L. J. (1995). Youth Risk Behavior Surveillance—United States. Division of Adolescent and School Health, National Center for Chronic Disease Prevention and Health Promotion, Centers for Disease Control and Prevention. *Journal of School Health, 65,* 163-171.

Kuhn, T. (1970). *The structure of scientific revolutions.* Chicago: University of Chicago Press.

Lewis, C. C., Pantell, R. H., & Sharp, L. (1991). Increasing patient knowledge, satisfaction, and involvement: Randomized trial of a communication intervention. *Pediatrics, 88*(2), 351-358.

Little, D. R. (1992). Health education programs in U.S. medical schools. *Academic Medicine, 67*(9), 596-598.

Lomas, J. (1994, July). Medicine in context: A neglected perspective in medical education. *Academic Medicine, 69* (Supplement), 95-100.

Moore-West, M., & O'Donnell, M. (1985). Program evaluation. In A. Kaufman (Ed.), *Implementing problem based medical education: Lessons from successful innovations* (pp. 180-206). New York: Springer.

Moore-West, M., Regan-Smith, M., Dietrich, A., & Kollisch, D. (1990). Enhancing humanism through the educational process. In H. Hendrie & C. Lloyd (Eds.), *Educating competent and humane physicians* (pp. 128-174). Bloomington: Indiana University Press.

Muller, S. (Chairman). (1984). Physicians for the twenty-first century: Report of the project panel on the general professional education of the physician and college preparation for medicine. *Journal of Medical Education, 59,* Part 2.

Novack, D. H., Volk, G., Drossman, D. A., & Lipkin, M. (1993). Medical interviewing and interpersonal skills teaching in U.S. medical schools: Progress, problems, and promise. *Journal of the American Medical Association, 269*(16), 2101-2105.

O'Donnell, J. (1992). Annual report to Charles E. Culpeper Foundation. Hanover, NH: Dartmouth Medical School.

Prochaska, J. O., & DiClemente, C. C. (1983). Stages and processes of self-change of smoking: Toward an integrative model of change. *Journal of Consulting and Clinical Psychology, 51,* 390-395.

42 PART I • PROFESSIONAL TRAINING AND PRACTICE

Rabinowitz, H. K. (1988). Evaluation of a selective medical school admissions policy to increase the number of family physicians in rural and underserved areas. *New England Journal of Medicine, 319*(8), 480–486.

Rabinowitz, H. K. (1990). The change in specialty preference by medical students over time: An analysis of students who prefer family medicine. *Family Medicine, 22*(1), 62–63.

Rappeleye, W. C. (1932). Medical education: Final report of the commission on medical education. New York: Association of American Medical Colleges.

Reed, V. A., & Jernstedt, G. C. (1994, October). *Meta-analytic assessment of the acquisition and retention of communication skills in medical education.* Poster presented at the Research in Medical Education Conference at the Annual Meeting of the American Association of Medical Colleges, Boston.

Reed, V. A., & Jernstedt, G. C. (1995, November). *Multidimensional assessment of medical student attributes and their changes over time.* Poster presented at the Research in Medical Education Conference at the Annual Meeting of the American Association of Medical Colleges, Washington, DC.

Reynolds, C., Adler, S., Kanter, S., Horn, J., Harvey, J., & Bernier, G. (1995). The undergraduate medical curriculum: Centralized vs. departmentalized. *Academic Medicine, 70,* 671–675.

Rivo, M., Mays, H., Katzoff, J., & King, D. (1995). Managed health care: Implications for the physician workforce and medical education. *Journal of the American Medical Association, 274,* 712–715.

Rosenthal, R. (1991). *Meta-analytic procedures for social research.* Newbury Park, CA: Sage.

Rosnow, R. L., & Rosenthal, R. (1989). Statistical procedures and the justification of knowledge in psychological science. *American Psychologist, 44*(10), 1276–1284.

Schmidt, F. L. (1992). What do data really mean? Research findings, meta-analysis, and cumulative knowledge in psychology. *American Psychologist, 47*(10), 1173–1181.

Schon, D. (1984). *The crisis of professional knowledge and the pursuit of an epistemology of practice.* Paper presented at the President and Fellows of Harvard College for the Harvard Business School 75th Anniversary Colloquium on Teaching the Case Method, Cambridge, MA.

Schon, D. (1987). *Educating the reflective practitioner.* San Francisco: Jossey-Bass.

Smith, S. (1994). *An educational blueprint for the Brown University School of Medicine competency based curriculum.* Providence, RI: Brown University Press.

Smith, S., Balint, J., Krause, K., Moore-West, M., & Viles, P. (1994). Performance based assessment of moral reasoning and ethical judgment among medical students. *Academic Medicine, 69,* 381–385.

Sox, H., Blatt, M., Higgins, M., & Marton, K. (1988). *Medical decision making.* Stoneham, MA: Butterworth.

Stillman, P. L., Burpeau-DiGregorio, M. Y., Nicholson, G. I., Sabers, D. L., & Stillman, A. E. (1983). Six years of experience using patient instructors to teach interviewing skills. *Journal of Medical Education, 58,* 941–946.

Stillman, P. L., Sabers, D. L., & Redfield, D. L. (1977). Use of trained mothers to teach interviewing skills to first-year medical students: A follow-up study. *Pediatrics, 60*(2), 165–169.

Straus, R. (1994). Departments and disciplines: Stasis and change. *Annals of the Association of Behavioral Sciences and Medical Education, 1,* 14–18.

Swanson, A., & Anderson, B. (1993, June). Educating medical students: Assessing change in medical education—The road to implementation. *Academic Medicine, 68*(Supplement), S1–46.

Tarallo-Falk, J. (1995). *The socialization of medical students in a preventive health community service learning experience.* Unpublished doctoral thesis. Cambridge, MA: Harvard Graduate School of Education.

Tarlov, A. R. (1992). The coming influence of social sciences perspective on medical education. *Academic Medicine, 67*(11), 724–731.

Tresolini, C., Shugars, D., & Lee, S. (1995). Teaching an integrated approach to health care: Lessons from five schools. *Academic Medicine, 70,* 665–670.

U.S. Preventive Services Task Force. (1989). Guide to clinical preventive services: An assessment of the effectiveness of 169 interventions. Report of the U.S. Preventive Services Task Force. Baltimore: Williams & Wilkins.

Walsh, J., Stevens, M., & Moore-West, M. (1994). *Glaxo pre med survey.* Unpublished manuscript. Hanover, NH: Dartmouth Medical School.

Wennberg, J. E. (1990). Outcomes research, cost containment, and the fear of health care rationing. *New England Journal of Medicine, 323,* 1202–1204.

Winett, R. A. (1995). A framework for health promotion and disease prevention programs. *American Psychologist, 50*(5), 341–350.

3

Health Behavior Research

What Physicians Must Know

Ann Randolph Flipse

INTRODUCTION

It would seem obvious that health behavior research is relevant to the training and practice of physicians. One might expect that a case need not be made for its relevancy and that the literature would substantiate the thesis. Interestingly, a search of the literature between 1985 and 1995 reveals no documentation of such claims or experiences. A case can be made for its importance by acknowledging some parameters.

Only consider, for example, the language in use: The physician, who ministers to the sick, is said to render "health care." There is the oxymoron "ill health." Health behavior has been defined to include illness behavior, which alone should make health behavior research a valued area of inquiry for physicians. In the absence of a body of literature to support the thesis, this chapter will focus on some of the reasons that physicians must know about health behavior research. Consideration of the relevance of health behav-

Ann Randolph Flipse • Clinical Skills Program, University of Miami School of Medicine, Miami, Florida 33101.

Handbook of Health Behavior Research IV: Relevance for Professionals and Issues for the Future, edited by David S. Gochman. Plenum Press, New York, 1997.

ior will be followed by a section on suggested future directions in medical training and sections on relevant knowledge, relevant conceptual frameworks, lessons from health behavior research, some of the problems in health behavior research, the complexity of issues, a model curriculum, and finally future research issues. It should be noted that the field is vast, the subject is far from exhausted, and this chapter is meant to be neither all-inclusive nor in any way exclusive.

RELEVANCE OF HEALTH BEHAVIOR

Without some knowledge of health behavior, the physician is unable to establish a valid and valued relationship with the patient. A physician who does not know the significance of illness to the patient, the patient's and family's belief systems, and how and by whom the decision-making process is being influenced will be unable to negotiate a treatment plan or assess how likely the patient is to respond to management or predict the likelihood of follow-up. The explanatory model of a patient often reflects a societal belief system, and it is increasingly believed that successful behavior modification must come at this level. Ethnocultural communities are strong determinants of when someone seeks help, from whom, and for what purpose: cure, care, relief. Expectations are often group-influenced, as is what constitutes a good result for the patient. For example, when Latino physicians with fatal diseases defer to their adult children, thus declining personal involvement in the decision-making process, they indicate that it is culturally determined. Our Hispanic students report this behavior in their own families, and many students report this in general in Hispanic patients. Additionally, physicians must know about their patients' belief systems in order to acknowledge, accept, and permit alternative treatments that may be very important to the well-being of patients.

It becomes especially important that the physician have this knowledge, given that at least 70% and perhaps as much as 90% of illnesses are treated by family and friends and only 10% by physicians, with the remaining receiving folk or alternative therapies from other healers. Kleinman (1980) refers to these overlapping sectors of health care as the "popular sector," the "professional sector," and the "folk sector." His work is instructive for physicians in that it can make them aware of how relatively little they participate in the global picture of health care. It also offers an explanation of why their participation is limited.

FUTURE DIRECTIONS IN MEDICAL TRAINING

According to Tarlov (1992), there are four health-related changes that will affect medical education. The first is the redefining of the term *health* that has taken place since the World Health Organization put the emphasis on a positive state of well-being. Tarlov's synthesis of many researchers' work reconceptualizes health as "an individual or group capacity relative to potential to function fully in the social and physical environment." The second change is an increase in disease prevention and health promotion. The third is an awareness of the paradox of the low health status and the high cost of health care in the United States. The final shift is from infectious causes of illness and death to chronic diseases with their multiple risk behaviors. Tarlov believes that the training of physicians will include the sociology as well as the biology of disease, health improvement as well as disease cure, training for population-based health care, and the assessing of medical outcomes by more than just medical results.

Like all other events in the positive socialization of students into the medical profession, incorporation of health behavior research into the learning of physicians and students has to be valued and utilized by educators and role models. Historically, since Johns Hopkins tied the founding of its medical school to a closely affiliated hospital, training of physicians has taken place in mostly tertiary care hospitals by subspecialists who are caring for the sickest of the sick and treating disease while 95% of the population receive care outside the traditional training venues for medical education.

With increased emphasis on education in ambulatory sites and the swing back to primary care, the behavioral sciences are becoming more important than ever. In order to treat the patient as a person—a member of a family with ethnocultural influences, of a community, and of a society—and not just "treat" the disease, the surgical specimen, the biochemical cascade, or the molecule, the physician must be trained to elicit, assess, and deal with very different patient stories that will be much more complex and inclusive than the traditional medical history. A larger, more diverse, more complex society will automatically bring more influences on health behavior. Demographic projections point toward more diversity in the physician population as well as in our patient populations in this country. Entering medical school classes now have more women, more blacks, more Latinos, more Asians, and more first-generation immigrants, in contrast to the predominantly white male classes of 20 years ago (Association of American Medical Colleges,

1995). These differences are especially pronounced in medical schools, which are attempting to enroll student bodies that mirror the very diverse patient populations for which they care. The greater the diversity in the patient population and in the student group, the greater the need to know and to understand the differences. The need to know begins with the students' being able to define their own families', their colleagues', and their patients' belief systems, of which health behavior is such an integral part.

Research on health behavior can be considered on a macro level as it pertains to groups and on a micro level as it pertains to a patient. Lifelong learners of medicine can conduct research and collect data in both spheres. A physician's research on the individual (the patient) has to be compared with the patient's population data in order to appreciate influences. Joseph et al. (1992) make a strong argument that physicians should themselves conduct research. Doing so would allow the physician to begin to understand the social, cultural, economic, and environmental causes of disease. The results will have more impact and therefore will be better remembered. The authors propose clinical–social discussions as opposed to the traditional clinical–pathological conferences. They also point out that the data can then be used for designing health education programs.

In making a case for change in medical education, Jonas (1984) states that "physicians have a special competence to discover risks that patients unwittingly run in their daily lives. They also have a special status and authority that can help them persuade individuals to alter their habits." He also suggests that coming changes in medical practice will include the importance of health rather than just disease and that the "extra time" resulting from the oversupply of physicians will allow them to communicate with and educate patients.

Brody (1980) writes that as physicians become more efficient at maintaining life, they will devote more time to quality of life and therefore become more oriented to the behavioral, psycho-

logical, and social components of a disorder. These components are reflected in compliance, psychiatric disturbances, and stressful life events, all of which are easily evaluated in a well-conducted interview. In discussing the subject of educating physicians for better patient health, Labonte (1986) states that people are demanding greater control over their health and want their physicians to advise them and not just prescribe medication.

RELEVANT KNOWLEDGE

The entire process of hypothesis generation that is at the center of clinical reasoning is facilitated by a knowledge of the health behavior of various demographic groups. Moreover, pattern recognition is dependent in large measure on such awareness.

Richard S. Schweiker (1982), the former Secretary of Health and Human Services, stated in his 1981 address to the Association of American Medical Colleges that "if we are to plant a strong prevention ethic in our country's health care system, then training physicians and other health care professionals is obviously the place to start."

In his 1979 report, the Surgeon General (U.S. Department of Health, Education and Welfare, 1979) stated:

> Medical care begins with the sick and seeks to keep them alive, make them well, or minimize their disability. Disease prevention begins with a threat to health—a disease or an environmental hazard—and seeks to protect as many people as possible from the harmful consequences of that threat. Health promotion begins with people who are basically healthy, and seeks the development of community and individual measures which can help them to develop lifestyles that can maintain and enhance the state of well-being.

Tarlov (1992) states that there are levels of health determinants, each with strategies for intervention: The first is biological–genetic–psychic and individual and involves medical care; the second is health behavior or lifestyle and involves disease prevention; the third is community environment and involves health promotion; the fourth is physical environment and involves health protection; finally, the fifth is the macro-social structure and involves adjustments in that social structure. Since medical care is a relatively late intervention for health improvement, other strategies are needed in order to influence morbidity, mortality, and life expectancy in more effective ways.

Repeated assessments of chronic illness cite data so disturbing that physicians in training and in practice should hear them as a call for both disease prevention and health promotion. Of the deaths in this country, 75% are due to cardiovascular disease, cancer, chronic obstructive pulmonary disease, and diabetes. The multiple risk factors of tobacco use, dietary factors, overeating, and alcohol abuse associated with these diseases become major determinants of health. Tarlov (1993) states that over 350,000 deaths per year are smoking-related and that more people die each year of alcohol-related deaths than died in the entire Vietnam war, and in so stating understandably attributes a major role to health behaviors, as well as to community environment and the macrosocial structure, in his health input–output model. The input side of Tarlov's model combines the external determinants already mentioned with the individual's inner genetic–biological makeup to result in a capacity and potential to function, to find role fulfillment, and to have a sense of well-being. In his model, these, then, are the key indicators of overall health and quality of life.

RELEVANT CONCEPTUAL FRAMEWORKS

Physicians' training should include familiarization with a number of health models in order to develop their own understanding of the multi-faceted concepts of health and illness and to acquire a framework for assessing research results. Disease is a relatively straightforward concept. The acknowledgment that the health belief model as proposed by Rosenstock (1960) and modified by Becker (1979) has received the widest theoretical and research attention makes it an especially important learning objective for physicians, as does its relationship with other models such as those of Kasl and Cobb (1966), Kosa and Robertson (1969), and Mechanic (1968). Cummings, Becker, and Maile (1980) brought 14 of the models together and provided an analysis of the variables. The Kasl and Cobb model of health and illness behavior hypothesizes that behavior is influenced by the perception of threat of disease and the benefit of the health action. The Kosa and Robertson model has four components: the assessment of disruption in the functioning of health, anxiety about symptoms, use of one's medical knowledge, and action to restore function and decrease anxiety. Mechanic's model focuses on the way patients perceive, evaluate, and respond to symptoms.

McLeroy, Bibeau, Steckler, and Glanz (1988) believe that Brofenbrenner's ecological model offers yet another framework, as does Belsky's combined individual development–ecological model. Although a detailed representation of these models is beyond the scope of this chapter, some mention should be made of Kasl and Cobb's (1966) theoretical framework of the likelihood that an individual will engage in a particular kind of health, illness, or sick role behavior. The variables involved are the perceived amount of threat and the attractiveness or value of the behavior. The former depends on the importance of health matters to the individual and the perceived susceptibility to and consequences of the disease. The latter depends on the perceived probability that the action will lead to the desired preventive results and the unpleasantness or cost of taking the action versus taking no action. Kasl and Cobb reviewed the literature concerning preventive health measures and concluded that perceived value of preventive action is the most important variable mediating the influence of perceived threat and that both are influenced by diverse demographic and background variables.

LESSONS FROM HEALTH
BEHAVIOR RESEARCH

Reviews such as those cited provide important lessons for physicians who must bridge the gap between their belief systems and those of their patients. There are variables most physicians are not aware of. As an example, the reviewers point to the correlations of level of education, income, race, high residential stability, being a veteran, or living in a rural area with the likelihood of participation in free health examinations. Another has to do with the participants' attitudes about health matters, their susceptibility, their preference for knowing whether they have an illness, and their belief that cure is possible.

Health behavior research by Rosenstock, Strecher, and Becker (1988) has shown correlations with concepts such as self-efficacy. Rosenstock also cautions that some behavior that seems to be health-related may in fact be determined by motives unrelated to health. Becker's (1979) review of health motivation has found relationships of health-related behaviors with locus of control, powerlessness, and alienation. Rakowski, Lasater, Wells, and Carleton (1991) found that past success at health habit change was the best predictor for future success and that optimism about future success placed individuals at an advantage for changing behavior. Interestingly, McGee and Cairns (1994) reported that unrealistic optimism appears to be a pervasive phenomenon that may prevent patients from changing their behavior because they believe there is little or no chance they will contract certain health problems.

Lomas (1994) speaks of the "patient's context" as a determinant of health, citing disability gradients between the rich and the poor, the better post–myocardial infarction survival rate of people with pets, and the extent of social support as a predictor of premature mortality. He also points out that in the United States individuals spend as much money on unconventional therapies such as those of acupuncturists and naturopaths as they do on hospital care.

PROBLEMS IN HEALTH
BEHAVIOR RESEARCH

For the physician, there are many other lessons to be learned about and from health behavior research. The health behaviors Tarlov lists in his model's risk profile are diet, physical fitness, tobacco, alcohol excess, drug abuse, recklessness, stress, and violence. A litany like this conjures up a perhaps overdrawn image of the American adolescent as a subject for research. Yet as Alexander and Natale (1994) point out, research with adolescents presents special problems that involve access to patients, research design, and the sensitive nature of questions related to behavioral issues such as sexuality and substance abuse. Other populations such as the underserved present additional problems for behavioral research. Chen (1994) reports that traditional sources for obtaining information are inadequate. While quantitative data may be collected through surveys and will tell us "how many" and "what kind," the "why" of qualitative data must be collected on the inside through focus groups and from key informants. This need mandates an ethnographic approach to health behavior research and should influence the physician's own research strategies as well as critical evaluation of others' reported data. The crossing over of AIDS into the heterosexual population brings regular reports that traditional ethnocultural roles prevent women from asking for "safe sex."

COMPLEXITY OF THE ISSUES

Physicians should know that disease prevention and health promotion are complex issues. For example, cautionary notes were sounded by Russell's (1986) study, which pointed out that hoped-for fiscal advantages may not materialize and that the costs of some prevention programs may exceed the costs of treating the diseases. Thomas (1983) suggested that the deluge of health promotion campaigns may have created an "epidemic of apprehension" about the seemingly omnipresent dangers in our lives. Regarding data, Becker (1993) pointed out that it is easy to get correlations and publish data, but far more difficult to attribute causal meaning. Becker has, however, a greater concern. He believes that the most disturbing aspect of health promotion is the tendency to assign the major responsibility for health problems to the individual. He attributes this tendency to the Western value system of personal responsibility for successes and failures and need for control. He argues that health habits are acquired within social groups; that health status is related, as Alonzo (1985) and Milio (1981) stated, to the broader societal components of economics, politics, and culture. Becker's final concern is that health has come to provide the measure of character and personal worth. By redefinition, "being ill is being guilty."

In a profession too long dominated by the relatively simplistic concepts of biomedicine, interest in health behavior research may best be stimulated by the social epidemiology of chronic diseases (Graham & Reeder, 1979). It is hard to resist the lure of the "why" when one first discovers such intriguing findings as soot, the chimney sweep, and scrotal cancer; socioeconomic status, hypertension, males, and blacks; the Japanese-Hawaiian-American heart study and acculturation; and the low risks of certain diseases in certain religious groups.

For physicians to understand health behavior, they should be aware of the diversity of elements other than just risk factors that may contribute to patients' explanations of health and illness. An example of such explanations is Pill and Stott's (1982) correlations of socioeconomic variables such as education and home ownership with patients' beliefs that their actions determine their health; attributions made to climate and invasions of the body by living entities from the natural world; the social world's witchcraft, sorcery, and evil eye; and the supernatural world's actions of gods, spirits, and shades.

Physicians must also understand what determines whether or not and when a patient will seek medical care. Some ill people consult physicians; some people with the same symptoms do not. Zola's (1973) "pathway to the doctor" involve the nonphysiological factors of availability of care, the affordability of care, the failure or success of care in the folk sector, and how the problem is perceived by the patient and by those around him. Zola's (1966) studies showed that the decision to seek care is largely determined by whatever is considered to be health in the patient's population. Zola noted that there are nonphysiological triggers for the decision to seek care that often varied with the ethnocultural group to which the patient belonged and might not correlate with the severity of the illness. These triggers are an interpersonal crisis or perceived interference with personal relationships, sanctioning by another individual of the decision to seek care, perceived interference with function, and the setting of external time criteria. Other studies involve what sign or symptom is considered normal or abnormal by groups of individuals and when it is so seen and therefore regarded as a reason to seek care. It is also significant that some patients go to physicians for relief of symptoms, but to folk healers for explanations and treatment by mystical means.

Kleinman's (1980) concept of explanatory models asserts that everyone in the clinical process has a belief about the meaning of sickness that involves a multitude of parameters. Kleinman notes that the physician–patient encounter is a meeting of lay and professional explanatory models, the success of which depends on a consensus between the two about etiology, diagnosis, pathophysiology, prognosis, and treatment. Research has shown that there are recurring problems in the physician–patient encounter, and they have been categorized by Helman (1984) as the misinterpretation of patients' "languages of distress" or the ethnocultural differences in how illness is communicated verbally and nonverbally, the incompatability of explanatory models, the case of disease without illness and of illness without disease, and problems of terminology and of treatment. He points out that interviews are conducted in a mixture of "everyday language and medical jargon" and that there is a danger of misunderstanding about the medical terms. The patient's use of folk terminology and self-labeled folk illnesses may also confuse the clinician, especially if patient and physician are from different cultures. For treatment to be accepted, it must make sense to patients in terms of their own explanatory models. Problems in this match surely account for the rush to judgment that a patient is noncompliant.

A MODEL CURRICULUM

Methodologies for incorporating the learning of health behavior into the curriculum include those utilized by the author in a year-long, first-year clinical skills course. The class is divided into groups as ethnoculturally diverse as possible. In the second week, the students are asked to draw their own genograms to share with a small group of their classmates and faculty. These genograms include data about countries of origin, ages, causes of death, households, and nurturing and disturbed relationships. At the next small-group meeting a month later, the students are asked to share information regarding their family's beliefs about health and illness; sickness; about the family's health behavior; and about how the family decides when a member is ill, who assigns the sick role, and to whom the family turns for care. They are also asked to tell about favorite home remedies, the use of alternative therapies, and the involvement of other healers. Self-study and self-awareness therefore form a basis for continued learning.

The students begin their weekly preceptorship experience in ambulatory sites, most of which are remote from the medical center. The first semester is devoted to the gathering of a complete history with specific assignments relating to family history and habits including diet, exercise, and caffeine, tobacco, alcohol, and drug use. Toward the end of the semester, the students do a health-risk appraisal on a patient and enter the data in a computer program in order to generate a risk profile. They also spend a session learning about how a patient has been educated about illness and counseled about behavior modification. In the course of their clinical encounters and as part of a home visit experience involving three visits to the home of the same patient with a chronic disease, the students are also asked to explore the patients' explanatory models.

Each student in the small group chooses one of the eight health issues that have been identified in the local south Florida community: women and children in poverty, AIDS, care for the terminally ill, substance abuse, domestic violence, the handicapped and disabled, homelessness, and the elderly. The students assigned to each topic develop a position paper that includes a definition of the problem, the local and the national picture, the costs to society, available community resources, and a proposal for a solution. Each group then hears a summary report of each problem. Since the research involves a comparison of the local extent of the problem with the national extent, it provides a framework for the students' assessment of their own experiences with patients.

Existing time constraints preclude incorporation into the course requirements of the obvious opportunities for collating the student's own patient data with those of classmates, for review of charts for a particular site, for participating in screening programs, for further study of the community's health behavior, and finally for comparison with the health of the public on a more global level. In the latter comparison are many lessons for providers of health care in this country to learn, including the reasons that United States citizens are not the healthiest in the world.

The rationale for including health behavior research in the training of the physician is basically to improve the physician's understanding of how a person becomes a patient. Clearly, the case has been made for the need to know about the diverse issues involved in health. Such knowledge should then facilitate several processes in patient care.

FUTURE RESEARCH ISSUES

The move toward more ambulatory-based and community-oriented medical care will require new skills of practicing physicians. With the identification of areas for modifying behavior, the physician should be able to increase prevention and improve intervention. A more valid picture of a community's needs and ethnocultural "demographic imperatives" will result from a knowledge of health behavior. It will also enable a more global approach to the health of the public by providing a perspective with longitudinal and horizontal dimensions. More knowledge of health behavior should improve the "economics" of health care. Even though the cost of care may not go down, other losses can be decreased. Among these losses are loss of contributions to society, diminishing of quality of life, and increasing of dependency. On a more individual basis, a knowledge of health behavior will permit physicians to ground diagnostic and therapeutic decisions for their patients in a reality-based framework that includes significant psychosocial data.

A legitimate goal for including health behavior research should be to encourage physicians' interest in undertaking research and study of their own patient population. The ultimate outcome should be delivery of care that will have much better and broader results. In primary care, the emphasis will then be, as that of health care should always have been, on the physician–patient encounter and the collection of data by the physician, not on the laboratory, and the generation of valid hypotheses. To achieve all these aims, the physician will need a better understanding of the behavioral, psychological, and social dimensions of the patient.

AUTHOR'S NOTE. For more information on the clinical skills course, write the author at: First Year Clinical Skills Program, University of Miami School of Medicine, PO Box 016960 (R-98), Miami, FL 33101.

REFERENCES

Alexander, E., & Natale, J. (1994). Consideration of venue and vehicle in health behavior research with adolescents. *Family Practice Research Journal, 14,* 379–388.

Alonzo, A. A. (1985). Health as situational adaptation: A social psychological perspective. *Social Science and Medicine, 21,* 1341–1344.

Association of American Medical Colleges. (1995). Trends, United States medical school applicants, matriculates and graduates, 1994. New York: Section for Educational Research, Division of Education Research, AAMC.

Becker, M. (1979). Psychosocial aspects of health-related behavior. In H. E. Freeman, S. Levine, & L. G. Reeder (Eds.), *Handbook of medical sociology* (pp. 253–274). Englewood Cliffs, NJ: Prentice-Hall.

Becker, M. (1993). A medical sociologist looks at health promotion. *Journal of Health and Social Behavior, 34,* 1–6.

Brody, D. S. (1980). Physician recognition of behavioral, psychological, and social aspects of medical care. *Archives of Internal Medicine, 140,* 1286–1289.

Chen, M. S., Jr. (1994). Behavioral and psychosocial cancer research in the underserved. *Cancer Supplement, 74*(4), 1503–1508.

Cummings, K., Becker, M., & Maile, M. (1980). Bringing the models together: An empirical approach to combining variables used to explain health actions. *Journal of Behavioral Medicine, 3*(2), 123–145.

Graham, S., & Reeder, L. (1979). Social epidemiology of chronic diseases. In H. E. Freeman, S. Levine, & L. G. Reeder (Eds.), *Handbook of medical sociology* (pp. 71–96). Englewood Cliffs, NJ: Prentice-Hall.

Helman, C. (1984). Doctor–patient interactions. In *Culture, health and illness* (pp. 65–94). Bristol, London, Boston: Wright-PSG.

Jonas, S. (1984, Aug. 25). The case for change in medical education in the United States. *Lancet,* 452–454.

Joseph, A., Abraham, S., Bhattacharji, S., Muliyil, J., John, K. R., Mathew, S., & Norman, G. (1992). The teaching of behavioral sciences. *Medical Education, 26,* 92–98.

Kasl, S. V., & Cobb, S. (1966). Health behavior, illness behavior and sick role behavior. *Archives of Environmental Health, 12,* 246–262.

Kleinman, A. (1980). *Patients and healers in the context of culture.* Berkeley: University of California Press.

Kosa, J., & Robertson, L. (1969). The social aspects of health and illness. In J. Kosa, A. Antonovsky, & I. K. Zola (Eds.), *Poverty and health: A sociological analysis* (pp. 35-68). Cambridge, MA: Harvard University Press.

Labonte, R. (1986). Educating physicians for better patient health. *Canadian Medical Association Journal, 134*, 390-395.

Lomas, J. (1994). Medicine in context: A neglected perspective in medical education. *Academic Medicine, 69*(10), S95-S101.

McGee, H. M., & Cairns, J. (1994). Unrealistic optimism: A behavioral sciences classroom demonstration project. *Medical Education, 28*, 513-516.

McLeroy K. R., Bibeau, D., Steckler, A., & Glanz, K. (1988). An ecological perspective on health promotion programs. *Health Education Quarterly, 15*(4), 351-377.

Mechanic, D. (1968). *Medical sociology: A selective view.* New York: Free Press.

Milio, N. (1981). *Promoting health through public policy.* Philadelphia: F. A. Davis.

Pill, R., & Stott, N. C. H. (1982). Concepts of illness causation and responsibility: Some preliminary data from a sample of working class mothers. *Social Science and Medicine, 16*, 43-52.

Rakowski, W., Lasater, T. M., Wells, B. L., & Carleton, R. A. (1991). Correlates of expected success at health habit change and its role as a predictor in health behavior research. *American Journal of Preventive Medicine, 7*(2), 89-94.

Rosenstock, I. M. (1960). What research in motivation suggests for public health. *American Journal of Public Health, 50*(3), 295-302.

Rosenstock, I. M., Strecher, V. J., & Becker, M. H. (1988). Social learning theory and the health belief model. *Health Education Quarterly, 15*(2), 175-183.

Russell, L. B. (1986). *Is prevention better than cure?* Washington, DC: Brookings Institution.

Schweiker, R. S. (1982). Disease prevention and health promotion. *Journal of Medical Education, 57*, 15-19.

Tarlov, A. R. (1922). The coming influence of a social sciences perspective on medical education. *Academic Medicine, 67*(11), 724-731.

Thomas, L. (1983). An epidemic of apprehension. *Discover, 4*, 78-80.

U.S. Department of Health, Education and Welfare. (1979). *Healthy people: The Surgeon General's report on health promotion and disease prevention.* Washington, DC: U.S. Government Printing Office.

Zola, I. K. (1966). Culture and symptoms: An analysis of patients' presenting complaints. *American Sociology Review, 31*, 615-630.

Zola, I. K. (1973). Pathways to the doctor: From person to patient. *Social Science and Medicine, 7*, 677-689.

4

Health Behavior Research and Medical Training and Practice

A Social Context

H. Jean C. Wiese and Eugene B. Gallagher

INTRODUCTION

The epidemiological profile of the United States has changed drastically over the last 70 years. The so-called "demographic transition" has been accomplished, with the shift from high birth and death rates to low birth and death rates. The population pyramid for this country has changed from the wide-based, sharp-peaked form characteristic of a rural, nonindustrialized country to the more nearly straight-sided, broad-topped form associated with industrialized, urbanized countries. This change in the shape of the population pyramid reflects a radical change in the demography and associated health concerns of the nation. The major health concerns of the United States are now chronic degenerative conditions, all of which have major behavioral com-

ponents in their etiology, treatment, and prevention. Advances in medical behavioral research focused on these conditions are being applied to the current changes in the training of health care professionals in the United States. This chapter addresses the application of these advances in medical behavioral research both to the curricular reforms of health education and to the specific training of medical students for patient care.

SOCIAL CONTEXT OF HEALTH CARE AND TRAINING

Ever since Louis Pasteur's doctrine of specific etiology was unveiled in 1873, this essentially machine model of medicine has been the "party line" of Western biomedical medicine and has heavily influenced the selection and training of physicians (Hamann, 1994). Its adoption was hastened by the overwhelming crisis of the newly industrialized population, which often made it impossible for a physician to know anything about the social context of the anonymous hordes of sick who swarmed the industrial cen-

H. Jean C. Wiese and Eugene B. Gallagher • Department of Behavioral Science, University of Kentucky College of Medicine, Lexington, Kentucky 40536-0086.

Handbook of Health Behavior Research IV: Relevance for Professionals and Issues for the Future, edited by David S. Gochman. Plenum Press, New York, 1997.

ters. Pasteur's pronouncement that for each illness there was a single, necessary, and sufficient pathogen suggested that there was, in fact, no need to know anything about the individual patient. The patient was merely an unwitting host and as such was potentially interchangeable with any other person. Once the pathogen was identified, the relatively impersonal administration of the pathogen-specific treatment was indicated. This approach appeared to work rather well, because the major killers at that time were acute infectious diseases, for most of which a specific pathogen was identified and a treatment developed. Medicine has basked ever since in the glory of its apparent success at stemming the massive epidemics of the early 20th century.

The ripple effects of Western medicine's adoption of the doctrine of specific etiology have influenced every facet of health care. Its adoption hastened the reorganization of medical education in the early 20th century, following the Flexner report (1910), from the existing apprenticeship system, whereby aspiring physicians lived and worked with an established physician, learning everything about the people of the community. This reorganization produced the current formal four-year system, which comprises two years of classroom and laboratory work memorizing the characteristics of the normal human organ systems and then the impacts on these systems of abnormal processes, followed by two years of patient crisis care, usually in a tertiary care setting, treating the abnormalities present in acute hospitalized patients. Use of the doctrine of specific etiology as the model for care has put the emphasis more on highly technical treatment of disease than on outpatient health maintenance and disease prevention.

This emphasis on technology and disease has influenced American medicine down to the very selection of candidates for medical school. Even beyond the threshold of adequate preparatory academic work and native ability, successful candidates are by tradition likely to come from a rigorous laboratory science background (MacLaren, 1995). Given the latitude of self-direction characteristic of American undergraduate programs, students interested in a particular type of work can largely insulate themselves from substantial exposure to other areas. Hence, students attracted to "hard science" can effectively minimize their exposure to "people sciences," i.e., the social sciences and humanities. The net effect, therefore, is the self-selection of medical school candidates to be more attracted to science than to people. With the undergraduate medical curriculum still largely geared to the memorization of scientific facts in a high-pressure environment, the students most likely to flourish are those with the strongest backgrounds in hard sciences. This phenomenon further culls those "people people" who chose broad undergraduate backgrounds in social sciences and humanities and who have only minimal prerequisite courses in laboratory sciences.

This unfortunate combination of self-selective forces can result in the brilliant but impatient and impersonal specialist who is intent on using the latest in technological medicine to "fix" the abnormal and who refers to the patient as "the acute abdomen in room 608." Such a physician is rapidly becoming not only decreasingly effective in dealing with today's major health issues, but also decreasingly acceptable to the American health care consumer (a term that, as explained later in the chapter, does not have the crass implications it may seem to). Changes in the American health scene make the practice of medicine a singularly unrewarding experience for such physicians, even though they are cast precisely in the traditional mold. There is evident need for a new mold in which to cast the next generation of physicians (Chi-Lum, 1995; Hickey, Kalishman, Skipper, Mennin, & Samet, 1994; Koop, 1993; Taylor & Moore, 1994; Walton, 1993; Wilkes, Slavin, & Usatine, 1994).

THE NEW HEALTH REALITY

Just as with any other significant initiatives for change, there are major forces vehemently both opposing and supporting changes in American medical training. Those who argue against changes are quite predictably those with the most invested in the status quo. The physicians who negotiated the gauntlet of medical school with least psychological discomfort and who are most comfortable practicing acute specialty care in a tertiary medical facility have little interest in decentralizing student clinical experiences or increasing student exposure to preventive medicine or epidemiology. From their vantage point in large urban tertiary care centers, their waiting rooms are always overflowing with critical patients in need of specialized care. Similarly, the administration of these large teaching hospitals has an enormous capital investment in the institution and the medical students, interns, and residents who train there. These "doctors in training" provide a great deal of relatively inexpensive patient care. They afford senior clinical faculty coveted respite from patient care, a luxury not possible in nonteaching institutions. The possibility of officially designated time and facilities to pursue one's personal research career is a major hiring incentive for clinical faculty.

In turn, such a clinical/research physician generates for the institution not only patient care income, but also salary reimbursement generated through externally funded research. The medical school and associated tertiary care teaching hospital, then, become almost a self-sustaining microcosm. The medical school–teaching hospital combination attracts research clinicians who generate revenue through highly technical patient care and buy research time by reimbursing the institution with research funds. In turn, the institution provides these attending physicians with clinical coverage by interns, residents, and medical students, all of whom are being trained in precisely the same tertiary care. Change, however, is coming to this apparently internally consistent system of medical education.

What are the forces propelling the current restructuring of American medical education and practice? The answer to this question lies in the changes both in this country's epidemiological

profile and in its social fabric and conscience. As early as the 1950s, the late great physician–epidemiologist John Cassel advocated a shift away from strict adherence to the narrow doctrine of specific etiology as a medical model toward a broader, more inclusive, multicausal model. He pointed out that the etiological concept of illness being caused by a single, necessary, and sufficient pathogen was patently antiquated. Hindsight has demonstrated that this model did not even predict accurately the occurrence of the epidemics of acute infectious diseases that fueled its adoption as Western medicine's "party line" (Dubos, 1965, p. 324). Cassel contended that the specter of rising rates of chronic degenerative conditions should move medical professionals to broaden the scope of their etiological model to encompass multiple dimensions. Cassel's thinking was visionary. At the end of the 20th century, momentum for change is building on several fronts.

First, populations throughout the world are more mobile than ever before in history. As a result, representatives of distinct ethnic groups from various corners of the globe appear throughout the developed world, carrying with them conditions and health beliefs unique to their cultures. These individuals are presenting themselves for care across all medical settings. Meeting their health care needs effectively requires consideration of a much broader spectrum of issues than simply the identification of the pathogen causing an infection. The very numbers of these patients have reached proportions such that they can no longer be dismissed as oddities, unlikely to be encountered in routine health care settings.

Second, the very philosophy underlying medical care has shifted in developed nations such as the United States. No longer is it considered morally acceptable for adequate health care to be available only to a small, wealthy elite. The current philosophy is that access to adequate health care is a moral if not a legal right of all citizens. In nations where attempts are being made to effect this mandate, the very nature of medical care is changing. No longer is the health care professional likely to tend only to patients quite similar in background to himself or herself in an essentially homogeneous cultural context. All modern medical care, from the retail pharmacist to the physician specializing in nuclear medicine, crosses cultural boundaries. The patients in any given care setting will represent an increasingly broad spectrum of ethnic and economic backgrounds. If the cross-cultural nature of the patient interaction is not recognized by health care professionals, the quality of care rendered is likely to suffer.

Third, with the advent of "consumerism" in some Western fee-for-service medical care systems, patients have come to actively resent having their medical conditions treated as disembodied entities with no relevant social ramifications. The "gallbladder in room 607" approach to patient care, whereby the disease process is considered devoid of a social experience, is a legacy of the doctrine of specific etiology. As the concept of the "informed consumer" has become popularized, patients have begun to seek out those medical facilities where they believe they are treated as "whole" people. Most recently, prevention of malpractice suits has been linked with issues of providers' sensitivity to and ability to communicate specifically with patients. In short, popular consensus about the ethical and medical importance of patient–professional interaction has become, at the very least, a sensitive economic point on which professionals are exerting pressure for curricular change.

Finally, the major health problems of the developed world are no longer the acute infectious epidemics of the last century. Rather, in societies such as the United States that have large and ever-increasing proportions of older citizens, the bulk of the health care dollar is spent on chronic degenerative conditions, such as hypertension, diabetes, coronary heart disease, and cancer, each of which has significant behavioral components in etiology, treatment, and prevention. Even HIV infection and AIDS, the most modern serious epidemic to sweep the world, has an insidious onset and degenerative quality unknown to previous world plagues. Optimal day-to-day maintenance of patients with chronic degenerative conditions cannot be managed by face-to-face interactions with physicians in an institutional setting. The routine management of such patients necessarily shifts from clinical to ambulatory home self-care. Physicians trained in traditional tertiary care settings increasingly feel frustrated and ill-equipped to practice preventive outpatient medicine and are questioning their own medical preparation. They realize only too well that the emphasis in medical education must necessarily shift from inpatient crisis care to outpatient community health maintenance and disease prevention. In order to make this change of focus, the doctrine of specific etiology must give way to a multicausal model, exactly what Cassel and others foresaw.

HEALTH BEHAVIOR RESEARCH AND MEDICAL TRAINING

Medical training must be brought into alignment with the proposed "product" of this process: a primary care physician finely tuned not only to render comprehensive care to patients in their community contexts, but also to devise and implement community health maintenance/disease prevention programs. The accumulated body of medical behavioral research is now being brought to bear on the restructuring of American medical training. The focus in this endeavor is a specific population under stress: physicians in training. What health behavior concepts can be brought to bear in preventing or reducing the stress in their learning environment?

Perhaps the research field being applied most widely to this curricular change is that of psychoneuroimmunology, the study of the pathways and mechanisms by which an organism's environment, and its behavioral, neural, and endocrine responses to that environment, interact with immune function (Bauer, 1994; McDaniel, 1992). The most direct application of this research is in the study of the deleterious or even toxic effects on human function, both mental and physical, of environments that are perceived as highly stressful physically or mentally or in both ways (Ader, 1992; Ader & Cohen, 1993; Justice, 1994).

The perception of stress by target populations is a core area of health behavior research. Since medical education has traditionally been perceived by participants as such a highly stressful experience, it is logical that stress perception is an area of health behavior research most heavily tapped in the reorganization of medical curricula. Burnout contributes significantly to high attrition rates in medical schools, and this attrition in turn is costly to the specific training program and to the profession in the loss of invested time and funds. The sheer prospect of mastering the total existing knowledge of human health and disease is by itself sufficiently daunting without being further complicated with potentially toxic stress levels generated by the design of the curriculum itself. In the current restructuring, efforts are being made to address several clearly identified sources of this "iatrogenic stress" on medical students (MacLaren, 1995).

One preventive measure implemented recently in many medical schools' "orientation" or prematriculation programs is active "burnout prevention." Firmly grounded in behavioral research on the importance to mental health of a sense of prediction and some semblance of control, these exercises take the form of not only laying out for incoming students common sources of stress imbedded in their training, but also delineating a wide range of appropriate coping strategies and emphasizing available formal and informal support services tailored for their particular needs. The general consensus among medical educators appears to be that if medical students are expected to consistently act with compassion toward their patients, then this quality must be modeled for them in their own preparation. For example, no longer are new students simply warned that a high percentage of their classmates will drop out or divorce. Instead, concerted efforts are made to identify for students the probable contributing factors to such distressing phenomena and what is known about preventing or coping with them. One routine stressor discussed is that these students have almost without exception self-selected to be competitive academic overachievers. It is pointed out to them that they are now part of a group all of whose academic abilities fall within a very narrow range on the top of the scale. Since many courses utilize a normal distribution curve in grading, this means that many of these students will experience their first grade lower than a B after the first round of medical school exams. This experience is frequently devastating to a student who has always derived much self-esteem from academic achievement and who has never received a grade below a B. Students are encouraged to support one another, especially around periods of examinations, and to consider the situation in its larger context; i.e., the competition is much stiffer at this level, and a B is therefore a more valuable grade.

Some programs go so far as to include small-group role playing and other exercises designed to facilitate the formation of social networking and mutual support systems within the class. In addition, many medical schools make extensive use of both basic science and clinical faculty as mentors/advisors for students. These advisors most often volunteer for this undertaking and invest much personal time and energy in the students they advise, serving not only as academic advisors but also as triage resources for a myriad of nonacademic crises, e.g., lost tuition checks, death of a loved one, relationships gone bad, and parent–student friction. These efforts are all part of a larger attempt to prevent or dilute the paralyzing sense of social isolation and helplessness so common to new students at any residential institution of higher learning, but greatly heightened by the pressure of the content-dense medical school curriculum.

Further measures to stress-proof medical students involve the presentation of the curriculum itself. In some medical schools, students can petition, with no stigmatization, for the option either of an "extended curriculum," which basically means extending one year of coursework over two years, or of a "leave of absence," simply dropping out of school for some specified period of time. Students who choose such alternatives feel that the increase in indebtedness is far outweighed by the improvement in the "quality of life" afforded by such decompression. Part of the reduction of stress achieved by these options is simply the student's perception of wielding some degree of control over the situation. The perception of control has such an empowering effect that sometimes simply counseling a student in crisis that such an option is available can afford enough stress reduction in the sense of helplessness that the student decides to soldier on and accomplishes the curriculum within the traditional time span. With the increasing numbers of "nontraditional" students entering medical school—older, financially independent students with family obligations—the use of crisis options such as the "extended curriculum" or "leaves of absence" may well increase (MacLaren, 1995).

Another curricular change intended to increase student coping abilities during their basic science or preclinical years is the "modular curriculum," in which courses are presented in brief but dense blocks, often containing only one or two subject areas. This approach enables students to concentrate all their attention and energy over a smaller number of areas and during a briefer period of time, rather than spreading the entire content of the eight or nine courses evenly over the entire semester or even the entire academic year. Students can focus and produce maximum effort and concentration, then disengage and change to a new focus. The approach is based firmly on the voluminous research into the negative psychological and physiological consequences of sustained vigilance, the very same general body of research that stimulated armies to rotate their front-line troops and hospitals to rotate clinical staff in and out of such high-intensity areas as neonatal intensive care units. Not only is the move toward a modular curriculum

lum, but also within these modules the very presentation of material is in accordance with behavioral research.

In order to lessen the potential for stressful dissonance in medical students between their training and the patients who await their care, module materials are "case-based"—centered around patient cases using knowledge generated by health behavior research. These "paper cases" are highly plausible fabrications designed to present all the types of complicating issues found in real patient care. The cases are woven such that care of the patient includes aspects from several different disciplines, e.g., microbiology, biochemistry, pharmacology, and physiology, not to mention issues of physician–patient confidentiality and of ethics. Not only is the organization of the material reality-based, i.e., an attempt to look at the illness of the patient within a socioeconomic context, but also the presentation of the modules is new. Much of the modular teaching is now done in small-group settings, utilizing a modified version of problem-based learning (PBL). The rationale in the research is that given the new health reality in the United States, i.e., outpatient care of multiple chronic degenerative conditions, there is a realization that physicians more than ever must learn how best to evaluate situations, identify crucial questions, and resolve these issues utilizing a wide array of resources; in short, they must learn to be "lifelong learners" (Friedman, Murphy, Smith, & Mattern, 1994).

Toward this end, the PBL groups work on each case as a team, with only modest input from a "tutor" whose main purpose is to shepherd the discussion along productive lines and to reasonably challenge each assumption. Such an approach represents a highly active, reality-based form of medical education, fostering a team approach to complex problem solving and a sense of confidence and efficacy. In the process, students become accustomed to approaching patient care utilizing a wide variety of resources, from other professionals to computer databases.

For both students and faculty, this new approach is a far cry from the passive lecture hall presentations that so dominated medical education, in which day after day for two years students were expected to sit for hours in large lecture halls furiously taking meticulous notes on intricate material presented by an authority in the field (Bernstein, Tipping, Bercovitz, & Skinner, 1995; Camp, Hollingsworth, Zaccaro, Cariaga-Lo, & Richards, 1994). This is not to say that lectures no longer occur. Large lecture presentations have a place, of course, but they are no longer the major teaching format in cutting-edge medical education. Students admitted to medical programs are extraordinarily bright, curious, and motivated to help patients. New medical curricula are being designed in part to nurture rather than extinguish these very characteristics by constantly encouraging the students to pursue their curiosity by giving them direction in problem solving and by letting them experience the reward of having successfully addressed the needs of a "patient."

In addition to the case-based nature of PBL, the sense of reality and immediacy sought in current medical education is heightened by several additional active learning procedures. First, standardized patients, hired actors or actresses trained to portray particular types of patient situations, are used increasingly in both teaching and evaluative settings. When well prepared and properly responsive, standardized patients render the student experience virtually real. Standardized patients are now widely used in teaching and evaluating both communication and physical examination skills (Anderson, Stillman, & Wang, 1994; Furman, Ross, Galofre, Heaney, & Mootz, 1994). They are the next best mode to having students deal with real patients.

Increasing use of off-site rotations is giving medical students earlier and more extensive experience with real, community-dwelling patients both in private practice sites and in community services, such as free clinics. Students are also being encouraged to further community medicine experience by participating in health education programs, such as AIDS education in the public schools and poster campaigns in liquor stores. In these programs, students are involved from the inception to the actual presentation of the materials, giving them extensive experience working with a variety of state, local, and community agencies and groups. By the time they complete their undergraduate medical training, medical students who have been active in such programs have first-hand experience with the real issues and problems involved in disseminating health information and care at the grassroots level. Even if they ultimately choose to go into research or a tertiary care specialty, because of this experience they are better able to appreciate the task faced by any health professional working at the community level. In this day of large numbers of patients suffering multiple chronic degenerative conditions, it is crucial that physicians realize the importance of a well-orchestrated interface between basic science and clinical inpatient and community-based care and professionals.

The importance of the interprofessional health care team is now being emphasized more in current medical training. It is stressed that in order to render optimal care to patients, physicians must function as part of a health care team that most often includes, among others, nurses, physical therapists, social workers, and pharmacists. Most PBL cases are written in such a way that mandates either coordination or consultation or both with other such professionals in order to identify and address the problems. Thus, the student is further exposed to and experienced in functioning as a real physician ministering to real patients who are trying to sustain function in a complex social network. A curriculum that gives students this type of rich reality experience makes less distressing and stressful their ultimate transition from "student" physician to practicing physician (Greenlick, 1992, 1995).

This general concern about the humanity and effectiveness of the system for training physicians has carried over into postgraduate education. There is mounting evidence that residency training programs are taking seriously the reformation efforts to improve student-physician preparation at all levels, even to the point of teaching house staff to teach (Dodek, Huang, & Chan-Yan, 1994). Following a court's determination that medical staff fatigue contributed to a patient death, the state of New York, in 1989, passed a law limiting the number of consecutive hours "on call" a medical intern/resident can be asked to perform (Bedrick, 1990; Petersdorf, 1991; Thorpe, 1990). The underlying concern was twofold: first, of course, for the well-being of the patients for whom exhausted, burned-out house staff might be caring and, second, the level of stress excessive hours imposes on physicians.

These, then, are the major ways in which health behavior research is being brought to bear on the current restructuring of American medical education. The overarching field applied is that of psychoneuroimmunology, most specifically in the area of attempting to prevent or reduce the stress put on medical students by the organization and presentation of their curriculum.

HEALTH BEHAVIOR RESEARCH AND MEDICAL PRACTICE

Other health behavior research is being applied to the preparation of medical students for their future practice as professionals. Along with the rise of chronic degenerative conditions as the nation's primary health concern and the general shift in emphasis from crisis care to prevention of both chronic degenerative and acute infectious diseases, such as HIV/AIDS, it has become apparent that in order to educate patients or render them optimal care, physicians must be thoroughly grounded in human health behavior. Within the first weeks of their training, medical students have impressed upon them the demonstrated links among patient satisfaction, rate of healing, cost of care, and their own sense of professional satisfaction and success, links they must be ever aware of.

For example, such grounding is essential for even the most basic comprehension of a patient's response to illness. An individual's assessment of a situation is a function of many factors, not

the least of which is the perceptual framework taught by that society. This culture-specific framework encompasses the society's entire health explanatory model, i.e., what is "known" about causes of ill health and what is "known" about preventing or treating it. Any characteristic associated in any way with health and ill health will thus be perceived according to its association. For example, if the use of condoms is thought to be associated only with illicit sexual activity, mention of condoms in any health education efforts may well elicit a hostile reaction from the public. Likewise, if breast-feeding is thought to be associated with poverty and ignorance, recommendations for breast-feeding may be perceived with revulsion by many families. To be truly "aware" of the reasoning behind a patient's behaviors, a physician must be able to assess accurately the context in which that patient lives. Furthermore, not only is perception heavily influenced by society's norms, but also these standards shift over time, so that perceptual patterning shifts from one generation to the next, even within the same sociocultural system. One need only consider briefly the changes in fashion and body weight preferences to realize the fickle nature of societal norms. It follows, then, that in order to comprehend the health behavior of patients from varying cohorts and backgrounds as well as one's own response to this behavior and the impact of that response on the health care one gives that patient, evidence from health behavior research is every bit as essential in medical training as is recent evidence from research in biomedical engineering (Wedding, 1995).

Medical technology is constantly changing, becoming ever more specific and powerful. Training medical students to utilize this technology therefore by definition fixes them in time to the technological cohort of their training years. Supplemented by their own capacity to keep abreast, through journals, of the technological advances of their trade, the most enduring preparation they can receive is an understanding of the basic common denominators of human response to illness—human health behavior. Armed with this flexible perspective, physicians can appreciate and accommodate their patients' behaviors regardless of the changes over time in the technology of medicine.

Given that American health care is moving toward outpatient self-care of long-term conditions, preparing physicians to most effectively facilitate patient compliance becomes a central issue in medical training. Some of the basic research in the field of health behavior stems from the health belief model (Hochbaum, 1958; Rosenstock, 1974; Rosenstock, Derryberry, & Carriger, 1959). This model attempts to account for the patient's illness behavior by delineating perceptions of the seriousness of the threat posed by the illness, as well as the feasibility of altering the course of the condition. Using such a model to scrutinize health behavior forces medical professionals to (1) admit the relativity of their personal health perceptions; (2) recognize at least some degree of face validity in patient behavior, even behavior they find apparently irrational; and (3) realize that any health program, whether preventative or curative, must take into account the discrepancies between the health information of the medical professional and that of the patient.

As a point of departure, health behavior research has shown that the entire notion of "normal" is a "floating set point," subject to varying interpretations depending on such individual and social factors as the number and salience of other sensory cues, the general prevalence of a given cue in the environment, and the general level of technical sophistication in the society's health data base. Goiter, for example, may be taken to be a "normal" condition in a group in which it is common due to iodine deficiency in the food and water. If nearly everyone has a goiter and it does not appear detrimental to their health, goiter will be considered "normal." A medical program aimed at goiter prevention in such a community will have few if any takers, because goiter is not defined as a threat and therefore does not warrant any remedial measure. Even morbid obesity, as long as it does not interfere markedly with routine function, will be

defined at least as "normal" in communities in which it is highly prevalent and not obviously threatening survival.

From this perspective, then, medical professionals who can step back and consider health behavior through a broad lens are best trained to meet the various health needs of today's communities. Now that every health care facility operates at least to some degree across socioeconomic if not cultural boundaries, an understanding of the health belief model and other cognitive models is basic to the preparation of any consummate medical professional. Arriving at a purely intellectual appreciation of the patient's perspective on the situation, however, is strictly academic unless the physician also has effective interpersonal skills to communicate this understanding to the patient and facilitate compliance.

The importance of good communication skills in the medical arena has long been widely recognized; in fact, formal courses in patient interviewing and communication have been standard fare in many medical schools since the early 1970s (Ong, de Haes, Hoos, & Lammes, 1995). It has long been recognized that patient satisfaction with physician interaction has direct bearing on recovery (Kaplan, Greenfield, & Ware, 1989). Recently, however, it has been argued that requiring medical students to practice interaction skills with their patients, with the implied increase in patient compliance and recovery, is in some sense a form of false advertising, because there is no time and little reward for such efforts out in "the real world of patient care." In the words of Werner (1995), "The fact-of-the-matter is that applying the knowledge and skills we teach in interviewing and doctor–patient relationships courses is hard under the best of circumstances and virtually impossible in many primary care settings today."

Thus far, the only rebuttal to this argument is that students are taught to aim for the highest level possible in patient care, knowing full well that such a level is usually unattainable in reality. Perhaps a more compelling point is that the very disincentives for pursuing good communication skills could be built into the standardized patient cases used in these interviewing courses. Besides giving students guidance in handling complicated medical situations and prickly patient presentations, why not prepare them to fend off encroachments that threaten the use of these skills? Simply having them practice such self-defense could help convince them of the ultimate importance of the doctor–patient interaction, much along the lines of the elaboration likelihood model of attitude change proposed by Petty and Cacioppo (1986). The major tenets of this model are that (1) the audience would be encouraged to process the message, (2) the topic must be important to the audience, and (3) the more actively involved audience members are in processing the message, the more persuasion takes place (Petty & Cacioppo, 1986).

The topic of physician–patient communication has acquired a heightened sense of urgency, however, because of evidence indicating a robust association between patient dissatisfaction and malpractice litigation (Goleman, 1991; Hickson, Clayton, Githens, & Sloan, 1992). The evidence points to patient perception of physician interest or competence as the pivotal issue, rather than demonstrated physician error. The patient who perceives the physician as disinterested, rude, incompetent, cavalier, or otherwise manifesting a negative attitude is the patient most likely to sue (Husserl, 1993; Moorhead, 1992). Medical insurance organizations are therefore also throwing their weight into the push for increased interaction/communication skills training for physicians.

The specter of managed care and rising patient consumerism is sharpening competition among health care facilities and providers. Even in the face of shrinking budgets, increasing attention is being paid to health behavior evidence about "patient-friendly" design and remodeling of both inpatient and outpatient facilities (Carpman & Grant, 1993; Gogorcena, Casajuana, & Jove, 1992). Designs are sought that actively address patient perceptions of waiting time, modesty and privacy measures, concern with child

care, and the need to explain "why." Part of the effort by health care facilities to slow the rush by patients to litigation is the creation of the "patient advocate" position now prominently visible on the roster of most major hospitals and clinics.

In the efforts to make health care more accessible and effective for all patients, special attention is being paid to high-risk, often stigmatized groups. One such group is the most rapidly growing segment of the American population, the elderly. This increased attention is important, because not only are the numbers of the elderly increasing rapidly, but also they are among the individuals most likely to need medical supervision for multiple conditions, both acute and chronic, at the same time that they experience a reduction in both physical and social coping resources. Medical curricula are now dedicating more time to various aspects of healthy aging and geriatric care, both inpatient and community-based. In courses on communication and physical examination, special attention is paid to the unique aspects of caring for the geriatric patient. One example is the effort expended to sensitize future physicians to the significant impact on geriatric practice of the normal transgenerational shift in norms, or the "generation gap." This "lack of fit" between the norms of two adjacent generations colors physician perception of patient competence, self-disclosure, and assertiveness, all of which in turn affect patient satisfaction, compliance, and recidivism rates. Geriatric medicine, of course, has no monopoly on perceptual differences between physician and patient.

Other large categories of patients considered specially in training physicians today are the physically and mentally disabled, the poor, and minorities. Improvements in medical technology enable greater numbers of severely limited or damaged individuals of all ages to survive and live with some degree of permanent limitation. Perhaps the most common health behavior issue that cuts across all these special categories of patients is that of stigma and its impact on both the patient and the caregiver.

The prime motivation for specifically addressing stigma in medical school communication courses is its direct link to stress and psycho-neuroimmunology in general (Elliott, 1995; Sigrun-Heide & Klauer, 1991). Especially in such a high-status setting as medicine, the patient is automatically less powerful. If the patient is then also stigmatized, the issue of power/powerlessness can subvert the entire therapeutic interaction (Collings, 1990). The problem of stigma is frequently addressed in the context of an interviewing course, usually in the first or second year of medical school. The culture-specific nature of stigma is emphasized. Stigma is a universal phenomenon—every human society stigmatizes something or someone—but the particular targets of this scorn vary among societies and even among segments within a single society. In fact, what is stigmatized by one group may well be highly prized by another. The stress experienced by a stigma victim is significant and therefore potentially detrimental to health. It is important that service professionals bear this in mind, because (1) all members of a society unconsciously apply their society's template to approved/disapproved characteristics; (2) health care facilities are being frequented by patients from an ever-broadening spectrum of sociocultural backgrounds; and, perhaps most serious, (3) the role of the physician is the most powerful professional role in American society, which heightens the potential for "abuse of power" in medical interactions.

Obesity is at once one of the most heavily stigmatized and also one of the most pervasive human characteristics cross-cutting the American health care scene. *Health United States, 1989,* indicated that 46.1% of the adult population would be clinically categorized as obese (U.S. Department of Health and Human Services, 1990, p. 174). Obesity has long been recognized in American culture as a stigmatizing personal quality (Richardson, Goodman, Hastorf, & Dornbusch, 1961). Medical students are not immune to the patterning of their culture. Medical students have been found to have negative attitudes toward obese patients before beginning their clinical experience, as have clinical faculty (Blumberg & Mellis, 1985; Kurtz, Johnson, Tomlinson, & Fiel, 1985). The physician may subtly communicate negative feelings to a patient and thereby preclude optimal care. The deleterious effects on interpersonal communication and therefore on medical care are well documented (Kleck, Ono, & Hastorf, 1966). A communication course for medical students is therefore an appropriate format in which to address the problem of stigma, using the characteristic of obesity as a prime example. In such a setting, it is possible to implement a program that alters medical students' stigma toward obesity and at the same time sensitizes them to the enormity of stigma in general and the plight of obese patients in particular (Wiese, Wilson, Jones, & Neises, 1992). If one considers stigma as a form of culture-specific negative placebo, with significant negative impact on patients' immune systems, the development and implementation of such stigma-reduction programs for all health professional students should be high-priority expenditures in the move toward health maintenance medicine.

A discussion of stigma and attitudes in general leads naturally to a consideration of the ethical dilemmas facing today's medical professionals (DiMatteo & DiNicola, 1982; McIntyre, 1992). Medical ethics is a rapidly evolving area of medical training. Since societal beliefs and attitudes develop largely on a system of "precedent," much in the way the American legal system develops, the explosive rate at which modern medical technology is developing subjects physicians increasingly to technologically perpetrated ethical dilemmas in which there are no solid precedents for guidance. One need only consider, for example, the potential of elaborate life support technology to sustain basic physical function nearly indefinitely, leaving the medical staff to grapple with such questions as: Which are they prolonging, life or dying? When does life end? This conundrum leads to agonizing struggles among health professionals, religious leaders, attorneys, and patient families over decisions such as fertility regulation, DNRs (do not resuscitate orders), living wills, organ donation, and patients' rights (Crimmins, 1993; Fitzgerald, Milzman, & Sulmasy, 1995; Landwirth, 1993; Muller, 1992; Rusin, 1992, Stelter, Elliott, & Bruno, 1992). As Califano (1995, p. 10) so aptly put it: "… the most challenging task for our society may be this: to deal with the confounding ethical and moral issues that medical science serves up almost daily."

Adequately preparing future physicians to cope effectively with these uncharted ethical issues mandates that they be well grounded in such areas of health behavior research as the basic formation of health perception, the relativity of attitudes and behavior norms differing among and within groups, and monitoring the influence of their personal values and attitudes on their clinical decisions. Toward this end, in the new medical curricula, these issues are all incorporated into most of the hypothetical patient cases utilized in small-group teaching. Rather than being given a fixed body of medical ethics with which to guide their clinical decisions, students are given training and practice in recognizing and monitoring their own and their patients' perceptions, both positive and negative. Here again, the explicit objective is to foster "lifelong learning," preparing the physician to be flexible and compassionate, able to assess the salient issues and tailor state-of-the-art clinical care to the patient's unique condition and personal circumstances.

Broadening the physician's frame of reference and perspective on human definition of and response to ill health will increase the physician's flexibility and resourcefulness. This should in turn significantly reduce potentially hazardous levels of stress frequently generated in both patient and physician by the medical interaction. Such preparation will greatly increase the physician's tolerance levels for the ambiguity and kaleidoscopic array of variables that affect human health (Merrill et al., 1994). This new approach to medical training will be especially fruitful in that it will free physicians of the need to cling to the crisis care model of medicine, which paralyzes efforts at effective and sweeping prevention campaigns so crucial in stemming both the rising

prevalence and cost of chronic degenerative conditions. These are the physicians who will step confidently into the hail of variables swirling around a major health issue and readily collaborate with other health professionals, behavioral scientists, educators, and community and religious figures to ultimately effect a unified approach that will include not only effective crisis care for those already afflicted, but also behavior-changing prevention programs and quality-of-life-enhancing long-term care options.

There is abundant evidence of this broader approach to disease, the "zooming back" of the lens through which physicians consider health. The inclusion of perceptual issues in the program is often the pivotal innovation. Chronic pain is being approached not only from the tissue damage/nerve impulse point of view, but also on a broader plane of modifying patient perception. There are now effective programs that target patient "pain maintenance" behaviors (Keefe & Van Horn, 1993; Scarinci, McDonald-Haile, Bradley, & Richter, 1994). Patients are taught to distinguish "pain sensation" from "pain distress." The newer intensive care units (ICUs) are taking into account the deleterious effect on patient perception, and therefore on health, of the older, harsher ICU environments, and the "ICU psychosis" from sensory deprivation. The newer units maintain technological surveillance but maximize patient privacy and "normalcy" by including, wherever possible, individual rooms and outside windows.

Physicians are prepared to address the powerful psychological and physical reactions to loss not only in dying patients and their families, but also on the much broader plane of loss encountered in such situations as loss of employment, loss of a limb, and "loss" of a "natural childbirth" by an emergency C-section. There is increasing hope of slowing the rising tide of teen pregnancies because medical professionals are considering a wider spectrum of behavioral and perceptual precursors. Even the "high tech" area of organ transplantation is paying increasing attention to the perceptual factors that affect the medical progress of patients, including such issues as depression experienced by a prospective live-donor family member whose tissue is found not to "match" and body image distortions plaguing patients on continuous ambulatory peritoneal dialysis. Perhaps the most visible and fortuitous application of health behavior research in clinical care is in the approach to the HIV/AIDS epidemic (Boyd, 1994; Lewis & Carlisle, 1994; Post, Botkin, & Headrick, 1995). In the facilities that minister to those stricken with this disease, behavioral issues are addressed with the same intensity as biomedical ones; the impact of diagnosis on the patient's social network and perception of self is evaluated for its effect on the individual's health with the same urgency and thoroughness as are the origins of a spiking fever.

Thus, there is ample evidence of the fruit being borne of this conscious application of health behavior research to and inclusion in medical training curricula.

PHYSICIAN BEHAVIOR IN THE HEALTH CARE SYSTEM

This chapter has shown two directions in which knowledge of health behavior is being applied in medical education. First, it is has considered the use of this knowledge in the design of new curricula and teaching formats, i.e., knowledge used "on" medical students to humanize and integrate the materials that they learn and to improve the learning milieu. Second, it has discussed the ways in which physicians are trained to use principles and skills of health behavior in their dealings with patients, i.e., knowledge used "by" them in helping patients with the prevention and management of illness. This body of knowledge is increasingly drawn upon and conveyed to students as part of their medical education.

The increasing application of health behavior research to the training of medical professionals is part of a general restructuring of American medicine. Medical education as a social institu-

tion possesses a high degree of autonomy and self-sufficiency that enables it to resist, or to respond selectively and slowly to, outside pressures and stimuli. Nevertheless, it does respond. The preceding discussion of new forces in medical education has linked the changes in it to other trends—in biomedical science, in the distribution of disease, in the demographic composition of the population, in the practice of medicine, and in the social conditions of modern life. The most salient of these trends are:

- Aging of the population and the predominance of chronic degenerative disease.
- The shift in medicine from small-scale practice to working in teams and more complex organizations.
- A new emphasis on prevention of illness.
- A multicausal model of disease etiology, displacing the earlier doctrine of specific etiology.
- Geographically mobile and diverse patient clienteles in an increasingly multicultural society.
- Adequate health care as a civic right, irrespective of one's ability to pay for it.
- The patient as an informed consumer of medical care.

What are the implications of these developments for health care delivery? How do physicians respond to them? How can knowledge of health behavior increase understanding of the professional dynamics of the health care system in the United States? Can it help to resolve problems that currently vex the system?

In order to deal with these questions, it is important to think about the tasks and functions of the health care system. This system has expanded a great deal in recent decades by virtually any index one might choose—the share of the gross national product represented by health care, the aggregate of health care providers as a fraction of the total labor force, the volume of services provided, and still other parameters (Himmelstein & Woolhandler, 1992; Mechanic, 1986; Rogers, 1986; Stoline, 1993). Some of the expansion is due to the rise in chronic illness. When an illness is incurable, i.e., chronic, the patient is likely to need continuing care—for adjustment of medications, monitoring of symptoms, and appropriate therapy to prevent or limit deterioration. The chronically ill patient thus contrasts strongly with the acutely ill patient, who most often needs brief, intensive medical care.

Another substantial cause of the expansion of medicine lies in American culture—its idealization of "health" as the supreme personal and social value, an extension of the "life" granted by right in the United States Constitution, a strong desire for protection against threats to health, and a fascination with biomedicine and almost blind faith in what medical technology can accomplish (Fox, 1988; Gochman, 1988; Knowles, 1977).

According to Fox (1988, p. 467):

> One indication of the scope that the "health–illness–medicine complex" has acquired in American society is the diffuse definition of health that has increasingly come to be advocated…. This conception of health extends beyond biological and psychological phenomena relevant to the functioning, equilibrium, and fulfillment of individuals, to include social and cultural conditions of communal as well as personal import. Such an inclusive perspective on health is reflected in the range of difficulties that persons now bring to physicians for their consideration and help…. Accompanying the increasingly comprehensive idea of what constitutes health and what is appropriate for medical professionals to deal with is the growing conviction that health and health care are rights rather than privileges, signs of grace, or lucky, chance happenings. In turn, these developments are connected with higher expectations about what medicine ideally ought to be able to accomplish and prevent.

The "higher expectations" that, according to Fox, are laid upon medicine pervade the health behavior, perceptions, beliefs, and hopes of patients concerning the power of medicine to cure disease and to restore health. Such expectations also indicate an ever-shrinking range of human experience that is acceptably "normal" and therefore requires no special attention or intervention. Discomforts, deviations, and anomalies that at one time were shrugged off as "part of life" now invite professional scrutiny instead of passive acquiescence.

This shift is fueled by advertising in the mass media about over-the-counter medications that promise quick relief from all manner of symptoms. No less, such expectations figure in the behavior and attitudes of physicians who share a common culture with patients and who are the pivotal actors in the health care system. These expectations imbue the self-conceptions and professional images that physicians acquire during medical training and hold up to themselves as standards of medical care.

As discussed earlier, the stress-proofing supports that have evolved in medical education are an early counterweight against the stresses of overexpectation to which physicians easily fall prey. Physicians in their later careers probably lack such supports. Two facets of the overexpectation phenomenon are, first, the drive toward perfection and, second, the accountability pressures on medicine.

A strain toward perfectionism has been noted by social scientists studying medicine. Searle (1981) noted "obsessive–compulsiveness" as deeply characteristic of medical behavior, especially in American medicine. Sharaf and Levinson (1964), in their study of psychiatric training, found that many psychiatrists yearn for omniscience concerning the patient's deep psychic life—as a way of penetrating the patient's resistance to self-disclosure and healing. Cassell (1991), in her study of surgeons, discovered that aging surgeons decide to curtail their practice not because of shakiness, failing eyesight, or other behavioral concomitants of aging, but because of the mental strain of making rapid, highly consequential decisions during surgery; a strong subjective sense of clinical accountability dominates their thinking about retirement.

Accountability pressures and perfectionism have been bearing down upon medicine in general like a quickening drumbeat for the past decade. They are of two main types. First are requirements emanating from third-party payers, government, and the internal administration of medical organizations for more uniform practice concerning diagnoses, treatments, and expenditures in relation to needed medical services (Ginzberg, 1991). The system of diagnostic related groups (DRGs) is a typical example: It establishes limits on length of stay for a hospitalized Medicare patient in relation to the patient's diagnosis; a hospital that prolongs a patient's stay beyond the stipulated limit receives no additional reimbursement and will therefore lose money on that patient.

Such requirements cannot be separated entirely from organizational innovations such as the continuous quality improvement (CQI) movement, which give administrators a stronger voice in the management of clinical affairs in hospitals (McLaughlin & Kaluzny, 1994; Shortell, Gillies, & Devers, 1995). These innovations are on the whole stronger in teaching hospitals than in nonteaching community hospitals. Both academic and nonacademic physicians have an ambivalent attitude toward the accumulating restraints on traditional medical authority. Many of them recognize that given the complexity of current medical care, better patient outcomes are often achieved when physicians consult with other health professionals. Others, however, resent seemingly extrinsic, gratuitous impositions by nonphysicians and by administration.

A second broad form of accountability pressure upon physicians comes from the ideals and traditions of medicine itself. Physicians, particularly medical educators, regularly hold meetings and forums to improve their knowledge and also to assess the accuracy of their diagnoses and the appropriateness of their treatments. So-called "M&M" conferences–morbidity and mortality conferences—are a familiar example. Although medicine has long monitored its own performance, however, the potential benefit from monitoring has greatly increased in recent decades. New technology has been developed for imaging the human body and analyzing human tissue. The burgeoning field of health services research systematically compiles evidence on the effective-

ness of medical treatments (Wennberg, 1991). Further, practice guidelines are being put forth by medical subfields and specialties as algorithms to guide physician decisions and behavior in common but highly specified clinical situations such as dealing with cataracts, diabetes, and depression (Agency for Health Care Policy and Research, 1993; Fishbein, 1993; Lee, 1993). Although the guidelines started out in a purely advisory, informative mode, they appear to be gathering prescriptive force.

It is more difficult for physicians to oppose these trends than those issuing from sheerly administrative or official sources; nevertheless, in the practice life of individual physicians, the rising profession-generated standards may lead to work dissatisfaction, low morale, and a diminshed sense of competence.

How can physicians protect themselves against the burdens implied by higher expectations in the health care system? What should they do? The remedies of their own devising focus upon technical proficiency, especially in "keeping up" with new knowledge and new techniques. Medical schools and specialty groups regularly offer courses on "What's New in ...." It is striking, however, that medical conferences and continuing education programs *virtually never* present material on doctor–patient relationships or communication skills in medical practice or on sources of stress in patients. Earlier, this chapter discussed the changes in medical education toward a focus on communication and on the student's ability to deal with the patient's problems in family and social context.

Once the undergraduate phase of medical education is over, however, these topics fade out of explicit medical awareness; physicians are on their own for maintaining and sharpening interpersonal skills. The lack of organized professional attention to this aspect of being a doctor is yet another vestige of the doctrine of specific etiology, namely, the prevailing theory that the practice of medicine is nothing but the straightforward, virtually automatic application of bioscientific knowledge to an anonymous patient:

The physician is an interpersonally "invisible," transparent agent of technique, and the patient is likewise an interpersonally invisible, compliant recipient of technique

A corollary to this theory is that the physician will, independently, in the course of practice, develop whatever competencies are needed for relating to patients. Actual experience is a good, indeed indispensable teacher; many of the innovations in medical education attempt, as with "standardized patients," to simulate the clinical reality of medical practice. Nevertheless, it is a fallacious theory. Medicine does not simply apply itself; even practicing physicians can benefit from more tutelage, feedback, and directed reflection on their approach and style with patients. Current demands for greater "cultural sensitivity" by doctors toward their patients—sensitivity across gaps of race and ethnicity—bring into clearer relief the fallacy of the theory; if medicine applied itself smoothly and transparently, why would anyone care about cultural sensitivity?

Medical practice, like other forms of complex human behavior, is a social–personal construction or achievement: it is not generated spontaneously from the font of biomedical knowledge. It does not simply "happen." Yet while the "medicine applies itself" theory is simplistic, it may accurately describe the detached, impersonal manner in which some physicians still deal with their patients. Patients' dissatisfaction with physicians who lack empathy and who "don't talk" or explain things runs like a fault line through the health care system, dividing physicians who recognize the relevance of behavioral factors to the optimal care of patients from those who resolutely ignore their relevance.

This intellectual blind spot takes on added significance in view of other, previously noted features of current medical care: the prevalence of chronic illness and the increasing consumer orientation of patients. "Consumer orientation" does not mean a predisposition to search for medical monetary "bargains," to doctor-shop, to collect medical services in an acquisitive mode,

or to regard medicine as a commercial enterprise. Rather it refers to the conception of an "activist" patient, as expressed by Pratt (1978):

> Consumers need to approach health care as a problem-solving endeavor that requires active coping effort, rather than as a situation calling for passivity and submission. This involves ... evaluating the results of medical services, and striving for increasingly greater mastery of personal health needs. Active problem-solving is more effective than passivity and unquestioning compliance, both in handling encounters with a particular physician and in managing lifelong health care.

The particular quality that the consumerist patient, as well as the chronic disease patient (obviously both can be the same person), seeks in the physician is the skill to teach—to describe, explain, and interpret disease and treatment on a clinical, one-to-one basis, in terms that the patient will understand. To do so, the physician must gauge the patient's capacity to absorb medical language and concepts and must tailor messages to the individual patient, making it more personally relevant and intellectually accessible than standardized brochures or pamphlets (it is a sign of the times, however, that many doctors' offices and clinic offices now provide such information, much of it rather inscrutable).

The clinical role transforms the physician into a health educator with patients. This component of the physician–patient relationship moves in a somewhat different direction from compassion, empathy, and emotional support. It empowers and activates the patient, shifting him from a sheerly passive-recipient, compliant plane to a stance of negotiation, self-management, and partnership with the doctor. This stance means one thing for chronic disease patients and another for consumerist patients. For the former, the disease is their disease, for life. That it is implies that whatever the physician's role, the day-in, day-out tasks of coping with monitoring and managing the illness, are primarily the responsibility of the patient, perhaps with assistance from family or other lay helpers. During phases of exacerbation, the physician may take an interventionist stance—the typical model of acute disease. Most of the time, however, the physician's most strategic contribution is from the sideline, as coach, tutor, mentor, guide, and teacher—the stance explicitly taught today in most medical school communication courses (Szasz & Hollender, 1956). In relation to the consumerist patient, the physician's task is to select and convey relevant portions from the daunting realms of health information (and health care information) available.

The abundance of health information in print and electronic media is a valid indicator of the extent to which American society has come to value health and to seek control over illness; the gradually increasing educational level of the population also means that it is capable of intelligent comprehension of the fundamentals of human bioscience (not, of course, the "cutting edge"), e.g., how the heart functions, the need for blood typing in transfusions, and the rationale for diabetic diets.

Despite its emerging importance in the contemporary practice of medicine, the teaching role of the physician receives little attention in medical education. As with so many other features of doctoring, it is assumed that what doctors need to know they will learn independently, or will acquire through latent learning from senior clinical mentors. This approach, however, is a haphazard one that fails to capitalize on the opportunities for "teaching the teacher." As compared with interviewing and history-taking skills, the training of physicians in how and what to teach patients is a low-order priority.

Symptomatic of its neglect is the fact that built-in opportunities for teaching patients are routinely rejected or resisted during medical training. For example, obtaining informed consent for surgery and other interventions is often viewed as a chore of getting the patient's signature in the right place with a minimum of effort ("consenting the patient"), whether or not the patient really understands what will happen. Thus, an apt opportunity for increasing the patient's knowledge in a highly relevant, person-alized mode is frequently reduced to a perfunctory legalism or delegated to nonmedical personnel. Similar opportunities for educating patients in simple pathology and pharmacology are frequently missed when medications are prescribed and dispensed.

Physicians could make better use of their opportunities within existing clinical medicine to educate and motivate patients toward their health and well-being. The ability of physicians to exploit these opportunities depends upon their ability to maintain control of their practice situations. Desirable elements of control include the appropriateness of their patient clientele in relation to their own skills; the availability of suitable technology and assisting personnel; a patient load that permits sufficient time to understand, and communicate with, the individual patient; and reimbursement mechanisms that do not limit the patient's access to optimum treatment.

As shown earlier, medicine as a *body of knowledge* has retained almost exclusive control of medical education, but does medicine as a *field of practice* have enough power to maintain control of its delivery modes? The counterpressures emanating from third-party payers and managed care are becoming very strong; the effect of health maintenance organization (HMO)-based practice on physician parameters such as job satisfaction and decision making has been little studied thus far. Its effect on "end-point" factors pertaining to patients—quality of care, patient satisfaction, and appropriate adherence to medical recommendations—has also been little studied. As HMOs increase their share in the total national scope of medical care, their impact will require thorough assessment. Public debate about HMOs and other features of health care reform has focused almost exclusively upon cost control, but as Emanuel and Dubler (1995) note, "little attention has been paid to how managed care might affect the physician–patient relationship."

Several existing studies point in troubling directions. Blendon, Knox, Brodie, Benson, and Chervinsky (1994) found that patients whose doctors worked on a fee-for-service basis had been with their doctors longer than patients in HMOs. The characteristic transience and staff turnover in HMOs do not foster the continuity of care that seems important for a sound and relatively enduring doctor–patient relationship. Further, employers, ever in search of ways to reduce their employee health care bills, are free to change their HMO affiliations annually within a competitive marketplace. Patients who are shifted from one plan to another lose contact with their previous doctor and must "start again." Having to change physicians involuntarily is inconvenient and distressing for patients in relatively good health; for patients with major problems, it can be profoundly upsetting. In addition to relating to a new medical face and interpersonal medical style, patients may worry greatly about the new doctor's competence to deal with their particular problems. An example is that of the protest of HIV-positive Medicaid patients in New York City against the city's plan to move them from their accustomed fee-for-service physicians into the city's managed care physician network; patient advocate groups expressed strong doubt that doctors enrolled in the network had much experience with HIV and AIDS treatment (Fein, 1995).

Another worrisome trend found at many points in the domain of managed care is the offering of financial rewards for doctors who order fewer tests and carry out fewer procedures (Hillman, Pauly, & Kerstein, 1989). In this format, the financial balance remaining at the end of a given budget period is distributed as a bonus to doctors who have been most sparing in claims upon the treatment fund during that period. Equally troubling, though it cannot be so readily identified as a perverse incentive, is that so-called "cognitive services"—talking to patients, exploring the background of symptoms, evaluating the patient's capacity to cope with various treatment alternatives—receive a lower scale of reimbursement than high-technology interventions. Another factor that significantly interferes with the doctor–patient relationship is the mounting claim of paperwork: Preprocedure permission, postprocedure justification, multiple reimbursement forms, and other administrative demands cut into the time that doctors could otherwise use to discuss care and treatment with patients (Woolhandler & Himmelstein, 1991).

The foregoing analysis of the potential intrusion of managed care into medical practice has many implications for the health behavior of patients—for their level of satisfaction with the doctor–patient relationship and for the responsibility that they take for their own care. These "real world" constraints are superadded to changes that are occurring in the major intellectual underpinnings of medicine as a set of evolving conceptions concerning health and disease.

IMPLICATIONS FOR FUTURE HEALTH BEHAVIOR RESEARCH

For medicine, there is no turning back, no realistic possibility of retreat into the secure boundaries defined by the doctrine of specific etiology. Clinical evidence supporting the need for health behavior research input into health care and health care planning is simply overwhelming. The ongoing pursuit of optimal health care and the resulting reformation in health care delivery systems dictate that the current boundaries of knowledge about human health behavior be continually extended. Unlike the quest for discrete "causal" agents at the heart of acute infectious epidemics during the last century, efforts in health behavior research are not really "causal" in nature. Rather, each significant finding identifies only another variable, not "the cause" (Finerman & Bennett, 1995). The distribution of every human health problem has a significant behavioral component, composed of potentially infinite numbers of discrete behaviors. The interrelationships among these behaviors and the impact of each on the ultimate health of the individual are currently understood only at a most rudimentary level. For example, in every human population about which there is some knowledge, the lowest socioeconomic stratum has the highest rates of poor health. Theories to explain this phenomenon abound. Is it accessibility? Or environment? Or genetics? Or levels of health care? Or psychological stress? Or some combination thereof? It is simply not yet known. There appears to be a factor of "general susceptibility," which only means that it takes all of the aforementioned factors to result in the observed rates, but no one has any idea of how they fit together or of the ratio in which they must be present (Syme & Berkman, 1990). Health behavior research is still operating in the plane of trying to identify all the pieces of the puzzle—and is not yet ready to try making directional inferences about the interrelationships among those variables. Teasing out "cause" in human behavior is almost impossible, because so few variables can be held constant or controlled.

The researcher who can flourish awash in variables is the true lifelong learner whose pleasure is in noting the changing images formed by the endless addition of new variables to the mix. For such an individual, fulfillment comes in watching new items float to the surface, even if their particular relationship to the others is still unclear. Health behavior research in the future demands researchers who have high thresholds of tolerance for ambiguity, for whom curiosity and not resolution is the driving intellectual force. These are the people who will be most effective in research/teaching careers within medical settings, working closely with physicians and other professionals in the design and implementation of preventive and treatment programs, realizing all the time that every program they propose is simply a hypothesis likely to fall to the next wave of significant new variables. These are the properties essential in the researchers, but what can be predicted about health behavior research itself?

Probably the most basic property of future health behavior research is going to be its increasingly interdisciplinary nature. As discipline-based fields of behavioral research expand, there is a tendency for them to become highly specialized and insular. A unique jargon develops that sometimes parallels jargon in another field. This process can make the cross-disciplinary sharing of information difficult, to say the least. It is but a symptom, however, of a much more pernicious and paralyzing process, intellectual isolationism. Health care costs are spiraling out of control, much of the American population is without even the most basic health care, the rates are rising for some of the most devastating diseases. There is continuing accrual of a larger and larger cohort of very elderly citizens with debilitating conditions that may have their etiological roots in these elderly citizens' early health habits. To reduce the rate of increase of health care costs, health professionals must stem the rising numbers of people who develop these conditions, convince those who do not have them to come for regular screening, and implement effective wide-scale prevention campaigns.

The productive future of health behavior research depends on the vision and flexibility of the researchers to specialize within their own discipline, but at the same time to collaborate with researchers in other disciplines—i.e., on their ability to "zoom" in and out on their subject. Without this vision, the highly specialized researcher investigating a tiny slice of behavior can hope only to discover ever more minute variables and relationships. The smaller the array of variables, and the more nearly "experimental" the study design can be made, the "cleaner" and more comfortable many researchers find the research and are thus encouraged to retreat into laboratory settings. Yes, variables can be identified and some basic significant relationships can be established. In order to unravel the tangle of relationships involved in any given human health condition, however, all disciplines must be brought to bear on the topic. The area of coronary heart disease is a prime example. Many discrete variables have been identified along the trajectory of this disease—e.g., heredity, diet, exercise, stress, weight, hypertension, smoking, gender, and age—and more will most likely appear. For all these data to be translated into any sweeping and effective prevention program, however, much more needs to be delineated about the impact on and relationship of each variable to the others and of all of them to behavior in free-roaming populations (Barefoot, Larsen, Von Der Lieth, & Schroll, 1995). For example, how do the culturally patterned preferences for certain body images play into the prevention of obesity, which in turn influences coronary load? Can prevention programs be designed to "teach" children a preference for an active lifestyle and a healthy diet? Even if theoretically possible, could such a program ever be implemented in a culture such as the United States, where individual free choice is so highly prized?

This discussion has now come full circle, back to the relevance of health behavior research to the training and practice of physicians. The reformation taking place in medical education bears directly on the issue of health behavior research. The accumulated knowledge gleaned from extant health behavior research is being applied directly to the reconstruction of medical education, from the selection process through to the design and evaluation of residency programs. Physicians in training are also being explicitly taught to utilize much health behavior information in their care of patients. The new physician, thus prepared, will be better equipped to collaborate readily with other professionals in both clinical care and research, will have a high tolerance for ambiguity, and will be comfortable working as a member of a team. The new physician, in short, will appreciate the kaleidoscopic beauty of human behavior without being frightened by its intricacies.

REFERENCES

Ader, R. (1992). On the clinical relevance of psychoneuroimmunology. *Clinical Immunology and Immunopathology, 64*(1), 6-8.

Ader, R., & Cohen, N. (1993). Psychoneuroimmunology: Conditioning and stress. *Annual Review of Psychology, 44,* 53-85.

Agency for Health Care Policy and Research. (1993). New federal guidelines seek to help primary care providers recognize and treat depression. *Hospital and Community Psychiatry, 44*(6), 598.

Anderson, M. B., Stillman, P. L., & Wang, Y. (1994). Growing use of standardized patients in teaching and evaluation in medical education. *Teaching and Learning in Medicine, 6*(1), 15-22.

Barefoot, J. C., Larsen, S., Von Der Lieth, L., & Schroll, M. (1995). Hostility, incidence of acute myocardial infarction, and mortality in a sample of older Danish men and women. *American Journal of Epidemiology, 142*(5), 477-484.

Bauer, S. M. (1994). Psychoneuroimmunology and cancer: An integrated review. *Journal of Advanced Nursing, 19,* 1114-1120.

Becker, M. H. (Ed.). (1974). *The health belief model and personal health behavior.* San Francisco: Society for Public Health Education.

Bedrick, A. (1990). The eighty-hour workweek. *American Journal of Diseases of Children, 144,* 857.

Bernstein, P., Tipping, J., Bercovitz, K., & Skinner, H. A. (1995). Shifting students and faculty to a PBL curriculum: Attitudes changed and lessons learned. *Academic Medicine, 70*(3), 245-247.

Blendon, R. J., Knox, R. A., Brodie, M., Benson, J. M., & Chervinsky, G. (1994). Americans compare managed care, Medicare, and fee for service. *Journal of American Health Policy, 4,* 42-47.

Blumberg, P., & Mellis, L. P. (1985). Medical students' attitudes toward the obese and morbidly obese. *International Journal of Eating Disorders, 4*(2), 169-175.

Boyd, K. M. (1994). Implications of HIV infection and AIDS for medical education. *Medical Education, 28,* 488-491.

Califano, J. A., Jr. (1995). Radical surgery: What's next for American's health care. *Carnegie Corporation Occasional Papers,* New York: Carnegie Corp.

Camp, D. L., Hollingsworth, M. A., Zaccaro, D. J., Cariaga-Lo, L. D., & Richards, B. F. (1994). Does a problem-based learning curriculum affect depression in medical students? *Academic Medicine, 69*(10), S25-S27.

Carpman, J. R., & Grant, M. A. (1993). *Design that cares: Planning health facilities for patients and visitors.* Chicago: American Hospital Publishers.

Cassell, J. (1991). *Expected miracles: Surgeons at work.* Philadelphia: Temple University Press.

Chi-Lum, B. (1995). Putting more prevention into medical training. *Journal of the American Medical Association, 273*(18), 1402-1403.

Collings, J. A. (1990). Epilepsy and well-being. *Social Science and Medicine, 31*(2), 165-170.

Crimmins, T. (1993). Ethical issues in adult resuscitation. *Annals of Emergency Medicine, 22,* 229-235.

DiMatteo, M. R., & DiNicola, D. D. (1982). *Achieving patient compliance: The psychology of the medical practitioner's role,* New York: Pergamon Press.

Dodek, P. M., Huang, S., & Chan-Yan, C. (1994). A lecturing skills course for residents. *Teaching and Learning in Medicine, 6*(2), 124-127.

Dubos, R. (1965). *Man adapting*. New Haven, CT: Yale University Press.

Elliott, S. J. (1995). Psychosocial stress, women and heart health: A critical review. *Social Science and Medicine*, *40*(1), 105-115.

Emanuel, E. J., & Dubler, N. N. (1995). Preserving the physician-patient relationship in the era of managed care. *Journal of the American Medical Association*, *273*, 323-329.

Fein, E. B. (1995). A report says medicaid plan would hurt AIDS care. *The New York Times*, Oct. 4, p. A15.

Finerman, R., & Bennett, L. A. (1995). Guilt, blame and shame: Responsibility in health and sickness. *Social Science and Medicine*, *40*(1), 1-3.

Fishbein, H. (1993). Patient outcomes research and type II diabetes. *Diabetes Care*, *16*(4), 656-657.

Fitzgerald, D., Milzman, D. P., & Sulmasy, D. P. (1995). Creating a dignified option: Ethical considerations in the formation of prehospital DNR protocol. *American Journal of Emergency Medicine*, *13*(2), 223-228.

Flexner, A. (1910). *Medical education in the Untied States and Canada*. Bulletin No. 4. New York: Carnegie Foundation for the Advancement of Teaching.

Fox, R. C. (1988). *Essays in medical sociology: Journeys into the field* (2nd ed.). New Brunswick, NJ: Transaction Books.

Friedman, C., Murphy, G. C., Smith, A. C., & Mattern, W. D. (1994). Exploratory study of an examination format for problem-based learning. *Teaching and Learning in Medicine*, *6*(3), 194-198.

Furman, G., Ross, L. R., Galofre, A., Heaney, R. M., & Mootz, W. C. (1994). A standardized patient clinical examination to assess clinical performance of medical students in an ambulatory care clerkship. *Teaching and Learning in Medicine*, *6*(3), 175-178.

Ginzberg, E. (Ed.). (1991). *Health services research: Key to health policy*. Cambridge, MA: Harvard University Press.

Gochman, D. S. (Ed.). 1988. *Health behavior: Emerging research perspectives*. New York: Plenum Press.

Gogorcena, M. A., Casajuana, C. M., & Jove, F. A. (1992). Accessibility to primary health care centers: Experience and evaluation of an appointment system program. *Quality Assurance Health Care*, *4*(1), 33-41.

Goleman, D. (1991). All too often, communicating is not a doctor's strong point. *The New York Times*, Nov. 13, p. C1.

Greenlick, M. R. (1992). Educating physicians for population-based clinical practice. *Journal of the American Medical Association*, *267*(12), 1645-1648.

Greenlick, M. R. (1995). Educating physicians for the twenty-first century. *Academic Medicine*, *70*(3), 179-185.

Hamann, B. P. (1994). *Disease: Identification, prevention, and control*. St. Louis, MO: C. V. Mosby.

Hickey, M. E., Kalishman, S., Skipper, B. J., Mennin, S. P., & Samet, J. M. (1994). Impact of a teaching strategy for health of the public. *Teaching and Learning in Medicine*, *6*(2), 108-113.

Hickson, G. B., Clayton, E. W., Githens, P. B., & Sloan, F. A. (1992). Factors that prompted families to file medical malpractice claims following perinatal injuries. *Journal of the American Medical Association*, *267*(10), 1359-1363.

Hillman, A. L., Pauly, M. V., & Kerstein, J. J. (1989). How do financial incentives affect physicians' clinical decisions and the financial performance of health maintenance organizations? *New England Journal of Medicine*, *321*, 86-92.

Himmelstein, D. U., & Woolhandler, S. (1992). *The national health program chartbook*. Cambridge, MA: Center for National Health Program Studies.

Hochbaum, G. M. (1958). *Public participation in medical screening programs: A sociopsychological study*. Public Health Service Publication 572. Washington, DC: U.S. Public Health Service.

Husserl, F. (1993). Effective communication: A powerful risk management tool. *Journal of the Louisiana State Medical Society*, *145*(1), 29-31.

Justice, B. (1994). Critical life events and the onset of illness. *Comprehensive Therapy*, *20*(4), 232-238.

Kaplan, S., Greenfield, S., & Ware, J. E., Jr. (1989). Assessing the effects of physician-patient interactions on the outcomes of chronic disease. *Medical Care*, *27*(3), S110-S127.

Keefe, F. J., & Van Horn, Y. (1993). Cognitive-behavioral treatment of rheumatoid arthritis pain: Maintaining treatment gains. *Arthritis Care Research*, *6*, 213-222.

Kleck, R. E., Ono, H., & Hastorf, A. H. (1966). The effects of physical deviance upon face-to-face interactions. *Human Relations*, *19*, 425-436.

Knowles, J. H. (Ed.). (1977). *Doing better and feeling worse: Health in the United States*. New York: Norton.

Koop, C. E. (1993, Oct. 15). Revitalizing primary care: A 10-point proposal. *Hospital Practice*, pp. 87-94.

Kurtz, M. E., Johnson, S. M., Tomlinson, T., & Fiel, N. J. (1985). Teaching medical students the effects of values and stereotyping on the doctor/patient relationship. *Social Science and Medicine*, *21*, 1043-1047.

Landwirth, J. (1993). Ethical issues in pediatric and neonatal resuscitation. *Annals of Emergency Medicine*, *22*, 236-241.

Lee, P. (1993). Guidelines: Cataract surgery and beyond. *Archives of Ophthalmology*, *222*(5), 597-598.

Lewis, C., & Carlisle, D. (1994). Continuing medical education about AIDS: A needs assessment. *Western Journal of Medicine*, *161*(1), 34-38.

MacLaren, C. (1995, Summer). From the National Chair. Association of American Medical Colleges. *GSA Reporter*, *25*(2), 1-2.

McDaniel, J. S. (1992). Psychoimmunology: Implications for future research. *Southern Medical Journal*, *85*(4), 388-396.

McIntyre, K. M. (1992). Implementation of advance directives: For physicians, a legal dilemma becomes an ethical imperative. *Archives of Internal Medicine*, *152*, 925-929.

McLaughlin, C. P., & Kaluzny, A. D. (1994). *Continuous quality improvement in health care*. Gaithersburg, MD: Aspen.

Mechanic, D. (1986). *From advocacy to allocation: The evolving American health care system.* New York: Free Press.

Merrill, J. M., Camacho, Z., Laux, L. F., Lorimor, R., Thornby, J. I., & Vallbona, C. (1994). Uncertainties and ambiguities: Measuring how medical students cope. *Medical Education, 28,* 316-322.

Moorhead, R. (1992). Communication skills training for general practice. *Australian Family Physician, 21*(4), 457-460.

Muller, J. H. (1992). Shades of blue: The negotiation of limited codes by medical residents. *Social Science and Medicine, 34*(8), 885-898.

Ong, L. M. L., de Haes, J. C. J. M., Hoos, A. M., & Lammes, F. B. (1995). Doctor-patient communication: A review of the literature. *Social Science and Medicine, 40*(7), 903-918.

Petersdorf, R. G. (1991). Regulation of residency training. *Bulletin of the New York Academy of Medicine, 67*(4), 330-337.

Petty, R. E., & Cacioppo, J. T. (1986). The elaboration likelihood model of persuasion. In L. Berkowitz (Ed.), *Advances in experimental social psychology 19.* New York: Academic Press.

Post, S. G., Botkin, J. R., & Headrick, L. A. (1995). Medical students in a time of HIV: Education and the duty to treat. *Medical Education, 29,* 128-132.

Pratt, L. V. (1978). Reshaping the consumer's posture in health care. In E. B. Gallagher (Ed.), *The doctor-patient relationship in the changing health scene* (pp. 197-226). Department of Health, Education and Welfare Publication No. 78-183. Washington, DC: U.S. Government Printing Office.

Richardson, S. A., Goodman, N., Hastorf, A. H., & Dornbusch, S. M. (1961). Cultural uniformity in reaction to physical disabilities. *American Sociological Review, 26,* 241-247.

Rogers, D. E. (1986). Where have we been? Where are we going? *Daedalus,* pp. 209-229.

Rosenstock, I. M., 1974. Historical origins of the health belief model. *Health Education Monographs, 2,* 328-335.

Rosenstock, I. M., Derryberry, M., & Carriger, B. K. (1959). Why people fail to seek poliomyelitis vaccination. *Public Health Reports, 74,* 98-103.

Rusin, M. (1992). Communicating with families of rehabilitation patients about "Do Not Resuscitate" decisions. *Archives of Physical Medicine and Rehabilitation, 73,* 922-925.

Scarinci, I. C., McDonald-Haile, J., Bradley, L. A., & Richter, J. F. (1994). Altered pain perception and psychosocial features among women with gastrointestinal disorders and history of abuse: A preliminary model. *American Journal of Medicine, 97,* 108-118.

Searle, M. (1981). Obsessive-compulsive behaviour in american medicine. *Social Science and Medicine, 15E,* 185-193.

Sharaf, M. R., & Levinson, D. J. (1964). The quest for omnipo-

tence in professional training. *Psychiatry, 27*(2), 135-149.

Shortell, S. M., Gillies, R. R., & Devers, K. J. (1995). Reinventing the American hospital. *Milbank Quarterly, 73*(2), 131-160.

Sigrun-Heide, P., & Klauer, T. (1991). Subjective well-being in the face of critical life events: The case of successful copers. In G. Strack, M. Argyle, & N. Schwarz (Eds.), *Subjective well-being—an interdisciplinary perspective* (pp. 213-234). New York: Pergamon Press.

Stelter, K., Elliott, B. A., & Bruno, C. A. (1992). Living will completion in older adults. *Archives of Internal Medicine, 152,* 954-959.

Stoline, A. (1993). *The new medical marketplace: A physician's guide to the health care system in the 1990s (revised).* Baltimore: Johns Hopkins University Press.

Syme, L. S., & Berkman, L. F. (1994). Social class, susceptibility, and sickness. In P. Conrad & R. Kern (Eds.), *The sociology of health and illness* (4th ed.). (pp. 29-35). New York: St. Martin's Press.

Szasz, T. S., & Hollender, M. H. (1956). The basic models of the doctor-patient relationship. *Archives of Internal Medicine, 97,* 585-592.

Taylor, W. C., & Moore, G. T. (1994). Health promotion and disease prevention: Integration into a medical school curriculum. *Medical Education, 28,* 481-487.

Thorpe, K. (1990). House staff supervision and working hours: Implications of regulatory change in New York State. *Journal of the American Medical Association, 263*(23), 3177-3181.

U.S. Department of Health and Human Services. (1990). *Health, United States, 1989,* DHHS Publication No. (PHS) 90-1232. (p. 174). Hyattsville, MD: U.S. Department of Health and Human Services.

Walton, H. (Ed.). (1993). *World summit on medical education: The changing medical profession.* Edinburgh, August 8-12. Proceedings published by the World Federation for Medical Education.

Wedding, D. (1995). *Behavior and medicine* (2nd ed.). St. Louis, MO: C. V. Mosby.

Wennberg, J. E. (1991). Outcomes research, patient preference and the primary care doctor. *Journal of the American Board of Family Practice, 4*(5), 327-330.

Werner, A. (1995). We are not telling our students the truth. *ABSAME Member Report,* Spring-Summer Issue, 1.

Wiese, H. J. C., Wilson, J. F., Jones, R. A., & Neises, M. (1992). Obesity stigma reduction in medical students. *International Journal of Obesity, 16,* 859-868.

Wilkes, M. S., Slavin, S. J., & Usatine, R. (1994). Doctoring: A longitudinal generalist curriculum. *Academic Medicine, 69*(3), 191-193.

Woolhandler, S., & Himmelstein, D. (1991). The deteriorating administrative efficiency of the U.S. health care system. *New England Journal of Medicine, 324,* 1253-1258.

5

Relevance of Health Behavior Research for Nursing

Carolyn L. Blue and Jo A. Brooks

Nursing is both an art and a science. The uniqueness of nursing is the ability to integrate factors of the nurse–client relationship and science in developing interventions that maintain or improve health. There are few nursing roles and tasks that, individually, could not be performed by another health care professional. Other health care professionals, however, do not have the generalized preparation that nurses have, and as a result cannot perform the broad spectrum of nursing activities. Information about the client and the client's environment is integrated with knowledge in a holistic way to tailor interventions for individuals and groups. Nursing has a much broader view of health promotion than other disciplines. Because nurses work with both well and ill clients, health promotion involves advancing a person's health along a health–illness continuum. The role of the nurse may encompass the roles of client/family/community advocate, educator, consultant, and coordinator of services as well as care provider.

Florence Nightingale (1859/1969), considered to be the founder of modern nursing, provided the earliest influence with respect to health promotion theory and interventions for nurses. Nightingale focused on changes in environmental conditions that could affect health (e.g., cleanliness, air, water, sunlight, diet). As early as 1909, the Metropolitan Life Insurance company supported a project aimed at improving the health of its policyholders. Working from the Henry Street Settlement House in New York City, nurses were successful in reducing mortality and improving the health of the community. Health education was a primary function of these nurses. They provided instruction so that mothers were better equipped to help with illness in the family. Health education and health promotion efforts of nurses soon advanced to schools and occupational settings. Nurses, especially those practicing in public and community health settings, have always encouraged behaviors that prevent or reduce the risk of illness and promote health.

In Nightingale's day and through the 1940s, nursing focused primarily on changing the environment to promote health. The 1950s and 1960s included a focus on client–nurse interactions

Carolyn L. Blue and Jo A. Brooks • School of Nursing, Purdue University, West Lafayette, Indiana 47907-1337.

Handbook of Health Behavior Research IV: Relevance for Professionals and Issues for the Future, edited by David S. Gochman. Plenum Press, New York, 1997.

(King, 1971; Orlando, 1961; Peplau, 1952). In the 1970s, nursing concentrated on assisting persons to supplement their own resources by making changes in themselves or the environment. The goal of nursing was to promote independence, assist the client in adapting to the present health or illness situation, and in maintaining self-care, with the purpose of moving the client to health (Henderson, 1966; Orem, 1971).

Nurses use a holistic approach that considers the totality of the person, including psychological, social, biological, and spiritual dimensions. While nursing care may be directed toward any one part of the person's identity, concern is for the effect on the whole person and the interaction of that person with cultural, behavioral, environmental, and other factors.

RELEVANCE OF HEALTH BEHAVIOR RESEARCH FOR NURSING PRACTICE

There are a number of ways in which health behavior research is relevant to nursing practice. Nursing has both an interdependent function (i.e., carrying out treatment regimens prescribed by physicians and other health care providers) and an independent function, including many nonmedical activities such as those aimed at behavior change, manipulation of the environment, and improving access to services. Interventions are aimed at promoting the factors that minimize poor outcomes and maximize health. Nursing research is needed in order to define client and environmental factors that lead to behaviors necessary for self-care and a higher level of health. Research addresses propositions of the discipline and the problems of practice. Since nursing practice is focused on factors that can be changed, there is a need for research that can help solve practical clinical problems.

That more than 2 million nurses are practicing in the United States in diverse institutional and community settings is another unique feature that has relevance to health behavior research. Nurses are involved with individuals and groups of diverse ages, ethnicity, and socioeconomic status. In addition, the persons with whom nurses come into contact are at different points along the health–illness continuum. Because nurses have knowledge that integrates concepts from the biological, sociocultural, and behavioral sciences, they are well suited not only to work with diverse populations, but also to conduct research focusing on behavioral interventions that recognize diversity.

In most health care environments, nurses have more frequent and longer face-to-face interactions with people than do other professionals. The nurse–client involvement provides insights that can be used to develop efficient and effective nursing care strategies, as well as valuable information for use by other health care professionals. The nurse–client relationship assumes that people are rational, perceiving, thinking beings who are competent and have the desire to care for themselves and others. Knowledge generated by health behavior research, such as information about perceptions of health and illness, belief structure, attitudes toward health practices and treatment regimens, general and explicit control factors, social support, and barriers to behavior, is used to develop individualized nursing interventions directed at improving self-care capabilities and health. Particularly, nursing is involved with maintaining and improving the health of well persons with primary and secondary health promotion interventions and with managing illness by facilitating self-monitoring, lifestyle changes, and evaluation of progress. In caring for ill persons, nurses work to bring about in their clients behavioral changes that will enable them to restructure their lifestyles, improve their level of functioning, and minimize their risk of exacerbating their illness. Nurses need research to build knowledge necessary to strategize their interventions and maximize the ultimate health benefits.

Historically, knowledge used by nurses has been derived from the physical and behavioral sciences. It is not surprising, then, that nursing research includes theoretical models from other disciplines to explain and predict health and health behavior. Most of the research using health behavior models has been done by community health nurses and reflects the health promotion role of the nurse. Although the models are appropriate for promoting health behaviors of ill clients, fewer studies have been done with these populations.

It is not surprising that no studies on supportive nursing care were found in a review of the literature on health behavior theories, since in the acute care setting, individuals assume the classic "patient" role and the focus is on implementing the medical regimen. Patients are in a very controlled environment and subject to a rigid schedule of activities (i.e., prescribed meals, medications, treatments at appointed times). Patients are passive recipients of care, and although nurses talk about involving patients in decisions about their care, in reality patients have few choices. This restriction on choices probably explains why there was little health behavior research related to in-hospital nursing practice. It is when patients are home that they regain higher levels of self-care. As individual responsibility for health behavior is critical for recovery, health behavior research becomes essential.

The health belief model (Rosenstock, 1966) has provided insight into reasons for using or not using preventive measures such as screening for early detection of cancer. Modified by Becker (Becker, 1974; Rosenstock, Strecher, & Becker, 1988) to include responses to illness, the health belief model includes individual perceptions concerning susceptibility, seriousness, benefits of and barriers to carrying out a particular action, modifying factors, other variables likely to affect initiating action, and self-efficacy. Nursing is frequently involved with teaching breast self-examination as a self-screening method for cancer; it is therefore not surprising that use of the health belief model to identify factors that promote or interfere with a woman's performance of monthly breast self-examination has been a popular focus in nursing research. For example, Champion and Scott (1993) found that nursing interventions tailored to health belief model variables positively affected women's perceptions of benefits, barriers, and seriousness of breast cancer. In addition, proficiency in or technique of breast self-examination improved after the nursing intervention.

Social cognitive theory (Bandura, 1977) proposes four sources of information persons use to develop self-efficacy expectations: performance attainment, vicarious experience, verbal persuasion, and emotional/physiological arousal. A number of nursing studies have examined self-efficacy and these four sources of information. Nurses continually work with clients and their families in fostering self-care abilities. For well persons, self-care includes health promotion activities that are aimed at keeping people well. For ill persons, self-care involves following treatment regimens, changing in appropriate health behaviors to those that restore a higher level of wellness, and assisting family members to provide the needed care.

For example, cardiac patients are often reluctant to increase their activity levels, and because families are also fearful of increased activity, on the patient's part, they frequently promote the patient's continuing in the sick role, fearing that activity will tax an already ailing cardiac system. In a randomized, controlled study, Gulanick (1991) compared home activity levels of three groups of post–myocardial infarction patients who were participating in a cardiac rehabilitation program under the direction of nurses. Cardiac patients who received exercise training and feedback had higher levels of self-efficacy and higher home activity. An intervention involving performance accomplishment and physical/emotional arousal influenced activity self-efficacy more than did verbal persuasion or vicarious experience alone.

This type of research is important to nurses in planning interventions, since it demonstrates the need to include a nurse–client interaction involving actual performance, nursing support, and feedback rather than just verbal interaction.

The theory of reasoned action (Fishbein & Ajzen, 1975) proposes that engaging in a specific behavior is a function of a person's intention to perform that behavior, which is determined by a person's attitude toward the behavior and by the person's subjective norm. Attitude toward a behavior is determined by a set of salient beliefs about the consequences of performing the behavior and the evaluation of the corresponding consequences. The subjective norm is a function of a person's perception that one or more referents think one should or should not perform the behavior and the motivation to comply with the referent(s).

The theory of planned behavior (Ajzen, 1988) is an extension of the theory of reasoned action that incorporates perceived behavioral control, or the person's perception of the ease or difficulty of carrying out the behavior. Nursing research can identify the client's specific beliefs that lead to the desired behavior. Nursing interventions, then, can be developed to address the beliefs that most influence the specific behavior needed for health promotion, health maintenance, or recovery from illness. The theory of reasoned action has been used to assess beliefs, attitudes, and subjective norms of hypertensive and cardiac patients that influence compliance with regimens. Nurses have used the research results to individualize rehabilitation programs (Miller, Wikoff, & Hiatt, 1992; Miller, Wikoff, McMahon, Garrett, & Ringel, 1988).

Social support has been a relevant concept for nurses studying health behaviors. Nurses regularly assess people's social support and social networks, since social support can increase a person's resources, enhance coping with change, and influence the course of ill health (Dean, 1986). Stewart (1993) made an important contribution to nursing with her research and integration of the plethora of social support literature. In *Integrating Social Support in Nursing*, Stewart (1993) concludes that the social support construct has unique relevance to the nursing profession and proposes a conceptual model that incorporates environment, nursing, health, and focal persons.

Although much research by nurses has been generated from health behavior models developed by other disciplines, the models do not reflect a holistic representation of the client or provide direction for nursing interventions that considers the nurse-client relationship and the use of problem solving to tailor interventions to individuals and groups. The nurse's role is to assist clients to identify factors that promote or prevent desirable behaviors and assist them to formalize an individual program and monitor their progress. Tailoring of interventions has long been a function of nursing, but nurses are just beginning to empirically document the relationships among nursing care, the client, the environment, and health outcomes. The relevance of health behavior research to advancing nursing knowledge and facilitating client care lies in the documentation of relationships and processes related to client uniqueness, the client-nurse interaction, and interventions.

HEALTH BEHAVIOR RESEARCH AND NURSING MODELS

Several behavioral models that have been advanced by nurse theorists incorporate variables from the health belief model (Rosenstock, 1966), theory of reasoned action (Fishbein & Ajzen, 1975), locus of control theory (Rotter, 1966), and social cognitive theory (Bandura, 1977). Original concepts have been further delineated and labeled where necessary, new concepts have been added, and relationships have been redefined.

Health Promotion Model

Pender (1982) recognized that a healthy lifestyle includes two complementary parts: health-protecting behaviors and health-promoting behaviors. Realizing that past behavioral research focused on the prevention of disease or injury, Pender (1982) developed the health promotion model (Figure 1), which is a wellness-oriented framework. Wellness is the realization of the opti-

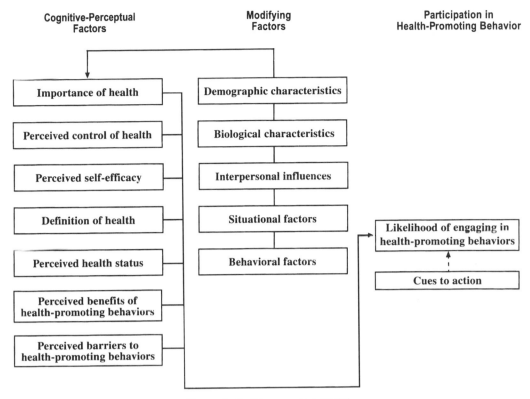

Figure 1. Health promotion model.

mum health potential of an individual, a family, or a community. Wellness is achieved by enhancing physical, psychological, and sociological well-being through activities aimed at the promotion of health. In congruence with nursing, Pender (1987) recognizes that levels of health exist along a continuum, and whatever a person's level of health, the person continues on a quest for optimum wellness. The health promotion model is similar to the health belief model (Rosenstock, 1966), the major difference being that the health promotion model is directed toward behaviors that optimize well-being, while the health belief model is directed toward behaviors that prevent disease.

Health-promoting behavior, which Pender (1982) views as an expression of the human actualizing tendency, is directed toward maintaining or improving the individual's level of well-being, personal fulfillment, and self-actualization. The health promotion model emphasizes seven cognitive–perceptual factors that directly affect the likelihood of engaging in health-promoting behaviors and five modifying factors that indirectly influence patterns of health behavior. Internal and external cues to action are transient stimuli that serve to prompt participation in health-promoting behaviors.

The cognitive–perceptual factors are (1) the importance of health, (2) perceived control of health, (3) perceived self-efficacy, (4) definition of health, (5) perceived health status, (6) perceived benefits of health-promoting behaviors, and (7) perceived barriers to health-promoting behaviors. The modifying factors include (1) demographic characteristics, (2) biological characteristics, (3) interpersonal influences, (4) situational factors, and (5) behavioral factors (Pender, 1987). While cognitive–perceptual and modifying factors constitute the decision-making phase of the model, cues to action are included in the taking-action phase. The level of readiness of the individual to engage in a health-promoting behavior, in conjunction with the intensity of internal or external cues, or both, required to trigger the behavior, determines whether the individual will perform the behavior (Pender, 1987). The concept of health promotion is popular in nursing practice, as evidenced by the number of nurse researchers using the health promotion model.

Although most studies have used health behavior models to examine the impact of nursing interventions on increasing exercise behavior or weight loss among ambulatory populations, the authors believe that the nursing models are broad enough to be applied by nurses working in an acute care setting. For example, a nurse may observe that a postoperative patient refuses to perform activities (e.g., ambulate or get up in a chair) that would promote earlier recuperation and hospital discharge. Using the health promotion model, the nurse assesses the patient's predisposition to engage in those behaviors necessary to restore health. Perhaps the patient perceives little benefit to what is anticipated to be a painful experience, or the patient may believe that health is so compromised that there is no chance of recovering to the former health status. The nurse assesses other model concepts that are known to influence the cognitive–perceptual factors (i.e., age, interpersonal factors, situational factors, and previous experience). Perhaps a friend has experienced a similar medical problem and did not survive, or the patient had a previous illness experience in which activity seemed to worsen the condition. At this point, it is crucial that the nurse identify the factors that can be changed by increasing the client's knowledge, changing the patient's perceptions, coaching, and supporting as the desired behavior is attempted. The goal of the nursing interventions

will be to increase planned physical activities that in turn will facilitate rehabilitation. Nursing knowledge of reasons for client behaviors (cognitive–perceptual factors) and selected nursing interventions that facilitate desired behaviors in various situations with groups of individuals having diverse modifying factors would be advanced by nursing research findings.

Interaction Model of Client Health Behavior

Believing that motivation is multidimensional, Cox (1982) developed the interaction model of client health behavior (Figure 2) to direct and document nursing assessment, plan of care, and evaluation of that care, as well as to explain and predict health-related behavior and to explore and document the effect of nursing interventions. The model can be used to examine the process of client health care, including client–professional interaction and the relationships among client needs, interventions, and client outcomes. Cox (1982) assumed that clients are capable of making informed, independent, and competent choices about their health care behaviors and that they should be given the maximum amount of control in making health care decisions. Cox (1982) postulated that clients are unique and that decisions about health care behavior are influenced by the singularity of the client and the relationship between the client and the caregiver.

The interaction model of client health behavior is comprised of elements of client singularity, client–professional interaction, and health outcome (Cox, 1982). Client singularity is determined by background variables, intrinsic motivation, cognitive appraisal of the health problem, and affective responses to it. Background variables include demographic characteristics, social influence, previous health care experience, and environmental resources. Motivation is the client's need to experience a sense of competence and self-determination in his or her health behavior. Cognitive appraisal involves the client's per-

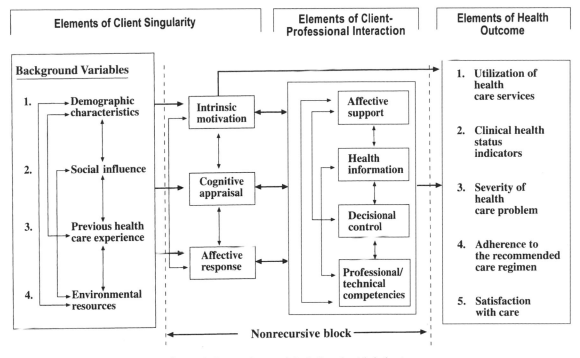

Figure 2. Interaction model of client health behavior.

ception and interpretation of the health state and choice of behavior. The client's affective response can disrupt cognitive appraisal and affect the behavior. The relationships among intrinsic motivation, cognitive appraisal, and affective responses are complex and are influenced by the background variables (Cox, 1982). Health outcomes include utilization of health care services, clinical health status indicators, severity of health care problems, adherence to the recommended care regimen, and client satisfaction with care (Cox, 1982). The model reflects the relevance of health behavior research by systematically including the client–professional relationship, considered by nurses to be a major influence on health care behavior.

The interaction model of client health behavior reflects the essence of nursing practice and is most relevant to nursing research. The targets of nursing care, the client and the client's family, can be assessed by examining background variables. Nursing care can be tailored to individuals, considering their uniqueness of culture, age, socioeconomic status, resources, and so forth. The model provides a method for identifying nursing problems (elements of client singularity), insights in terms of interventions and intervention guidelines (elements of client–professional interaction), and evaluation of nursing care (elements of health outcome). A unique characteristic of the model, and a characteristic of nursing, is the reciprocal relationship between client and health care provider.

A typical nursing problem might involve working with a diabetic client who is learning how to self-administer insulin, follow a prescribed diet, and self-monitor blood glucose levels. The nurse assesses elements of client singularity such as age, educational level, social support, past dietary habits, and experience with administering medications. An assessment of anxiety, knowledge, and food preferences would also be included. On the basis of this initial assessment, the nurse interacts with the client to provide education appropriate to the client's cognitive ability and psychomotor skill and offers emotional support as needed. Assisting the client in self-administering insulin and assessing blood glucose, the nurse provides feedback that promotes correct continuance of the procedures and builds confidence to continue the behavior. The nurse also assists the client in meal planning and reading food labels. As the nurse–client interaction continues, the client's anxiety decreases and feelings of adequacy increase. Upon assessment of client characteristics, the nurse may find that certain cultural beliefs influence the client's motivation to follow the dietary prescription. The interaction between nurse and client would then address the beliefs, and the nurse and client together would find a workable solution to the problem. The process of nursing care is evaluated by examining elements of health outcome such as adherence to the medical regimen, indicators that the blood sugar is staying within the normal range, and satisfaction with the care received. Nursing research is used to examine elements of the client–nurse interaction with aspects of client uniqueness that lead to positive health outcomes.

The interaction model of client health behavior is in its early stages of development, and most of the research has focused on developing the instrument and determining the empirical validity of the theory's propositions (for a review, see Carter & Kulbok, 1995). The model parallels, however, the metaparadigm concepts of person, health, environment, and nursing. More comprehensive and complex than previous models of client behavior, the interaction model offers a framework for examining client uniqueness and the process by which the client interacts with health care professionals to make behavioral decisions. The model also reflects the philosophy of nursing practice that the client is holistic and unique, capable of actively reacting with health professionals in making decisions.

Theory of Care-Seeking Behavior

Believing that the health belief model and the theory of reasoned action had limitations with respect to variables needed for health promotion behaviors and inconsistencies in the variance in behavior explained by the model concepts, Lauver (1992a) developed the theory of care-seeking behavior (Figure 3) to explain and predict preventive health behaviors (primary and secondary), as opposed to illness-related behaviors. The model draws from concepts in the health belief model, the theory of reasoned action, and Triandis's (1977) theory of intrapersonal behavior. The theory of care-seeking behavior is modeled after Triandis's (1977) theory, but differs in that behavioral intention and physiological arousal concepts are not included. Lauver (1992a) feels that physiological arousal associated with health behaviors (as opposed to illness behaviors) is difficult to measure and that the affect concept is an indicator of arousal. Affective variables (e.g., anxiety, fear, denial), utility (referring to beliefs about the worth of care seeking), social norms, and habits have a direct influence on care-seeking behavior. Facilitating conditions such as having health insurance or a regular health care provider are expected to interact with other variables in the model (Lauver, 1992a).

Lauver (1992b) tested the theory of care-seeking behavior to examine racial influence on intention to care for breast cancer symptoms promptly. Utility and social norms were significantly associated with intention and were contingent on race. Although utility was significantly associated with intention, the positive influence of utility was stronger among Caucasians than among African-Americans. The positive influence of social norms on intention was significant only for Caucasians.

Positive affective responses, such as feelings of reducing worry or of reassurance or relief, were a primary expectation of seeking or not seeking treatment for breast symptoms (Lauver & Angerame, 1993). An assessment of optimism may indicate the level of emotional distress and outcome expectations involved in making care-

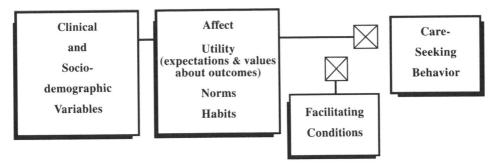

Figure 3. Theory of care-seeking behavior.

seeking decisions (Lauver & Tak, 1995). Although the effect of interventions on care-seeking behaviors has not been tested, findings from Lauver's research suggest that nursing interventions that support positive emotions and other affective responses may improve the likelihood of prompt care-seeking behavior.

Lauver's model is particularly important for nurses working with clients who have not entered the health care system for medical care. Since nurses are accessible in community settings, it is the nurse who frequently discovers symptomatology and provides reinforcement of positive outcomes and emotional support when clients need to seek care.

Health-Promoting Self-Care System Model

Simmons (1990a) proposed the health-promoting self-care system model (Figure 4) as an integration of three nursing frameworks: the self-care deficit nursing theory (Orem, 1985), the interaction model of client health behavior (Cox, 1982), and the health promotion model (Pender, 1987). The health-promoting self-care system model includes the link of nursing to health states and behaviors of individuals. There are seven major concepts: (1) basic conditioning factors, (2) self-care requisites, (3) therapeutic self-care demand, (4) exercise of self-care agency, (5) nursing system, (6) health-promoting self-

care, and (7) health outcomes. Orem (1985, p. 123) defined self-care agency as "the developed or developing capability to engage in the investigative and decision-making phase of self-care (phase one) and the capability to engage in the production phase of self-care (phase two)." Self-care agency reflects the human control to perform self-care in the promotion and maintenance of health as well as in the prevention and treatment of illness. Simmons (1990a) uses Orem's (1985) conceptualization of a supportive–educative nursing system to represent nursing interaction with the client to affect perceptions, motivation, values, and psychomotor skills of self-care and to encourage health-promoting self-care. Basic conditioning factors and universal and developmental factors influence a person's total requirement for health-promoting self-care demand. The model is intended to explain cumulative and interactive relationships among the concepts (Simmons, 1990a).

Simmons (1990b) examined the effect of exercise of self-care agency on health-promoting self-care among active duty military personnel. Although self-care agency predicted health-promoting lifestyle, the combination of basic conditioning factors (demographics, military rank, duty type, and perceived health state) and self-care agency was more explanatory of health-promoting behaviors (Simmons, 1990b).

Nursing research using the health-promoting self-care system model will be valuable in answering questions concerning the kinds, frequency,

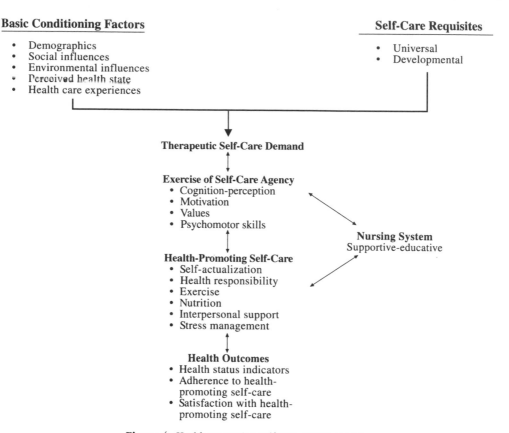

Figure 4. Health-promoting self-care system model.

and length of supportive and educational nursing interventions that affect aspects of self-care agency and behaviors. Examining health outcomes would demonstrate the health effectiveness of the nursing interventions and client behaviors.

Resource Model of Preventive Health Behavior

Kulbok (1985) proposed the resource model of preventive health behavior, in which people act to maximize their investment of resources in health. The model proposes that the greater the perceptions of better health and social resources, the more frequent will be the performance of health behaviors. Resource model variables are

(1) social resources, including educational level and income; (2) health resources, including perceived health status and energy level, concern about health and feelings about capability of taking care of one's own health, participation in social groups and religious services, number and closeness of friends and relatives, and general psychological well-being; and (3) health behaviors, including diet and exercise, physical activity, sleeping, smoking, alcohol and caffeine consumption, dental hygiene, seat belt use, use of professional health services, and behaviors necessary to control hypertension.

Using secondary data from Wave 1 of the National Survey of Personal Health Practices and Consequences, Kulbok (1985) revealed the dimensionality of preventive health behaviors. Health resources factored into activity level, general well-being, and health comparison. Preventive health behavior factored into dental hygiene, medical checkups, harmful consumption, health protection, and physical fitness. Social and health resources explained dental and physical fitness, but not other preventive health behaviors. In addition, Kulbok (1985) reported several different patterns for the prediction of preventive health behavior factors. Although the model concepts need further refinement, the resource model of preventive health behaviors appears potentially useful in the future study of health behaviors.

Nursing Priorities

The variety of research settings and foci included in the nursing research literature reflects the practice of nursing. Because nursing is a practice-oriented discipline, the objective of nursing research is to understand basic phenomena that can be used to monitor and promote health along the health–illness continuum and to care for and assist persons to care for themselves. Thus, nursing research mirrors all the many practice settings in the domain. Since nurses work in a number of health care settings with persons who have a variety of behavioral needs, the kaleidoscopic nature of nursing research is not surprising.

Of the 11 priorities identified by the American Nurses Association Cabinet on Nursing Research (1985), the following 3 directly address the involvement of nursing with health-promoting behavior:

1. Promote health, well-being, and the ability to care for oneself among all age, social, and cultural groups.
2. Minimize or prevent behavioral and environmentally induced health problems that compromise the quality of life and reduce productivity.
3. Develop integrative methodologies for the holistic study of human beings as they relate to their families and lifestyles.

The establishment of the National Center for Nursing Research (now the National Institute for Nursing Research) in 1986 has provided additional federal support for research in nursing. The National Institute for Nursing Research funding priority for health promotion research reflects not only the focus of nursing but also the national health care objectives for interventions that foster and promote health among well and ill populations.

RESEARCH AND METHODOLOGICAL ISSUES

Nurses have taken an active role in health behavior research through their efforts to refine the models and operationalize definitions of the concepts. Nurse researchers have contributed to health behavior research through systematically and carefully defining and operationalizing concepts. Evaluation of models for their reliability and validity will be further advanced when concepts can be measured with standardized instruments.

Instruments Developed by Nurse Researchers

This section reviews 16 reliable and valid instruments developed by nurse researchers to measure theoretical constructs for specific health-related behaviors (Table 1).

Health Belief Model Constructs. Champion (1984) developed an instrument to measure health belief model constructs in the context of breast self-examination (BSE). Self-efficacy items were developed to include magnitude (i.e., level of difficulty), generality (relevance to BSE), and strength. The original instrument consisted of 39 items representing five subscales: susceptibility, seriousness, benefits, barriers, and health mo-

Table 1. Instruments Developed by Nurses to Measure Constructs Relevant to Health Behavior Research

| Instrument | Author(s) | Sample | Reliability | | | Validity | |
			Internal consistency?	Test/retest?	Content	Construct	Criterion
Champion Health Belief Model Scale	Champion (1984, 1993)	Healthy women 35 years and older	Yes	Yes	Literature Experts	Factor analysis	BSE frequency and proficiency.
Osteoporosis Health Belief Scale	Kim, Horan, Gendler, & Patel (1991)	Elderly adults	Yes	—	Adapted from Champion's scale	Factor analysis	Discriminated low and high levels of calcium intake and exercise.
Exercise Benefits/Barriers Scale	Sechrist, Walker, & Pender (1987)	Healthy adults	Yes	Yes	Interview Literature Experts	Factor analysis	—
Miller Attitude Scale	Miller, Wikoff, McMahon, Garrett, & Johnson (1982)	Cardiac patients	Yes	—	Interview Literature Experts	Factor analysis	Correlated with adherence behaviors.
Interpersonal Relationship Inventory	Tilden, Nelson, & May (1990)	Adults under life stresses Nursing students	Yes	Yes	Experts	—	—
Norbeck Social Support Questionnaire	Norbeck, Lindsey, & Carrieri (1981)	Nursing students	Yes	Yes	Literature	Negative relationship with psychiatric symptomatology and life stresses	Correlated with other measures of social support. Not related to social desirability.
Personal Resource Questionnaire—Part 2	Weinert (1988)	Adults with multiple sclerosis Healthy adults	Yes	—	Experts	Factor analysis	Correlated with Family Adjustment Scale.

Instrument	Author (year)	Population			Source	Method	Validity
Insulin Management Diabetes Self-Efficacy Scale	Hurley (1990)	Diabetic adults	Yes	Yes	Literature Experts Diabetic patients	Factor analysis	Correlated with diabetes self-care and subsequent behavior 1 month later.
Cardiac Exercise Self-Efficacy Instrument	Hickey, Owen, & Froman (1992)	Cardiac patients	Yes	Yes	Literature Experts	Factor analysis	Correlated with diet and exercise goal attainment and with marathon runners.
Epilepsy Management Self-Efficacy Scale	Dilorio, Faherty, & Manteuffel (1992)	Adults with epilepsy	Yes	Yes	Literature Experts Epileptics	Factor analysis	Correlated with self-management of epilepsy and social support.
Self-Rated Abilities for Health Practices Scale	Becker, Stuifbergen, Oh, & Hall (1993)	Healthy adults Nursing students Adults with disabilities	Yes	Yes	Literature	Factor analysis	Correlated with general ratings of self-efficacy and Health-Promoting Lifestyle Profile.
Health-Promoting Lifestyle Profile	Walker, Sechrist, & Pender (1987)	Adults from the general population	Yes	Yes	Literature Experts	Factor analysis	—
Laffrey Health Conception Scale	Laffrey (1986)	Nursing students Adults from the general population Participants in adult education classes	Yes	Yes	Interview Literature Experts	Factor analysis	Correlated with health-promoting behavior choices and creativity.
Health Self-Determinism Index	Cox (1985)	Adults from the general population	Yes	—	Literature Experts	Factor analysis	—
Health Self-Determinism Index for Children	Cox, Cowell, Marion, & Miller (1990)	Children aged 7–13 years	Yes	Yes	Adapted from Cox's Health Self-Determinism Index for Adults	Factor analysis	Correlated with healthy behaviors and children with known exceptional health behaviors.

tivation. Each concept scale is measured on a 5-point Likert format with responses ranging from "Strongly agree" to "Strongly disagree." Champion (1993) refined the original instrument by developing a scale to measure confidence in performing BSE. Extensive validity and reliability analyses have been completed. The instrument has been used with samples of various ages and ethnic groups and has been modified to measure theoretical concepts with respect to mammography and professional breast examination.

Champion's (1984) BSE instrument was modified for measuring osteoporosis health beliefs (Kim et al., 1991). This 35-item scale focuses on two behaviors relevant to osteoporosis prevention: calcium intake and physical exercise. The instrument consists of 15 common items measuring susceptibility, seriousness, and health motivation, and 10 unique items, each related to calcium and exercise. Although the instrument has not been tested with a variety of samples, there is initial evidence that it is valid and reliable.

An Exercise Benefits Barriers Scale was developed to measure physical, psychological, and social benefits of and barriers to habitual exercise (Sechrist et al., 1987). The instrument includes 44 items relevant to benefits and 17 items relevant to barriers, measured on a 4-point forced-choice Likert format. The instrument was developed to evaluate the role of cognition and perception within Pender's (1987) health promotion model.

Attitude. The Miller Attitude Scale (MAS) (Miller et al., 1982) was constructed to measure attitude toward health behaviors that would be consistent with recovery form myocardial infarction and cardiac surgery (i.e., taking medication, managing stress, engaging in physical activity, eliminating smoking, and following a prescribed diet). The MAS includes a 12-item, 7-point semantic differential scale for each compliance health behavior. The instrument was developed for and has been used extensively with cardiac patients, and so may not be appropriate for use with samples of well persons.

Social Support. Although nurses have contributed a number of instruments for the measurement of social support, only three of these instruments have been thoroughly examined for psychometric properties (Stewart, 1993). The Interpersonal Relationship Inventory (IPRI) came from a revision of the Cost and Reciprocity of Social Support scale (Tilden, 1985). Tilden et al. (1990) interviewed 44 adults in the community who were experiencing life stresses (e.g., cancer, homelessness) to develop 140 items representing interpersonal support, reciprocity, and conflict. Three subscales (social support, reciprocity, and conflict) emanate from social exchange theory (Cook, 1987) and equity theory (Burgess & Huston, 1979). The final scale consists of 39 Likert-type items. Construct validity was determined with a sample of 235 subjects experiencing a variety of stressful situations (e.g., students, cancer patients, obesity program participants). Criterion validity was established with the Personal Resource Questionnaire (Weinert, 1988) (described below).

The Norbeck Social Support Questionnaire (NSSQ) is based on Kahn's (1979) definition of support (Norbeck et al., 1981). The NSSQ measures three functional properties (affect, affirmation, and aid) and four network properties of support (network numbers, duration of relationships, frequency of contact with network members, and recent losses) (Norbeck, Lindsey, & Carrieri, 1983). Scores for the functional and network properties are derived from ratings for each person in the personal network. Evidence for concurrent validity was found with other measures of social support (Norbeck et al., 1983). The measure has also been found to have acceptable levels of predictive validity and appears to be free of social-desirability response bias (Norbeck, 1984).

The Personal Resource Questionnaire (PRQ) is a 25-item, 7-point Likert-type scale that was developed from Weiss's (1974) five dimensions of social support and includes a description of resources and their perceived adequacy (Brandt & Weinert, 1981). The questionnaire emphasizes the multidimensional nature of social support with subscales representing worth, intimacy, social integration, nurturance, and assistance. The PRQ has undergone refinement and modification (Weinert, 1988). Although the instrument has been used in a number of studies, Higgins and Dicharry (1991) found the content validity to be culturally unacceptable for use with a sample of Navajo women.

Self-Efficacy. Self-efficacy has been found to predict subsequent behavior that promotes health behavior and lifestyle changes in areas that have implications for nurses and other health care professionals. Although research on self-efficacy and health behavior is promising, the behavioral specificity of the construct makes it necessary to develop behavior-specific measures in order to test the empirical and practical merit of self-efficacy. Several nurse researchers have contributed to the study of self-efficacy in health behavior research, developing behavior-specific self-efficacy scales.

Hurley (1990) developed the Insulin Management Diabetes Self-Efficacy Scale (IMDSES), which includes dimensions of self-efficacy pertaining to perceived confidence in one's ability to manage diabetes. Although the instrument includes three subscales (general diabetes, diet, and insulin), factor analysis determined nine factors (confidence to follow diet, to make insulin decisions, to exercise regularly, to adjust insulin, to manage foot care, and to detect changes in blood glucose; general confidence; insecurity in changing usual routines; and overall insecurity). The IMDSES was related with diabetes self-care and metabolic control and predicted self-care behavior 1 month later, and the variance in behavior explained by the addition of the health belief model variables increased only slightly (Hurley, 1990).

The Cardiac Exercise Self-Efficacy Instrument (CESEI) was developed to determine self-efficacy perceptions for behaviors related to lifestyle improvements in persons with cardiac conditions (Hickey et al., 1992). The CESEI consists of 16 items related to diet self-efficacy and 16 items related to exercise self-efficacy. Items are scaled

on a 5-point format. A relationship was found between diet self-efficacy and subsequent diet goal attainment and between exercise self-efficacy and exercise goal attainment. Marathon runners were found to have high levels of exercise self-efficacy.

Dilorio et al. (1992) developed the Epilepsy Management Self-Efficacy Scale (EMSS) to encompass three dimensions: medication management, seizure management, and general management. The EMSS consists of 25 items scaled on a 5-point Likert scale. A positive relationship was found between the EMSS and self-management of epilepsy and social support.

Significant to the study of a variety of health-promoting behaviors, Becker et al. (1993) developed and tested the Self-Rated Abilities for Health Practices Scale (SRAHPS) from three samples of well and ill adults (health fair attenders, students, and persons with disabilities). The instrument was designed to measure perceived self-efficacy with respect to exercise, nutrition, psychological well-being, and responsible health practices, the same behaviors addressed in the Health-Promoting Lifestyle Profile (Walker et al., 1987) (described below). The instrument consists of 28 items asking for a rating of how well the respondent is able to perform each health practice on a 5-point scale. The SRAHPS was related with total scores on the Health-Promotion Lifestyle Profile.

Health-Promoting Lifestyle Profile. Walker et al. (1987) made an important contribution to health behavior research by developing the Health-Promoting Lifestyle Profile (HPLP). The HPLP measures six hypothesized dimensions of health-promoting lifestyle: self-actualization, health responsibility, exercise, nutrition, interpersonal support, and stress management. The HPLP reflects Pender's (1982) view that health-promoting lifestyle is a multidimensional pattern of behaviors directed toward the maintenance or enhancement of wellness, self-actualization, and personal fulfillment. Pender (1982) developed the Lifestyle and Health Habits Assessment (LHHA) from literature sources, and the HPLP was developed from the LHHA. The HPLP contains 70

4-point additive scale items. Evidence of reliability and validity of the scale has been obtained in a number of studies involving both well (Duffy, 1988; Pender, Walker, Sechrist, & Frank-Stromborg, 1990) and ill (Frank-Stromborg, Pender, Walker, & Sechrist, 1990; Stuifbergen & Becker, 1994) young, middle-aged, and elderly adults. The HPLP was also found to be reliable in studies with samples of low-socioeconomic-status Spanish-speaking adults (Kuster & Fong, 1993), African-American women (Ahijevych & Bernhard, 1994), and blue-collar workers (Lusk, Ronis, Kerr, & Atwood, 1994). The HPLP and its subscales have been used extensively by nurses in studies of behaviors related to health promotion behaviors and has been an important factor in the examination of Pender's health promotion model.

Laffrey Health Conception Scale. Laffrey (1985a) views health promotion from the viewpoint of the person's health care potential; i.e., individuals perform health-related behaviors to achieve their own life goals rather than to achieve the goals of preventing a particular illness state or of promoting general health. Unlike definitions of health promotion from other disciplines, Laffrey's definition involves behaviors "taken for the purpose of achieving a higher level of health and well being, however these are defined by the individual" (Laffrey, 1985a, p. 37).

Laffrey (1986) felt that instruments used in prior health behavior research either represented health as the absence of disease or viewed health as a unidimensional concept. Laffrey's multidimensional view of health is appropriate for nursing, since the discipline aims to assist a person to achieve higher levels of health even when that person has an acute or chronic medical condition. If health is viewed as a multidimensional concept, nurses have more information from client assessments to develop meaningful interventions. Health conception is described by Laffrey (1985b) as a manifestation of the value attributed to health by an individual. The Laffrey (1986) Health Conception Scale (LHCS) follows Smith's (1981) definition of health and measures

four dimensions of health: clinical (the absence of disease, illness, or symptoms), functional/role performance (one's capacity to carry out usual roles in a satisfactory manner), adaptive (flexible adjustment and adaptation), and eudamonistic (the ability to excel in or complete life achievements). The LHCS is composed of 28 Likert-type scale items. Health conception was associated with health-promoting behavior choices (Laffrey, 1985b). In addition, wellness (clinical) health conception was an important predictor of health-promoting behaviors measured by the HPLP (Frank-Stromborg et al., 1990; Pender et al., 1990; Stuifbergen & Becker, 1994). Volden, Langemo, Adamson, and Oechsle (1990) found gender differences concerning the meaning of health, with females scoring higher than males.

Health Self-Determinism Index. Motivation in health behavior research has been measured as a global trait (e.g., locus of control) or as health beliefs (e.g., belief of vulnerability to a health problem in the health belief model). Cox (1985), believing that the process of choosing (i.e., intrinsic motivation) between behaviors is the primary source of energy for setting goals and behaving in accordance with those goals, developed the Health Self-Determinism Index (HSDI). The HSDI, based on Deci's (1975) theoretical framework of intrinsic motivation, is a multidimensional instrument comprised of four subscales: self-determined health judgments, self-determined health behavior, perceived competency in health matters, and internal and external cue responsiveness. The HSDI consists of 17 items and results in highly acceptable internal consistency and test–retest reliability (Cox, Miller, & Mull, 1987).

Cox et al. (1990) adapted the HSDI for use with children (HSDI-C). The 27-item HSDI-C measures intrinsic motivation and the strength of intrinsic–extrinsic motivation within each of the four dimensions of the original scale. Internal consistency and test–retest reliabilities have been adequate. Factor analysis resulted in four unique scales: behavior and goals, competency, internal–external cue responsiveness, and judgment. Children with known exceptional positive health behaviors scored significantly higher on the HSDI-C than did a general sample of children.

From a theoretical perspective, the HSDI and HSDI-C are useful in theory development for examining the intrinsic motivation concept in Cox's (1982) interaction model of client health behavior. After the HSDI undergoes further testing for reliability and validity, its practical application for nursing will be to offer a short assessment tool for use in clinical settings to facilitate interventions tailored to individual and group health motivation orientations.

Study Designs and Threats to Internal and External Validity

Research reviewed in the nursing literature has revealed a variety of psychosocial determinants of health-promoting behaviors. The impact of the various concepts on single behaviors or lifestyle indices, however, is far from conclusive. The difficulty in drawing conclusions about which variables are most critical to behavior is most likely due to the variety of theoretical approaches, operational definitions, and research methods used to study these variables.

Nurse researchers have focused primarily on explaining the influence of a variety of beliefs and perceptions on singular behaviors. Although these efforts have produced additional information with respect to the impact of these variables, there has been little explanation of the variance in behavior. Future research should be directed to other factors outside the individual that influence behavior and incorporate concepts that appear to facilitate health behaviors, eliminating those concepts that do not appear to facilitate healthy behaviors. For example, questions have been raised concerning whether to retain the health value variable (Pender, 1987). Interpersonal influence and social support, however, have been important variables in health behavior research. Nurses and other health professionals may need to consider complementary theories.

Nursing research may be advanced more by synthesizing models that show promise for nursing interventions. The authors are not suggesting simply that large numbers of concepts be included in behavior models to increase the explained variance. There are problems associated with models containing large numbers of variables (Wallston & Wallston, 1984), one being that the number of subjects needed to test such models is generally prohibitive from a statistical perspective as well as from a practical point of view. Instead, researchers need to select variables carefully to determine what proportion of variance in health behavior is explained by which variables and by which combinations of variables.

Although nurse researchers acknowledge that in designing and implementing nursing interventions, it is important to understand factors that facilitate health-related behaviors, few studies examining theoretical concepts, interventions, and the resulting changes in behavior have been done. In addition, even though nursing interventions have been shown to have an effect on positive behavior change, there is no evidence that change holds over time. There is initial empirical evidence that nursing interventions (especially those tailored to conceptual characteristics) have an effect on conceptual variables and positive behavior change. As yet, however, there is no evidence that behavior change holds over time. Although the authors acknowledge that before interventions can be planned, the model must be carefully tested, there is much evidence that some concepts such as self-efficacy, barriers, and social support have an effect on health-related behaviors. More research, especially case–control studies, should be conducted to determine what kind of nursing support and interventions are needed to produce behavior change and positive health outcomes. The interaction model of client health behavior appears to be promising for nurses, since the model emphasizes not only the structure and outcomes of interventions but also the process by which interventions are developed and implemented.

Most nursing studies using models and concepts relevant to health behavior have used cross-sectional study designs with convenience samples. Researchers examined the models in a variety of settings with a variety of samples. Generalizability to the population being studied is limited. In addition, in a convenience sample, volunteers may be those who are most interested in and most actively practicing healthful behaviors. Most of the samples for descriptive studies were large. In many studies in which participants were randomly selected, however, response rates were quite low, so that the subjects were of somewhat "volunteer" disposition. In both situations (i.e., volunteer selection and random selection with low response rates), the participants are self-selected and may indeed represent persons who are most interested in health. Better sampling efforts must be used to include persons who are not interested in health, hold negative beliefs (or no beliefs), and do not practice positive health behaviors. To avoid selection bias, studies might include the solicitation of information from non-participants to discern their beliefs, attitudes, perceptions, and behaviors.

Unfortunately, sample sizes were small in many of the quasi-experimental and experimental studies. The resulting low statistical power probably contributed to nonsignificant findings in many of the outcomes from nursing interventions.

Although the simplest statistic used by the researchers to determine relationships among variables was the correlation coefficient, most researchers examined model variables using multiple regression and canonical correlation analysis. The problem with bivariate correlations is that they represent total correlation without sorting out the potential effects of a third variable on one or both variables considered in the bivariate relationship. Since examining different variables provides information about different partial relationships, it was difficult to examine the effects of any one model variable on health behavior. Fewer researchers used path analysis or structural equation modeling to estimate both the direct and indirect effects of each variable on the others in the model being studied. Cluster analysis such as the ordering of lifestyle patterns of older adults (Walker, Volkan, Sechrist, & Pender, 1988) provides information about diversity of variables among identifiable sample subgroups. In addition, interactions among variables and the influence of combinations of variables on health behavior need to be examined. Using statistical techniques to examine complex relationships among model variables would add more to our knowledge of beliefs, psychosocial predictors, and other predictors of health-promoting behaviors.

Summary

Nurse researchers have made valuable contributions to health behavior research by developing valid and reliable instruments for measuring theoretical concepts according to their defining properties. Measures have maintained behavior specificity. Concepts have been measured on an ordinal or ratio level so that parametric statistical operations can be used. Since nurses work with diverse populations and with both well and ill persons, instruments need to be further tested for use with special populations (e.g., disabled persons, ethnic groups, children).

RELEVANCE OF HEALTH BEHAVIOR RESEARCH FOR NURSING EDUCATION

The following ad, which appeared on the front page of the June 1993 issue of *American Nurse*, chronicles the changes that are occurring in the health care delivery system and the kind of nurse that nursing education is being expected to produce:

> Help wanted: RNs to work with leading Western world power to carry out ambitious plan to overhaul the way health care is delivered to 260 million individuals. Desirable applicants will have versatile abilities and flexibility to meet ever-growing needs of diverse population. Must have vision for future of health care that draws on rich experience of the past.

Nursing is moving from a system that was centered on hospital-based illness care with an emphasis on acute care to a reformed health care delivery system that in contrast will focus on person-centered care with an emphasis on wellness. There will be a full continuum of coordinated care. The new system will require increased responsibility for health promotion behaviors of individuals and groups. Because nurses are in strategic positions to assess, plan, intervene in, monitor, and evaluate health behaviors of the consumer, it is essential that nursing students acquire knowledge of factors that are demonstrated to influence health-related behavior.

Because nursing is a practice profession, changes in practice (i.e., new technology, organizational changes) have an impact on nursing education, and changes in education (advance of nursing knowledge) have an impact on nursing practice. Neither one drives the other, but each influences the other. This symbiotic relationship makes it difficult to separate the relevance of health behavior research for education from its relevance for practice.

In the 1970s, the United States was experiencing a nursing shortage. The federal government made funding available to increase the number of both entry-level practitioners and nurses with graduate preparation. As registered nurses returned to colleges and universities to pursue graduate studies, many were exposed to the health behavior theories of Rosenstock (1966), Fishbein and Ajzen (1975), and Bandura (1977). For many, this was an "aha" moment when they suddenly realized this was the piece of knowledge that was missing as they attempted to figure out why their patients returned to their hospital units with additional acute episodes or why clients they were working with to lose weight were in fact continuing to eat high-caloric foods.

Many of those nurses who now had graduate degrees moved on to roles as clinical nurse specialists, administrators, and educators. Those who became nursing faculty began to incorporate health behavior models and concepts into their teaching.

By the mid-1980s, health promotion and disease prevention was a thread in the majority of undergraduate curricula. By the time health care reform became front page news, many nursing curricula had already begun the shift from institutional care to community-based care. In a study of nursing programs, 93% of the baccalaureate nurse educators reported that health behavior concepts were included in the nursing curriculum, although only 69% reported that they felt these concepts were critical to nursing education (Valiga & Bruderle, 1994). While nurses at the graduate educational level receive instruction in health behavior models and frameworks, it is the generalist preparation at the baccalaureate level that needs to incorporate more health behavior model concepts as the basis for the professional practice of nursing. Nurse educators must concern themselves with incorporating models of health behavior in nursing curricula. Nurses at all educational levels are involved with behavior changes (e.g., following medical regimens, altering activity levels, increasing coping behaviors), yet strategies to teach health behavior change interventions as a nursing role have not completely been formulated. Although nursing students are taught behavior-focused strategies in educating, counseling, and managing, these skills are not always taught from a health promotion theory perspective.

One of the problems in incorporating health behavior content in undergraduate courses has been the lag in textbooks in terms of including health behavior concepts and theories. A survey of the most popular nursing texts currently used in baccalaureate programs in the United States showed that all of the community health texts and three of the pediatric texts included one or more of the health behavior models or concepts. The health belief model was presented in 10 of the 25 texts surveyed: 6 community health, 2 pediatric, and 2 of the major medical-surgical texts. Pender's (1987) health promotion model was described in 5 community health texts. Of the texts reviewed, 19 mentioned one or more of the concepts/variables used in the various health behavior models, including susceptibility, barriers, benefits, beliefs, values, expectancies, individual characteristics, knowledge, locus of control, self-efficacy, and social support.

It is not surprising that this content is included in depth in the community health nursing texts. Community health nursing has from its inception focused on health promotion and disease prevention. From Lillian Wald and the nurses in the Henry Street Settlement in 1893 to today's community health nurse, health education has been a traditional nursing function. Health education activities are designed to promote wellness and to prevent illness. Changing health beliefs and ultimately behaviors is the purpose of the health teaching these nurses do. The goal is to promote health behaviors that foster optimal health. The client bears the major responsibility for his or her health behavior, and the role of the community health nurse is one of consultant and facilitator in the process.

Rationale for Specific Nursing Diagnoses

The unique practice of nursing in health promotion comes from the blending of behavioral theories and the practice or activities that have developed from those theories and concepts. One way nursing operationalizes components of theory for practice is through the development of the nursing process and nursing diagnosis. Nursing diagnosis is a classification system for structuring nursing knowledge, guiding nursing research, and directing nursing care (Carpenito, 1993).

The development of nursing diagnoses involves an initial literature review to derive implications for practice. Relevant concepts are examined for the adequacy of supporting health outcomes and for implications for practice (i.e., for phenomena that can be manipulated independently by nurses). Assessment criteria and behavioral norms are developed from relevant conceptual indicators. In fact, the research instruments developed by nurses can be used in the practice

setting as assessment tools. Nursing diagnoses and problems are defined and theory-specific interventions are developed. Finally, the planning of nursing care is based on specific observations that come from empirical evidence of conceptual relationships. The nursing process can be used as a format for deducing theoretically based nursing interventions.

Each nursing diagnosis established by the North American Nursing Diagnosis Association (Carpenito, 1993) represents a concept to be used in nursing practice and research. Although to date many nursing diagnoses are too abstract and are not all-inclusive or mutually exhaustive, the classification system offers a way for nurses to use research findings to develop interventions that are unique to nursing and are efficient for promoting optimal health of individuals and groups.

Selected nursing diagnostic categories that have a direct link with health behavior theory include (1) altered health maintenance, (2) health-seeking behavior, (3) high risk for injury, (4) ineffective management of therapeutic regimen, and (5) noncompliance. Table 2 summarizes theoretical concepts that have been influential in promoting health behavior within each category.

It is important to note that some theoretical concepts shown in Table 2 underlie all of the selected diagnostic categories relevant to health promotion/illness prevention. Client–professional interaction and knowledge are addressed in all diagnostic categories, since nursing interventions are directed to the person and to the circumstances contributing to the problem. Knowledge is believed to be a basic factor in promoting behaviors that lead to positive health outcomes. If one does not have knowledge and understanding of the risks and benefits of a behavior, or of the seriousness of the outcomes of a behavior, or does not know and understand that one is susceptible to a particular outcome, it is unlikely that interventions aimed at changing one's beliefs or self-efficacy perceptions will be successful.

Although it may appear that some diagnostic categories are the same, they are not. For exam-

Table 2. Inclusion of Major Health Behavior Theoretical Concepts in Selected Nursing Diagnostic Categories

Theoretical concepts	Diagnostic categories				
	Altered health maintenance	Health-seeking behavior	High risk for injury	Ineffective management of therapeutic regimen	Noncompliance
Barriers	X	X		X	X
Benefits	X	X		X	
Client–professional interaction	X	X	X	X	X
Health values/beliefs	X	X		X	X
Expectancies	X	X		X	
Individual characteristics	X		X	X	X
Knowledge	X	X	X	X	X
Locus of control	X			X	X
Perceived control			X	X	
Self-efficacy			X	X	X
Seriousness		X	X	X	X
Social influence	X	X			X
Social support	X	X		X	X
Susceptibility	X	X	X	X	X
Cue response	X				

ple, while "altered health maintenance" applies to the individual seeking lifestyle change, the diagnostic category "health-seeking behavior" refers to an individual or group desiring the promotion of a higher level of wellness. Both diagnostic categories require motivation on the part of the individual. Health-seeking behaviors, however, include prevention of illness through screening such as the practice of breast self-examination. Nursing interventions listed under "altered health maintenance" include benefits of changing the behavior, knowledge of negative and positive aspects of the behavior in question for the client (e.g., health risks of tobacco use), social influence, and social support. Nursing interventions listed under "health-seeking behavior" include the benefits of positive health behaviors in preventing the disease, knowledge of the disease and preventive behaviors, and the seriousness of and susceptibility to the disease.

The foci for "high risk for injury" include individual characteristics that may lead to physical injury, such as physical impairments or knowl-edge deficit. Interventions give considerable attention to knowledge concerning injury prevention.

"Ineffective management of therapeutic regimen" and "noncompliance" are similar diagnostic categories in that one may have difficulty fitting a treatment for illness into one's lifestyle. Control factors such as self-efficacy and locus of control are important concepts included in these diagnostic categories, since nonadherence to treatment is often accompanied by barriers such as complex regimens and treatment cost. The self-efficacy concept has important implications for nursing interventions, including pointing out past successes, telling the client about others' successes, proceeding with change slowly, and pointing out the client's own successes during the behavior change period. For noncompliance, the intervention focuses on the reduction or elimination of contributing factors such as negative experiences with the health care system or assistance to reduce side effects of medications. Knowledge and client–professional interaction concepts are most emphasized for noncompliance.

The nursing process is used for developing the curriculum, identifying clinical experiences, and evaluating students' clinical performance. Students learn to function independently by using the methodology of the nursing process. Since nursing takes a holistic approach to providing nursing care to individuals, the physically, psychologically, and sociologically related concepts are utilized in building nursing curricula.

Assessing the Client.   Nursing students are taught to collect data relevant to the medical diagnosis, physiological characteristics, psychosocial and cultural factors, developmental characteristics, and environmental conditions in which the person lives and relates to others. Both physical and psychosocial assessment skills are developed in basic nursing education programs. For example, the nursing student assesses an obese client and inquires about exercise and nutrition, family risk for heart diseases and hypertension, and smoking history, observes the person's cholesterol and triglyceride levels, and inquires about stress management and social networks. From this initial assessment, the student chooses an appropriate nursing diagnostic category ("health-seeking behavior" in this example).

Planning and Implementing Nursing Care. Nursing interventions include the theoretical concepts specified under each diagnostic category. To continue this example, under "health-seeking behavior," the interventions would include knowledge or perception of the value of early detection and of the seriousness of an susceptibility to the disease. Past individual and family patterns of health, including expectations; client–provider interactions; influences of family, cultural group, peer group, and mass media; the benefits of regular exercise; elements of stress management; and development of social networks would also be included in working with this obese client.

Nursing students learn to work in collaboration with individuals and groups in areas in which the individual or the group feels a change can be made. When stress management is identified as the underlying factor associated with overeating, for example, the student is advised to include more specific interventions such as assertiveness training, problem solving, or relaxation techniques. Since the nursing student (or practicing nurse) is not always the best professional to carry out all interventions, students learn to make referrals when the intervention can best be addressed by other professionals.

Evaluation.   Outcome criteria are developed by the student to compare actual client outcomes to the predicted outcomes determined in the planning step of the nursing process. The statement includes achievement of client goals, since nurses are socialized to work in a partnership relationship with the consumer.

The nursing process is an organizing framework whereby nurses learn to assess, plan, intervene in, and evaluate problems, including the need for health behavior change. The nursing process and interventions included in the process reflect empirical support from health behavior theory. To appreciate the rationale behind each nursing diagnostic category, however, it is necessary that students be educated in specific health behavior theories. To these authors' knowledge, nursing curricula have not been empirically evaluated for content that teaches nurses health behavior theory.

Roles within Nursing.   Nursing students are socialized into several roles that require knowledge of health behavior theory and concepts. For example, the health educator role of the nurse requires that students learn to focus on clients' learning needs and readiness to learn. Health education includes both health promotion of well persons and education necessary for following medical regimens. As the health care system changes and the consumers of health care demand more choices concerning health care, there has been an escalation in health promotion activities among nurses. Implementation of teaching reflects the principles of social cognitive theory (Bandura, 1977). The focus of the counselor role of the nurse is helping the client develop new attitudes and perceptions. Students learn to assist individuals to examine alternative behaviors, recognize choices, and increase their sense of control. Nurses as advocates and change agents learn to assist clients to modify health-destructive behaviors and to assume health-promotive behaviors, which requires students to have the relevant knowledge to assist clients in decision making. Although principles are taught to students, the theory is not examined fully at the undergraduate level. Client beliefs, values, benefits, and barriers are emphasized in the socialization process, but specific theories may not be taught to undergraduate students.

The American Association of Colleges of Nursing (AACN) (1993) charges nursing leaders in education and practice to work together to meet the challenges of *Addressing Nursing Education's Agenda for the 21st Century*. Preparation for the entry-level professional nurse will require an orientation to community-based practice within an emphasis on health promotion and maintenance in relation to acute and chronic conditions and infectious diseases. In addition, an emphasis on health promotion activities of well persons will include the promotion of such behaviors as good nutrition, mental health, family planning, age-related health screening, substance abuse prevention, environmental and occupational health, and prevention of family and social violence.

The positions of the National League for Nursing (NLN) and the AACN provide guidance to nursing faculty as they reexamine the curricula and clinical experiences utilized for student learning to prepare students for practice in this reformed health care system. Both the NLN and the AACN recognize that since nursing is a practice profession, faculty need to serve as role models who reflect the knowledge, skills, and attitudes of the practitioner for 2005 (AACN, 1993).

Didactic Focus for Nursing Students

Although some nurse educators have identified the need for a course in health promotion at the undergraduate level, the authors believe that health promotion and health behavior theories are of such importance that they should be integrated throughout the curriculum and should be introduced early and reinforced at every level of the educational process. Currently, most undergraduate students are oriented to the concepts of illness behavior and sick role behavior, with little emphasis placed on behaviors that maximize health (Pender, 1987). For the didactic portion, selected content foci could include:

- Theories relevant to health behavior research with examples specific to nursing.
- The relevance of health behavior research for professional nursing.
- Health behavior concepts as a basis for client teaching and other nursing interventions.
- Appropriate nursing interventions to promote healthful behaviors on the part of individuals, families, and communities.
- Theoretical and empirical contributions of nurse researchers to the health behavior knowledge base.

Students could assess their own health behaviors utilizing one of the conceptual frameworks, identify the relevant concepts, then plan an intervention that would facilitate their changing some unhealthy behavior.

Clinical Focus for Nursing Students

Learning experiences will need to be expanded to provide opportunities that will prepare students for community-based practice with a focus on health promotion and disease prevention. Students need to understand the factors that influence their clients' health, and they need to recognize that the community is not just a setting for their practice, but the environment in which their clients live and work.

Concrete experiences throughout the students' educational program will be needed to prepare them for practice in community-based systems. Faculty need to shift from hospitals and other traditional sites to neighborhood health centers, nurse-managed clinics, outpatient facilities, day care centers, homeless shelters, rehabilitation centers, schools, and occupational settings. This shift of clinical learning to the community provides opportunities for greater depth and diversity of learning with respect to health promotion assessment, planning, and interventions. Table 3 outlines suggested experiential learning assignments.

The curriculum at the School of Nursing at Purdue University has been moving toward a community-based setting for several years, in part in response to the low occupancy rates and subsequent downsizing of local and regional hospitals. The school also has one of the first academic nursing centers in the country. The Nursing Center for Family Health (NCFH), which opened in 1981, has grown and expanded throughout the years. It provides a full range of primary care services and has contracted with the university to provide health screening and counseling services to all of the university employees and retirees. All of the students who graduate from the school of nursing have at least one experience in the NCFH; many are involved in the health fairs and have the opportunity to do health promotion counseling with a diverse employee group. Practical experiences such as these assist students in developing the knowledge and skills needed to promote health and prevent disease. Several of the faculty supervise students in this setting. Faculty and NCFH staff facilitate the students' learning by role modeling the nursing role in health promotion.

Table 3. Suggested Experiential Learning Assignments for the Baccalaureate Nursing Student

- Discuss nurse–client partnership in the promotion and maintenance of client health.
- Prepare a simple teaching plan for a simulated client situation.
- Discuss the application of the health promotion model to individual clients.
- Reinforce clients' personal and family health-promoting behaviors.
- Participate in teaching client and family members methods to eliminate tobacco use.
- Participate in teaching sessions for client and family members in ways to reduce coronary risk factors.
- Assist individuals, families, and communities to develop and choose health-promoting options.
- List various behavioral science theories applicable as conceptual frameworks for nursing research problems.
- Examine the health belief model and the health promotion model and discuss the strengths and weaknesses of each.
- Plan and implement a group teaching project that incorporates behavioral objectives and teaching strategies in the assigned community.
- Analyze essential components of health promotion as they relate to the pediatric/adolescent population.

Graduate Nursing Education

Given the changes in health care delivery that are affecting undergraduate nursing programs, it was inevitable that there would be changes in the purposes and goals of graduate programs. The AACN is in the process of developing consensus concerning the essential knowledge and competencies required for advanced nursing practice in the 21st century. Although much work remains to be done, it is clear that health promotion and health protection will be a function of nurses at this level.

Pender (1987) believes that specialists in health promotion should be prepared at the graduate level. She also points out, however, that given the current emphasis on health promotion embodied in health care reform, no graduate student should receive an advanced degree in nursing without at least some understanding of the major health promotion concepts. All graduate students should be introduced to the theoretical models that underpin health-promoting and health-protecting behavior. The authors believe that discrete courses that cover this content are appropriate at the graduate level, but that the theories and concepts must also be integrated throughout the graduate curriculum. For some programs, health behavior theories could provide a framework for the curriculum; others may see health behavior theories as curricular threads.

In some graduate programs, students seeking specialization in health promotion are guided toward the community health nursing track. Regardless of the approach, it is essential that students at this level have opportunities to develop skills in planning and implementing interventions directed toward health promotion at the systems level at which they will be functioning (i.e., individual, family, or community).

Clinical experiences must be provided that will enable graduate students to develop skills in the application of health promotion strategies. Such experiences could include working with individuals, families, and communities to develop health promotion plans, teach lifestyle modification techniques, and provide health education and counseling. It is also essential that students have opportunities to practice and learn in settings in which health professions are functioning in collaborative relationships that recognize the contribution of professional nurses to the health promotion team.

Doctoral education prepares nurse scholars who are competent in theory development, instrument development, and health behavior research. Currently, several doctoral programs in nursing offer advanced preparation in the area of health promotion. A cursory review of dissertations listed in CINAHL for 1991 and 1992, searching under the headings of health beliefs, health behaviors, health belief model, health knowledge, and health promotion, identified 120 dissertations. Of the 746 nursing doctorates awarded during that period, the latest for which figures are available (NLN, 1994), it is clear that health behavior research was a major emphasis. Between 1990 and 1995, 1155 journal articles related to health promotion, health behaviors, and health beliefs were published in the nursing literature. Clearly, health behaviors are relevant for nurse scholars.

The need to increase the number of nurses with graduate preparation will increase greatly as the nation moves to a community-based health care system that emphasizes health promotion, disease prevention, self-care, and interventions that promote an optimal level of wellness in a shorter amount of time. Since nurses interact with large numbers of persons in diverse populations and at various levels of wellness, nursing research must continue to focus on health behavior interventions that maximize health.

Summary

As nursing shifts from an acute care/cure focus to a disease prevention/health promotion model, nurses will become increasingly more concerned with client–nurse interactions in the process of changing behaviors. It will be essential that students understand the determinants of health behaviors. Although nursing has a history of being involved in changing individual and group behaviors to promote higher levels of health, it appears that nursing education is just beginning to include specific teaching with respect to the theoretical concepts and their relationships as a basis for interventions as part of the basic education for the profession. It is essential to the practice of nursing that undergraduate students have relevant learning experiences to practice skills based on theoretical concepts.

While health care reform and the shift to community-based health promotion and disease prevention services present a major challenge to nurses, they also represent a significant opportunity for the profession. As Donna Shalala, U.S. Secretary of Health and Human Services, stated in her keynote address to the NLN's 20th biennial convention (Shalala, 1993, p. 290):

> Nurses were the handmaids of the medical profession. And now, through gallant and sometimes arduous efforts of men and women, nursing has redefined itself. It has staked out its territory and that territory is health: prevention, self-sufficiency and mobility for the elderly,... women's health, health education.

Progressive nursing education programs provide competent professionals to assume health promotion responsibilities not only in community settings, but also in acute care settings. Through research, practice, and education, nurses are making valuable contributions to the nation's health promotion objectives.

REFERENCES

Ahijevych, K., & Bernhard, L. (1994). Health-promoting behaviors of African American women. *Nursing Research, 43,* 86-89.

Ajzen, I. (1988). *Attitudes, personality, and behavior.* Chicago: Dorsey Press.

American Association of Colleges of Nursing. (1993). *Addressing nursing education's agenda for the 21st century* [position statement]. Washington, DC: AACN.

American Nurses Association Cabinet on Nursing Research. (1985). *Directions for nursing research: Toward the twenty-first century.* Kansas City MO: ANA.

Bandura, A. (1977). Self-efficacy: Toward a unifying theory of behavioral change. *Psychological Review, 84,* 191-215.

Becker, H., Stuifbergen, A., Oh, H. S., & Hall, S. (1993). Self-Rated Abilities for Health Practices: A health self-efficacy measure. *Health Values, 17,* 42-50.

Becker, M. H. (Ed.). (1974). The health belief model and personal health behavior (special issue). *Health Education Monographs, 2*(4), 324-473.

Brandt, P. A., & Weinert, C. (1981). The PRQ: A social support measure. *Nursing Research, 30,* 277-280.

Burgess, R., & Huston, T. (1979). *Social exchange in developing relationships.* New York: Academic Press.

Carpenito, L. J. (1993). *Nursing diagnosis: Application to clinical practice* (5th ed.). Philadelphia: J. B. Lippincott.

Carter, K. F., & Kulbok, P. A. (1995). Evaluation of the interaction model of client health behavior through the first decade of research. *Advances in Nursing Science, 18,* 62-73.

Champion, V. L. (1984). Instrument development for health belief model constructs. *Advances in Nursing Science, 6,* 73-85.

Champion, V. L. (1993). Instrument refinement for breast cancer screening. *Nursing Research, 42,* 139-143.

Champion, V., & Scott, C. (1993). Effects of a procedural/belief intervention on breast self-examination performance. *Research in Nursing and Health, 16,* 163-170.

Cook, K. S. (1987). *Social exchange theory.* Beverly Hills, CA: Sage.

Cox, C. L. (1982). An interaction model of client health behavior. Theoretical prescription for nursing. *Advances in Nursing Science, 5,* 41-56.

Cox, C. L. (1985). The Health Self-Determinism Index. *Nursing Research, 34,* 177-183.

Cox, C. L., Cowell, J. M., Marion, L. N., & Miller, E. H. (1990). The Health Self-Determinism Index for children. *Research in Nursing and Health, 13,* 237-246.

Cox, C. L., Miller, E. H., & Mull, C. S. (1987). Motivation in health behavior: Measurement, antecedents, and correlates. *Advances in Nursing Science, 9,* 1-15.

Danchik, K. M., Schoenborn, C. A., & Elinson, J. (1981). Highlights from Wave 1 of the National Survey of Personal Health Practices and Consequences: United States, 1979. National Center for Health Statistics, *Vital and health statistics,* Series 15, No. 1. DHHS PHS Publication No. 81-1162. Washington, DC: U.S. Government Printing Office.

Dean, P. G. (1986). Expanding our sights to include social networks. *Nursing and Health Care, 12,* 545-550.

Deci, E. (1975). *Intrinsic motivation.* New York: Plenum Press.

Dilorio, C., Faherty, B., & Manteuffel, B. (1992). Self-efficacy and social support in self-management of epilepsy. *Western Journal of Nursing Research, 14,* 292-307.

Duffy, M. E. (1988). Determinants of health promotion in midlife women. *Nursing Research, 37,* 358-362.

Fishbein, M., & Ajzen, I. (1975). *Belief, attitude, intention and behavior.* Reading, MA: Addison-Wesley.

Frank-Stromborg, M., Pender, N. J., Walker, S. N., & Sechrist, K. R. (1990). Determinants of health-promoting lifestyle in ambulatory cancer patients. *Social Science and Medicine, 31,* 1159-1168.

Gulanick, M. (1991). Is phase 2 cardiac rehabilitation necessary for early recovery of patients with cardiac disease? A randomized, controlled study. *Heart and Lung, 20,* 9-15.

Henderson, V. (1966). *The nature of nursing: A definition and its implications for practice, research, and education.* New York: Macmillan.

Hickey, M. L., Owen, S. V., & Froman, R. D. (1992). Instrument development: Cardiac diet and exercise self-efficacy. *Nursing Research, 41,* 347-351.

Higgins, P. G., & Dicharry, E. K. (1991). Measurement issues addressing social support with Navajo women. *Western Journal of Nursing Research, 13,* 242-255.

Hurley, A. C. (1990). Measuring self-care ability with diabetes: the Insulin Management Self-Efficacy Scale. In O. L. Strickland & C. F. Waltz (Eds.), *Measurement of nursing outcomes: Vol. 4. Measuring client self-care and coping skills* (pp. 28-44). New York: Springer.

Kahn, R. L. (1979). Aging and social support. In M. W. Riley (Ed.), *Aging from birth to death: Interdisciplinary perspectives* (pp. 77-91). Boulder, CO: Westview Press.

Kim, K. K., Horan, M. L., Gendler, P., & Patel, M. K. (1991). Development and evaluation of the Osteoporosis Health Belief Scale. *Research in Nursing and Health, 14,* 155-163.

King, I. M. (1971). *Toward a theory for nursing: General concepts of human behavior.* New York: Wiley.

Kulbok, P. P. (1985). Social resources, health resources, and preventive health behavior: Patterns and predictions. *Public Health Nursing, 2*, 67-81.

Kuster, A. E., & Fong, C. M. (1993). Further psychometric evaluation of the Spanish language Health-Promoting Lifestyle Profile. *Nursing Research, 42*, 266-269.

Laffrey, S. C. (1985a). Health promotion: Relevance for nursing. *Topics in Clinical Nursing, 7*, 29-38.

Laffrey, S. C. (1985b). Health behavior choice as related to self-actualization and health conception. *Western Journal of Nursing Research, 7*, 179-295.

Laffrey, S. C. (1986). Development of a Health Conception Scale. *Research in Nursing and Health, 9*, 107-113.

Lauver, D. (1992a). A theory of care-seeking behavior. *Image: Journal of Nursing Scholarship, 24*, 281-287.

Lauver, D. (1992b). Psychosocial variables, race, and intention to seek care for breast cancer symptoms. *Nursing Research, 41*, 236-241.

Lauver, D., & Angerame, M. (1993). Women's expectations about seeking care for breast cancer symptoms. *Oncology Nursing Forum, 20*, 519-525.

Lauver, D., & Tak, Y. (1995). Optimism and coping with a breast cancer symptom. *Nursing Research, 44*, 202-207.

Lusk, S. L., Ronis, D. L., Kerr, M. J., & Atwood, J. R. (1994). Test of the health promotion model as a causal model of workers' use of hearing protection. *Nursing Research, 43*, 151-157.

Miller, P., Wikoff, R., & Hiatt, A. (1992). Fishbein's model of reasoned action and compliance behavior of hypertensive patients. *Nursing Research, 41*, 104-109.

Miller, P., Wikoff, R., McMahon, M., Garrett, M. J., & Johnson, N. (1982). Development of a health Attitude Scale. *Nursing Research, 31*, 132-137.

Miller, P., Wikoff, R., McMahon, M., Garrett, M. J., & Ringel, K. (1988). Influence of a nursing intervention on regimen adherence and societal adjustments postmyocardial infarction. *Nursing Research, 37*, 297-302.

National League for Nursing. (1994). *Nursing data review: 1994.* Division of Research. New York: National League for Nursing Press.

Nightingale, F. (1859/1969). *Notes on nursing: What it is and what it is not* [facsimile of the First Edition, printed in London, 1859]. New York: Dover.

Norbeck, J. S. (1984). The Norbeck Social Support Questionnaire. *Birth Defects: Original Article Series, 20*, 45-55.

Norbeck, J. S., Lindsey, A. M., & Carrieri, V. L. (1981). The development of an instrument to measure social support. *Nursing Research, 30*, 264-269.

Norbeck, J. S., Lindsey, A. M., & Carrieri, V. L. (1983). Further development of the Norbeck Social Support Questionnaire: Normative data and validity testing. *Nursing Research, 32*, 4-9.

Orem, D. E. (1971). *Nursing: Concepts of practice.* Scarborough, Ontario: McGraw-Hill.

Orem, D. E. (1985). *Nursing: Concepts of practice* (3rd ed.). New York: McGraw-Hill.

Orlando, I. (1961). The dynamic nurse-patient relationship. New York: G. P. Putnam.

Pender, N. J. (1982). *Health promotion in nursing practice.* Norwalk, CT: Appleton-Century-Crofts.

Pender, N. J. (1987). *Health promotion in nursing practice* (2nd ed.). Norwalk, CT: Appleton & Lange.

Pender, N. J., Walker, S. N., Sechrist, K. R., & Frank-Stromborg, M. (1990). Predicting health-promoting lifestyles in the workplace. *Nursing Research, 39*, 326-332.

Peplau, H. E. (1952). *Interpersonal relations in nursing.* New York: G. P. Putnam.

Rosenstock, I. M. (1966). Why people use health services. *Milbank Memorial Fund Quarterly, 44*, 94-127.

Rosenstock, I. M., Strecher, V. J., & Becker, M. H. (1988). Social learning theory and the health belief model. *Health Education Quarterly, 15*, 175-183.

Rotter, J. B. (1966). Generalized expectancies for internal versus external control of reinforcement. *Psychological Monographs, 80*, 1-28.

Sechrist, K. R., Walker, S. N., & Pender, N. J. (1987). Development and psychometric evaluation of the Exercise Benefits/Barriers Scale. *Research in Nursing & Health, 10*, 357-365.

Shalala, D. E. (1993). Nursing and society: The unfinished agenda for the 21st century. *Nursing and Health Care, 14*, 289-291.

Simmons, S. J. (1990a). The health-promoting self-care system model: Directions for nursing research and practice. *Journal of Advanced Nursing, 15*, 1162-1166.

Simmons, S. J. (1990b). *Self-care agency and health-promoting behavior of a military population.* Ann Arbor, MI: University Microfilms Dissertation Services, No. PUZ9027683.

Smith, J. A. (1981). The idea of health: A philosophical inquiry. *Advances in Nursing Science, 3*, 43-50.

Stewart, M. J. (1993). *Integrating social support in nursing.* Newbury Park, CA: Sage.

Stuifbergen, A. K., & Becker, H. A. (1994). Predictors of health-promoting lifestyles in persons with disabilities. *Research in Nursing and Health, 17*, 3-13.

Tilden, V. P. (1985). Issues of conceptualization and measurement of social support in the construction of nursing theory. *Research in Nursing and Health, 8*, 199-206.

Tilden, V. P., Nelson, C. A., & May, B. A. (1990). The IPR Inventory: Development and psychometric characteristics. *Nursing Research, 39*, 337-343.

Triandis, H. (1977). *Intrapersonal behavior.* Monterey, CA: Brooks/Cole.

Valiga, T. M., & Bruderle, E. (1994). Concepts included in and critical to nursing curricula: An analysis. *Journal of Nursing Education, 33*, 118-124.

Volden, C., Langemo, D., Adamson, M., & Oechsle, L. (1990). The relationship of age, gender, and exercise practices to measures of health, life-style, and self-esteem. *Applied Nursing Research, 3*, 20–26.

Walker, S. N., Sechrist, K. R., & Pender, N. J. (1987). The Health-Promoting Lifestyle Profile: Development and psychometric characteristics. *Nursing Research, 36*, 76–81.

Walker, S. N., Volkan, K., Sechrist, K. R., & Pender, N. J. (1988). Health-promoting life styles of older adults: Comparisons with young and middle-aged adults, correlates and patterns. *Advances in Nursing Science, 11*, 76–90.

Wallston, K. A., & Wallston, B. S. (1984). Social psychological models of health behavior: An examination and integra-tion. In A. Baum, S. E. Taylor, & J. Singer (Eds.), *Handbook of psychology and health, Vol. 4* (pp. 23–53). Hillsdale, NJ: Erlbaum.

Weinert, C. (1988). Measuring social support: Revision and further development of the Personal Resource Question-naire. In C. Waltz & O. Strickland (Eds.), *Measurement of nursing outcomes: Vol. 1* (pp. 309–327). New York: Springer.

Weiss, R. (1974). The provision of social relationships. In Z. Rubin (Ed.), *Doing unto others* (pp. 17–26). Englewood Cliffs, NJ: Prentice-Hall.

6

Health Behavior Research and Social Work

Rona L. Levy

The distinctiveness of social work in health care settings is that people served are clients rather than
patients; that the focus of work is on the social effects
of illness, not illness; that problem formulation and
intervention rests on clear understanding of social
cause, social manifestation, and social intervention as
group phenomena. (Falck, 1984, p. 167)

SOCIAL WORK IN HEALTH CARE

The 1980s produced a virtual explosion of
research and texts in social work and health care.
There is considerable commonality in the titles of

Rona L. Levy • School of Social Work, University of Washington, Seattle, Washington 98105-6299.

This chapter is dedicated to Professor Zeev Ben-Sira
(1925–1995), late of the Hebrew University of Jerusalem, Jerusalem, Israel, whose lifetime career of critical
scholarship in health research and commitment to
social work values has set the standard for social work
and health behavior research. His comments on this
chapter are very much appreciated. He was a wonderful
colleague and close friend who is very much missed.

*Handbook of Health Behavior Research IV: Relevance for
Professionals and Issues for the Future*, edited by David S.
Gochman. Plenum Press, New York, 1997.

many of these books, some of which are: *Social
Work Issues in Health Care* (Miller & Rehr,
1983); *Health Care Social Work Practice* (Schlesinger, 1985), *Clinical Social Work in Health
Settings* (Carlton, 1984), *Social Work Practice in
Health Care* (Germain, 1984), *Clinical Social
Work in Health Care* (Wallace, Goldberg, &
Slaby, 1984), *Social Work in Health Settings* (Kerson, 1989), and *Social Work in Hospitals* (Ratliff,
Timberlake, & Jentsch, 1982). All of these works
seek, in one way or another, to describe the roles,
activities, and work settings of social workers in
the health and medical care arenas.

The activities of social workers in the health
care field are changing along with those of all health
care professionals. In this sense, now is both an extremely difficult and an ideal time to be writing this
chapter. It is difficult because anything said about
what social work is doing in health care may be outdated by the time this volume is published. It is
ideal because now is a key time to look at potentially
new directions and make appropriate changes.

Settings for Social Work Practice

It would be difficult to identify health settings in which social work is not active. Social

workers practice in a wide range of medical services in acute settings, including the emergency room, burn centers, pediatrics, oncology, neurology, spinal cord injury centers, discharge planning units, obstetrics, surgery, and so on (Kerson, 1989). Social workers have worked in dental settings (Levy, Lambert, & Davis, 1979), public and mental health care services, and long-term care facilities (Kerson, 1989; Schlesinger, 1985). In fact, it would be fair to say that if there is any setting associated with health care in which social workers are not currently involved, there are many social workers who could explain why social workers should be in that setting.

The current shift in health care delivery away from increasing reliance on medical specializations and toward prevention, primary care, and community-based services provides more setting opportunities for social work. Simons (1994) argues that social work has a great deal to offer within this new context.

Practice and Research

To begin to address the question of how health behavior research is relevant to social work, one must first consider the broader question of how *any* research is relevant to social work practice. Many social work writers have lamented the minimal attention paid to research in social work practice. The tone was set decades ago by a classic social work author, Hollis (1968, p. 7):

> Is casework just a coldly intellectual process? Heaven forbid! Casework is in essence an experience between two people—a totality that rests upon delicate nuances of interaction that can only be described as art rather than science.

While this attitude still represents a strong sentiment in the profession, changes have occurred. In a text published by the National Association of Social Workers (NASW), Hess and Mullen (1995) noted that many social work practitioners study their own practice, serve as consultants in research programs, and serve as principal investigators and co-investigators in research. Hess and

Mullen highlight many factors that affect these activities, including individual interests and needs, roles and responsibility, power issues, and philosophical, organizational, political, and ethical considerations. Covering all these points is beyond the scope of this chapter and in fact could constitute another volume. It is a sufficient summary, however, to note that the acceptance of research by social work practitioners and the participation of social workers in research are products of a complex process. This chapter will highlight some of these factors specifically as they relate to health behavior research.

Social Work Activities

The Code of Ethics developed by the NASW (1990), and Rosenberg's (1978) value guidelines for social work professionals provide a good introduction to the defining characteristics of social work. Many of these principles are directly or indirectly linked to key issues in health behavior research. Excerpted below are some of the major points in the NASW Code (NASW, 1990):

• The social worker should regard as primary the service obligation of the social work profession.
• Primacy of clients' interest—the social worker's primary responsibility is to clients.
• Rights and prerogatives of clients—the social worker should make every effort to foster maximum self-determination on the part of clients.
• Community service—social workers should assist the profession in making social services available to the general public.
• Development of knowledge—the social worker should take responsibility for identifying, developing, and fully utilizing knowledge for professional practice.
• Promoting the general welfare—the social worker should promote the general welfare of society.
• The social worker should act to insure that all persons have access to the resources,

services, and opportunities which they require.

- The social worker should act to expand choice and opportunity for all persons, with special regard for disadvantaged or oppressed groups or persons.
- The social worker should promote conditions that encourage respect for the diversity of cultures which constitute American society.
- The social worker should advocate changes in policy and legislation to improve social conditions, and to promote social justice.

Rosenberg's value guidelines for social workers in health care settings include (Rosenberg, 1978, p. 123):

1. Total health care is a right.
2. Access to what is already in existence is a right.
3. Quality of life is to be striven for, as contrasted with an emphasis purely on the prolongation of life.
4. The concepts of caring and coping need to be stressed more than continued investments in already sophisticated technological systems.
5. Any new system must emphasize the positives of social health, rather than follow a disease-focused model, for example, use people's strengths, educate for health maintenance, and prevent illness.

Several of the points in the ethical code and guidelines are directly compatible with specific recommendations that can be derived from health behavior research. For example, it is obvious that individuals without access to health care cannot receive this care. Equally important, individuals who do not perceive that they have the opportunity to improve their health or a right to access health care (Fishbein and Ajzen, 1975) will also not take appropriate health care action. Social workers are encouraged by their profession to work toward changing this access for the individual and even society as a whole, if necessary. This

encouragement by the profession for system-level goals also would lead social workers to address negative attitudes on the part of professionals that could affect health behavior. For example, if professionals convey a lack of caring to patients (Maslach, 1978), patients are not likely to follow health care recommendations. Furthermore, health behavior research has shown the necessity to "tailor" health recommendations to the unique characteristics of the individual, such as educational level and cultural background (Fink, 1976). Again, social workers are strongly encouraged to emphasize issues of diversity in their work.

Another major emphasis in health behavior research has recognized the importance of prevention and health maintenance. Once again, the guidelines for social workers are on target.

Health behavior research has also demonstrated the importance of individuals participating in their own treatment plans as a way of maximizing behavior change (Schulman, 1979). The social work ethic of self-determination encourages social workers in this direction.

Quality of life is recognized as important in health behavior research, and thus is frequently studied. Social workers also place significant emphasis on quality of life issues.

Finally, the Code of Ethics encourages social workers to participate in knowledge building and utilization. Doing so legitimizes social workers' participation in and utilization of research, which could be generalized to health behavior research.

This chapter will next focus on some of the activities in which social workers have been involved. For simplicity, social work activities will be broadly separated into individual assessment; individual intervention; needs assessment, outreach, and case finding; and community intervention.

Individual Assessment. Social workers are often the professionals who can best obtain detailed information from clients. The social worker is typically the professional whose role it is to gather from the patient pertinent non-medical background information that health behavior research has shown may have a significant impact on the patient's health. Some relevant information typically obtained would include information on support systems, such as family or friends, who might be able to help support a person's health. Financial aspects of a client's life are also important. Relevant cultural factors, including norms, values, goals, and attitudes toward illness, would be other important areas for social exploration. Finally, any relevant psychological factors, e.g., coping skills, anxiety, depression, guilt, would all be appropriate for social work assessment activities (Germain, 1984).

There is an extensive body of health behavior research that demonstrates the importance of the social, familial, institutional, and cultural influences on an individual's health beliefs and health behavior. Social supports are critical in determining access to health care opportunities for compliance with treatment regimens. Social groups, families, institutions, and culture affect how an individual defines, and thus acts, regarding, health, illness, and disability. These factors affect where, and if, an individual seeks treatment and who is listened to once treatment is sought. For example, some cultures may encourage "toughing it out" or "suffering in silence." Others may socialize against even the *perception* of suffering. Cultural determinants of health behavior are covered extensively in Volume I of this *Handbook*, and this chapter will therefore not discuss these issues in detail. The key focus here is on some of the specific assessment information social workers already obtain, or are encouraged by their profession to obtain, that health behavior research has indicated is critical.

Hepworth and Larsen's (1993) text on direct practice in social work is used extensively in many social work training programs in the United States. Several chapters are devoted exclusively to recommendations to social workers concerning information that should be obtained during assessment. While these chapters focus primarily on generic social work practice, a consideration

of many of their recommendations demonstrated how consistent they are with factors shown by health behavior research to be critical determinants of health behavior. Health behavior research would recognize a thorough assessment to include these factors to maximize obtaining useful information for health care intervention.

Selected recommendations from Hepworth and Larsen of key factors to be addressed in assessment are listed in italics below, followed by descriptions of their health behavior research:

- *Developmental stage and/or life transition* (p. 214): A significant body of health behavior research has demonstrated that an individual's developmental stage will have an impact on, for example, compliance behavior (Krasnegor, Epstein, Johnson, & Yaffe, 1993).
- *Meanings clients ascribe to problems* (p. 217): An extensive body of health behavior research, such as the work on health beliefs and self-efficacy (Bandura, 1982, 1989; Becker, 1974; Becker & Maiman, 1975), has demonstrated that health actions will be determined by individuals' belief about their conditions. Individuals who believe that they cannot change, or that there is no benefit in changing, are less likely to alter health-related behaviors than are those who hold different beliefs.
- *Cultural, societal, and social class factors* (p. 225): The emphasis social work places on cultural, societal, and social class factors is a repeated theme throughout this chapter. Modeling provides one example of how health behavior research has demonstrated their importance. Bandura (1969) stated that much learning occurs vicariously through observation. Keefe and Blumenthal (1982, p. 11) point out how "many of the sick-role behaviors displayed by patients who are ill are acquired via a modeling process." Similarly, cultural norms may affect where and how an individual seeks care. Is a healing elder or medicine man preferred to a physi-

cian or health clinic? Is medicine thought to be dangerous?

- *Family myths and cognitive patterns* (p. 310): Family myths and cognitive patterns have impacts on health behavior similar to those of cultural, societal, and social class factors.
- *Social support systems* (p. 270) and *negative social support systems* (p. 272): The social worker should determine how social support will facilitate the individual in following through on health care recommendations or deter the individual from doing so. Often, for example, a social worker may not discharge a patient back to the patient's environment if the worker's home assessment is that the home environment will not support needed medical regimes. The extent of social support may even be a factor in a health care provider's selection of treatment. If it is determined, for example, that the social support does not exist for compliance with highly demanding post-treatment regimens, alternate regimens may be selected.

In summary, the assessment part of a social worker's job is one that emphasizes obtaining information on perceptions and perspectives and on social networks and supports, as well as on the environmental context in which health behavior occurs. Health behavior research informs social workers that these are critical factors in determining an individual's health beliefs and behavior.

Individual Intervention. There are many directions for social work activities that come directly from health behavior research recommendations. Again, there is an easy "fit" between social work intervention strategies and health behavior knowledge. Social workers, trained and encouraged to be sensitive to and to respect cultural diversity, adapt their interventions to the client group being addressed. An example of this approach is evident in a paper on the social work

treatment of women with alcoholism. Wilke (1994, p. 31) noted that "many differences in the psychosocial histories of alcoholic women directly affect the treatment process." Similarly, Zambrana, Ell, Dorrington, Wachsman, and Hodge (1994) looked at the underutilization of pediatric emergency services by Latino immigrants. They pointed out the importance of investigating maternal factors such as the "perception of [the] seriousness of [the] child's illness" (p. 101).

Education and counseling directed at changing beliefs about such lifestyle behaviors as nutrition, smoking, and exercise are recommended by Simmons (1994). She sees these interventions as appropriate for social work in the new health care environment, in which the goal of optimizing self-care is critical. These and other risk factors are key concepts in health behavior research (Davidson & Davidson, 1980). In fact, a significant percentage of all health behavior research consists of efforts to reduce these risk factors in different groups (Milsum, 1980).

Social workers are traditionally associated with a variety of activities that may fall in the general category of networking—connecting clients to the people and services they need. Discharge planning is the common function for social workers that involves, in large measure, networking activities. Some medical social workers see this activity as the core of social work in medical settings. Findings from health behavior research on social support could inform such social work interventions. Clients need to be connected with financial resources, day care facilities, job opportunities, services for those with physical challenges, follow-up medical care, home health care, nursing homes, mental health outpatient services, and so on. All of this assistance must be rendered in a context of social and cultural sensitivity.

Health behavior research has also provided several specific recommendations concerning methods for enhancing compliance and reducing barriers to compliance (Haynes, Taylor, & Sackett, 1979). Since appropriateness of social work involvement in compliance enhancement has been discussed elsewhere (Levy, 1978; Schultz, 1980), barriers to compliance will be considered first. Social workers may be helpful in explaining to other health care providers how certain features of the individual's life, such as a time-consuming job, financial limitations, or difficulty in obtaining transportation, might interfere with a particular regimen as prescribed. The social worker may be able to explore different regimens with health care providers who can then provide the patient with alternate treatment strategies from which to choose. A lack of understanding may also interfere with compliance (Kellaway & MacRae, 1975), and the social worker might inform other professionals about a patient's limited ability to understand medical directives. Terry (1981) discusses a different role for social workers as part of a professional team trying to enhance parental compliance. As a "team buffer," the social worker might be the primary target of parental anger toward and frustration with treatment regimens. Having the social worker as a buffer provides the parent with a single specific person to communicate difficulties to, one who will in turn pass this information on to others. Obviously, having a social worker as buffer also reduces difficulties for nutritionists, pediatricians, and others who must make unpopular recommendations.

Health behavior research also informs social workers of several barriers to compliance and compliance enhancers (Shelton & Levy, 1981) that especially affect the elderly, a population that social work is committed to serving. One of these barriers is adverse side effects (Hemminki & Heikkila, 1975). In discussing the social worker's role in enhancing compliance of elderly patients, Giannetti (1983) noted that older people in the community may be particularly susceptible to drug interaction problems because they are under the care of multiple health care providers. This problem of drug interactions can occur as a result of interactions between prescription drugs and over-the-counter (OTC) drugs. OTC drugs are heavily used by the elderly population (Giannetti, 1983), and this use may not be known to

their physicians. Giannetti also suggests that social workers encourage their elderly patients to utilize pharmacies that maintain medication profiles of their elderly clients. With patient consent, the social worker could even be involved in reviewing these profiles and discussing them with the patient and the prescriber, if appropriate.

The elderly may also face financial constraints, which may be another barrier to compliance (Kincey, Bradshaw, & Ley, 1975). To save money, patients may delay in filling prescriptions, discontinue treatment early, and save or share medication from one acute episode to another.

Working with the individual in the community, the social worker may have the best opportunity of any health care provider to observe and try to alleviate these problems and improve compliance. The social worker can provide reinforcement, an important compliance enhancer (Shelton & Levy, 1981). If there is family contact (which is an important asset for effective social work intervention), the social worker may involve family members to provide support for compliance.

Social workers are also familiar with resources in the community and should know how to make referrals to community groups that can provide needed monitoring and praise for regimen compliance.

With their knowledge of the individual's environment, social workers can be helpful in addressing the problem of forgetting, another common reason for noncompliance, by setting up a reminder system for the patient. This may involve helping the individual set up his or her own system, having the worker actually do the reminding, or again enlisting available sources of support, e.g., family and community resources.

Several problems such as grieving, depression, anxiety, and so forth are linked to health behaviors (Frazier, Davis, & Dahl, 1994). Two professions that are very active in addressing these problems in health care, in addition to social work, are psychosocial nursing and psychology. Both of these professions, along with social work, can justify their interventions as appropriate activities for which they are trained and as logical components of their job-related roles. Unfortunately, there are no clear training and performance criteria for the treatment of these problems. One potentially useful research direction would produce empirical evidence demonstrating any differential effectiveness of the professions on criteria such as compliance, satisfaction, patient decision-making, and so on. In the absence of such data, decisions on who will treat these problems in health care will remain a political issue. The individuals who will engage in these activities will belong to whichever profession that chooses to define itself as the rightful occupant of these roles and that also has the ability to hold onto these roles in a multidisciplinary health care setting. The competition to define oneself in specific ways increases as department administrators need to justify their staff in a more fiscally conservative health care market. This competition is similar to what is also going on in the broader health care arena, where a number of health care providers are competing to provide primary care services to patients.

Needs Assessment, Outreach, and Case Finding. The recognition in health behavior research of the importance of behavioral risk factors to an individual's well-being should encourage social workers to assess client needs and risk factors, so that this information can be utilized in case finding and outreach programs. Hepworth and Larsen (1993, p. 643) state that "both public and private human service organizations often engage in outreach efforts aimed at people who are unaware of or do not voluntarily seek service or resources that could improve their life situations."

Intervention at the Community Level and Beyond. Health behavior research has demonstrated that interventions at the institutional, community, or social policy level will produce change in individuals' health beliefs and behavior. For example, individuals often are accurate

in their recognition of such barriers to compliance as finances, child care, and the like (Owens, 1995). A systemwide response to these problems can be beneficial. Similarly, clients may accurately perceive that health care workers are hostile or uninformed, and system-level intervention aimed at health care workers may be appropriate. The attitudes of family and friends may support health care beliefs that do not maximize the chances for desirable outcomes, and health behavior research has demonstrated the effectiveness of large-scale health education and health promotion interventions (Maccoby & Alexander, 1980). As Ewart (1993, p. 270) states, "It is well known that one's ability to engage in health protective activities is affected by one's cultural environment [among other factors]."

These areas are again examples of ones in which social workers are trained and encouraged to participate. The Code of Ethics specifically calls for social workers to assure access to services and "advocate changes in policy and legislation to improve social conditions, and to promote social justice" (NASW, 1990). Similarly, Hepworth and Larsen (1993) devote considerable time to topics such as "supplementing resources in the home environment," "moving clients to a different environment," "improving institutional environments," "employing advocacy and social action," and "social planning/community organization." Finally, nearly all schools of social work allow students at the master's level to specialize in something often called "macro practice," in which the focus of intervention activity is large groups, such as an institution, community, or society.

TRAINING OF SOCIAL WORKERS

Overall Structure: Classroom and Practicum Experience

Social work educators have long believed that students should receive their training both in the classroom and in the field. The exact formula for providing such training varies from school to school, but not uncommonly, first year master's students spend approximately two days a week in the field and second year master's students spend three days. A minimum of nine credit hours of total field time is required by the Council of Social Work Education ([CSWE], 1992b), the accrediting body for programs in social work. At the University of Washington, undergraduate students may choose their social work major during their junior year, and during their senior year they spend one day a week in the field. A minimum of 400 hours is required by the CSWE (1992a) for baccalaureate students. Doctoral students typically are not required to have a practicum experience.

Students in the field are placed with a practicum supervisor, who must have an MSW degree and two years of post-master's experience. Often, students are given the opportunity to choose either a specific practicum site or at least a type of site, such as a hospital or an AIDS service center. Ideally, the practicum supervisor receives some general guidelines from the school on field instruction content. At the University of Washington, these guidelines are provided through a learning contract, which each student helps develop, and through seminars held by the school and written materials. In actuality, however, field instruction is determined by each site choosing to teach whatever content it feels is appropriate for its particular client group and field setting. This instruction may be daily or infrequent; may be in a behavioral, psychodynamic, or other theoretical orientation; may or may not include reading; may or may not include content on health behavior research; or may otherwise differ in any conceivable variable or instruction method. The fact is that there is little standardization in field instruction in many schools of social work.

Course Content

The CSWE has a written policy statement for content at both the baccalaureate and the master's level, over and above the hours in the field as discussed above. At the baccalaureate level,

course content is expected to include both a liberal arts perspective and content in "professional foundation." Specifically, this professional foundation is to include content on social work values and ethics, diversity, social and economic justice, populations-at-risk, human behavior and the social environment, social welfare policy and services, social work practice, research, and field practicum (CSWE, 1992a, p. 5). The master's foundation is expected to include the same content, with additional concentration content for advanced practice in an identifiable area (CSWE, 1992b). One option often available to students for advanced practice is social work in health care.

Content specifically relevant to health behavior research may be found throughout much of the required foundation. For example, knowledge about sensitivity to diverse cultures may convey useful knowledge about different cognitive and behavioral aspects of health and illness. The human behavior and social environment curriculum is described as providing "content about theories and knowledge of human-bio-psycho-social development, including theories and knowledge about the range of social symptoms in which individuals live" (CSWE, 1992b, p. 8). This content *may* be highly relevant to health behavior research—the key word in this statement being "may." The exact direction all of these courses take is determined in a fairly individualistic manner by faculty in each program.

The place for health behavior research in an advanced practice concentration is also unclear. A 1975 position statement by the house of delegates of CSWE and the Board of Directors of the Society of Hospital Social Work Directors encouraged a biological and physiological knowledge base, as well as training in epidemiology, program planning, collaboration, and prevention (CSWE, 1975). Again, however, details about how this training is to be implemented are lacking.

In the absence of a single agreed-upon set of recommendations for advanced practice, there is considerable variety in the operationalization of course content. A survey of 72 out of 85 graduate schools of social work (Caroff & Mailick, 1985) found that 42 had a concentration in health care. Major course groupings included direct practice, policy planning, psychosocial aspects of health and illness, "platform skills" (introductory courses in health), and miscellaneous specialty courses, such as genetics, human sexuality, and the like.

Numerous authors have provided their own sets of specific curriculum recommendations, although none of these sets provides a single agreed-upon standard. Wallace et al. (1984) encouraged a biomedical dimension in social work health care training. Specific recommended content includes information on medical disorders that masquerade as psychosocial symptoms (e.g., a brain tumor or thyroid problem resembling depression), as well as information on commonly used drugs that produce psychiatric symptoms. Berkman (Berkman, 1981; Berkman, Kemler, Marcus, & Silverman, 1985) has provided the most comprehensive list available for a recommended knowledge base. She outlines the following areas (Berkman, 1981, pp. 86–88):

- Effect of the illness or disease on the psychosocial, economic, and physical functioning of the patient and family.
- Impact of illness on the social worker.
- Legal and ethical dilemmas.
- Epidemiology of disease, including social and environmental risk factors.
- Organization of health care systems.
- Health policy and legislative measures, as well as the financing of health care.
- Interprofessional and intraprofessional collaboration and practice.
- Consultation within the framework of multi-disciplinary practice.
- Accountability measures.
- Consumerism.
- Teaching [of other professionals].
- Scientific inquiry.

Nearly all of these topics either provide recommendations for future health behavior research or are areas in which research already exists. For example, several aspects of a chronic problem, such as pain, are all legitimate topics for health behavior research. These aspects could include how the pain affects all parts of an individual's life, how individuals respond differently to pain, and which risk factors are associated with greater disability from pain, among others. Health behavior researchers have also looked at the less obvious topic of the effects of their findings on health care professionals (Coady, Kent, & Davis, 1990; Maslach, 1978). Furthermore, while research is not extensive in this area, Stone (1979) points out that there are several legitimate and important health behavior research questions that should be addressed regarding topics such as organizations or policies. For example, one question he poses is: "How do health attitudes and health values affect voting for health facilities or contributions to health organizations?" (p. 65)

Some interesting additional content has been recommended. Recognizing the litigious nature of American health care, Miller and Rehr (1983, p. 16) point out the need for social workers to have information about risk management "to assist the patient and the family to set aside intentions to sue the institution for assumed personal damage as a result of care." Finally, Collins and Shannon (1988) add a recommended course in self-evaluation methods, including biofeedback, relaxation, and hypnosis. It is likely that political issues are as present in the selection of health training curricula as they are in role differentiation in health care settings. One social work administrator told the author ("off the record") that his university does not include content on health behavior research because the school sees it as being within the domain of health education, a program that is included in the school's public health program.

SCHOLARLY ACTIVITIES IN SOCIAL WORK

Social Work Journals in Health Care

Social work has two primary journals that focus exclusively on social work in the health care field. A review of papers published in these journals in 1994 includes a range of topics that may fit under broad guidelines for health behavior research given in this volume. A sampling of titles gives an idea of breadth of treatment areas in which social work is involved:

- "Treatment Issues for Alcohol-and-Drug Dependent Pregnant and Parenting Women (Finkelstein, 1994) examined history, access, and other issues in drug treatment problems.
- "The Relationship between Psychosocial Status of Immigrant Latino Mothers and Use of Emergency Pediatric Services (Zambrana et al., 1994) surveyed factors related to the use of emergency room care by Latino immigrant mothers.
- "Factors Contributing to the Early Rehospitalization of Elderly People (Lockery, Dunkle, Kart, & Coulton, 1994) utilized path analysis to look at a longitudinal sample of persons over 60 and the factors associated with rehospitalization in this sample.
- "Estimating Rates of Psychosocial Problems in Urban and Poor Children with Sickle Cell Anemia" (Barbarin, Whitten, & Bonds, 1994).
- "Health Problems of Sheltered Homeless Women and Their Dependent Children" (Burg, 1994). This conceptual article suggested that a categorization system for the homeless could be utilized as a basis for, for example, the testing of differential preventive health behavior strategies with this clientele.
- "A Closer Look at Social Support as a Moderator of Stress in Breast Cancer" (Roberts, Cot, Shannon, & Wells, 1994). This paper reported a study of psychological adjustment of newly diagnosed breast cancer patients, a topic that is also consistent with health behavior research. First, much of health behavior research has focused on social support. Second, behavior affects stress levels, and researchers suspect that stress may have an impact on health directly, such as by not allowing time for self-

care, or indirectly, through an impact on the immune system (Fox, 1976).
- "The Ethics of Assisted Suicide" (Callahan, 1994) If suicide is conceptualized as a health behavior, researchers testing strategies to prevent suicide should consider points raised in this article.
- "Community Based Care: The New Health Social Work Paradigm" (Simmons, 1994) outlines new directions social work should address as treatment moves out of traditional settings.
- "Impact of Social Work on Recidivism and Non-medical Complaints in the Emergency Department" (Keehn, Roglitz, & Bowden, 1994) studied patients seen by social workers in emergency rooms for a variety of problems and attempted to discern reasons for differences in recidivism rates.
- "African-American Women and AIDS: A Public Health/Social Work Challenge" (Dicks, 1994) utilized an epidemiological analysis to make a case for suggested intervention strategies within the African-American community. Since strategies to alter health behavior should be tailored to the recipients' backgrounds, this article offers a valuable perspective to researchers in this area.

Some interesting themes for health behavior emerge from this sampling. First, social workers are involved in a broad range of medical areas, including substance abuse, emergency rooms, maternal and child health, stress and cancer, AIDS, community health care delivery, and ethical issues. Health behavior occurs in all of these arenas, may be assessed, and is an appropriate target for intervention. Second, articles published in these social work journals in 1994 addressed the concerns of many individuals who would be labeled as disenfranchised in American society: Latinos, the elderly, urban and poor children, the homeless, and African-American women with AIDS. An understanding of health cognitions, actions, and adherence behavior must take into account an individual's unique characteristics and the family, community, or other group context. As an example, assessment of and intervention to change health behaviors should also be appropriate for the specific age group of interest to achieve maximum effectiveness (Agras, 1993; Herman & Barnes, 1982). The focus of social work on many groups that have extensive health problems potentially altered by behavior change can help all health behavior researchers recognize many unique characteristics that will increase social workers' ability to do assessment and intervention in health behavior.

The types of articles published in these journals are also interesting: The vast majority of the articles are either conceptual or some form of survey research. There is very little in the way of health behavior research that involves experimental manipulation of interventions. This is not to say, however, that social work researchers do not conduct this type of research. As will be shown subsequently by looking at selected lines of social work scholarship, social workers in fact often do this type of intervention research. Their research, however, is often published in non-social work journals. There are many possible reasons that it is. Most likely, intervention researchers hope to reach a larger audience than social workers. The success of a technique, for example, may be viewed as knowledge valuable not just to social work but valuable in general. Thus, the information may be conveyed to the "parent" medical field—e.g., oncology, urology, pediatrics—or to other disciplines such as psychology or sociology or to multidisciplinary arenas such as *The Journal of Behavioral Medicine* or *Pain*. Some researchers may also believe that publication of their work in journals other than social work journals confers more status. This may not be the view of a tenure review committee in a school of social work, but the researcher may have a professional reference group beyond that school.

Selected Lines of Social Work Research in Health Behavior

Some social work scholars would argue that there are core themes that identify the writings

of social workers whether they are found in social work or not. These core themes reflect basic social work values: concern for the context of an individual's life, not just the individual in isolation; a focus on the society's disenfranchised, beginning with the client's preferences in selecting intervention goals, not predetermining these goals; and so on. Others would counter that many professions take these positions—that they are not unique to social work.

Instead of attempting to resolve this debate, this chapter will present a summary of three lines of health behavior research conducted by social work scholars. These summaries should provide the reader with a good sampling of social work research in health behavior. For purposes of this illustration, I have chosen to summarize my own work and that of two of my social work colleagues: Roger Roffman and Lewayne Gilchrist.

Health Promotion in Children and Adolescents. Gilchrist has combined cognitive–behavioral methods with theories from social psychology and child/adolescent development to devise and test health promotion and problem prevention for adolescents and youths. A series of studies, many with Schinke, have focused on contraception motivation and prevention of early and unwanted pregnancy (e.g., Blythe, Gilchrist, & Schinke, 1981; Gilchrist & Schinke, 1983; Gilchrist, Schinke, & Blythe, 1979, 1985; Schinke, Blythe, & Gilchrist, 1981; Schinke & Gilchrist, 1977; Schinke, Gilchrist, & Blythe, 1980; Schinke, Gilchrist, & Small, 1979/1983), preventing initiation and habitual drug use (e.g., Gilchrist, 1990, 1991; Gilchrist & Gillmore, 1992; Gilchrist, Gillmore & Lohr, 1990; Lohr, Gillmore, Gilchrist, & Butler, 1992; Schinke & Gilchrist, 1985; Schinke, Gilchrist, et al., 1985; Schinke, Schilling, et al., 1985), and stress management and reduction for young adolescents, with particular emphasis on young women (e.g., Bobo, Gilchrist, Elmer, Snow, & Schinke, 1986; Schinke, Barth, Gilchrist, & Maxwell, 1986; Schinke, Schilling, Kirkham, et al., 1986; Schinke, Schilling, Barth, Gilchrist, & Maxwell, 1986). In summary, the majority of Gilchrist's research has investigated factors related to the development of effective models of social skills training to alter a range of health promotion behaviors.

In addition, her research group is conducting a 9-year natural history of low-income women who become pregnant at 17 or younger and the transition of these young women to adulthood. This research includes an emphasis on mental health, social relationships, and economic/financial variables. The study traces and attempts to explain these mothers' movement in and out of drug use; the physical and psychological consequences of violence in their lives and interpersonal relationships; their reproductive histories and health incidence of sexually transmitted diseases; and finally the health and development of the children they bore as adolescent mothers.

Risk Behavior Research. Several studies have applied Marlatt and Gordon's (1985) relapse prevention work to chronic marijuana users who wished to stop smoking (Roffman, 1994; Roffman & Barnhart, 1987; Roffman & Stephens, 1993; Roffman, Stephens, Simpson & Whitaker, 1988, 1989). Since the early 1980s, Roffman's work has shifted to reducing high-risk sexual behavior, particularly in gay men. After conducting a needs assessment of this problem (Roffman, Gillmore, Gilchrist, Mathias, & Krueger, 1990), Roffman designed and assessed a 17-session in-person treatment program (Roffman, Beadnell, Downey, & Ryan, 1992; Roffman, Gilchrist, Stephens, & Kirkman, 1988; Stephens, Stern, & Roffman, 1990) combining Marlatt and Gordon's model with cognitive behavioral principles. He also began a lengthy series of studies to assess the effectiveness of an intervention conducted entirely by telephone (Roffman, Beadnell, & Ryan, 1992; Roffman, Beadnell, Ryan, & Downey, in press; Roffman, Ryan, Downey, & Beadnell, 1993).

Roffman has also been involved in a community intervention research program to reduce AIDS risk behavior (Beckman et al., 1995; Kelly et al., 1990, in press; Perry et al., 1994). Finally, he is currently working on a study focusing on AIDS risk reduction and low-income women of color who live in public housing projects.

In summary, throughout his career, Roffman has utilized innovative methodologies to study and develop interventions to alter undesirable repetitive health practices that operate in an addictive pattern.

Compliance and Women's Health. Much of the author's work has focused on issues of compliance with health care regimens. This work has included a model to organize compliance enhancement recommendations in general (Shelton & Levy, 1979; Levy, 1987a) and also specifically in social work in health care practice (Levy, 1978, 1986–1987, 1987b). A number of studies have demonstrated the effectiveness of some components of this model, such as specificity, reminders, and a public commitment (Levy & Claravell, 1977; Levy & Clark, 1980; Levy, Yamashita, & Pow, 1979). Working with a population of low-income families in a community clinic, social workers expanded into a different setting by training dentists to work with this community and patients in preventive care (Davis, Domoto, & Levy, 1979; Levy & Domoto, 1979; Levy, Domoto, Olson, Lertora, & Charney, 1980; Levy, Lambert, & Davis, 1979; Levy, Lodish, & Pawlak, 1982; Levy, Weinstein, & Milgrom, 1977; Levy & Yoshida, 1980; Olson, Levy, Evans, & Olson, 1981). In this work, the use of compliance enhancement procedures by dentists and dental students was both studied and encouraged.

A review was also conducted of a series of federally funded compliance studies investigating the effectiveness of social support in enhancing compliance. As a result of this review, several methodological problems, including the operational definition of social support, were highlighted in the literature (Haynes et al., 1982; Levy, 1980, 1983, 1985, 1986).

Current research again includes testing the application of compliance enhancement techniques to areas of women's health care. One of these areas addresses the concern that many women urology patients undergo unnecessary medical procedures or take unnecessary medications. One study found that an alteration in certain health behaviors produced a desired health effect by reducing unpleasant symptoms (Levy & Bavendam, 1995).

Irritable bowel syndrome (IBS) is another health problem faced by many women that can often be altered with behavior change.

The author and her colleagues have most recently been studying behavioral and psychological factors that may be related to IBS as well as the effect of intervention strategies on symptoms (Heitkemper, Levy, Jarrett, & Bond, 1995; Jarrett, Cain, Heitkemper, & Levy, 1996; Levy, Cain, Jarrett, & Heitkemper, 1997).

This work in urology and gastroenterology has been conducted in collaboration with colleagues in the School of Medicine and the School of Nursing's Center for Women's Health Research. These colleagues' physiological backgrounds complement the knowledge base of psychology and social work. Such collaboration in health behavior research is highly beneficial when social workers are involved in the medical arena.

In conclusion, Levy's research has combined theory and methodology from a social psychological and cognitive–behavioral perspective to develop techniques for maximizing patient compliance and understanding behavior across a broad range of health issues.

SUMMARY AND CONCLUSION

Health behavior research clearly is relevant to the professional activities of social workers. Whether in dealing with individuals on a one-to-one basis or working to change the attitudes or behaviors of families or communities, much of what social workers are most concerned with is directly tied to some of the major themes of this research: personal, familial, and cultural cognitions about health and health-related behaviors, including compliance, and the impact of these influences on these behaviors. Unfortunately, there is little agreement among social workers on what health behavior research findings should be applied in their practice. This lack of agreement is evidenced by the ongoing effort to define the appropriate educational basis for social workers

in the health field. The problem is compounded by the fact that many social workers are not enthusiastic about research and do not naturally turn to research findings either to guide their practice or to educate student social workers. Thus, as noted earlier, convention may dictate assessment and practice activities as much as (or more than) research findings.

Social work would benefit by improving the socialization of its students in recognizing the value of research findings in all areas, including that of health behavior. If the utilization of these findings were to be generally valued, the profession would have taken a major step toward defining the specifics of what findings would form an appropriate educational basis for its students.

Social workers are found throughout the health care field in a variety of settings, and thus are well situated to participate in health behavior research activities consistent with their profession's ethical guidelines. Social worker researchers have been involved in many areas of health behavior research, although these activities may not be immediately obvious because social workers often publish their research in non–social work journals. While most research comes from doctoral-level social workers who are typically associated with an educational institution, there have been efforts in the profession to encourage clinicians to participate more in research through the use of the single-subject methodology (Jayaratne & Levy, 1979; Levy & Olson, 1979). With social work so well placed throughout the health care arena, the challenge to the profession is to go beyond academic social work researchers and generate increased enthusiasm for health behavior research activities among front-line social work practitioners.

REFERENCES

Agras, W. S. (1993). Adherence intervention research: The need for a multilevel approach. In N. A. Krasnegor, L. Epstein, S. B. Johnson, S. J. Johnson, & S. J. Yaffe (Eds.), *Developmental aspects of compliance behavior*, (pp. 285–302). Hillsdale, NJ: Erlbaum.

Bandura, A. (1969). *Principles of behavior modification*. New York: Holt, Rinehart & Winston.

Bandura, A. (1982). Self-efficacy mechanism in human agency. *American Psychologist, 37*, 122–147.

Bandura, A. (1989). Human agency in social cognitive theory. *American Psychologist, 44*, 1175–1184.

Barbarin, O. A., Whitten, C. F., & Bonds, S. M. (1994). Estimating rates of psychosocial problems in urban and poor children with sickle cell anemia. *Health and Social Work, 19*(2), 112–119.

Becker, M. H. (Ed.). (1974). *The health belief model and personal health behavior*. Thorofare, NJ: Slack.

Becker, M. H., & Maiman, L. A. (1975). Sociobehavioral determinants of compliance with health and medical care recommendations. *Medical Care, 13*, 10–24.

Beckman, T. G., Kelly, J. A., Roffman, R. A., Solomon, L. J., Winett, R. A., Stevenson, Y. L., Perry, M. J., Norman, A. D., & Disiderato, L. J. (1995). Differences in HIV risk characteristics between bisexual and exclusively gay men. *AIDS Education and Prevention, 7*, 504–512.

Berkman, B. (1981). Knowledge base needs for effective social work practice in health. *Journal of Education for Social Work, 17*(2), 85–90.

Berkman, B., Kemler, B., Marcus, L., & Silverman, D. (1985). Course content for social work practice in health care. *Journal of Education for Social Work, 21*(3), 43–51.

Blythe, B. J., Gilchrist, L. D., & Schinke, S. P. (1981). Pregnancy-prevention groups for adolescents. *Social Work, 26*, 503–504.

Bobo, J. K., Gilchrist, L. D., Elmer, J. F., Snow, W. H., & Schinke, S. P. (1986). Hassles, role strain, and peer relations in young adolescents. *Journal of Early Adolescence, 6*, 339–352.

Burg, M. A. (1994). Health problems of sheltered homeless women and their dependent children. *Health and Social Work, 19*(2), 125–131.

Callahan, J. (1994). The ethics of assisted suicide. *Health and Social Work, 19*(4), 237–244.

Carlton, T. O., with contributors. (1984). *Clinical social work in health settings: A guide to professional practice with exemplars*. New York: Springer.

Caroff, P., & Mailick, M. D. (1985). Health concentrations in schools of social work: The state of the art. *Health and Social Work, 10*(1), 5–14.

Coady, C. A., Kent, V. D. & Davis, P. W. (1990). Burnout among social workers working with patients with cystic fibrosis. *Health and Social Work, 15*(2), 116–124.

Collins, S. K., & Shannon, C. (1988). Teaching beyond the medical model: What social workers in health care need to know. *Journal of Teaching in Social Work, 2*(2), 131–144.

Council on Social Work Education. (1975). Position statement on preparation for the practice of social work in the health field jointly approved by the Society of Hospital Social Work, Directors of the American Hospital Association, Chicago. Mimeographed.

Council on Social Work Education. (1992a). *A curriculum policy statement for baccalaureate degree programs in social work education*. Mimeographed.

Council on Social Work Education. (1992b). *A curriculum policy statement for master's degree programs in social work education*. Mimeographed.

Davidson, P. O., & Davidson, S. M. (Eds.). (1980). *Behavioral medicine: Changing health lifestyles*. New York: Brunner/Mazel.

Davis, G. R., Domoto, P. K., & Levy, R. L. (1979, May-June). The dentist's role in child abuse and neglect. *Journal of Dentistry for Children*, 1–8.

Dicks, B. A. (1994). African-American women and AIDS: A public health/social work challenge. *Social Work in Health Care, 19*(3/4), 123–143.

Ewart, C. K. (1993). Health promotion and disease prevention: A social action conception of compliance behavior. In N. A. Krasnegor, L. Epstein, S. B. Johnson, & S. J. Yaffe (Eds.), *Developmental aspects of health compliance behavior* (pp. 251–280). Hillsdale, NJ: Erlbaum.

Falck, H. S. (1984). *Social work in health settings*. In T. O. Carlton (Ed.), *Clinical social work in health settings: A guide to professional practice with exemplars* (pp. 167–175). New York: Springer.

Fink, D. L. (1976). Tailoring the consensual regimen. In D. L. Sackett & R. B. Haynes (Eds.), *Compliance with therapeutic regimens* (pp. 110–118). Baltimore: Johns Hopkins University Press.

Finkelstein, N. (1984). Treatment issues for alcohol-and-drug dependent pregnant and parenting women. *Health and Social Work, 19*(1), 7–16.

Fishbein, M., & Ajzen, I. (1975). *Belief, attitude, intention and behavior*. Reading, MA: Addison-Wesley.

Fox, B. H. (1976). The psychosocial epidemiology of cancer. In J. W. Cullen, B. H. Fox, & R. N. Isom (Eds.), *Cancer: The behavioral dimensions* (pp. 11–22). New York: Raven Press.

Frazier, P. A., Davis, A. S., & Dahl, K. E. (1994). Correlates of non-compliance among renal transplant recipients. *Clinical Transplants, 8*(6), 550–557.

Germain, C. B. (1984). *Social work practice in health care: An ecological perspective*. New York: Free Press.

Giannetti, V. J. (1983). Medication utilization problems among the elderly. *Health and Social Work, 8*, 262–270.

Gilchrist, L. D. (1990). The role of schools in community-based approaches to prevention of AIDS and intravenous drug use. In C. G. Leukefeld, B. J. Battjes, & Z. Amsel (Eds.), *AIDS and intravenous drug use: Future directions for community-based prevention research* (pp. 150–166). NIDA Research Monograph 93. Washington, DC: U.S. Government Printing Office.

Gilchrist, L. D. (1991). Defining the interventions and the target population. In C. Leukefeld & W. Bukowski (Eds.), *Drug abuse prevention intervention research: Methodological issues* (pp. 110–122). NIDA RAUS Monograph 107. Washington, DC: U.S. Government Printing Office.

Gilchrist, L. D., & Gillmore, M. R. (1992). Methodological issues in prevention research on drug use and pregnancy.

In M. M. Kilbey & K. Asghar (Eds.), *Methodological issues in epidemiological, prevention, and treatment research on drug-exposed women and their children* (pp. 1–17). NIDA RAUS Monograph 107. Washington, DC: U.S. Government Printing Office.

Gilchrist, L. D., Gillmore, M. R., & Lohr, M. J. (1990). Drug use among pregnant adolescents. *Journal of Consulting and Clinical Psychology, 58*(4), 402–407.

Gilchrist, L. D., & Schinke, S. P. (1983). Coping with contraception: Cognitive and behavioral methods with adolescents. *Cognitive Therapy and Research, 7,* 379–388. [Reprinted in French in *Fertilité-Sexualité-Contraception,* 1985, *13,* 795–800.]

Gilchrist, L. D., Schinke, S. P., & Blythe, B. J. (1979). Primary prevention services for children and youth. *Children and Youth Services Review, 1,* 379–391. [Abstracted in Stein, M. D., & Davis, J. K. (1982). *Therapies for adolescents* (pp. 309–310). San Francisco: Jossey-Bass.]

Gilchrist, L. D., Schinke, S. P., & Blythe, B. J. (1985). Preventing unwanted adolescent pregnancies. In L. D. Gilchrist & S. P. Schinke (Eds.), *Preventing social and health problems through life skills training* (pp. 55–62). Seattle: University of Washington Center for Social Welfare Research.

Haynes, R. B., Mattson, M. E., Chobanian, A. V., Dunbar, S. M., Engebretson, T. O. Garrity, T. F., Leventhal, H., Levine, R. J., & Levy, R. L. (1982). Management of patient compliance in the treatment of hypertension. *Hypertension, 4,* 415–423.

Haynes, R. B., Taylor, D. W., & Sackett, D. L. (1979). *Compliance in health care.* Baltimore: Johns Hopkins University Press.

Heitkemper, M., Levy, R. L., Jarrett, M., & Bond, S. I. (1995). Interventions for irritable bowel syndrome: A nursing model. *Gastroenterology Nursing, 18*(6), 224–230.

Hemminki, E., & Heikkila, J. (1975). Elderly people's compliance with prescriptions and quality of medication. *Scandinavian Journal of Social Medicine, 3,* 87–92.

Hepworth, D. H., & Larsen, J. (1993). *Direct social work practice* (4th ed.). Pacific Grove, CA: Brooks/Cole.

Herman, S., & Barnes, D. (1982). Behavioral assessment in geriatrics. In F. J. Keefe & J. A. Blumenthal (Eds.), *Assessment strategies in behavioral medicine* (pp. 473–500). Washington, DC: American Psychological Association.

Hess, P. M., & Mullen, E. J. (1995). *Practitioner-researcher partnerships.* Washington, DC: NASW Press.

Hollis, F. (1968). *A typology of casework treatment.* New York: Family Service Association of America.

Jarrett, M., Cain, K. C., Heitkemper, M., & Levy, R. L. (in press). Relationship between gastrointestinal and dysmenorrheic symptoms at menses. *Research in Nursing and Health, 19,* 45–91.

Jayaratne, S., & Levy, R. L. (1979). *Empirical clinical practice.* New York: Columbia University Press.

Keefe, F. J., & Blumenthal, J. A. (1982). Behavioral medicine: Basic principles and theoretical foundations. In F. J. Keefe & J. A. Blumenthal (Eds.), *Assessment strategies in behav-ioral medicine* (pp. 3–18). Washington, DC: American Psychological Association.

Keehn, D. S., Roglitz, C., & Bowden, M. L. (1994). Impact of social work on recidivism and non-medical complaints in the emergency department. *Social Work in Health Care, 20*(1), 65–76.

Kellaway, G., & MaCrae. (1975). Non-compliance and errors of drug administration in patients discharged from acute medical wards. *New Zealand Medical Journal, 81,* 508–512.

Kelly, J. A., St. Lawrence, J. S., Brasfield, T. L., Lemke, A., Amdei, T., Roffman, R., Hood, H. V., Smith, J. E., Kilgore, H., & McNeill, C. S. (1990). Psychological factors that predict AIDS high-risk versus AIDS precautionary behavior. *Journal of Consulting and Clinical Psychology, 58*(1), 117–120.

Kelly, J. A., Sikkema, K. J., Winett, R. A. Solomon, L. J., Roffman, R. A., Heckman, T. G. Stevenson, L. Y., Perry, M. J., Norman, A. D., & Disiderato, L. J. (1995). Factors predicting continued high risk behavior among gay men in small cities: Psychological, behavioral, and demographic characteristics related to unsafe sex. *Journal of Consulting and Clinical Psychology, 63,* 101–107.

Kerson, T. S. (1989). *Social work in health settings.* New York: Haworth Press.

Kincey, J., Bradshaw, P., & Ley, P. (1975). Patients' satisfaction and reported acceptance of advice in general practice. *Journal of the Royal College of General Practitioners, 25,* 558–566.

Krasnegor, N. A., Epstein, L., Johnson, S. B., & Yaffe, S. J. (Eds.). (1993). *Developmental aspects of compliance behavior.* Hillsdale, NJ: Erlbaum.

Levy, R. L. (1978). Facilitating patient compliance with medical regimens: An area for social work research and intervention. In N. Bracht (Ed.), *Social work in health care: A guide to professional practice* (pp. 281–292). New York: Haworth Press.

Levy, R. L. (1980). The role of social support in patient compliance: A selective review. In R. B. Haynes, M. E. Mattson, & T. O. Engebretson (Eds.), *Patient compliance to prescribed antihypertensive regimens* (pp. 139–164). NIH Publication No. 81-2102. Bethesda, MD: National Institutes of Health.

Levy, R. L. (1983). Social support and compliance: A selective review and critique of treatment integrity and outcome measurement. *Social Science and Medicine, 17,* 1329–1338.

Levy, R. L. (1985). Social support and compliance: Update. *Journal of Hypertension* (Supplement 1), *3,* 45–49.

Levy, R. L. (1986). Social support and compliance: Salient methodological problems in compliance research. *Journal of Compliance in Health Care, 1,* 189–198.

Levy, R. L. (1986–1987). Treatment compliance in social work. *Journal of Social Service Research, 10,* 85–103.

Levy, R. L. (1987a). Compliance and medical practice. In J. Blumenthal & D. McKee (Eds.), *Applications in behavioral medicine* (pp. 567–587). Sarasota, FL: Professional Resource Exchange.

Levy, R. L. (1987b). Treatment compliance in social work. In B. A. Thyer & W. W. Hudson (Eds.), *Progress in behavioral social work* (pp. 85–103). New York: Haworth Press.

Levy, R. L., & Bavendam, T. (1995). Promoting women's urologic self-care: Five single-case evaluations. *Research on Social Work Practice, 5*(4), 430–441.

Levy, R. L., Cain, K. C., Jarrett, M., & Heitkemper, M. M. (1997). The relationship between daily life stress and gastrointestinal symptoms in women with irritable bowel syndrome. *Journal of Behavioral Medicine.*

Levy, R. L., & Claravell, V. (1977). Differential effects of a phone reminder on patients with long and short between-visit intervals. *Medical Care, 15,* 435–438.

Levy, R. L., & Clark, H. (1980). The use of an overt commitment to enhance compliance: A cautionary note. *Journal of Behavior Therapy and Experimental Psychiatry, 11,* 105–107.

Levy, R. L., & Domoto, P. K. (1979). Current techniques for behavior management: A survey. *Pediatric Dentistry, 1,* 160–164.

Levy, R. L., Domoto, P. K., Olson, D. G., Lertora, A. K., & Charney, C. (1980). Evaluation of one-to-one behavioral training. *Journal of Dental Education, 44,* 221–222.

Levy, R. L., Lambert, R., & Davis, G. (1979). Social work and dentistry in clinical, training and research collaboration. *Social Work in Health Care, 5,* 177–185.

Levy, R. L., Lodish, D., & Pawlak, F. C. (1982). Teaching children to take more responsibility for their own dental treatment. *Social Work in Health Care, 7,* 69–76.

Levy, R. L., & Olson, D. G. (1979). The single subject methodology in clinical practice. *Journal of Social Science Research, 3,* 25–49.

Levy, R. L., Weinstein, P., & Milgrom, P. (1977). Behavioral guidelines for plaque control programs. *Dental Hygiene, 51,* 13–18.

Levy, R. L., Yamashita, D., & Pow, G. (1979). Relationship of an overt commitment to the frequency and speed of compliance with symptom reporting. *Medical Care, 17*(3), 281–284.

Levy, R. L., & Yoshida, B. (1980). The measurement of the effect of social work on the enhancement of dental student training. *Social Work in Health Care, 6,* 33–38.

Lockery, S. A., Dunkle, R. E., Kart, C. S., & Coulton, C. J. (1994). Factors contributing to the early rehospitalization of elderly people. *Health and Social Work, 19*(3), 182–191.

Lohr, M. J., Gillmore, M. R., Gilchrist, L. D., & Butler, S. S. (1992). Factors related to substance use by pregnant, school-aged adolescents. *Journal of Adolescent Health, 13,* 475–482.

Maccoby, N., & Alexander, J. (1980). Use of media in lifestyle programs. In P. O. Davidson & S. M. Davidson (Eds.), *Behavioral medicine: Changing health lifestyles* (pp. 307–370). New York: Brunner/Mazel.

Marlatt, G. A., & Gordon, J. R. (1985). *Relapse prevention: Maintenance strategies in addictive behavior change.* New York: Guilford Press.

Maslach, C. (1978). The burn-out syndrome and patient care. In C. Garfield (Ed.), *Psychosocial care of the dying.* New York: McGraw-Hill.

Miller, R. S., & Rehr, H. (Eds.) (1983). *Social work issues in health care.* Englewood Cliffs, NJ: Prentice-Hall.

Milsum, J. H. (1980). Lifestyle changes for the whole person: Stimulation through health hazard appraisal. In P. O. Davidson & S. M. Davidson (Eds.), *Behavioral medicine: Changing health lifestyles* (pp. 116–150). New York: Brunner/Mazel.

National Association of Social Workers. (1990). The NASW Code of Ethics. Passed by the 1979 delegate assembly, implemented July 1, 1990.

Olson, D. G., Levy, R. L., Evans, C. A., & Olson, S. K. (1981). Enhancement of high-risk children's utilization of dental services. *American Journal of Public Health, 71,* 631–634.

Owens, S. (1995). Attitudes toward and knowledge of AIDS among African-American social work students. *Health and social work, 20*(2), 110–115.

Perry, M. J., Solomon, L. J., Winett, R. A., Kelly, J. A., Roffman, R. A., Disiderato, L. L., Kalichman, S. C., Sikkema, K. J., Norman, A. D., Short, B., & Stevenson, L. Y. (1994). High risk sexual behavior and alcohol consumption among bar-going gay men. *AIDS, 8*(9), 1321–1324.

Ratliff, B. W., Timberlake, E. M., & Jentsch, D. P. (1982). *Social work in hospitals.* Springfield, IL: Charles C. Thomas.

Roberts, C. S., Cot, C. E., Shannon, V. J., & Wells, N. E. (1994). A closer look at social support as a moderator of stress in breast cancer. *Health and Social Work, 19*(3), 157–164.

Roffman, R. A. (1994). *Motivational enhancement interventions in substance abuse.* Paper presented at the Seventh Annual Northwest Conference on Addictions, Seattle, WA, May 13.

Roffman, R. A., & Barnhart, R. (1987). Assessing need for marijuana dependence treatment through an anonymous telephone interview. *International Journal of the Addictions, 22*(7), 639–651.

Roffman, R. A., Beadnell, B., Downey, L., & Ryan, R. (1992). *Preventing relapse to unsafe sex in gay and bisexual males.* Poster presented at the annual meeting of the American Public Health Association, Washington, DC, November.

Roffman, R. A., Beadnell, B., & Ryan, R. (1992). *Telephone counseling in the reduction of barriers to AIDS prevention.* Paper presented at the Second International Congress of Behavioral Medicine, Hamburg, Germany, July.

Roffman, R. A., Beadnell, B., Ryan, R., & Downey, L. (1995). Telephone group counseling in reducing AIDS risk in gay and bisexual males. *Journal of Gay and Lesbian Social Services, 2,* 145–157.

Roffman, R. A., Gilchrist, L. D., Stephens, R. S., & Kirkman, M. A. (1988). Relapse prevention with gay or bisexual males at risk of AIDS due to ongoing unsafe sexual behavior. In J. A. Kelly (Chair), *Behavioral interventions to prevent AIDS: Current status and future directions.* Symposium conducted at the annual meeting of the Association for Advancement of Behavior Therapy, New York, November.

Roffman, R. A., Gillmore, M. R., Gilchrist, L. D., Mathias, S. A., & Krueger, L. (1990, March-April). Continuing unsafe sex: Assessing need for AIDS-prevention counseling. *Public Health Reports, 105*(2), 202-208.

Roffman, R. A., Ryan, R., Downey, L., & Beadnell, B. (1993). *A telephone group intervention can overcome barriers to enrolling isolated gay and bisexual males in AIDS risk-reduction counseling.* Paper presented at the Annual Meeting of the American Public Health Association, San Francisco, October.

Roffman, R. A., & Stephens, R. S. (1993). Cannabis dependence. In D. L. Dunner (Ed.), *Current psychiatric therapy* (pp. 105-109). Orlando, FL: W. B. Saunders.

Roffman, R. A., Stephens, R. S., Simpson, E. E., & Whitaker, D. L. (1988). Treatment of marijuana dependence: Preliminary results. *Journal of Psychoactive Drugs, 20,* 129-137.

Roffman, R. A., Stephens, R. S., Simpson, E. E., & Whitaker, D. L. (1989). Relapse prevention with adult chronic marijuana smokers. *Journal of Chemical Dependencies Treatment, 2,* 241-257.

Rosenberg, G. (1978). Practice roles and functions of the health social worker. In R. S. Miller & H. Rehr (Eds.), *Social work issues in health care* (pp. 121-180). Englewood Cliffs, NJ: Prentice-Hall.

Schinke, S. P., Barth, R. P., Gilchrist, L. D., & Maxwell, J. S. (1986). Adolescent mothers, stress, and prevention. *Journal of Human Stress, 12,* 162-167.

Schinke, S. P., Blythe, B. J., & Gilchrist, L. D. (1981). Cognitive-behavioral prevention of adolescent pregnancy. *Journal of Counseling Psychology, 28,* 451-454. [Reprinted in M. Bloom (Ed.). (1983). *Life span development* (2nd ed.). New York: Macmillan.]

Schinke, S. P. & Gilchrist, L. D. (1977). Adolescent pregnancy. An interpersonal skill training approach to prevention. *Social Work in Health Care, 3,* 159-167.

Schinke, S. P. & Gilchrist, L. D. (1985). Preventing substance abuse with children and adolescents. *Journal of Consulting and Clinical Psychology, 53,* 596-602.

Schinke, S. P., Gilchrist, L. D., & Blythe, B. J. (1980). Role of communication in the prevention of teenage pregnancy. *Health and Social Work, 5*(3), 54-59.

Schinke, S. P., Gilchrist, L. D., Schilling, R. F., Walker, R. D., Kirkham, M. A., Bobo, J. K., Trimble, J. E., Cvetkovich, G. T., & Richardson, S. S. (1985). Strategies for preventing substance abuse with American Indian youth. *White Cloud Journal, 3*(4), 12-18.

Schinke, S. P., Gilchrist, L. D., & Small, R. W. (1979/1983). Preventing unwanted adolescent pregnancy: A cognitive-

behavioral approach. *American Journal of Orthopsychiatry, 49,* 81-88. [Reprinted in M. Bloom (Ed.). (1983). *Life span development* (2nd ed.) (pp. 44-52). New York: Macmillan.]

Schinke, S. P., Schilling, R. F., Barth, R. P., Gilchrist, L. D., & Maxwell, J. S. (1986). Stress-management intervention to prevent family violence. *Journal of Family Violence, 1,* 13-26.

Schinke, S. P., Schilling, R. F., Gilchrist, L. D., Barth, R. P., Bobo, J. K., Trimble, J. E., & Cvetkovich, G. T. (1985). Preventing substance abuse with American Indian youth. *Social Casework, 66,* 213-217.

Schinke, S. P., Schilling, R. F., Kirkham, M. A., Gilchrist, L. D., Barth, R. P., & Blythe, B. J. (1986). Stress management skills for parents. *Journal of Child and Adolescent Psychotherapy, 3,* 293-298.

Schlesinger, E. G. (1985). *Health care social work practice: Concepts and strategies.* St. Louis, MO: Times Mirror/C. V. Mosby.

Schulman, B. (1979) Active patient orientation and outcomes in hypertensive treatment. *Medical Care, 17,* 267-280.

Schultz, S. K. (1980). Compliance with therapeutic regimens in pediatrics: A review of implications for social work practice. *Social Work in Health Care, 5,* 267-278.

Shelton, J. L., & Levy, R. L. (1979). Home practice activities and compliance: Two sources of error variance in behavior research. *Journal of Applied Behavior Analysis, 12,* 324.

Shelton, J. L., & Levy, R. L. (1981). *Behavioral assignments and treatment compliance: A handbook of clinical strategies.* Champaign, IL: Research Press.

Simmons, J. (1994). Community based care: The new health social work paradigm. *Social Work in Health Care, 20*(1), 35-46.

Stephens, R. S., Stern, M., & Roffman, R. A. (1990). Utility of the self-efficacy construct in the reduction of unsafe sexual behavior in gay men. In B. S. McCann (Chair), *Self-efficacy and health behavior change.* Symposium conducted at the Annual Meeting of the Society of Behavioral Medicine, Chicago, April.

Stone, G. C. (1979). Psychology and the health system. In G. C. Stone, F. Cohen, & N. E. Adler (Eds.), *Health psychology* (pp. 47-75). San Francisco: Jossey-Bass.

Terry, P. O. (1981). Clinical social work roles and an integrative, interdisciplinary team: Enhancing parental compliance. *Social Work in Health Care, 6,* 1-15.

Wallace, S. R., Goldberg, R. J., & Slaby, A. E. (1984). *Clinical social work in health care: New biopsychosocial approaches.* New York: Praeger.

Wilke, D. V. (1994). Women and alcoholism: How a male-as-norm bias affects research, assessment and treatment. *Health and Social Work, 19*(1), 29-36.

Zambrana, R. E., Ell, K., Dorrington, C., Wachsman, L., & Hodge, D. (1994). The relationship between psychosocial status of immigrant Latino mothers and use of emergency pediatric services. *Health and Social Work, 19*(2), 93-102.

7

Health Behavior Research and Oral Health

Helen C. Gift and B. Alexander White

INTRODUCTION

For over four decades, health behavior research has been an important tool in understanding the actions of dental practitioners, patients, and administrators of oral health services. Early investigations of fluoridation of public water supplies provided information on health behaviors of organizers and policy makers at the community level. Following World War II, there was increased interest in the characteristics of dentists and their practice activities and in the impact of practitioner behavior on oral health status, access, and cost. With the increasing availability of additional preventive strategies, such as topical fluoride applications and dental sealants, compliance with these new regimens on the part of the public, patients, and health care professionals was the object of considerable behavioral research (Richards & Cohen, 1971). The evolution

of the profession from a treatment to a prevention orientation in the 1960s and 1970s brought increased interest in the organization of dental practices and the types of services provided, the employment of dental hygienists and auxiliary personnel, and dentist–patient interactions. Concurrently, as the population of the United States increased, there was a surge of interest in estimating the size and composition of the dental workforce. This increasing interest resulted in other thrusts for behavior research: understanding what type of health professional was attracted to dentistry, training the ideal dentist, assuring that appropriate practice strategies were developed and used, and expanding the function of dental auxiliaries.

The growth of dental insurance in the 1970s set the stage for yet another series of studies on the behaviors of dental professionals, patients, and the public. The issues of dental services utilization, treatment alternatives, who pays for services, quality assurance, and fees were addressed extensively in studies of the public and patients during this period (Cohen & Bryant, 1984; Gift, Gerbert, Kress, & Reisine, 1990). The 1980s witnessed the emergence of issues in dentists' behaviors associated with infection control, special

Helen C. Gift • National Institute of Dental Research, National Institutes of Health, Bethesda, Maryland 20892-6401. B. Alexander White • Kaiser Permanente, Portland, Oregon 97227-1098.

Handbook of Health Behavior Research IV: Relevance for Professionals and Issues for the Future, edited by David S. Gochman. Plenum Press, New York, 1997.

121

care patients, and access for underserved populations (Gift, 1988, 1993; Gift et al., 1990; White, 1994). Further, changes in the epidemiology of oral diseases—declining prevalence of dental caries among schoolchildren and less tooth loss—have resulted in pressures to change the dental education curriculum and dental practice behaviors (Tedesco, 1995; White, 1994).

Health behavior research has been increasingly interpreted within the context of the organizational structure of the practice, the community, and the society, since much of what is unique about behaviors in dentistry is associated with these contexts as well as with the changing patterns of oral diseases and conditions. During the 1990s, researchers have made increasing efforts to understand (1) what sets the dental profession apart from other health care professions (e.g., almost all oral diseases are preventable; the dental care system is reasonably isolated; the treatment approach restricts verbal exchanges) as well as (2) the responses of the profession to increasing regulations and other pressures from outside its unique system.

Almost all people experience oral diseases and conditions at some time or other. The progressive consequences are not only physical, but also economic, social, and psychological (Gift, 1993; Reisine & Locker, 1995; White, 1994). At the physical or biological level, oral diseases and conditions may compromise host resistance to systemic infection, and limitations in oral function may impair chewing of certain foods and ability to swallow. At the social and psychological levels, oral diseases, disorders, and conditions (including impaired function) may adversely affect self-esteem, self-expression, communication, and personal appearance.

Most oral diseases and conditions are preventable through an appropriate combination of behaviors at some or all of the individual, health care professional, organizational, and societal levels. The availability and use of preventive strategies, improved restorative approaches, and changing norms, attitudes, and expectations have resulted in extraordinary declines in the

major indicator of oral diseases—total tooth loss—over the past several decades. Nevertheless, there are still considerable amounts of oral diseases and conditions, all too often among people who are socially and economically disadvantaged or who suffer concurrent burdens of systemic illnesses (Chen, 1995). Continued progress in prevention of oral diseases and conditions requires attention to these special populations and a range of these individual, professional, organizational, and societal behaviors. The challenges of studying these behaviors are considerable, since often the behaviors occur in settings in which they cannot be readily observed and studied, e.g., the privacy of the home or the dental operatory.

The purpose of this chapter is to review the relationships of health behaviors and health behavior research to the education, training, and practice activities of oral health professionals. The contexts within which health behaviors occur in dentistry are summarized. The health behavior research relevant to the education and training of oral health professionals and to the practice activities of these professionals is then presented, and the applications and interpretations of sociobehavioral research to dental education and practice are discussed. Finally, recommendations are made.

THE ENVIRONMENT AND ORAL HEALTH CARE DELIVERY SYSTEMS: CONTEXTS FOR BEHAVIORS

Cultural, social, political, and economic conditions establish opportunities for obtaining information or utilizing resources and influence individual values, beliefs, and behaviors associated with self-care and seeking or using professional or community services. Individual behaviors are established and influenced in family, school, peer, and health professional settings. Dental professional behaviors are influenced by social systems of education and training, professional organizations, and the general environment.

Alterations in cultural norms, social and organizational structures and policies, socioeconomic trends, and changes in oral disease patterns, can influence oral health behaviors. Some of the changing environmental conditions that have influenced behaviors in the oral care system during the past several decades are: (1) the demographic structure of the United States population (older and more diverse ethnically and racially); (2) slower United States population growth than projected in 1970; (3) changing patterns of oral diseases and conditions: declining dental caries, lower than expected prevalence of periodontal diseases, decreases in the amount of tooth loss; (4) increases in conditions associated with aging, immune deficiencies, and multiple chronic diseases and associated medications; and (5) more evidence of selective occurrence of oral diseases and conditions among disadvantaged populations, including low socioeconomic and certain racial and ethnic groups, the chronically ill, and those with HIV/AIDS (Gerbert, 1989; Gift, 1988, 1993; Gift ct al., 1990; Nowjack-Raymer & Gift, 1990; White, 1994).

Dental care delivery systems have been examined in terms of, among other characteristics, the availability and accessibility of professionals; appropriateness and acceptability of organizations; interactions among oral health professionals, the public, and administrators; and activities of dentists in the larger community (Andersen, Marcus, & Mahshigan, 1995; Cohen & Bryant, 1984; Gift et al., 1990; Petersen & Holst, 1995). While these system factors are critical to understanding dentist and patient behaviors, they have seldom been interpreted as such in research. For the purposes of this chapter, systems are seen as the contexts within which public, patient, and professional behaviors occur.

Dental care delivery in the United States has different historic roots than does medical care and remains a unique system of care. In the United States, dental services essentially are available on demand for those who can afford care,

have private dental insurance, or have some form of public coverage. Dental services are delivered predominantly in private dental practices. Over 85% of dentists practice alone or with one or two other dentists, directly supervising a small number of staff, which may include any or all of dental hygienists (60% of dentists employ this prevention staff), dental assistants, receptionists, and bookkeepers. In 1991, there were approximately 151,000 practicing dentists in the United States, of whom about 21% were specialists (Neenan, Paunovich, Solomon, & Watkins, 1993).

Typically, dental practices are located throughout communities, as opposed to being concentrated in medical centers or hospitals. Most offices have all the necessary equipment for the diagnosis of diseases and provision of routine preventive and restorative services. Large-group, multispecialty, and multiprofessional practices are few. Emergency dental care is also provided in hospitals and other institutional settings. Few nursing homes or chronic care facilities employ permanent dental staff. Delivery of dental care in worksites and schools is almost nonexistent. Some community and migrant health centers provide dental services, though only about half provide basic dental care services; moreover, these centers are not found in every community (Neenan et al., 1993). Dental services are also available through the Indian Health Service and the Veterans Administration.

Payment for dental services is different from that for ambulatory physician services. Generally, there are lower levels of dental insurance than of physician or hospital insurance. Approximately 95 million people, or 40.5% of the United States civilian population, have private dental insurance of some kind, but it is often limited by copayments and deductibles. Less than 4% of dental expenditures comes from public sources. Medicare does not cover routine dental care. Thus, many elderly have no assistance with dental payments unless they carry their private insurance forward as part of their retirement package. Dental services for adults under the Medicaid program are optional, although services for children are required in each state. Fewer than 17% of all Medicaid-eligible people in 1991 received dental services, and these expenditures represented less than 1% of the Medicaid bill (White, 1994).

EDUCATION OF ORAL HEALTH PROFESSIONALS: FOUNDATIONS FOR BEHAVIORS

Dental schools most often are affiliated with universities in academic medical centers. Of the 54 United States dental schools, 35 are public and 19 are private institutions. With the exception of basic sciences in some academic health centers, dental school curriculum is independent of medical education. Clinical training experiences are provided almost exclusively within the dental school; experiences in community settings or hospitals are limited. Dentists are educated, trained, and licensed to provide comprehensive oral health services as general practitioners. Internships and residencies are not required, but approximately one third of graduating dentists enroll in these 1- to 2-year programs. Graduates of dental schools may go beyond general education and obtain additional in-depth training in areas of specialization in one of the eight recognized dental specialties. Education and training of dental auxiliary personnel, which is not addressed in this chapter, is provided through apprenticeships, junior college certificate programs, and baccalaureate degree programs in universities. Each state has different requirements for the education and licensing of specific auxiliary personnel.

Dental Student Characteristics

The career paths of dentists have been studied extensively, examining the associations of aptitude tests, predental academic standing, demographic and socioeconomic status, personality, and role orientation in the selection of dentistry as a career and the success of individuals in dental school and practice (Grogono & Lancaster, 1988; Richards & Cohen, 1971). Common reasons

given for choosing dentistry as a career are desire to be one's own boss, flexibility of schedule, income potential, working with people, working with one's hands, and perceived prestige. Diversity of motivations shows up again in the interpersonal conflict between professional and proprietary orientations throughout the dental career (Nash, 1994).

Dental students have been observed to be conventional, conforming, compulsive, more practical than theoretical, and technologically oriented rather than oriented toward knowledge as an end in itself (Richards & Cohen, 1971). The dental school environment enhances these characteristics by focusing on technical competence rather than problem-solving and interaction skills (Tedesco, 1995). Thus, those students with these predominant traits have more self-esteem, higher ability to cope with dental school, lower psychological distress, and higher satisfaction with dentistry (Mozer, Lloyd, & Puente, 1990). While these dominant personality traits fit well with the current technical orientation in most dental schools, they are not as appropriate for the development of adequate communication and related interpersonal skills. A critical step between the classroom and the clinical setting is the application and integration of didactic principles in patient care and communication. Students need faculty assistance to be successful in this process, but since the dental faculty are products of the same educational system, these instructors may not have the skills to provide the necessary guidance.

Dental School Education and Training

A major goal of professional education is to assure that appropriate and necessary quality dental care is provided to the public. Over the years, changing technologies, disease patterns, and population demographics have placed pressures on the dental education system to evaluate educational content, processes, and outcomes. Often, these evaluations have been accomplished by increasing the number of specific technical requirements that must be met to receive a degree and a license (Jeffcoat & Clark, 1995; Tedesco, 1995). Since the traditional external outcome measures reflecting the success of training have been state and national dental board exams, often the curriculum is justified in terms of the material included on the licensing examinations. These examinations include little that evaluates behavioral competencies in patient care; thus, this focus remains underrepresented in the dental school curriculum (Kress, 1995).

The practice of clinical dentistry has remained essentially the same for several decades, with high values placed on restorative treatment. Despite increases in the number of dental schools with behavioral sciences and prevention in the curriculum during the past two decades, and the addition of a behavioral sciences section to the national boards a decade ago, the behavioral sciences curriculum, which includes health behavior, represents only about 3% of the hours. The actual number of hours offered has decreased in the past 20 years, and there is little evidence showing integration of behavioral sciences into clinical training (Jeffcoat & Clark, 1995; Kress, 1995; Tedesco, 1995).

Lack of focus and time spent on health behavior in dental schools does not result from a lack of guidelines. Professional associations and some dental schools have issued guidelines over the past two decades. These guidelines provide competency expectations and curricular goals for a wide range of topics, including the psychology of the dental practitioner, the dynamics of dentist–patient interactions, characteristics of patient behaviors, protective health behaviors, special conditions/special patients, staff development, and office management (Tedesco, 1995).

The value of a health behavior component in dental education has been established in several studies. Approaches are being tested to improve dentist–patient interaction in dental schools, notably in the history-taking experience, e.g., patient-instructors who give feedback to students (Stilwell & Reisine, 1992). Graduates who received training for behavioral approaches with fearful patients versus those who had received only exposure to pharmaceutical strategies saw a greater number of fearful patients and reported greater effort directed toward fear reduction in the initial contact with patients (Tay, Winn, Milgrom, & Hann, 1993). When treating geriatric patients, dental students are learning to recognize stereotypes they themselves may hold. Students are being trained to recognize patients' limits in sensory and motor skills and physical mobility, the time intensiveness of dental procedures, differential socialization of the patient and the dentist, and the presence of major chronic illnesses common among the elderly (Kiyak & Brudvik, 1992).

Continuing education programs, which could help address the gaps in training, have met with varying degrees of success. Courses with disabled patients have demonstrated gains in knowledge and confidence by dental care professionals and have resulted in participants applying their training (Stiefel & Truelove, 1995). In contrast, following a demonstration research project conducted to increase awareness of the role dentists must play in facilitating dental visits among nonusers of dental services, the dentists "blamed the patients" and, if willing to address the problems at all, wanted quick fixes, not professional development courses (Anderson & Morgan, 1992). Often, courses that address communication and behavior management skills are not selected by those dentists most in need of the training (Amstutz & Shulman, 1994).

Assessments are under way to determine whether dental schools, working within the changing environment, can effect institutional changes to improve the education of dental students and, ultimately, the behavioral and technical skills, appropriate health delivery behaviors, and collaborative efforts working with patients and the general public (Tedesco, 1995). A major concern is that of enhancing dentists' skills in acknowledging, interpreting, and acting on patient information and motivations, as well as their ability to look at their own behaviors, motivations, and roles in achieving positive patient behaviors and treatment outcomes. These recent evaluations have revitalized attention to the importance of behavioral research in the education of oral health professionals throughout the career cycle. The following sections present contributions of research on behavior within these larger contexts.

ORAL HEALTH BEHAVIORS

Despite the long history of behavioral research in dentistry, there is still much to be learned about what leads to or influences behaviors of professionals, patients, and the public. All too often, oral health behaviors have been examined on a short-term basis, cross-sectionally, and without assessing health outcomes. Also, clinical and field trials have often tested only the adoption of a therapeutic regimen in the absence of influencing behavioral and contextual factors.

Many theoretical and conceptual approaches described in other volumes of this *Handbook* have been used to examine and explain behaviors of dental professionals, patients, and the public in regard to oral health. Theories that address developmental learning and socialization have been particularly valuable, since so many routine oral health behaviors are initiated at early ages. Also, developmental approaches have been used to establish the appropriateness of targeting program interventions (Krasnegor, Epstein, Johnson, & Jaffe, 1993). For example, children between the ages of 6 and 12 can master skills and competence for self-care practices such as personal oral hygiene. By the time they reach adolescence, these children will have established a set of routines begun during childhood and will have experienced a set, unique to each child, of family, peer, and environmental pressures and several years of influence from gender, family, cultural, and socioeconomic factors. During adolescence, oral health behaviors may range from habits (tooth brushing) to preventive behaviors (using headgear for sports) to problem behaviors (tobacco and alcohol or trauma), each requiring

different approaches that adapt to these influences. Youths begin to accept individual responsibility and respond to rules and conformity to receive the "rewards" of future oral health or orofacial changes (Albino & Lawrence, 1993). There has been successful implementation in this age range of orthodontic procedures (Albino, 1984), oral hygiene procedures focused on reduced gingival bleeding (Nowjack-Raymer et al., 1995), and the elimination of oral soft tissue lesions as a motivation for changes in tobacco behaviors (Mecklenburg et al., 1990).

Comprehensive analytical models, envisioning behaviors as interactive processes involving the individual, social group, society, and environmental factors, have been used extensively in studies of oral health status, dental visits, and other oral health behaviors. These models include health services utilization models that focus on social-structural and environmental factors, lifestyles, individual values, norms, and attitudes, and other characteristics leading to illness, health, or behaviors (Andersen et al., 1995; Maizels, Maizels, & Sheiham, 1991; Petersen & Holst, 1995); economic, decision, and utility models that focus on patient preferences, trade-offs between benefits and risks, and quality and quantity of health in the receipt of care (Antczak-Bouckoms & Tulloch, 1995); and community approaches that focus on institutional strategies to alter the context in which oral health behaviors occur (Drury & Snowden, 1995).

Preventive Behaviors

The oral health behaviors of an individual that are intended to prevent oral diseases and conditions are not random events, but are structured by a variety of demographic, social status, organizational, and environmental resources. Preventive orientations appear to manifest themselves in a variety of consistent behaviors (Gift, 1986); having a given preventive behavior in one's repertoire is usually related to having another (Krasnegor et al., 1993). Preventive oral health behaviors that are corollary to health-promoting behaviors (e.g., improved diet, exercise, seeking diagnosis rather than treatment) occur at the individual, professional, and societal levels. At the individual level, preventive oral health behaviors include self-care (oral hygiene, use of fluoride), use of trauma protection, avoidance of alcohol and tobacco, and dental visits for asymptomatic purposes. At the professional level, it is reflected in a preventive orientation and by provision of preventive services such as topical fluorides or dental sealants. At the community level, public policies and regulations, such as for community water fluoridation, may be instituted.

Self-Care Behaviors

Tooth brushing and use of fluoride dentifrice are nearly universal in the United States and many other industrialized countries, yet frequent brushing provides no assurance of efficient cleaning (Gift, 1986). Other self-care measures, such as flossing, therapeutic mouth rinses, and other fluoride products, are less frequently used (Gift, 1986; Gift, Corbin, & Nowjack-Raymer, 1994). Optimal oral health is usually correlated with the receipt of adequate oral hygiene instruction from dental care professionals and of brushing assistance and instruction from parents (Blinkhorn, 1993; Gift, 1986). No data provide a clear indication of whether oral hygiene behaviors emanate from oral health motivation alone or derive from socially acceptable norms.

In a variety of studies, a complex of individual attitudes, beliefs, and attributed meanings, as well as lifestyle, behavioral, social, and cultural factors, are associated with these self-care behaviors and ultimately with oral health status (Frazier & Horowitz, 1995; Gift, 1986). Many approaches have been tested to encourage or enhance oral hygiene behaviors, with short-term successes. Perhaps because of the diversity of related factors or the difficulty in conducting longitudinal trials, few behavioral interventions have demonstrated sustained, long-term success.

There is a considerable history of research on preventive behaviors in dentistry beginning with large surveys that captured data on knowledge, attitudes, and behaviors in the 1950s and 1960s (Richards & Cohen, 1971). These early surveys reflected the state of the science, with a focus on tooth brushing, use of fluoride, and care of dentures. During these time periods, several important observations were made: General oral health education alone is insufficient to improve preventive behaviors; positive attitudes toward oral health do not necessarily translate to appropriate behaviors, but need to be considered in terms of an individual's social and psychological characteristics and motivations; uniform approaches might not be appropriate to change oral health behaviors; interventions with rewards can have negative results for compliance with new preventive habits if the reward rather than the behavior is the driving force; and past behaviors, social support in primary social groups, and pervasive social norms (e.g., oral health is not a life-or-death issue) may outweigh perceived susceptibility and seriousness in decisions about oral health behaviors. These basic premises still prevail and form the foundations of many intervention studies (Tedesco, Keffer, Davis, & Christersson, 1992).

Habits and behaviors are difficult to change if they require the individual to assume an active, continuous role, if they are part of a larger complex of habits or behaviors, or if they are difficult or intrusive. An appropriate home self-care program is difficult to achieve, being time-consuming and intrusive and requiring action, persistence, and attention to detail. Behaviors that are to be pursued long-term and with long-range outcomes are inherently more problematic, resulting in noncompliance, and are more difficult to observe than are behaviors with positive, immediate, and certain outcomes.

Dental professionals have been slow to acknowledge that oral hygiene practices are complex and require much reinforcement and too ready to assume that single training sessions are sufficient. Studies of oral hygiene interventions illustrate that regardless of approach, if more time is spent on instructing in oral hygiene, there are more sustained improvements (Nowjack-Raymer et al., 1995). Almost all dentists report providing regular oral hygiene education to all or most of their patients, yet the public more often reports little instruction from the dentist, perhaps reflecting different perspectives on the amount of time spent on, or the absence of individualized attention to, instruction (Gift, 1986, 1991b, 1993).

Research on oral health behaviors has focused on developing knowledge, motivation, and skills. Many of the strategies to alter self-care behaviors are applied in the dental office, and it is in that environment that the research on behavior change and compliance has been conducted.

Dental Visits

Access. Dental visits are the most frequently studied behavior in dentistry. During the 1980s, between 55% and 57% of the United States population visited a dentist in a 12-month period. Despite increases in dental utilization since 1964, socioeconomic differences in use persist (White, 1994). Those individuals with the fewest resources and the lowest utilization rates are the same groups who have experienced the most disease. In 1989, African-Americans, Hispanics, persons with low educational attainment, and members of low-income families were less likely to have had a dental visit during the past year when compared to whites, non-Hispanics, persons with high educational attainment, and those in higher-income families. Dentate status influences dental visits more than does socioeconomic status and appears to be the basis of attitudes that affect visit behaviors (Petersen & Holst, 1995; White, 1994).

Many reasons are given for not visiting a dentist. The relative impact of the complex of influencing factors appears to have changed over the past decades. The decline in dental caries and tooth loss, improvements in dental restorative treatment techniques, and the presence of dental insurance have been significant factors in these changes. For example, in the 1950s, hopelessness regarding teeth was a reason for not visiting the dentist—a response that would not be given today. With improvements in oral health and techniques to treat diseases, fear and poor attitudes toward dental care have declined. With increased numbers of dentists and availability of dental insurance, limited access and cost are less significant factors, but improved accessibility or reduced cost alone does not increase dental visits. Similarly, when payment for dental services is provided through public programs, dental utilization does not increase dramatically. Factors most commonly associated with dental care utilization continue to be related to a combination of perceived need (observed symptoms, presence of teeth), culture (ethnicity, race), knowledge of the oral health care system (education, ethnicity, routine source of care), ability to pay (insurance, public program, income, size of family), physical limitation (transportation, location, disabilities, age), characteristics of the system (practice styles, fees), lifestyle, and attitudes (toward oral health, dentists) (Petersen & Holst, 1995; Syrjala, Knuuttila, & Syrjala, 1994; ter Horst & de Wit, 1993).

Going to a dentist in a given year provides no information on pattern of care. A regular pattern of dental care appears to increase the likelihood that a person will receive primary care, e.g., exposure to oral hygiene instruction and professionally provided preventive services. Approximately one half of the United States population has a regular pattern of care (visit in the past 2 years for a checkup or preventive purpose and a routine source of care). Persons with resources (as measured by more years of education and an ability to pay for care), an attitude of self-efficacy, with no perceived symptoms, and who are dentate are more likely to have a regular pattern of care (Attwood, West, & Blinkhorn, 1993; Newman & Gift, 1992; Syrjala et al., 1994).

What actually happens during a dental visit is even more important in understanding oral health behaviors. It is in the dental operatory that individuals become patients.

Nature of a Dental Visit. While there is little doubt that the diagnostic and therapeutic procedures conducted in the dental office represent a class of professional behaviors, what actually happens during dental visits (the behaviors of the dental professional and the patient) is not frequently studied. Most procedures occur in the privacy of the dental office, and the prevailing philosophy is that individuals are not able to self-report information about services provided. Most people assess their experiences with dentists as satisfactory (Andersen et al., 1995; Petersen & Holst, 1995), yet when the interactions are observed in the research setting, the treatment process is evaluated less positively.

The provision of preventive dental services in dental offices has increased dramatically over the past several decades. In 1957, only 20% of dentists were considered highly preventive, using topical fluorides, prophylaxes, x-rays, lab tests for dental caries, and a recall system (Gift & Milton, 1975). By 1982, substantially more dentists employed hygienists, and 54% of dentists reported being highly preventive, providing diet and nutrition counseling, plaque control and fluoride education, prophylaxes, dental sealants, and topical fluoride applications. Approximately three-fourths of dentists perceive a problem with patient compliance with oral hygiene education, rather than any shortcoming in the time devoted to patient education or their own instructional skills (Gift, 1986).

Despite the reported provision of these preventive services, the extent and appropriateness of their use for specific patients are unknown. For example, in addition to information on teeth, dental records should include information on medications, social habits, periodontal conditions, and informed consent (Workshop on Quality Assurance in Dentistry, 1994); yet there is little evidence that such complete records are kept. Also, periodontal examinations and reinforcement advice to patients about taking care of their gums are provided less than necessary to improve oral hygiene behaviors and oral health status. All too often, preventive education and topical fluoride applications are provided without regard to individual patient needs and in fact are often provided to those with the least need. Also,

despite evidence of effectiveness, the use of dental sealants as a preventive strategy dependent on provider behavior remains low (Frazier & Horowitz, 1995; Gift et al., 1994).

Research on dentists' treatment decisions has documented significant variation in the diagnosis and treatment of oral diseases (Bader & Shugars, 1992). Patient factors—such as risk for disease, preferences for alternative treatments, age, dental insurance status, and care-seeking behavior—and dentist factors—including preferences for alternative treatments, beliefs about the effectiveness of preventive and restorative therapies, clinical skills, style of practice (preventive versus restorative orientation), and past clinical experiences—are important components of the decision process. Dentists vary in their assessment of the presence of dental caries, in their decision to intervene, and in their selection of which treatment to recommend to the patient (Bader & Shugars, 1992).

Dentist–Patient Interactions. Effective communication facilitates decision making and improves not only patient and dentist understanding and satisfaction with outcome, but also the quality of the work and patient health (Gerbert, Bleecker, & Saub, 1995; Neidle, 1994). In contrast, lack of communication or inappropriate communication may have a negative effect on satisfaction, cooperation, and resolution of problems. Obtaining informed consent, discussing potential outcomes of major procedures, determining need for antibiotics, and assessing interactions of medical–dental conditions and medications are all part of communication (Gift, 1991a).

Theory suggests that cultural expectations, social systems, and social roles are very different for dentists and patients, and these very factors form the basis of the interactions that exist (Parsons, 1951). Traditionally, the dentist has been characterized as active, powerful, and expert, while the patient has been described as passive and cooperative. The dental operatory, in which the patient is in a submissive position with procedures limiting speech and the dentist is in a controlling position with exclusive access to clinical records and verbal communication, supports these traditional roles. These different orientations set the stage for inappropriate use of influence and power on the part of the dentist or apathy on the part of the patient and for consequent lack of communication and less than desirable treatment outcomes.

Realizing that communication is important is one issue, but facilitating communication is another issue. With a focus on technical expertise, a dentist often believes that interactions with the patient are based on common sense or are less important to successful treatment. Often, dentists lack interviewing skills, miscalculate how much information should be transferred, have difficulty detecting and resolving problems with patient cooperation, and have few skills in interpreting nonverbal behaviors. Dentists do not make the best use of written communications in the form of records and history taking, nor do they devote time to developing behavioral skills. Dentists are often equally unaware of how communication and behavioral principles extend to working with staff: interviewing prospective employees, reviewing their performance, evaluating interaction with patients, and general professional interactions (Silversin, 1989).

Dentists must recognize and deal with their own personal characteristics and emotions. One of the most important characteristics is being a good listener, which in turn translates into warmth, empathy, and respect for the patient (Gift, 1991a; Weinstein, 1984). Defensive, placatory, and conciliatory behaviors are vestiges of inappropriately expressed power and do not facilitate positive dentist–patient interactions. A dentist's own health is affected by poor communication. For example, a dentist's stress goes up with anxious patients and the appointment consequently takes more time. A patient whose expectations were not assessed is more likely to return with a complaint about a treatment than a patient whose expectations were identified and addressed (Silversin, 1989).

Dentists' ability to deal with their own and their patients' emotions and anxiety is a valuable asset. It is also important that dentists learn the effective use of the range of communication distances—personal, social, public—in a care situation in which the professional relationship necessitates intrusion on personal space in a social, public setting (Silverstein, 1989; Weinstein, 1984). For example, touching the patient on the shoulder can improve the dentist–patient relationship. This issue has not been examined, however, in the more recent environment of concerns about child or sexual abuse.

Patients often do not initiate interactions, express interests, provide information, or describe all symptoms, any of which would help the dentist determine potential expectations or compliance with recommendations. All too often, the dentist blames the patient for an inappropriate attitude, silence, or unreasonable expectations, but has done little to facilitate involvement. Rather than examine the patient side of the communication equation in isolation, one should also consider the dentist's response to the patient (Rouse & Hamilton, 1991; Silversin, 1989).

Assuring compliance by patients with oral hygiene and treatment instructions is often cited as a major justification for improved dentist–patient communication (Croucher, 1993). Dental professionals need to be specifically trained in ways to encourage acceptance of instructions and to alter nonresponsiveness. It is essential that dentists and their staff have perceptions and behaviors that incorporate sufficient time to instruct and reward patients, using appropriate information and behavior modification approaches. Compliance with oral hygiene and other recommendations is an often-studied topic in dentistry, and many conceptual models have been tested (Blinkhorn, 1993). It is perhaps this focus on patient compliance, which implies a superior–subordinate relationship rather than collaboration, that has reduced successes in cooperation.

Oral health education is particularly dependent on dentist–patient interaction and cooperative interaction. Oral health education needs to be conducted in a favorable environment and to be made relevant to individual patients with regard to prevailing norms in their lifestyle (Blinkhorn, 1993). Communication and education regarding oral hygiene appear not to be associated with patient need or risk, and dental health professionals often are more involved with compliant patients with less disease (Frazier & Horowitz, 1995).

Patient acceptance of preventive and treatment regimens and satisfaction with dental experience can be improved with a variety of approaches (Corah, 1988). Many strategies have been tested, including recorded relaxation instructions and active distraction (e.g., video games). Beyond specific techniques, characteristics of the dentists (listening skills, empathy, friendliness, calmness, competence, avoidance of generalizations, and stereotypes) improve communication, resulting in increased compliance (Corah, 1988).

Community Preventive Behaviors

A major component of health behavior research in dentistry is the intersection of individual, professional, and community behaviors. Health care policies—as represented by laws, regulations, and official actions—and mass media communications, are behaviors at the society level and are important in determining knowledge of, availability of, access to, and acceptance of preventive strategies. Supportive or adversarial actions of individual advocates, health professionals, the corporate private sector, the press, and public officials constitute behaviors that can influence oral health decisions of individuals or groups.

Oral health can be improved if dental professionals work with peers, within their professional organizations, with other oral health professionals, with other health professionals, and in communities to influence policies, laws, and regulations (Drury & Snowden, 1995; Reisine, 1993; Silversin, 1989). Career satisfaction has been shown to improve with professional and community involvement (Reisine, 1993). Unfortunately,

this involvement is not always encouraged or facilitated in schools of the health professionals, and few dentists are trained in community organization methods and techniques for carrying out community oral health promotion programs. Consequently, the dentist is ill prepared to participate effectively.

With fluoridation of public water supplies, oral health offers a unique experiment in health behaviors at the community level (Frazier & Horowitz, 1995). Behavioral research on water fluoridation helped to demonstrate the importance of health consumerism in politics, a force not well seen in other areas (e.g., smoking) until later. Research on this public health issue illustrates the complexity of the phenomena, showing how the combination of population characteristics, attitudes, ideologies, social movements, decision-making processes, community leaders, and voting behaviors, among other factors, can influence a community's health behaviors. Behaviors related to the institution of water fluoridation are not dissimilar to other behaviors; e.g., attitudes do not necessarily correlate with behaviors, nor does existence of a technology assure knowledge and use of it.

One of the major outcomes of years of research on oral health behaviors has been the development of extensive programs to educate the public and professions to provide motivation to change behaviors (Croucher, 1993; Frazier & Horowitz, 1995). Years of commercial advertising and marketing of dentifrices and oral hygiene aids with recommendations for brushing with fluoride toothpaste and visiting a dentist regularly have had a considerable impact on oral health in the United States, yet improving knowledge of oral disease symptoms and appropriate approaches to prevention is still a challenge. After decades of normative education, many people do not readily identify the symptoms of oral diseases and cannot recall the purpose of community water fluoridation or specify actions they can take to prevent dental caries, periodontal diseases, or oral cancers (Frazier & Horowitz, 1995; Gift et al., 1994; Horowitz, Nourjah, & Gift,

1995). It appears that the norm to visit the dentist and brush daily are understood, but these behaviors may be influenced by family and peers as much as or more than by health care providers.

Sick Role Behaviors, Anxiety and Fear, and Behavioral Responses to Chronic Conditions

Sick Role Behaviors

In dentistry, sick role behaviors are most commonly exhibited in relation to pain or other chronic conditions, iatrogenic conditions resulting from complex treatments, and compliance with recommendations following surgery or other complex restorative procedures. Such illness behavior is in response to perceived symptoms related to some condition or treatment. Since the oral cavity is the center of multiple nerves, symptoms are frequently manifested as feelings of general pain or discomfort (Bell, 1989; Corah, 1988; Rugh & Lemke, 1984).

Anxiety and Fear

The oral cavity and face are psychologically important to individuals. Fear and anxiety are not uncommon reactions to general discomfort or pain and, in and of themselves, become symptoms and chronic conditions (Corah, 1988). Because individuals cannot see inside their mouths, their perceived or actual control may be limited, leading to increased anxiety and stress. Under such uncertain conditions, people may postpone action, assuming that symptoms will go away, and are highly motivated to seek causal attributions to explain unfamiliar or difficult-to-evaluate symptoms. Such speculations may result in unwarranted inferences and increased fear and distress.

In dentistry, postponement in dealing with a symptom may be encouraged by the perception that the solution will be more painful than the symptom and that no matter when the condition is addressed, the tooth may be lost anyway. Anxiety about visits to a dental care provider and potentially painful dental treatment is socially acceptable and is the topic of many humorists. Often, anxiety or fear is based on perceptions or previous experiences and may have little to do with the current treatment experience. Anxiety, attitudes, and care-seeking behaviors interact. Anxiety often progresses to other symptoms and behaviors: additional anxiety and fear, discomfort and distress, tension resulting in more sensitivity to treatment procedures, and postponement of needed care resulting in even more extensive treatments and more actual discomfort. Individuals with previous painful experiences and perceptions of a dentist's inappropriate behavior are more likely to be anxious and fearful and to report pain (Corah, 1994).

There are cultural, sociodemographic, and psychosocial differences in individual perception and expression of anxiety and stress that make treating these conditions challenging (Corah, 1988). Symptoms of anxiety are more common among females, among individuals who visit the dentist less regularly or need treatment, among those with perceived poor oral health, and among individuals with other psychological attributes, including neurotic behaviors, lack of well-being, indecisiveness, lower self-esteem, and pessimism.

A combination of behavioral approaches to anxiety reduction appears to be the most successful, starting with the most practical, least expensive, and least invasive strategy. Hypnosis, distraction, systematic desensitization, muscular exercise, counseling, contingent aversive reinforcement, pain charting, assertiveness training, general relaxation, biofeedback, self-monitoring, behavioral instructions, cognitive coping training, provision of procedural and sensation information, modeling, and habit reversal have been used successfully with selected patients (Corah, 1988). Therapy may require selection from a variety of alternate approaches suitable to the patient.

Dentists are often less than confident in understanding and managing anxiety (Corah, 1988).

The role of auxiliary personnel is important, but dentists may be less than sure about facilitating this role because of lack of training in working with team members on other than technical clinical activities. Despite the reported inadequacy of these skills, training in both pharmaceuticals and behavioral techniques for anxiety and pain reduction remains insufficient in most dental schools (Dionne & Gift, 1988; Gift, 1991a).

Behavioral Responses to Chronic Conditions

Essentially, all oral diseases are chronic, but with appropriate treatment and supportive behaviors and environments, outcomes are considered as healthy rather than as persistent chronic conditions. Some oral habits such as bruxism (spasmodic grinding of the teeth in other than chewing movements) or thumb sucking may lead to severe chronic pain and destruction of oral tissue. These habits can be responsive to behavioral interventions, such as patient education and motivation, habit modification, monitoring, stress-reduction activities, and cognitive conditioning, if they are not due to morphological or iatrogenic conditions (Rugh & Lemke, 1984). Oral conditions that are conceptualized as chronic include cleft lip and palate, orofacial pain, and malocclusion.

Pain. Pain is a multifaceted experience involving sensory, cognitive, and emotional dimensions. Pain in the oral cavity is unique, since there are so many nerves in the facial areas. Perceptions of, tolerance of, and response to pain are modified by beliefs, anxiety, personality, culture, and experience, among other factors (Bell, 1989).

It is not uncommon for patients to visit oral health care professionals with complaints of pain for which there are no apparent causes. Evidence suggests that absence of organic pathology does not mean there is no pain, nor does absence of complaints or grimaces mean there is no pain. Expressions of pain influence clinical judgment (Locker & Gruskha, 1987). How the oral care professional treats orofacial pain is largely dependent on the training received in professional school. All too often, that training focused exclusively on the physiological level, approaching pain reduction from the disease model. This approach can result in considerable overtreatment, surgery, and medications for chronic pain conditions. Psychological components are increasingly recognized, particularly when the pain has no defined source. Behavioral scientists have demonstrated that approaches such as distractions, anxiety reduction techniques, patient self-control techniques, relaxation, hypnosis, suggestion, and placebo can be successful in reducing chronic orofacial pain (Dionne & Gift, 1988).

Malocclusion. Whether or not the occlusion of teeth is defined as malocclusion is in large part driven by cultural, social, peer, and family norms. Scales have been developed to evaluate perceptions of self and others in terms of need for orthodontic care or aesthetics, neither of which is directly related to function. It appears that malocclusion has more psychosocial impact than other oral conditions, and that orthodontic treatments to alter malocclusions have more impact on dental facial aesthetics and self-esteem than on general health or clinical function (Albino, 1984; Cons et al., 1994).

Malocclusion may affect psychosocial functioning: Unattractive orofacial appearance may have debilitating social and psychological consequences; children with severe malocclusion often may suffer from teasing and harassment; some individuals may translate negative feedback into withdrawal, isolation, depression, or other psychological and behavior responses; and perceptions may drive care seeking more than actual biological malocclusion, on the part of both the parent and the child (Albino, 1984).

Adherence to regimens (compliance) has been examined among orthodontic patients. Patients (mostly adolescents) who are the most compliant with orthodontic recommendations (office visits, wearing appliances, and self-care) have been identified as highly motivated, treated by well-trained dentists, having adequate oral health status, perceiving the value of treatment, being cognitively competent, having some knowledge of oral health, having nonfearful parents with positive attitudes, and being privately insured. No one study has examined comprehensively all of these factors; there remains considerable disagreement concerning which are the most important factors (Albino, 1984; ter Horst & de Wit, 1993). The patient is often "blamed" for noncompliance. Few studies have examined the role of dental professionals in assuring appropriate patient responsiveness.

Self-Destructive Behaviors

Oral health is seldom associated with self-destructive behaviors, yet certain such behaviors can lead to death or seriously complicating medical conditions. Just as tobacco use, excessive use of alcohol, inappropriate diet, absence of protective devices, and occupational hazards drive much of the research agenda for destructive behavior in health, these same factors are critical in the dental care environment.

Smoking and Alcohol

Approaches in general health for altering tobacco and alcohol use behaviors (described elsewhere in this *Handbook*) and excessive exposure to the sun have been applied using oral outcomes such as oral cancer, other soft tissue lesions, and periodontal diseases. The level of knowledge regarding risk factors for oral cancer is exceptionally low (Horowitz et al., 1995). Oral cancers occur many years after the implicated behaviors began, making it more difficult to establish relevance in behavior change programs. Conversely, periodontal conditions and other soft tissue lesions are observable more quickly and have been used in clinical and educational settings to illustrate the impact of tobacco use (Mecklenburg et al., 1990).

Advice and counseling from health care professionals are helpful in cessation efforts, yet oral health care professionals have limited training in cessation techniques. Nearly all dentists believe they should be good role models, as well as help patients quit, yet they are less certain of appropriate strategies (Severson, Eakin, Stevens, & Lichtenstein, 1990). Few oral health care providers track tobacco and alcohol use in medical histories or provide specific counseling on these behaviors in relation to oral health (Horowitz et al., 1995).

Behaviors at the social level make a difference in risk factors for tobacco use. A major public health initiative was undertaken with major league baseball to reduce the media exposure of children to sports heros who use chewing tobacco (National Institute of Dental Research, 1994). This application of role theory has resulted in a considerable reduction of media exposure to this life-threatening behavior.

Occupational Hazards

Serious consequences may result from unsafe practices in dental offices. Inappropriate professional behaviors, such as handling mercury-containing dental amalgam (filling material) and other hazardous materials in the dental operatory, may affect the professionals' biological processes. Long-term exposure of dental personnel to trace anesthetics, resulting from inappropriate use in dental procedures, is associated with increased general health problems such as neurological diseases and spontaneous abortions (Neidle, 1994; Gerbert, Bleecker, & Saub, 1995).

Dental professionals are at risk for contracting and spreading infectious diseases through contact with bodily fluids (hepatitis B, HIV) or airborne microorganisms (tuberculosis, respiratory diseases, colds). Behaviors related to office procedures have changed over the past decade to accommodate minimum safety guidelines: vaccinations and revaccinations for hepatitis B, improved sterilization procedures, new equipment, increased use of disposable materials, and increased use of body protection, e.g., gloves, masks, and glasses. In comparison to the introduction of other technologies, the acceptance of infection control was rapid, in part due to extensive professional education programs and imposed regulations, but largely attributed to the threat to the dentist's livelihood when patients perceived that precautions were not being taken to protect the transmission of diseases. Yet this process was not as readily accomplished as might be expected, given the life-threatening nature of some of the diseases (Neidle, 1994).

The impact of HIV/AIDS on dental practices has been examined extensively (Gerbert, 1989; Kunzel & Sadowsky, 1993). A 1990 survey of general dentists in the United States illustrates the concerns expressed about treating patients with HIV/AIDS (Kunzel & Sadowsky, 1993). Nearly one third of the dentists surveyed did not believe that HIV/AIDS patients could be treated safely in dental offices. The highest levels of perceived risk were attributed to needle sticks (75%) and being bitten (45%). Differences in levels of perceived risks are predicted largely by concerns for the economic viability of the practice, perceptions of ethical obligations to threat these patients, and experiences with HIV/AIDS patients. These justifications are not very different from considerations given in decisions to care for other subgroups of the population, such as those who cannot pay for services.

Continued inappropriate behaviors with potential occupational risks result from inadequate knowledge on the part of the dental professional, lack of attention to regulations and guidelines for practice, and insufficient sterilizing and scavenging techniques (Neidle, 1994). Many factors, including irrational fear of disease, denial of personal responsibility, and expense of altering practice procedures, have resulted in less than universal use of these protection procedures (Diehnelt, 1993) and continued need for education of dental personnel and patients.

Occupational Stress

The impact of occupational stress on dental professionals has received considerable attention in the mass media and in research (Gerbert, Bleecker, & Saub, 1994; Gerbert et al., 1995; Gift, 1977; Richards & Cohen, 1971). Historically, dentists have been rated reasonably high among oc-

cupations by the public on characteristics such as prestige, skill, and fairness, yet many people express some discomfort about going to a dentist (Richards & Cohen, 1971). This public image of going to a dentist appears to cause some dissonance and stress within the profession (Gift, 1977; Richards & Cohen, 1971). As a result of these public/patient perceptions and pressure associated with delivering dental care, the media have reported perceptions that dentists are more inclined to general malaise, depression, and suicide. Dentists themselves believe their occupation is stressful, the major sources for this belief being lack of patient cooperation, pain and anxiety of patients, interpersonal relations, lack of respect received for being a dentist, lack of control of treatment environment, process of delivering care, level of income, amount of personal time, physical strain, economic pressures, third-party constraints, and perfectionism (Gerbert et al., 1995; Humphris & Peacock, 1993). Rather, available data indicate that dentists do not experience more stress than do other professionals and that they commit suicide at about the same rate as the average white male in the United States (Gift, 1977). Despite efforts to alter this belief and counter erroneous mass media messages, the myth continues to prevail.

SPECIAL POPULATIONS

More and more, the dental professional needs to be involved in the provision of comprehensive medical care and social services to patients. Oral manifestations of medical conditions and dental treatment of special care patients constitute major links between medical and dental care professionals.

Medically Compromised Individuals

Among the major reasons for examining the dentist's diagnostic and treatment decision behaviors are the oral symptoms and conditions associated with underlying medical or handicapping conditions, ranging from very rare genetic diseases to congenital anomalies to compromised immune systems to more common chronic diseases such as arthritis and diabetes. These symptoms and conditions include severe facial deformity, limited mouth opening, high risk of fracture, limited ability to chew and swallow, reduction in essential body fluids, and secondary infections, among others. The individuals who are at high risk for medically compromising conditions are all too often the same ones who receive less dental care. This situation results in a risk, unmeasured but assumed to be high, of oral complications because of limited access to dental care. Among persons with compromised immune systems, the presence of oral diseases has been linked to opportunistic infections, oral complications, and compromised nutritional status (Feigal, 1991; Gift, 1988).

Routine dental examinations can play an important role in initial diagnosis of chronic diseases and opportunistic infections as well as in the management, care, and referral of special care populations. But much of dentists' current orientation, as well as their positions in the medical and social system, limit their contributions. It appears that the separation of the medical and dental systems hinders patients from receiving full and appropriate treatment for many chronic and handicapping conditions.

Chronically Ill

With an increasingly older population and encouragement of chronically ill persons to remain active, many ambulatory persons are on multiple medications. These persons seek dental care, and dentists' appreciation of pharmacology and drug interactions affects their care. Dental schools need to ensure that students move from the focus on didactic information to clinical experiences with pharmaceuticals. Because of constant changes, dental professionals need to engage in formal continuing education on pharmaceuticals in relation to dental procedures (Dionne & Gift, 1988).

Prophylaxes and antibiotics are being used to prevent infective endocarditis among at-risk patients undergoing dental surgeries (Gould & Buckingham, 1993). Appropriate behaviors on the part of dentists require that they know the association between dental procedures and infective endocarditis and be informed that the patient is at risk. Similarly, individuals with prosthetic joints are at risk for joint infections from oral bacteria if dental care is provided without antibiotics (Tsevat, Durand-Zaleski, & Pauker, 1989). Oral complications of radiation, chemotherapy, and bone marrow transplants for cancer patients require specific approaches to oral hygiene and dental treatment (Lockhart & Clark, 1994).

HIV/AIDS Patients

Oral symptoms are among the first signs of HIV infection, and regular oral examinations are particularly important (Feigal, 1991). The care-seeking patterns of HIV-infected individuals change, however, because of the perceived attitudes of dental personnel, concerns about confidentiality, or refusal of treatment by dentists (Robinson, Zakrzewska, Maini, Williamson, & Croucher, 1994). Common behaviors are to refrain from revealing HIV status, change dentists, or avoid seeking dental care.

Older Adults

The increasing number of older adults has provided many research challenges. Throughout life, individuals have been exposed to a variety of lifestyle, environmental, and health risks, resulting in a range of oral health status in the older age group (Gift, 1988; Kiyak, 1993; Schou, 1995). For example, use of tobacco and alcohol over a lifetime has a progressive impact on oral health status, specifically soft tissue lesions and oral cancer. Behaviors set in values established 50–60 years ago are challenges to address.

Edentulism (toothlessness) is more common among older adults and though it is declining, remains a critical concern in addressing oral health behaviors. Typically, edentulous people do not visit a dentist regularly despite potential problems with ill-fitting dentures and related lesions, oral cancer, medications or systemic diseases, limited saliva flow, or poor oral hygiene.

Interventions using behavioral approaches in institutional and community settings have provided both short- and long-term improvements in oral health among older adults. These adaptations of behavioral approaches to specific cognitive and physical skills of older adults in alternative settings will help determine which strategies, or what combination of strategies, will alter attitudes and behaviors and reduce and prevent oral diseases (Kiyak, 1993).

Disabled Patients

Historically, dentistry has been relatively nonresponsive to care for the disabled. Problems in dealing with disabled patients are associated with lack of experience and knowledge of treatment (Russell & Kinirons, 1993). Perceived patient behavior problems, locations of patient — institutions, homebound — and finances are the basis of the disparity. It is difficult for these patients to schedule appointments in the fixed dental private practice; private dental offices provide little physical accommodation for disabled individuals; concerns exist regarding treatment planning, consent to care, and consultation with caregivers; and dentists have historically had limited affiliations with formal social and health care professionals who treat these patients (Soto-Rojas & Cushing, 1992).

Young Children

Dental visits are uncommon among children under the age of 2. Oral hygiene, use of fluoride, and dietary habits are a function of the parent's knowledge and behaviors, advice received from friends and neighbors, commercial messages, and physicians. Assuring appropriate combinations of therapies is a challenge (Nowjack-Raymer & Gift, 1990). Neither parents nor physicians may

have sufficient knowledge regarding multiple regimens of fluoride, particularly using dietary fluorides in areas with community water fluoridation or problems with ingesting toothpaste. Additionally, many parents and physicians have limited knowledge about the impact on severe infant caries of insufficient fluorides, nutrition, and poor dietary habits of the mother and child (Nourjah, Horowitz, & Wagener, 1994).

When children do start visiting a dentist, many factors affect the success of the visit. Because of social, family, and medical conditions, some children have been inadequately socialized for experiences in the dental office. Often, these children are defined as problem patients, and inappropriate communications between the dentist and patient result in long-term avoidance of appropriate dental care (Blinkhorn, 1993).

There is an extensive literature on the interaction of dentists with pediatric patients, particularly problem children (Allen, Loiben, Allen, & Stanley, 1992; Weinstein, 1984). Many times, these children are treated as anxious or fearful patients, when in fact they may be uncomfortable with their role in the dentist–patient interaction. Therapeutic control mechanisms such as nitrous oxide and hypnosis have been used extensively with problem children. Various behavioral approaches have been tried over the years, ranging from hand-over-mouth restraint to loud voice commands to distraction. No support has been found for a punitive approach, and mixed results have been found using rewards and sedation with problem children.

The typical dental office is not well suited to many of the techniques tested with problem children. Most dentists will not have a large number of such children as patients and would therefore not be justified in organizing their practices to accommodate those who do visit. Many dentists have only limited training using nitrous oxide, and the typical private dental office is not environmentally suited for the use of this approach. Approaches with more child involvement and respect, such as modeling, empathy, some physical contact, and conversations with the child, have been emphasized since the mid-1980s (Weinstein, 1984).

RESEARCH ISSUES

Over the past two decades, the oral health status of the United States population has improved dramatically. Dental caries rates have declined, particularly among schoolchildren. Among adults, the number of teeth lost has declined, and the percentage of individuals having lost all their teeth has decreased. In part, these improvements are the result of preventive behaviors at the personal, professional, and community levels. More people are brushing and flossing, and the use of dentifrices containing fluoride is almost universal. Preventive procedures, including education, comprise a greater proportion of all services provided in the dental office. Water fluoridation, seat belt use, warning labels on smokeless tobacco products, and protective sports equipment contribute to oral health at the community level.

Despite these advances, significant challenges remain for the dental profession to ensure that these improvements are realized by all segments of the population. Increased life expectancy and greater tooth retention places many people at risk for oral diseases for more years. Individuals and groups with extensive oral diseases or challenging life situations require special attention to benefit from preventive and therapeutic strategies. Special categories of patients, such as the aged, the medically, physically, or mentally challenged, the socioeconomically disadvantaged, and minorities, have differential expressions of oral diseases. Access to, availability of, and acceptability of dental services are critical barriers that need to be identified for many of these individuals and addressed in dental education and practice.

The role of social, ethnic, racial, geographic, age, and other sociobehavioral differences in values placed on oral health and care-seeking behaviors must be better understood by dental professionals. While dentists are trained to recognize diseases and to provide therapeutic care and primary prevention, they are not well trained in approaches that recognize and interpret cognitive or social development, cultural meanings, or situational and social constraints. Since oral diseases, perceptions of need for care, risk factors and behaviors, and the ability to comply with recommended preventive therapies vary across social and environmental conditions and throughout the life span, oral health behaviors cannot be generalized. Approaches to altering behaviors must take these variations into account. The applications of the principles generalized from oral health behavior research suggest targeting to specific groups and their care providers. Current dental education and practice strategies may need to be altered.

Oral health professionals must increase their collaborations with other health and social professionals. Interventions that address all systems and multiple risk behaviors with underlying similarities increase the likelihood of substituting health-enhancing behaviors for risk activities. Notable areas in which collaborations are required are for tobacco cessation, trauma prevention, and complications associated with systemic diseases and medications.

Much of what has been learned in health behavior research can be used by oral health care professionals. Applying this knowledge successfully, however, requires a more complex model of disease and prevention than is typically embraced. Most of what oral health care professionals do to prevent and treat disease is procedure-based and is directed primarily toward the dentition. Dental education focuses on the oral cavity, biological principles, and technical clinical skills. Lesser focus on the interaction among systemic diseases, prevention, and behavioral skills, and the limited experience with patients outside a small operatory, lead to dentists who are ill prepared to effect a productive treatment planning process collaboratively working with the patient or the community. More directive approaches are required in dental schools to enhance the skills needed to optimize public and patient behaviors.

Changes in dental professional behaviors, in education or practice, typically have been accomplished only slowly unless they are regulated or have a considerable impact on livelihood. While health behavior research has improved the understanding of dentist–patient interactions and other critical issues surrounding provision of care, more often than not the research findings have not been applied in professional education, training, or practice. Unfortunately, there is limited understanding of the ways in which dental professionals obtain new information about behaviors and the barriers to the incorporation of this knowledge into clinical practice. Until ways are found to translate research findings into action, few changes in behavioral skills will be seen in the dental profession.

What has been learned in health behavior research must be tested and demonstrated in social and environmental contexts in which oral health behaviors of the public occur and in which professionals are educated, work, and continue to learn. To augment the role of health behavior in improving oral health, additional research is necessary. Expanded conceptual models, improved methodologies, sampling strategies, and analytical approaches are needed to enhance understanding of oral health behavior.

The current debate about dental education is addressing issues that will produce a graduate who has the intellectual, physical, technical, and interpersonal skills to become a competent professional who will continue to develop throughout a career in both the practice and the community. Application of health behavior research can help effect these needed changes.

REFERENCES

Albino, J. E. (1984). Psychosocial aspects of malocclusion. In J. D. Matarazzo, S. M. Weiss, & J. A. Herd (Eds.), *Behavioral health: Handbook of health enhancement and disease prevention* (pp. 918–929). New York: Wiley.

Albino, J. E. N., & Lawrence, S. D. (1993). Promoting oral health in adolescents. In S. G. Millstein, A. C. Petersen, & E. O. Nightingale (Eds.), *Promoting the health of adolescents: New directions for the twenty-first century* (pp. 242–259). New York: Oxford University Press.

Allen, K. D., Loiben, T., Allen, S. J., & Stanley, R. T. (1992). Dentist-implemented contingent escape for management of disruptive child behavior. *Journal of Applied Behavior Analysis, 25*(3), 629–636.

Amstutz, R. D., & Shulman, J. D. (1994). Perceived needs for dental continuing education within the Army dental care system. *Military Medicine, 159*(1), 1–4.

Andersen, R., Marcus, M., & Mahshigan, M. (1995). A comparative systems perspective on oral health promotion and disease prevention. In L. K. Cohen & H. C. Gift (Eds.), *Disease prevention and oral health promotion: Socio-dental sciences in action* (pp. 307–340). Copenhagen: Munksgaard.

Anderson, R. J. & Morgan, J. D. (1992). Marketing dentistry: A pilot study in Dudley. *Community Dental Health, 9*(Supplement 1), 1–220.

Antczak-Bouckoms, A. A., & Tulloch, J. F. C. (1995). Clinical decision analysis. In L. K. Cohen & H. C. Gift (Eds.), *Disease prevention and oral health promotion: Socio-dental sciences in action* (pp. 427–453). Copenhagen: Munksgaard.

Attwood, D., West, P., & Blinkhorn, A. S. (1993). Factors associated with the dental visiting habits of adolescents in the west of Scotland. *Community Dental Health, 10*(4), 365–373.

Bader, J. D., & Shugars, D. A. (1992). Understanding dentists' restorative treatment decisions. *Journal of Public Health Dentistry, 52*(2), 102–110.

Bell, W. E. (1989). *Orofacial pains: Classifications, diagnosis, management,* (4th ed.). Chicago: Year Book Medical Publishers.

Blinkhorn, A. S. (1993). Factors affecting the compliance of patients with preventive dental regimens. *International Dental Journal, 43*(Supplement 1), 294–298.

Chen, M-s. (1995). Oral health of disadvantaged populations. In L. K. Cohen & H. C. Gift (Eds.), *Disease prevention and oral health promotion: Socio-dental sciences in action* (pp. 153–212). Copenhagen: Munksgaard.

Cohen, L. K. & Bryant, P. S. (Eds.) (1984). *Social sciences in dentistry: A critical bibliography: Vol. II.* London: Quintessence Publishing for the Federation Dentaire Internationale.

Cons, N. C., Jenny, J., Kohout, F. J., Jakobsen, J., Shi, Y., Ying, W. H., & Pakains, G. (1994). Comparing ethnic group-specific DAI equations with the standard DAI. *International Dental Journal, 44*, 153–158.

Corah, N. L. (1988). Dental anxiety: Assessment, reduction, and increasing patient satisfaction. *Dental Clinics of North America, 32*(4), 779–790.

Croucher, F. (1993). General dental practice, health education, and promotion: A critical reappraisal. In L. Schou & A. S. Blinkhorn (Eds.), *Oral health promotion* (pp. 153-168). New York: Oxford University Press.

Diehnelt, D. E. (1993). The cost of infection control in dental clinics: A comprehensive case study. *Compendium of Continuing Education in Dentistry*, *14*(10), 1329-1335.

Dionne, R. A., & Gift, H. C. (1988). Drugs used for parenteral sedation in dental practice. *Anesthesia Progress*, *35*, 199-205.

Drury, T. F. & Snowden, C. B. (1995). Community oral health promotion: Organizational, methodological, and statistical issues. In L. K. Cohen & H. C. Gift (Eds.), *Disease prevention and oral health promotion: Socio-dental sciences in action* (pp. 505-584). Copenhagen: Munksgaard.

Feigal, D. W. (1991). The prevalence of oral lesions in HIV-infected homosexual and bisexual men: Three San Francisco epidemiological cohorts. *AIDS*, *5*, 519-525.

Frazier, P. J. & Horowitz, A. M. (1995). Prevention: A public health perspective. In L. K. Cohen & H. C. Gift (Eds.), *Disease prevention and oral health promotion: Socio-dental sciences in action* (pp. 109-152). Copenhagen: Munksgaard.

Gerbert, B. (1989). The impact of AIDS on dental practice: Update 1989. *Journal of Dental Education*, *53*(9), 529-530.

Gerbert, B., Bleecker, T., & Saub, E. (1994). Dentists and the patients who love them: Professional and patient views of dentistry. *Journal of the American Dental Association*, *125*(3), 264-272.

Gerbert, B., Bleecker, T., & Saub E. (1995). Risk perception and risk communication: Benefits of dentist-patient discussions. *Journal of the American Dental Association*, *126*, 333-339.

Gift, H. C. (1977). The occupation of dentistry: Its relation to illness and death: A review of and comment on published research. *Journal of the American Dental Association*, *95*, 606-613.

Gift, H. C. (1986), Current utilization patterns of oral hygiene practices: State-of-the-science review. In H. Löe & D. V. Kleinman (Eds.), *Dental plaque control measure and oral hygiene practices* (pp. 39-71). Oxford: IRL Press.

Gift, H. C. (1988). Issues of aging and oral health promotion. *Gerodontics*, *4*, 194-206.

Gift, H. C. (1991a). Issues to consider in the control of acute pain, fear and anxiety. In R. A. Dionne & J. C. Phero (Eds.), *Management of pain and anxiety in dental practice* (pp. 1-15). New York: Elsevier.

Gift, H. C. (1991b). Prevention of oral diseases and oral health promotion. *Current Opinion in Dentistry*, *1*, 337-347.

Gift, H. C. (1993). Social factors in oral health promotion. In L. Schou & A. S. Blinkhorn (Eds.), *Oral health promotion* (pp. 65-102). London: Oxford University Press.

Gift, H. C., Corbin, S. B., & Nowjack-Raymer, R. E. (1994). Public knowledge of prevention of dental diseases. *Public Health Reports*, *109*(3), 397-404.

Gift, H. C., Gerbert, B., Kress, G. C., & Reisine, S. T. (1990). Social, economic, and professional dimensions of the oral health care delivery system. *Annals of Behavioral Medicine*, *12*(4), 161-169.

Gift, H. C., & Milton, B. B. (1975, Fall). Comparison of two national preventive dentistry surveys: 1957-1974. *Journal of Preventive Dentistry*, 25-27.

Gould, I. M. & Buckingham, J. K. (1993). Cost effectiveness of prophylaxis in dental practice to prevent infective endocarditis. *British Heart Journal*, *70*(1), 79-83.

Grogono, A. L. & Lancaster, D. M. (1988). Factors influencing dental career choice—A survey of currently-enrolled students and implications for recruitment. *Journal of the American College of Dentists*, *55*(4), 30-35.

Horowitz, A. M., Nourjah, P., & Gift, H. C. (1995). U. S. adult knowledge of risk factors and signs of oral cancers: 1990. *Journal of the American Dental Association*, *126*, 39-45.

Humphris, G. M., & Peacock, L. (1993). Occupational stress and job satisfaction in the community dental service of North Wales: A pilot study. *Community Dental Health*, *10*(1), 73-82.

Jeffcoat, M. K. & Clark, W. B. (1995). Research, technology transfer, and dentistry. *Journal of Dental Education*, *59*(1), 169-184.

Kiyak, H. A. (1993). Age and culture: Influences on oral health behavior. *International Dental Journal*, *43*(1), 9-16.

Kiyak, H. A. & Brudvik, J. (1992). Dental students' self-assessed competence in geriatric dentistry. *Journal of Dental Education*, *56*(11), 728-734.

Krasnegor, N. A., Epstein, L., Johnson, S. B., & Jaffe, S. J. (Eds.). (1993). *Developmental aspects of health compliance behavior*. Hillsdale, NJ: Erlbaum.

Kress, G. C. (1995). Dental education in transition. In L. K. Cohen & H. C. Gift (Eds.), *Disease prevention and oral health promotion: Socio-dental sciences in action* (pp. 387-425). Copenhagen: Munksgaard.

Kunzel, C. & Sadowsky, D. (1993). Predicting dentists' perceived occupational risk for HIV infection. *Social Sciences in Medicine*, *36*(12), 1579-1586.

Locker, D. & Grushka, M. (1987). The impact of dental and facial pain. *Journal of Dental Research*, *66*(9), 1414-1417.

Lockhart, P. B. & Clark, J. (1994). Pretherapy dental status of patients with malignant conditions of the head and neck. *Oral Surgery, Oral Medicine, and Oral Pathology*, *77*(3), 236-241.

Maizels, J., Maizels, A., & Sheiham, A. (1991). Dental disease and health behaviour: The development of an interactional model. *Community Dental Health*, *8*, 340-346.

Mecklenburg, R. E., Christen, A. G., Gerbert, B., Gift, H. C., Glynn, T. J., Jones, R. B., Lindsay, E., Manley, M. W., & Severson, H. (1990). *How to help your patients stop using tobacco*. NIH Publication No. 91-3191. Bethesda, MD: National Cancer Institute.

Mozer, J. E., Lloyd, C., & Puente, E. S. (1990). The relationship of bi/polar personality patterns with self esteem, stress, and satisfaction in dental school. *Journal of Dental Education*, *54*(2), 153–157.

Nash, D. A. (1994). A tension between *two cultures* … Dentistry as a profession and dentistry as proprietary. *Journal of Dental Education*, *58*(4), 301–306.

National Institute of Dental Research. (1994). Office of Communication Activities. *Annual Report of the National Institute of Dental Research*.

Neenan, M. E. Paunovich, E., Solomon, E. S., & Watkins, R. T. (1993). The primary dental care workforce. *Journal of Dental Education*, *57*(12), 863–875.

Neidle, E. A. (1994). Infectious disease in dental practice—Professional opportunities and obligations. *Journal of the American College of Dentists*, *61*(1), 12–17.

Newman, J. F., & Gift, H. C. (1992). Regular pattern of preventive dental services—A measure of access. *Social Sciences in Medicine*, *35*(8), 997–1001.

Nourjah, P., Horowitz, A. M., & Wagener, D. K. (1994). Factors associated with the use of fluoride supplements and fluoride dentifrice by infants and toddlers. *Journal of Public Health Dentistry*, *54*(1), 47–54.

Nowjack-Raymer, R. E., Ainamo, J., Suomi, J. D., Kingman, A., Driscoll, W. S., & Brown, L. J. (1995). Improved periodontal status through self-assessment: A 2-year longitudinal study in teenagers. *Journal of Clinical Periodontology*, *22*, 603–608.

Nowjack-Raymer, R., & Gift, H. C. (1990). Contributing factors to maternal and child oral health. *Journal of Public Health Dentistry*, *50*(6), 370–378.

Parsons, T. (1951). Illness and the role of the physician: A sociological perspective. *American Journal of Orthopsychiatry*, *21*, 452–460.

Petersen, P. E., & Holst, D. (1995). Utilization of dental health services. In L. K. Cohen & H. C. Gift (Eds.), *Disease prevention and oral health promotion: Socio-dental sciences in action* (pp. 341–386). Copenhagen: Munksgaard.

Reisine, S. (1993). The role of the decision maker in oral health promotion. In L. Schou & A. S. Blinkhorn (Eds.), *Oral health promotion* (pp. 103–120). New York: Oxford University Press.

Reisine, S., & Locker, D. (1995). Social, psychological, and economic impacts of oral conditions and treatments. In L. K. Cohen & H. C. Gift (Eds.), *Disease prevention and oral health promotion: Socio-dental sciences in action* (pp. 33–71). Copenhagen: Munksgaard.

Richards, N. D., & Cohen, L. K. (Eds.) (1971). *Social sciences and dentistry: A critical bibliography*. The Hague, Netherlands: A Sijthoff for the Federation Dentaire Internationale.

Robinson, P., Zakrzewska, J. M., Maini, M., Williamson, D., & Croucher, R. (1994). Dental visiting behaviour and experiences of men with HIV. *British Dental Journal*, *176*(5), 175–179.

Rouse, R. A., & Hamilton, M. A. (1991). Dentists evaluate their patients: An empirical investigation of preferences. *Journal of Behavioral Medicine*, *14*(6), 637–648.

Rugh, J. D., & Lemke, R. R. (1984). Significance of oral habits. In J. D. Matarazzo, S. M. Weiss, J. A. Herd, & N. E. Miller (Eds.), *Behavioral health: Handbook of health enhancement and disease prevention* (pp. 947–966). New York: Wiley.

Russell, G. M., & Kinirons, M. J. (1993). The attitudes and experience of community dental officers in North Ireland in treating disabled people. *Community Dental Health*, *10*(4), 327–333.

Schou, L. (1995). Oral health, oral health care, and oral health promotion among older adults: Social and behavioral dimensions. In L. K. Cohen & H. C. Gift (Eds.), *Disease prevention and oral health promotion: Socio-dental sciences in action* (pp. 213–270). Copenhagen: Munksgaard.

Severson, H. H., Eakin, E. G., Stevens, V. J., & Lichtenstein, E. (1990). Dental office practices for tobacco users: Independent practice and HMO clinics. *American Journal of Public Health*, *80*(12), 1503–1505.

Silversin, J. (1989). Communicating with each other. *International Dental Journal*, *39*(4), 258–262.

Soto-Rojas, A. E., & Cushing, A. (1992). Assessment of the need for education and/or training in the dental care of people with handicaps. *Community Dental Health*, *9*(2), 165–170.

Stiefel, D. J., & Truelove, E. L. (1995). A postgraduate dental training program for treatment of persons with disabilities. *Journal of Dental Education*, *49*(2), 85–90.

Stilwell, N. A., & Reisine, S. (1992). Using patient-instructors to teach and evaluate interviewing skills. *Journal of Dental Education*, *56*(2), 118–122.

Syrjala, A. M., Knuuttila, M. L., & Syrjala, L. K. (1994). Obstacles to regular dental care related to extrinsic and intrinsic motivation. *Community Dentistry and Oral Epidemiology*, *22*(4), 269–272.

Tay, K. M., Winn, W., Milgrom, P., & Hann, J. (1993). The effect of instruction on dentists' motivation to manage fearful patients. *Journal of Dental Education*, *57*(6), 444–448.

Tedesco, L. A. (1995). Issues in dental curriculum development and change. *Journal of Dental Education*, *59*(1), 97–147.

Tedesco, L. A., Keffer, M. A., Davis, E. L., & Christersson, L. A. (1992). Effect of a social cognitive intervention on oral health status, behavior reports, and cognitions. *Journal of Periodontology*, *63*(7), 567–575.

ter Horst, G., & de Wit, C. A. (1993). Review of behavioural research in dentistry 1987–1992: Dental anxiety, dentist-patient relationship, compliance and dental attendance. *International Dental Journal*, *43*(3 Supplement 1), 265–278.

Tsevat, J., Duran-Zaleski, I., & Pauker, S. G. (1989). Cost-effectiveness of antibiotic prophylaxis for dental procedures in patients with artificial joints. *American Journal of Public Health*, *79*, 739–743.

Weinstein, P. (1984). Influence of dentist variables on patient behavior: Managing child behavior in the operatory. In J. D. Matarazzo, S. M. Weiss, J. A. Herd, & N. E. Miller (Eds.), *Behavioral health: Handbook of health enhancement and disease prevention* (pp. 930–946). New York: Wiley.

White, B. A. (1994). An overview of oral health status, re-sources, and care delivery. *Journal of Dental Education, 58*(4), 285–290.

Workshop on Quality Assurance in Dentistry. (1994). Model clinical guidelines for primary dental health care providers for managing patients with adult periodontitis. *Journal of Dental Education, 58*(8), 659–662.

8

Relevance of Health Behavior Research to Health Promotion and Health Education

Karen Glanz and Brian Oldenburg

INTRODUCTION

Many professionals who work in health promotion and health education would agree that health behavior research is a core foundation for both research and practice. In fact, it has been suggested that "the central concern of health education is health behavior" (Glanz, Lewis, & Rimer, 1990, p. 9). If this is so, then the short answer to the question of whether health behavior research is relevant to health promotion and health education is simple: It is highly relevant, pervasive, and almost always woven into work in the field. This short answer, however, does not convey a complex story very well. Health promotion and health education are eclectic, rapidly evolving, and reflect a conglomeration of approaches, methods, and strategies from social and health sciences.

The purpose of this chapter is to examine how concepts, methods, and findings from health behavior research influence health promotion and health education. Three domains of health promotion and health education are examined: professional training, practice, and research. The analysis of each area draws on relevant research literature, published policy and viewpoint statements, and the authors' personal experiences over two decades of teaching, research, and practice in health promotion and health education.

Because this examination is a broad, challenging, and sometimes controversial task, we first wish to acknowledge our limitations and biases. One author (KG) completed her graduate training in a department of health behavior and health education; the other (BO) completed his graduate work in clinical psychology. Both authors are currently active in teaching, program development, and research in health promotion and health education. They live in two different countries (the United States and Australia), however, and recognize major differences between

Karen Glanz • Cancer Research Center of Hawaii, University of Hawaii, Honolulu, Hawaii 96813. **Brian Oldenburg** • School of Public Health, Queensland University of Technology, Red Hill, Queensland 4059, Australia.

Handbook of Health Behavior Research IV: Relevance for Professionals and Issues for the Future, edited by David S. Gochman. Plenum Press, New York, 1997.

the systems of higher education in these nations. Thus, this discussion of professional preparation is limited to the United States, where university-level health education programs have the longest history, dating back nearly 60 years (Simonds, 1984). The coverage of research and practice is based primarily on the state of the art in industrialized nations, the authors having collaborated with colleagues in several countries other than their own (e.g., the Netherlands, United Kingdom, Spain, Scandinavia). Both dominant and evolving approaches to health promotion practice and research in these developed countries are more similar than different, but the situation in developing countries is too different to do it justice in this chapter.

To provide a point of reference, the chapter begins with a brief profile of the evolution of the professional practice of health promotion and health education (HP/HE), including definitions of the field, dominant scientific foundations, and the scope of professional training, practice, and research activities and settings. This profile is followed by observations about the extent of health behavior knowledge in professional training for HP/HE. The next section examines major themes, concepts, and findings in the empirical and theoretical bases of HP/HE practice, dominant theoretical models, and current trends. A synthesis of some of our own research is then presented to illustrate applications of health behavior theory and research to HP/HE in the areas of lifestyle change and worksite mammography promotion. The chapter concludes with a discussion of major research and methodological issues and future directions for health behavior research in health promotion and health education.

EVOLUTION OF THE PROFESSIONAL PRACTICE OF HEALTH PROMOTION AND HEALTH EDUCATION

Many types of professionals contribute to and conduct health promotion and health education programs. The primary specialists in the field, however, are those trained in the profession of health education (Simonds, 1984). Health education in the United States has evolved over more than six decades from a small number of training programs to include more than 150 graduate-level training programs, role delineation, guidelines for professional preparation, and certification of health education specialists beginning in 1988 (Breckon, Harvey, & Lancaster, 1994).

Health education and health promotion are defined in many ways. Most definitions of *health education* emphasize efforts to bring about behavior change for improved health (Breckon et al., 1994; Glanz et al., 1990; Simonds, 1984). A widely accepted definition proposed by Green in 1980 suggests that "health education is any combination of learning experiences designed to facilitate voluntary adaptations of behavior conducive to health" (Green, Kreuter, Deeds, & Partridge, 1980, p. 7). The Role Delineation Project defined health education as "the process of assisting individuals, acting separately or collectively, to make informed decisions about matters affecting their personal health and that of others" (National Task Force, 1985, p. 50).

Definitions of *health promotion*,[1] include one suggested by Green: "any combination of health education and related organizational, economic, and environmental supports for behavior of individuals, groups or communities conducive to health" (Green & Kreuter, 1991). Another, slightly different definition is suggested by O'Donnell (1989): "Health promotion is the science and art of helping people change their lifestyle to move toward a state of optimal health.... Lifestyle change can be facilitated by a combination of efforts to enhance awareness, change behavior, and create environments that support good health practices." Definitions arising in Europe and Canada have yet other emphases (Hawe, Degeling, & Hall, 1990; Kolbe, 1988). For example, the Ottawa Charter for Health Promotion defines

---

[1]The term "health promotion" was seldom used before 1980, so most of the development of the field occurred under the label of "health education."

health promotion as "the process of enabling people to increase control over, and to improve, their health ... a commitment to dealing with the challenges of reducing inequities, extending the scope of prevention, and helping people to cope with their circumstances ... creating environments conducive to health, in which people are better able to take care of themselves" (Epp, 1986).

Although some may argue that health promotion is a broader endeavor than health education because it includes health education *and* related environmental and advocacy approaches, health educators have always used more than "educational" strategies (Glanz et al., 1990). In fact, the terms "health promotion" and "health education" are often used interchangeably in the United States (Breckon et al., 1994). In some countries, such as Australia, *health education* is considered a much narrower endeavor. Nevertheless, although the term *health promotion* emphasizes efforts to influence the broader social context of health behavior, the two terms remain closely linked and overlapping. Increasingly, they are being used in combination, as in the title of this chapter. The term "health education" is used specifically in this chapter when discussing historical developments in the field, but otherwise the two terms are considered too closely related to distinguish.

Interdisciplinary Scientific Foundations

By its very nature, health promotion and education (HP/HE) is eclectic and inclusive. It is strengthened by being inclusive rather than exclusive. HP/HE is at the intersection of biological and behavioral sciences and, as Kolbe (1988) notes, is based on knowledge generated by behavioral epidemiology and basic health behavior research. HP/HE draws on theoretical perspectives, research, and practice tools of such diverse disciplines as psychology, sociology, anthropology, communications, economics, and marketing. At the same time, HP/HE is dependent on

epidemiology, statistics, and medicine as a basis for defining optimal health practices and identifying populations in need (Glanz et al., 1990, p. 4). Further, HP/HE activities focus on behaviors along the health continuum from primary prevention to treatment, rehabilitation, and palliative care. As the field of practice has grown and diversified, so too has its research tradition.

This varied mix of disciplines makes the task of analyzing the relevance of health behavior research in HP/HE somewhat more complex: For example, while both authors of this chapter consider health promotion and health education to be the core of our professional endeavors, we proactively seek significant ties to other "fields" We serve on editorial boards of journals in nutrition education, health psychology, patient education, and public health and publish in journals as diverse as the *Journal of Occupational Medicine, International Review of Health Psychology, Journal of General Internal Medicine, Annals of Epidemiology, Psychology and Health, Preventive Medicine, Ethnicity and Disease, Transfusion, Chest, Behaviour Change*, and *Academic Medicine*. In availing ourselves of this array of outlets, we are encouraged that our ideas and findings can reach audiences outside "mainstream" health promotion and health education.

Spectrum of Professional Training and Roles

Early health education evolved from three primary settings: communities, schools, and patient care settings (Green, 1984). Today, health promotion and health education are delivered in many and varied settings—universities, schools, pharmacies, grocery stores, shopping centers, houses of worship and religious institutions, worksites, prisons, health maintenance organizations, voluntary health agencies, migrant labor camps, and homeless shelters. They are disseminated through the mass media, in the development of public policy, and at all levels of government (Glanz et al., 1990). Increasingly, HP/HE occur without the direct involvement of health professionals and outside the health care system. In fact, many of the great health promotion and public health achievements of the past generation have occurred primarily as a result of efforts outside the health care system. Legislation, policy, and advocacy efforts have made dramatic differences in areas as diverse as tobacco control, seat belt use, early cancer detection, and AIDS education.

Because of the growing marketplace interest in and demand for health promotion and health education, more positions identified as "health educator" have been created. One result of this demand has been the increased tendency of persons without specific training to call themselves or their staff members "health educators" (Breckon et al., 1994, p. 6). During this same period, professional organizations of health educators in the United States became more concerned with professional standards, leading to the creation of the Certified Health Education Specialist (C.H.E.S.) by the National Commission for Health Education Credentialing in 1988. The commission administers examinations based on specified competencies for health education specialists and monitors continuing professional development in the form of approved continuing education programs (Breckon et al., 1994, pp. 9–10).

Professional training opportunities for health educators at the baccalaureate, master's, and doctoral level in the United States and other developed countries have increased markedly over the past 60 years, with the number of programs growing from fewer than 50 in 1940 to more than 260 in the 1980s (Simonds, 1984). An estimated 25,000 qualified health educators were in the United States in 1982 (U.S. Department of Health and Human Services [USDHHS], 1982) (this is the most recent available figure). In addition, persons with other types of training—nurses, dietitians, psychologists, industrial hygienists—often work as health educators. Also, many previously trained health educators, especially those with doctoral degrees or active in research, are leaders in the field but have not sought certification.

Thus, it will probably take a generation or so until the reach and impact of the credentialing movement can be evaluated.

Concern about what type of training should be required for the practice of health promotion and health education has drawn considerable attention, particularly in Australia, where most health promotion (and public health) activity is conducted by professionals with other titles (e.g., general practitioners, dietitians, psychologists). Further, efforts to disseminate many health education innovations, such as brief counseling for smoking cessation, have resulted in projects that aim specifically to improve the quality of smoking interventions conducted by physicians (Oldenburg, 1994). In addition, the authors are aware of no studies that test the relative effectiveness of health promotion and health education activities when delivered by "professional health educators" compared to persons with other types of professional training.

Health Behavior Knowledge in Professional Training

Before the credentialing movement, over a decade of effort from hundreds of health educators in the 1970s and 1980s contributed to developing a competency-based curriculum framework for entry-level health educators (National Task Force, 1985; Simonds, 1984). The key responsibilities and competencies in this framework (see Table 1) are the basis for review and accreditation of undergraduate-level health education training programs. The main thrusts of the framework are assessing needs, planning, implementing, and evaluating health education programs, coordinating services, and acting as a resource person in health education (National Task Force, 1985).

For the first four responsibilities, the subcompetencies (not shown in Table 1) do not explicitly refer to the systematic acquisition and application of health behavior knowledge based on research or theory, though this might be considered implicit in skills such as "Investigate

Table 1. Key Responsibilities and Competencies for Entry-Level Health Educators[a]

Responsibility I.	Assessing individual and community needs for health education
Competency A.	Obtain health-related data about social and cultural environments, growth and development factors, needs, and interests.
Competency B.	Distinguish between behaviors that foster, and those that hinder, well-being.
Competency C.	Infer needs for health education on the basis of obtained data.
Responsibility II.	Planning effective health education programs.
Competency A.	Recruit community organizations, resource people, and potential participants for support and assistance with program planning.
Competency B.	Develop a logical scope and sequence plan for a health education program.
Competency C.	Formulate appropriate and measurable program objectives.
Competency D.	Design educational programs consistent with specified program objectives.
Responsibility III.	Implementing health education programs
Competency A.	Exhibit competence in carrying out planned educational programs.
Competency B.	Infer enabling objectives as needed to implement instructional programs in specified settings.
Competency C.	Select methods and media best suited to implement program plans for specified learners.
Competency D.	Monitor educational programs, adjusting objectives and activities as necessary.
Responsibility IV.	Evaluating effectiveness of health education programs.
Competency A.	Develop plans to assess achievement of program objectives.
Competency B.	Carry out evaluation plans.
Competency C.	Interpret results of program evaluation.
Competency D.	Infer implications from findings for future program planning.
Responsibility V.	Coordinating provision of health education services.
Competency A.	Develop a plan for coordinating health education services.
Competency B.	Facilitate cooperation between and among levels of program personnel.
Competency C.	Formulate practical modes of collaboration among health agencies and organizations.
Competency D.	Organize inservice training programs for teachers, volunteers, and other interested personnel.
Responsibility VI.	Acting as a resource person in health education
Competency A.	Utilize computerized health information retrieval systems effectively.
Competency B.	Establish effective consultative relationships with those requesting assistance in solving health-related problems.
Competency C.	Interpret and respond to requests for health information.
Competency D.	Select effective educational resource materials for dissemination.
Responsibility VII.	Communicating health and health education needs, concerns, and resources
Competency A.	Interpret concepts, purposes, and theories of health education.
Competency B.	Predict the impact of societal value systems on health education programs.
Competency C.	Select a variety of communication methods and techniques in providing health information.
Competency D.	Foster communication between health care providers and consumers.

[a]From National Task Force on the Preparation and Practice of Health Educators (1985).

physical, social, emotional, and intellectual factors influencing health behaviors" (Responsibility I, Competency B, Sub-Competency 1) and "Recognize the role of learning and affective experiences in shaping patterns of behavior" (Responsibility I, Competency B, Sub-Competency 3). Responsibility VII, Communicating health and health education needs, concerns, and resources includes Competency A: "Interpret key concepts, purposes, and theories of health education." Thus, at least for undergraduate professional training, health behavior knowledge may either be pervasive throughout training or be minimal. The authors' observations suggest that the actual situation is somewhere between these two extremes, with "concrete knowledge" such as specific facts about health, disease, and behavioral factors that affect health as probably a stronger and more consistent focus than knowledge related to theory, research, and data about health behavior.

There is no framework analogous to these key responsibilities and competencies for graduate-level training in health education, although the Council on Education for Public Health (CEPH) has requirements for accreditation of master's degree programs in community health education and health education programs in schools of public health. The CEPH clearly requires that students complete coursework in health behavior theory and research methods relevant to health behavior (CEPH, 1994). However, a survey of master's level programs in 22 schools of public health and 128 programs located outside schools of public health found that only 31% of the public health programs and 12% of those outside schools of public health required a course in program planning, in which one would logically expect coverage of theories and models (Speers, 1994). These findings may underestimate the extent of health behavior coverage in graduate programs, as some programs have full courses in health behavior (theory and research). In addition, several large departments that offer training HP/HE have even added "health behavior and ..." to their department names. Further, it might be necessary to conduct a thorough content analysis of curricula and course syllabi to accurately estimate the degree to which health behavior knowledge is included in professional training in health promotion and health education training programs.

Despite the difficulty of making precise estimates, it appears that coverage of health behavior knowledge in HP/HE training programs has increased since the early 1980s (Breckon et al., 1994). This phenomenon can be observed not only in North America, but also in Australia and a number of European countries, particularly the Netherlands (Kok, 1993). A key factor in this growth may be the wide adoption of Green et al.'s (1980) book on program planning in the 1980s. This book, now in its second edition (Green & Kreuter, 1991), advocates and instructs in the use of a systematic model for planning health education programs. This model, known as the PRE-CEDE (Predisposing, Reinforcing and Enabling Causes in Educational Diagnosis and Evaluation)/PROCEED (Policy, Regulatory and Organizational Constructs for Educational and Environmental Development) model, places substantial emphasis on the use of theory and data from health behavior throughout the planning and evaluation process (Green & Kreuter, 1991). A second important contribution to stronger coverage of health behavior knowledge was the publication of a text that covers a broad range of theories and their application in both research and practice (Glanz et al., 1990). This book has been widely adopted and is generally considered the main textbook for teaching theory in health promotion and health education (Breckon et al., 1994; Green et al., 1994).

Health behavior knowledge should be a central component of professional training in HP/HE at both the undergraduate and graduate levels. Because health promotion and health education are based on such diverse interdisciplinary orientations, students cannot possibly master all disciplines. Rather, the rich and growing body of work in health behavior theory and research can be used to give clear, specific examples of their application to HP/HE. As suggested, the most logical context for conveying health behavior to students is in courses on program planning and (if available) those on theory and research. Further, if an internship or field experience is provided, this is an ideal time to teach the application of health behavior concepts and methods systematically.

HEALTH PROMOTION AND HEALTH EDUCATION PRACTICE

The rationale for examining the role of health behavior knowledge in professional training for HP/HE is the assumption that this training will carry over into professional practice. Of course, this assumption frequently is not borne out, due to job requirements, time and resource pressures, administrators' orientations, and numerous other real-world obstacles. This section attempts a partial answer to the question of whether health behavior knowledge affects professional practice, this answer being based primarily on trends in the literature and on the authors' observations as active practitioners, researchers, and speakers in the field.

It is first necessary to offer two humbling disclaimers: (1) To date, no full empirical assessment of these matters has been attempted; (2) observations of the published literature probably reflect innovations in practice, and related research, rather than the normative practices.

Theoretical and Empirical Foundations

To what degree are professional health education and health promotion activities based on empiricism and/or theory? The multidisciplinary nature of health promotion and health education requires practitioners to master, integrate, and collaborate with experts from several scientific and professional disciplines (Green & Kreuter, 1991, p. 31). Efforts to synthesize literature from the biomedical sciences and the behavioral sciences in the context of program administration can be both challenging and discouraging. The question of whether health educators do in fact base their work on a systematic analysis of theory and data, which is called for in using the PRECEDE/PROCEED model for planning, is a difficult one. Speers (1994) contends that practitioners often select models or intervention activities on the basis of their perception of what works, based on limited direct exposure and selective exposure to a range of theories during their training. She suggests that most health educators lack the skills to utilize a variety of models and theories and that the field lacks the resources to assist them in doing so (Speers, 1994).

Our observations suggest that much of this argument (but not all of it) is correct. The deficiencies may be due to a combination of factors: Most practicing health educators were trained more than a decade ago and have not been required to obtain continuing professional education despite the field's rapid progress. The state of the art of knowledge in health education has many gaps (Simonds, 1984). Some have criticized the way theory is taught (Burdine & McLeroy, 1992), claiming that concepts are not sufficiently linked to real-world problems. Other barriers cited—which may be far more influential—include inadequate planning, inadequate research on theories and models, and underestimation of the barriers to diffusion and implementation (Green et al., 1994). Indeed, the path of least resistance may be to work with what is most familiar, most "popular," and easiest to implement.

As to whether health promotion and health education activities are based on empiricism, they appear to be so only to a limited extent. Many practitioners have insufficient time and motivation to keep up with the literature (Kling, 1984), which is growing so rapidly that doing so is a difficult challenge even for the most dedicated scholars. More likely, only a small segment of professionals routinely seek empirical data on the determinants of health behavior and the effectiveness of HP/HE interventions. Specialized electronic databases and publications that synthesize the state of the art are increasingly available, however, and should prove helpful in coming years.

To what degree are professional health promotion and health education activities based on *theory?* Again, we observe that many practitioners are most comfortable regarding "theory and practice as separate realms" (D'Onofrio, 1992). Practitioners may find the abstract thinking involved in applying theoretical constructs too demanding for their fast-paced work environments. Nevertheless, there is likely a small proportion of HP/HE professionals who consistently aim to use theory as a tool to untangle and simplify the complexities of human nature (and we hope some of them are our former students!) (Green et al., 1994). In this area, too, there are increasing resources to make theory accessible to practitioners (Glanz et al., 1990) and to introduce and reinforce it in a clear, usable, problem-based format (Glanz & Rimer, 1995).

An important distinction should be made between theoretical models and the data that they have generated. The preceding paragraph concerns primarily the more or less direct application of theoretical constructs for practice, not their acceptance or rejection based on research findings. As to whether HP/HE professionals base their work on data generated in theoretically based health behavior research, we think this question is still more complicated: Do they principally use the *findings*, or do they interpret the findings in light of theory testing? The former is probably more likely, with the latter done principally by association. This may be partly a function of the frequent only superficial mention of theory in published research literature.

One example of a resource to promote the use of empirical findings and theory is the *Pathways to Better Health* report released in Australia (Department of Health, 1993). The report reviewed health promotion practice in Australia, highlighted examples of successful programs that had been evaluated, analyzed mechanisms for strengthening practice, and also analyzed evidence concerning the cost-effectiveness of health promotion. In light of the recent expansion of professional training programs in Australia, the document also provides a cornerstone for strengthening professional preparation (Oldenburg, Wise, Nutbeam, Leeder, & Watson, 1994).

A different type of example illustrates the dilemmas involved in applying theory, research, and theory-testing research in health promotion and health education practice in the United States. In the late 1970s and early 1980s, three large community cardiovascular disease intervention studies were begun in California, Minnesota, and Rhode Island (Matarazzo, Weiss, Herd, Miller, & Weiss, 1984; Winkleby, 1994). Each study was a multimillion-dollar undertaking and integrated epidemiological and behavioral research methods and intervention strategies. The studies addressed smoking, hypertension, high-fat diets, obesity, and physical inactivity—all widespread risk factors that many practitioners were tackling. The multicomponent risk reduc-

tion education programs in these trials used mass media, and interpersonal education programs for the public, professionals, and those at high risk. Community organization strategies were used to create institutional and environmental support for the programs, and theoretically derived program-planning strategies emphasized community participation (Winkleby, 1994).

During the 1980s, many professionals in the field of HP/HE came to view these programs as models for the state of the art, striving to copy their activities even without comparable funding (and often without evaluation). This trend could only be considered one of using *precedent*, combined with some direct application of conceptual frameworks. Two of the three studies have now reported their findings for risk factor changes. The Stanford Five-City Project in California found strong positive secular trends—i.e., changes in control communities that could not be attributed to intervention—and significant improvements in blood pressure and smoking favoring the treatment communities (Farquhar et al., 1990). Findings from the Minnesota Heart Health Program were released in 1994, and they also document strong secular trends in risk factors in all communities, but only modest, short-lived, and nonsignificant positive changes in risk factors in the intervention communities (Luepker et al., 1994).

These studies produced a wealth of knowledge about health behavior, and many of the short-term targeted interventions were found to be effective (Winkleby, 1994). Nevertheless, the results cast doubt on the wisdom of widespread adoption of population-based intervention strategies as "optimal" in the absence of data. At the same time, the lack of significant long-term community-wide impact in these studies in no way "disproves" the conceptual foundations of the intervention methods. Another important lesson relates to the tremendous limitations of such large, complex, multicomponent trials as definitive arbiters of how practice should be conducted. An alternative view is to regard the interventions used in these studies as contributors to the substantial secular trend in cardiovascular disease prevention (Winkleby, 1994).

Multilevel Perspective on Health Behavior

The upswing in attention to *health promotion* and its defining concepts since the early 1980s has coincided with at least one major influence on health promotion and health education: the widespread acknowledgment of the importance of a multilevel perspective on health behavior. This can be considered either as a new paradigm or as a revival of a long-standing philosophy: that the determinants of health and health behavior are multifactorial and are both intrapersonal and structural (Epp, 1986; Green & Kreuter, 1991; Glanz et al., 1990). The notion of an ecological perspective, whereby attention is given to intrapersonal, interpersonal, institutional, community, and public policy factors (McLeroy, Bibeau, Steckler, & Glanz, 1988), has become widely accepted. This perspective, not a theory per se, stresses the inclusiveness of health promotion and health education (McLeroy et al., 1988; Stokols, 1992; Winett, King, & Altman, 1989). Although it seems that individual and interpersonal-level strategies still dominate professional activities in HP/HE, the multilevel approach has begun to take root.

Nevertheless, it appears that both practice and research will gradually evolve toward the multilevel model over time. An important distinction in programs to reduce smoking and encourage dietary change is between clinical approaches and public health approaches (Oldenburg, 1994; Rogers & Glanz, 1991). As one example, the traditional clinical approach to the problem of smoking has focused on developing and delivering relatively intensive programs under reasonably controlled conditions to highly motivated individuals. These high-exposure programs serve individuals and small groups effectively, but have limited reach. At the other end of the spectrum are some strong public health approaches—notably tobacco taxes, and smoking policies in

workplaces and public settings. These public health approaches reach more people with deterrents to smoking, but are less intensive, and they may not help addicted smokers to quit. Ideally, clinical and public health approaches should be integrated for maximum impact and broad reach (Oldenburg, 1994). In practice, however, many efforts to disseminate health promotion and health education to broad populations consist of little more than implementing clinical approaches in new settings such as worksites (Rogers & Glanz, 1991).

Dominant Theoretical Models

An initial review of the use of theory in major health education journals in 1988 found 51 distinct theoretical formulations discussed or applied in 116 theory-based articles. The theories employed most often were social learning theory (23 articles), the theory of reasoned action (19 articles), and the health belief model (16 articles) (Glanz et al., 1990, p. 25). It was apparent that no single model dominated the field and, as others have noted (Preston & Mansfield, 1991), that a substantial proportion of published work lacks any explicit theoretical underpinning.

The review is currently in the process of being repeated (in preparation for a second edition of *Health Behavior and Health Education: Theory, Research, and Practice*) and expanded to include articles relevant to HP/HE in 20 different journals in health promotion and education, preventive medicine, and health psychology between the years 1992 and 1994. Although the review is not yet complete, we note that almost half the articles lack identification of any type of theoretical framework. Some shift has been noted in the most frequently discussed models, which now appear to be social learning theory/ social cognitive theory, social marketing, the health belief model, and the stages of change construct from the transtheoretical model of change. The latter model has rapidly gained attention, with its focus on readiness to change and its position that behavior change is a process rather than an event (Prochaska, DiClemente, & Norcross, 1992).

Again, it is important to recognize the multitude of available theoretical frameworks and to avoid using a model simply because it is the "flavor of the month." It is further essential to fit the theory to the problem, setting, and population, rather than simply to follow the precedent of others.

Populations with Special Needs

Because health promotion and health education are applied endeavors, they remain continually responsive to the changing social and health environment. Cultural diversity is a central focus of society in industrialized nations today, and so HP/HE has turned its attention to diverse populations. Further, in the United States (and Australia), ethnic minority groups are often socioeconomically disadvantaged, underserved by health and health promotion services, and suffering disproportionately from preventable or manageable health problems (USDHHS, 1991). Thus, it is natural that public health policy and funding priorities have turned the attention of health educators to underserved populations.

While health educators in the 1990s have vigorously begun to address the needs of these special populations, they are discovering how little we really know about them. For example, Asians are the fastest growing ethnic minority in the United States, but there is little health behavior research and there are few evaluated health promotion programs for Asian-Americans. The emphasis on special populations will most likely be a major force in application of health behavior knowledge to health promotion and health education in the future.

THEORY, RESEARCH, AND PRACTICE: MULTIPLE FOUNDATIONS AND APPLICATIONS

This section is a synthesis of some of our own research, to illustrate applications of health behavior theory and research to HP/HE in the

areas of lifestyle change and mammography promotion. Our commitment to theory-based interventions and the analysis and testing of innovative strategies for solving highly prevalent health problems demonstrates how health promotion and health education is well positioned to utilize health behavior knowledge to maximize success and cumulative development of the field—in effect, how health behavior research is unquestionably relevant and useful to health promotion and health education. Common themes and crosscutting methodological issues in these studies will be addressed in the following section.

Changing Lifestyles: Dietary Practices and Physical Activity

Worksite Nutrition Research: The Working Well Trial. There is considerable and growing evidence that certain dietary practices are significant contributors to chronic diseases in developed countries. Five of the ten leading causes of death for American adults are associated with nutritional practices: heart disease, some cancers, stroke, diabetes, and atherosclerosis (USDHHS, 1988). These findings and similar ones in other industrialized nations have led to the development of consensus statements and guidelines for health promotion through diet, focusing principally on reducing dietary fat, avoiding overweight, and increasing fiber and fruit and vegetable intake (National Research Council, 1989; U. S. Department of Agriculture/USDHHS, 1990).

Worksites are an important setting for health promotion programs addressing nutrition. Worksites enable programs to reach large groups, thus making a greater public health impact possible (Glanz & Eriksen, 1993). The workplace provides unique opportunities for reinforcement and environmental support for health-promoting behaviors. Program convenience, social support from coworkers, and existing communications networks can facilitate program implementation and effectiveness (Glanz, Sorensen, & Farmer, 1996). The Working Well Trial, a randomized, controlled multicenter trial of worksite health promotion in 114 worksites in four regions of the United States, addresses multiple risk factors including nutrition, tobacco use, physical inactivity, and sun exposure (Abrams et al., 1994). This discussion summarizes the application of health behavior theory and research methods to the nutrition component of the Working Well Trial. The central objectives of the nutrition intervention are to decrease dietary fat intake to no more than 30% of calories, increase the intake of dietary fiber to 20–30 grams or more per day, and to increase fruit and vegetable intake to an average of five servings per day (Abrams et al., 1994; Glanz & Eriksen, 1993). These objectives are based on the NCI Dietary Guidelines (Butrum, Clifford, & Lanza, 1988). Additional worksite-level objectives include increasing the availability of healthful foods in food service operations.

The Working Well Trial nutrition intervention involves application of a combination of four theoretical models: consumer information processing (CIP), stages of change, social cognitive theory, and the diffusion of innovations (Glanz & Eriksen, 1993). It simultaneously focuses on individuals and worksite environments and aims to produce change, during a 2- to 3-year program, in three stages: awareness, action, and maintenance (Abrams et al., 1994). This overall sequencing of interventions is based on the stages of change model, which proposes that people are at various points along a continuum of readiness to change (Prochaska et al., 1992). The emphasis on both individuals and the environment reflects the broad approach of social cognitive theory (Bandura, 1986). The informational content of the nutrition intervention is influenced by CIP concepts (Glanz & Rudd, 1991). A key example of this is the translation of the project's nutrient objectives into food-focused eating pattern messages (Glanz & Eriksen, 1993). Finally, the use of liaisons and employee advisory boards at each worksite to disseminate the programs is an example of the application of the diffusion of innovations (Rogers, 1983). Most of the educational materials (print media, posters, videos, and so on) are "off the shelf" materials that are widely available through government and voluntary health organizations, thus assuring the ready adoptability of the program if it is found effective.

Because the intervention was based on an integration of theoretical perspectives, it was important to develop research methods that would capture not only the main results of the trial but also information about whether and how the interventions affected the presumed determinants of dietary behavior (based on theory). The major nutrition end points of fat, fiber, and fruit and vegetable intake were assessed by a validated food frequency questionnaire; however, practical instruments to assess determinants of dietary practices, or mediating factors, were not available at the beginning of the trial. The challenge of developing such a measurement tool was addressed by defining the central domains and variables, creating a catalogue of items, and developing, pretesting, and refining an instrument (Glanz et al., 1993). Baseline findings provided criterion validation for algorithms used to measure the stages of change (Glanz, Patterson, Kristal, et al., 1994) and also revealed that predisposing factors (e.g., motivation, perceived benefits) were more significant determinants of diet than were enabling factors (e.g., social supports, norms) (Kristal et al., 1995).

Results of the Working Well Trial showed a significant trend toward dietary improvement in both control and treatment sites and a small, statistically significant change in the desired direction in dietary fat and fruit and vegetable intake (Sorensen et al., 1996). There was a small but nonsignificant trend toward increased fiber intake. In addition, the treatment worksites adopted more environmental and structural changes to increase availability and visibility of healthful food (Sorensen et al., 1996). Analyses are now in progress to examine the impact of the intervention on stage of change and other psychosocial factors, and the relationships of these factors to dietary endpoints.

Physical Activity Promotion in Primary Health Care Settings. Physical inactivity is a risk factor for a number of chronic diseases, including cardiovascular diseases. Although the health benefits of regular exercise are well established, a large percentage of adults in Australia, as in most industrialized countries, do not engage in sufficient physical activity to improve or maintain their health (Owen & Bauman, 1992). Primary health care settings offer an excellent venue to reach sedentary persons with programs to advise and encourage patients to exercise. The Fresh Start program, designed to be used by primary care physicians, has been developed and evaluated in Australia. It was part of a program for physicians to use with their patients to influence tobacco use, dietary behaviors, and physical activity (Graham-Clarke & Oldenburg, 1994). The physicians are trained in the use of lifestyle change strategies and provided with audiovisual and other educational aids. This description is limited to the physical activity component.

The program is intended to help individuals achieve long-term lifestyle changes and is based on social learning theory (Bandura, 1986) and an adaptation of the stages of change construct (Prochaska et al., 1992), suggesting that change can be accomplished in three basic stages (Brownell, Marlatt, Lichtenstein, & Wilson, 1986). Stage I involves motivating, preparing, and advising the person to change (Preparation stage). Stage II, the Action stage, involves the initial lifestyle change efforts. Stage III, the Maintenance stage, is characterized by attempts to help the person consolidate initial changes and build on these changes for the longer term (Oldenburg, 1994).

Methods used in the Preparation stage include self-instructional print and video materials. discussions with the patient to weigh the "pros" and "cons" of increasing physical activity, and strategies to make exercise personally relevant by emphasizing the short-term or immediate benefits of exercising. In the Action stage, already motivated patients receive help in setting attainable goals, individualizing the exercise plan, and warming up and cooling down. This is accomplished using professionally produced and targeted printed and audiovisual materials that the physician gives the patient to use at home. These materials, developed specially for the project, reinforce the physician's support for lifestyle change efforts and allow for flexible use (Graham-Clarke & Oldenburg, 1994). The focus of the Maintenance stage strategies is to prevent and/or

manage relapse using theoretically derived strategies (Marlatt & Gordon, 1985) that are also practical, affordable, and feasible to deliver from a primary care setting. The program provides ongoing contact with health professionals at a reduced frequency, for the purposes of monitoring, feedback, and revision of strategies if necessary. The contacts are made by a combination of telephone and mail contacts (Graham-Clarke & Oldenburg, 1994).

The Fresh Start program was evaluated in a randomized, controlled trial conducted in three regions surrounding Sydney, Australia, between January 1991 and January 1993. In the trial, 80 volunteer general practitioners (physicians) in 75 medical practices were randomly assigned to one of three conditions: routine care, lifestyle counseling using video, and lifestyle counseling using videos and self-instructional materials. The practice was the unit of randomization. Each general practitioner enrolled up to 20 patients in the trial, and physical activity was measured by questionnaire at baseline, and at 4-month and 12-month follow-up (Graham-Clarke & Oldenburg, 1994).

Results of the trial showed no difference between groups in physical activity over time. The least active patients, however, were more likely to respond to physician-based advice by an increase in *intention to change* toward becoming more physically active, among about 20% of the patients in the study. The results of this trial were subject to a number of limitations, including barriers to implementing the intervention in a general practice setting, statistical and methodological considerations, and the apparent limitations of a staged approach to encouraging physical activity in the health care setting. Further studies may reveal whether similar approaches are efficacious in achieving similar goals.

Improving Adherence to Mammography at Worksites

Foundations. Breast cancer is the most common women's cancer and the second most common cause of cancer mortality in women (American Cancer Society, 1994). Despite remarkable progress in early detection and treatment, there remains no proven strategy for *preventing* breast cancer. Early detection can decrease breast cancer deaths and increase the quality and length of women's survival after diagnosis. Regular screening mammography, in particular, has been shown to reduce mortality from breast cancer between 20% and 39% in women aged 50 years or older (Kerlikowske, Grady, Rubin, Sandrock, & Ernster, 1995). Currently, the evidence to support the efficacy of screening mammography in women aged 40–49 years is less convincing (Fletcher, Black, Harris, Rimer, & Shapiro, 1993); until a few years ago, however, several scientific and medical organizations were recommending mammograms at 1 to 2-year intervals for women in this age group (National Medical Roundtable, 1989).

Given the growing workforce presence of women, and the prevalence of breast cancer and its impact on employed women, workplace mammography programs have great potential for improving health, preventing unnecessary expense and suffering, prolonging life, and improving the quality of life. Between 1988 and 1993, while developing a field experiment to improve the adherence of employed women to mammography on a mobile unit, we drew on theories and past research in health behavior. To better understand why some women do not adhere to mammography guidelines for their age group, we first developed a conceptual framework based on an ecological, multilevel perspective. Four levels of influence were considered: (1) individual factors, including demographics, awareness, knowledge, attitudes, symptom status, and family history; (2) environmental influences, such as exposure to mass media; (3) health care factors, e.g., physician recommendations, and the out-of-pocket cost of mammography; and (4) employer factors and available worksite health promotion programs (Glanz, Rimer, Lerman, & Gorchov, 1992).

The next step in developing our intervention was to conduct focus groups with employed

women, using a social marketing assessment approach and drawing on what we knew from previous research and theory. Quantitative and qualitative data were collected from 45 women in four focus groups, using a structured questionnaire and informal group discussions. Our findings revealed several positive beliefs about mammography and its potential effectiveness, but also indicated the women's concerns about radiation exposure, fear of receiving positive results, transient discomfort from the exam, and possible embarrassment about disrobing for a mammogram at or near the workplace. Some of the women had previously used the mobile mammography unit and described the experience as convenient, careful, confidential, and low in cost (Glanz, Rimer, et al., 1992). These findings were used to develop tailored educational and promotional materials for an intervention trial at worksites in southeastern Pennsylvania and New Jersey.

The study was a randomized field experiment conducted at worksites with female employees aged 40 and older who were members of an individual practice association–model health maintenance organization (HMO). The study had 74 participating worksites, and worksites were the unit of randomization. Control sites had access to a mobile mammography unit (van) and information. Treatment sites received the mobile unit, tailored health education, and special promotion (described below). Data sources included telephone surveys at baseline and 1 month and 1 year after the van visit, worksite characteristics surveys, process evaluation, and mammography records (Glanz & Resch, 1994).

The intervention was a multicomponent, theory-based set of strategies drawing on the health belief model, stages of change, social cognitive theory, and social marketing methods. It included group education with a tailored video, discussion period, and incentive gift; enhanced publicity; encouragement of employer cost-sharing; alternative sign-up opportunities; and reminder letters. The health belief model was applied in crafting messages emphasizing women's susceptibility to breast cancer and the net benefits of regular mammograms (Glanz, Resch, Lerman, & Rimer, 1992; Kirscht, 1988). The stages of change construct was operationalized in a simplified form, promoting three types of action in stages: increased awareness and motivation, an opportunity for action (a mammogram on the mobile unit at the worksite), and promotion of subsequent screening mammograms at regular intervals. Social cognitive theory (Bandura, 1986) was a foundation for efforts to influence both individual women and the environment, to increase convenience, and to assist women by informing them clearly about what to expect during mammography. Social marketing methods (Novelli, 1990) were used to develop the intervention content and methods (as described above) and to evaluate and refine the program during the study.

The telephone surveys conducted at baseline and on two follow-up occasions measured concepts from the health belief model and social cognitive theory. These surveys yielded data not only to assess the main behavioral end point (adherence to age-based mammography guidelines), but also to examine whether the intervention influenced factors hypothesized to contribute to mammography utilization. Analysis of telephone interviews conducted with 798 women at the first 39 worksites in the trial provided some support for the theoretical foundations of the interventions using cross-sectional data. Logistic regression analyses indicated that a doctor's advice to have a mammogram, knowledge of screening guidelines, knowing someone with breast cancer, and the belief that mammography is effective and necessary in the absence of symptoms were associated independently with past use of mammography (Glanz, Resch, et al., 1992).

Racial Differences. Subsequent analyses provided an opportunity to examine racial differences in knowledge, attitudes, and practices related to breast cancer screening of black and white women HMO members participating in the study (Glanz, Resch, Lerman, & Rimer, 1996). This analysis provided an opportunity to exam-

ine racial/ethnic correlates of women's beliefs and behaviors about early cancer detection while controlling for much of the variance in socioeconomic status (all subjects were employed and entitled to mammograms at no extra cost under their HMO coverage). The analysis focused primarily on health belief model variables. Data from baseline interviews of 1677 women (20% black) over age 40 who were employed at 75 worksites showed that black and white women did not differ in terms of self-reported mammography use (86% ever had a mammogram and 69% were in compliance with age-based guidelines). Compared to whites, however, blacks were more likely to underestimate their cancer risk and to fear radiation and less likely to have had a doctor advise them to get a mammogram (72% of whites versus 57% of blacks). In addition, the results of multivariate modeling suggested that different sets of knowledge and belief variables may explain mammography adherence among black and white women (Glanz, Resch, et al., 1992). This last finding suggests broader implications—that concepts from a theoretical model that was developed and tested primarily with data from nonminority populations (the health belief model) may be less useful in explaining the health behavior of nonwhite populations. This notion warrants further examination in other populations and with other health behaviors.

Impact. The impact of the worksite intervention to improve mammography adherence was evaluated using both worksite-level and individual-level data analyses. Individual-level analyses were based on survey data, and statistical adjustment for the cluster design and intracluster correlation was done on the individual-level analyses of impact (Snedecor & Cochran, 1980). The individual-level analysis is the least conservative, and if the study groups do not differ on the basis of individual-level analyses, they will not be found to differ with worksite-level analysis.

The sample used for the individual-level analyses from the baseline and 1-month follow-up surveys included 1742 and 1580 women, respectively. There were slight improvements in beliefs between baseline and follow-up, but no differences between treatment and control groups. There were significant increases in knowledge of age-specific guidelines for mammography, but again, treatment and control groups did not differ. Attendance at the health education program was associated with improvements in beliefs about the benefits of mammography. Both treatment and control group adherence rates improved by approximately 11% from baseline to 1-month follow-up (from 71% to 82%), but again, no significant treatment effect was found. The worksite-level results using HMO records of mammography utilization also showed no treatment impact on mammography adherence. These data did show that having higher proportions of women attending the education session was associated with lower proportions adherent at baseline ($r = -.040$, $p = .0003$) and higher proportions adherent at follow-up ($p = .048$, $p = .00002$) (Glanz & Resch, 1994).

Cost-Effectiveness. The findings from this trial showed a strong secular trend in mammography adherence among working women, but indicated no additional impact due to the tailored worksite health promotion and education interventions. These results parallel the findings from the Stanford (Farquhar et al., 1990) and Minnesota (Luepker et al., 1994) community cardiovascular trials. Despite the limitations of the main study findings, we were able to use the research situation to evaluate a related, important health policy question: What is the relative cost-effectiveness of a mobile mammography program at the workplace compared to screening mammography for employed women at a dedicated stationary facility? To address this question, we analyzed survey data from the trial, survey data from a random sample of employed women in the community whose worksites did not have mobile unit screening, and program cost and operations data in the region of the study (Hill, Glanz, & Rimer, 1993). The estimated cost per mammo-

gram was higher for the mobile program than for the stationary program ($68.21 versus $51.24), but this difference was minimized to a difference of only $3–$8 when women's time and travel costs were included in the calculations. Adherence to guidelines for screening was 26% higher at worksites with the mobile program. The cost of life-years saved was then estimated on the basis of findings from randomized trials of mammography applied to a hypothetical cohort of 100,000 women like those in the study. Estimated cost per additional life-year saved of between $15,303 and $23,154 suggests that the mobile program is a cost-effective method for achieving the benefits of increased adherence. Hence, although unit costs are slightly higher for a program of mobile mammography at the worksite than for mammography in a stationary office setting, the higher costs can be justified by higher adherence rates and hence lives saved by the mobile program (Hill et al., 1993).

This study of improving adherence to mammography at worksites exemplifies many uses of health behavior theory and research methods in health promotion and health education. It used a broad public health approach to reach a clearly defined target group, using rigorous experimental design in a real-world setting. The quantitative and qualitative data collected during the study permitted the authors to address both conceptual and practical questions with public health and health policy significance. The findings underscored the limits of brief health education programs in affecting behavior change in times of rapid secular change in cancer control practices.

MAJOR RESEARCH AND METHODOLOGICAL ISSUES

Several major research and methodological issues cut across the topics discussed thus far, beginning with the role of health behavior research in training health promotion and health education professionals and the application of theory-based research findings in health promotion and health education practice. First and foremost among these issues is the matter of making research relevant to practice, with clear practice implications. This is a challenging endeavor, given that the demands of rigorous research often inherently require greater control than is reasonable in most HP/HE programs in the field. A companion issue is the ongoing need to evaluate programs in the field, to bring research and practice closer together. Various creative evaluation designs are feasible in community and clinical settings, to provide some degree of control in the evaluation; simple before-and-after designs are usually too weak to permit even cautious inferences of causality.

A related concern is the diffusion of programs and strategies that are found successful in controlled research settings. Diffusion requires timely publication and dissemination of findings, appropriate adaptations for different populations and settings, and the distribution of resources developed for intervention research. At present, such practices are more the exception than the rule in health promotion and health education.

The question of the appropriate unit of study and randomization raises conceptual, scientific, and practical questions. If HP/HE professionals are to implement and test ecological approaches, then environmental and structural interventions must be a prominent component of health promotion strategies. Note the worksite and primary care intervention studies described in this chapter that address nutrition, smoking, and mammography use. When structural/environmental interventions are tested, and efforts to change organizational environments are attempted, it is not feasible to randomize individuals to treatment and control conditions. When organizations are the unit of randomization and analysis, however, sample size requirements mandate extremely large samples and very costly studies. The most extreme example of this is the community cardiovascular risk reduction trials (Winkleby, 1994), in which entire communities are randomized to treatment or control conditions. An important challenge will be to test environmental interventions without dedicating disproportionately great resources to any one study or set of studies.

The natural environments in which HP/HE research occur also present difficulties in obtaining measurement that is psychometrically and biologically sound, yet not overly burdensome for research subjects. A related concern is how to handle attrition in data analyses and in interpreting research findings.

In the community cardiovascular disease risk reduction trials, the Working Well Trial, and the worksite mammography study, investigators and practitioners are faced with the difficulty of interpreting equivocal results. How should one treat results that are minimized or masked due to secular trends toward improving health practices? Should significant effects, even those that are small in magnitude, be seen as successes in the context of public health approaches?

One final research issue involves opening up the "black box" of experimental research so that practitioners and scientists alike can learn from the depth of experience in descriptive and intervention research. This approach requires routine efforts to blend qualitative and quantitative methods. While many current and recent studies take this approach, they are often limited by time and funding so that qualitative data cannot be fully analyzed. Although there is no easy answer to the question of how to accomplish this blending, the issue deserves attention now and in the future.

FUTURE DIRECTIONS

Future advances in health promotion and health education will depend on conceptual advances, improved application of creative research methodologies, and improved training for practitioners in health behavior theory and research. In the face of shrinking federal research budgets, partnerships between practicing HP/

HE professionals and scientists will become ever more important to advancements in the field.

New scientific discoveries and medical technologies will create new areas of interest for health educators and new demands for health behavior research. Among the areas of imminent development are genetic discoveries and the resultant growth in medical diagnostics related to genetic testing, and treatments based on gene therapy. The informational, psychological, ethical, and social implications of these technologies will require the attention of health educators as the products of this scientific work enter the public health and clinical arenas. In addition, biobehavioral technology will create new tools for health behavior change that health educators will have to evaluate, consider, and perhaps adopt.

Health promotion and health education are broad endeavors that involve multidisciplinary and multisectoral perspectives. Ultimately, the most important question will not be whether professional health educators alone should provide programs, but the question of how to assure quality in helping people to make important health decisions to improve both the quality and quantity of their lives. Insofar as health promotion and health education professionals seek to lead and collaborate with clinicians and other professionals whose work focuses on health behavior, the health of the public will ultimately benefit.

REFERENCES

Abrams, D. B., Boutwell, W. B., Grizzle, J., Heimendinger, J., Sorensen, G., & Varnes, J. (1994). Cancer control at the workplace: The Working Well Trial. *Preventive Medicine, 23*, 15–27.

American Cancer Society. (1994). *Cancer facts and figures*. Atlanta: Author.

Bandura, A. (1986). *Social foundations of thought and action: A social cognitive theory*. Englewood Cliffs, NJ: Prentice-Hall.

Breckon, D. J., Harvey, J. R., & Lancaster, R. B. (1994). *Community health education: Settings, roles and skills for the 21st century*. Gaithersburg, MD: Aspen.

Brownell, K. D., Marlatt, G. A., Lichtenstein, E., & Wilson, G. T. (1986). Understanding and preventing relapse. *American Psychologist, 41*, 765–782.

Burdine, J. N., & McLeroy, K. R. (1992). Practitioners' use of theory: Examples from a workgroup. *Health Education Quarterly, 19*, 331–340.

Butrum, R., Clifford, C. K., & Lanza, E. (1988). NCI dietary guidelines: Rationale. *American Journal of Clinical Nutrition, 48*, 888–895.

Council on Education for Public Health. (1994). Requirements for master's degree programs in community health education. Washington, DC: CEPH.

Department of Health, Housing and Community Service National Health Strategy Unit. (1993). *Pathways to better health*. Issues paper No. 7. Melbourne, Australia: Department of Health, Housing and Community Service National Health Strategy Unit.

D'Onofrio, C. N. (1992). Theory and the empowerment of health education practitioners. *Health Education Quarterly, 19*, 385–403.

Epp, L. (1986). *Achieving health for all. A framework for health promotion in Canada*. Toronto: Health and Welfare, Canada.

Farquhar, J. W., Fortmann, S. P., Flora, J. A., Taylor, B., Haskell, W., Williams, P., Maccoby, N., & Wood, P. (1990). Effects of communitywide education on cardiovascular disease risk factors: The Stanford Five-City Project. *Journal of the American Medical Association, 264*, 359–365.

Fletcher, S. W., Black, W., Harris, R., Rimer, B. K., & Shapiro, S. (1993). Report of the International Workshop on Screening for Breast Cancer. *Journal of the National Cancer Institute, 85*, 1644–1656.

Glanz, K., & Eriksen, M. P. (1993). Individual and community models for dietary behavior change. *Journal of Nutrition Education, 25*, 80–86.

Glanz, K., Kristal, A. R., Sorensen, G., Palombo, R., Heimendinger, J., & Probart, C. (1993). Development and validation of measures of psychosocial factors influencing fat- and fiber-related dietary behavior. *Preventive Medicine, 22*, 373–387.

Glanz, K., Lewis, F. M., & Rimer, B. K. (Eds.). (1990). *Health behavior and health education: Theory, research, and practice*. San Francisco: Jossey-Bass. (2nd Ed., 1996).

Glanz, K., Patterson, R. E., Kristal, A. R., DiClemente, C., Heimendinger, J., Probart, C., & McLerran, D. (1994). Stages of change in adopting healthy diets: Fat, fiber, and correlates of nutrient intake. *Health Education Quarterly, 21*, 499–519.

Glanz, K., & Resch, N. (1994). Final progress report: Mobile mammography—Improving adherence at the worksite. Philadelphia: Fox Chase Cancer Center.

Glanz, K., Resch, N., Lerman, C., & Rimer, B. K. (1992). Factors associated with adherence to breast cancer screening among working women. *Journal of Occupational Medicine, 34*, 1071–1078.

Glanz, K., Resch, N., Lerman, C., & Rimer, B. K. (1996). Black–white differences in factors influencing mammography use among employed women HMO members. *Ethnicity and Health, 1*(3), 217–230.

Glanz, K., & Rimer, B. K. (1996). *Theory at a glance: A guide to health promotion practice.* Bethesda, Md,: National Cancer Institute.

Glanz, K., Rimer, B. K., Lerman, C., & Gorchov, P. M. (1992). Factors influencing acceptance of mammography: Implications for worksite cancer control. *American Journal of Health Promotion, 7,* 28–36.

Glanz, K., & Rudd, J. (1991). Consumer information on the quality of medical care: A health education and health information policy review. In W. B. Ward & F. M. Lewis (Eds.), *Advances in health promotion and education: Vol. 3* (pp. 15–43). London: Jessica Kingsley.

Glanz, K., Sorensen, G., & Farmer, A. (1996). The health impact of worksite nutrition and cholesterol programs. *American Journal of Health Promotion, 10,* 453–470.

Graham-Clarke, P., & Oldenburg, B. (1994). The effectiveness of a general-practice-based physical activity intervention on patient physical activity status. *Behaviour Change, 11,* 132–144.

Green, L. W. (1984). Health education models. In J. D. Matarazzo, S. M. Weiss, J. A. Herd, N. E. Miller, & S. M. Weiss (Eds.), *Behavioral health: A handbook of health enhancement and disease prevention* (pp. 181–198). New York: Wiley.

Green, L. W., Glanz, K., Hochbaum, G., Kok, G., Kreuter, M., Lewis, F. M., Lorig, K., Morisky, D., Rimer, B. K., & Rosenstock, I. M. (1994). Can we build on, or must we replace, the theories and models in health education? *Health Education Research, 9,* 397–404.

Green, L. W., & Kreuter, M. W. (1991). *Health promotion planning: An educational and environmental approach* (2nd Ed.). Mountain View, Cal: Mayfield.

Green, L. W., Kreuter, M. W., Deeds, S. G., & Partridge, K. B. (1980). *Health education planning: A diagnostic approach.* Palo Alto, CA: Mayfield.

Hawe, P., Degeling, D., & Hall, J. (1990). *Evaluating health promotion: A health worker's guide.* Sydney, Australia: MacLennan & Petty.

Hill, J., Glanz, K., & Rimer, B. K. (1993). *Selecting the cost-effective setting for screening mammography: A comparison of mobile and stationary facilities.* Paper presented at the American Society for Preventive Oncology Annual Meeting, Tucson.

Kerlikowske, K., Grady, D., Rubin, S. M., Sandrock, C., & Ernster, V. L. (1995). Efficacy of screening mammography: A meta-analysis. *Journal of the American Medical Association, 273,* 149–154.

Kirscht, J. P. (1988). The health belief model and predictions of health actions. In D. S. Gochman (Ed.), *Health behavior: Emerging research perspectives* (pp. 27–41). New York: Plenum Press.

Kling, B. (1984). Health education practice and the literature. *Health Education Quarterly, 11,* 341–347.

Kok, G. J. (1993). Theorieen van verandering (Theories of change). In B. Damoiseaux & G. J. Kok (Eds.), *Gezondheidsvoorlichting en gedragsverandering* (pp. 221–236). Assen, The Netherlands: Van Gorcum.

Kolbe, L. J. (1988). The application of health behavior research: Health education and health promotion. In D. S. Gochman (Ed.), *Health behavior: Emerging research perspectives* (pp. 381–396). New York: Plenum Press.

Kristal, A. R., Patterson, R. E., Glanz, K., Heimendinger, J., Hebert, J., Feng, Z., & Probart, C. (1995). Psychosocial correlates of healthful diets: Baseline results from the Working Well Study. *Preventive Medicine, 24,* 221–228.

Luepker, R. V., Murray, D. M., Jacobs, D. R., et al. (1994). Community education for cardiovascular disease prevention: Risk factor changes in the Minnesota Heart Health Program. *American Journal of Public Health, 84,* 1383–1393.

Marlatt, A., & Gordon, J. (1985). *Relapse prevention.* New York: Guilford Press.

Matarazzo, J. D., Weiss, S. M., Herd, J. A., Miller, N. E., & Weiss, S. M. (Eds.) (1984). *Behavioral health: A handbook of health enhancement and disease prevention.* New York: Wiley.

McLeroy, K. R., Bibeau, D., Steckler, A., & Glanz, K. (1988). An ecological perspective on health promotion programs. *Health Education Quarterly, 15,* 351–377.

National Medical Roundtable. (1989, June 29). National organizations agree on joint mammography guidelines. *News from the National Medical Roundtable,* 4 p. Chicago: American Medical News.

National Research Council, National Academy of Sciences. (1989). *Diet and health: Implications for reducing chronic disease risk.* Washington, DC: National Academy Press.

National Task Force on the Preparation and Practice of Health Educators, Inc. (1985). *A framework for the development of competency-based curricula.* New York: National Task Force.

Novelli, W. D. (1990). Applying social marketing to health promotion and disease prevention. In K. Glanz, F. M. Lewis, & B. K. Rimer, (Eds.), *Health behavior and health education: Theory, research and practice* (pp. 342–369). San Francisco: Jossey-Bass.

O'Donnell, M. P. (1989). Definition of health promotion. Part III. Expanding the definition. *American Journal of Health Promotion, 3,* 5.

Oldenburg, B. (1994). Promotion of health: Integrating the clinical and public health approaches. In S. Maes, H. Leventhal, & M. Johnston (Eds.), *International Review of Health Psychology, 3,* 121–143.

Oldenburg, B., Wise, M., Nutbeam, D., Leeder, S., & Watson, C. (1994). Pathways to enhancing Australia's health. *Health Promotion Journal of Australia, 4,* 15–20.

Owen, N., & Bauman, A. (1992). The descriptive epidemiology of physical inactivity in adult Australians. *International Journal of Epidemiology, 21,* 305-310.

Preston, D. B. & Mansfield, P. K. (1991). Assessing the health status of rural people: An analysis of American studies, 1980-1985. In W. B. Ward & F. M. Lewis (Eds.), *Advances in health promotion and education: Vol. 3* (pp. 241-287). London: Jessica Kingsley.

Prochaska, J. O., DiClemente, C. C., & Norcross, J. C. (1992). In search of how people change: Applications to addictive behaviors. *American Psychologist, 47,* 1102-1114.

Rogers, E. (1983) *Diffusion of innovations (3rd ed.).* New York: Free Press.

Rogers, T., & Glanz, K. (1991). Worksite nutrition programs: A review. In J. P. Mayer & J. K. David (Eds.), *Worksite health promotion: Needs, approaches and effectiveness* (pp. 112-151). Lansing: Michigan Department of Health.

Simonds, S. K. (1984). Health education. In J. D. Matarazzo, S. M. Weiss, J. A. Herd, N. E. Miller, & S. M. Weiss (Eds.), *Behavioral health: A handbook of health enhancement and disease prevention* (pp. 1223-1229). New York: Wiley.

Snedecor, G., & Cochran, W. G. (1980). *Statistical methods.* Ames: Iowa State University Press.

Sorensen, G., Thompson, B., Glanz, K., Feng, Z., Kinne, S., DiClemente, C., Emmons, K., Heimendinger, J., Probart, C. & Lichtenstein, E. (1996) Working Well: Results from a worksite-based cancer prevention trial. *American Journal of Public Health, 86,* 939-947.

Speers, M. (1994). *Community health promotion models: A resource for practice.* Paper presented at the Annual Meeting of the American Public Health Association, Washington, DC., Oct. 31.

Stokols, D. (1992). Establishing and maintaining healthy environments: Toward a social ecology of health promotion. *American Psychologist, 47,* 6-22.

U.S. Department of Agriculture, U.S. Department of Health and Human Services. (1990). *Nutrition and your health: Dietary, guidelines for Americans* (3rd ed.). Washington, DC: U.S. Government Printing Office.

U.S. Department of Health and Human Services. (1982). *Public health personnel in the United States, 1980.* DHHS Publication No. (HRA) 82-6. Washington, DC: U.S. Government Printing Office.

U.S. Department of Health and Human Services. (1988). *The Surgeon General's report on nutrition and health.* Washington, DC: U.S. Government Printing Office.

U.S. Department of Health and Human Services. (1991). *Healthy people 2000: National health promotion and disease prevention objectives.* DHHS Publication No. PHS 91-50213. Washington, DC: U.S. Government Printing Office.

Winett, R., King, A., & Altman, D. (1989). *Health psychology and public health: An integrated approach.* New York: Pergamon Press.

Winkleby, M. A. (1994). The future of community-based cardiovascular disease intervention studies. *American Journal of Public Health, 84,* 1369-1372.

9

Relevance of Health Behavior Research to Public Health Professionals

David R. Buchanan

THE HISTORICAL CONTEXT

Public health has historically viewed health and disease as the product of three interacting factors: the host, the agent, and the environment. As classically captured in Hippocrates' *Airs, Waters, Places*, the major emphasis of public health interventions until modern times was focused on changing the environment to prevent illness: building sewage systems, assuring clean water supplies, draining swamps. In one of the best-known legends of public health, a medical practitioner and anesthetist named John Snow plotted the locations of an outbreak of cholera cases in London in the year 1854 (Rosen, 1958). On the basis of his scatterplot, he deduced that one well, the Broad Street pump, was responsible for the outbreak. He then marched down and removed

David R. Buchanan • School of Public Health and Health Sciences, University of Massachusetts, Amherst, Massachusetts 01003.

Handbook of Health Behavior Research IV: Relevance for Professionals and Issues for the Future, edited by David S. Gochman. Plenum Press, New York, 1997.

the handle from the pump, thus interrupting further spread of the epidemic—an effective environmental intervention enacted 30 years before the discovery of bacterial agents.

With the rise of modern science, a shift in the emphasis of public health interventions occurred toward the end of the 19th century. Based on the pioneering work of Koch, Pasteur, Jenner, and others, an explosion of scientific discoveries led to the identification of virtually all known infectious disease-causing bacteria—including typhoid, malaria, leprosy, tuberculosis, streptococcus, cholera, diphtheria, staphylococcus, tetanus, pneumococcus, and the plague—within a 20-year span, 1880–1900. Koch's Postulates set the necessary and sufficient criteria for identifying causal agents.

Koch's Postulates specify four principles to establish a causal relationship between a suspected agent and the disease: (1) The organism is always found with the disease; (2) the organism is not found with any other disease; (3) the isolated organism reproduces the disease in experimental animals; and (4) even where an infectious disease cannot be transmitted to animals, the "regular" and "exclusive" presence of the organism proves the relationship.

In light of the discovery of these many microorganisms, the focus of attention in public health shifted to the role of agents in disease prevention. This shift is sometimes referred to as the "first revolution" in public health.

With the development of immunizations and, later, antibiotics, public health and medicine possessed the tools for preventing microbial agents from causing infectious diseases or for treating the diseases. Thereafter, sometime in the period between 1920 and 1940, infectious diseases, such as tuberculosis, pneumonia, and smallpox, declined as the leading causes of death in the United States and were eclipsed by "chronic diseases," health problems such as heart attacks, cancer, and strokes (see Figure 1).

The etiology of chronic diseases was initially puzzling to researchers. On the basis of the paradigm defined by Koch's Postulates, scientists continued the search for disease-causing agents as the underlying basis for cancer and heart disease until well into the 1960s. They wanted to find the "germ" that caused cancer and then, heading down what was by then a well-worn path, develop an immunization or antibiotic that could prevent these new diseases. Their search proved unsuccessful.

As investigators grew frustrated in their search for causal agents in the development of cancer and heart disease, a new set of public health studies laid the groundwork for a major rethinking of the etiology of chronic diseases. The pioneering and landmark Framingham heart disease study was initiated in the early 1950s. Centered in a small town in Massachusetts, the Framingham study is now one of the best known and

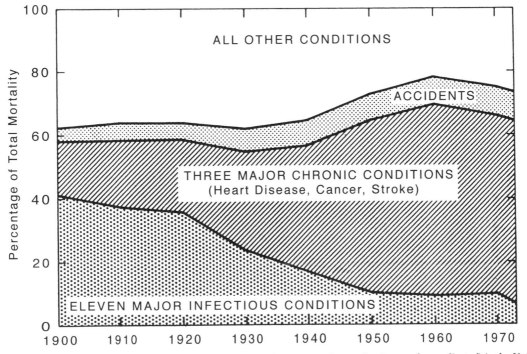

Figure 1. Changing contribution of chronic and infectious conditions to total mortality (age- and sex-adjusted) in the United States, 1900–1973. Reprinted with permission from McKinlay and McKinlay (1977).

widely published studies in public health history. Using a prospective, longitudinal research design, Dawber, Kannel, and others collected a wealth of clinical, behavioral, and demographic information on a group of 6507 men between the ages of 30 and 60 (Dawber, Meadors, & Moore, 1951; Kannel, Dawber, Kagan, Revotskie, & Stokes, 1961). The researchers followed these men over time and looked for commonalities among those suffering heart attacks. The results of this study (and of similar ones, such as the Alameda County Population Laboratory studies [see Belloc & Breslow, 1972]) are now part of the stock of common knowledge: The three leading risk factors for heart disease are smoking, cholesterol, and high blood pressure.

The significance of the Framingham study lies in two areas. First, the unsuccessful search for direct causal agents in the development of chronic diseases forced the field to abandon the paradigm defined by Koch's Postulates of searching for a one-to-one, cause-and-effect relationship between agent and disease. Where the cause-and-effect model had enjoyed stunning success in explaining the genesis of infectious diseases, the explanation of the "cause" of chronic diseases required a shift to a probabilistic model: The presence of "risk factors" made the onset of chronic diseases more likely, but the risk factors could no longer be seen as necessary and sufficient causes.

The second major import of the Framingham study lies in marking the "second revolution" in public health—the shift in attention from the agent to the role of the host in the etiology of chronic diseases (Neubrauer & Pratt, 1981). As smoking, diet, weight control, and so forth were voluntary behaviors that could not be controlled by immunizations or antibiotics, attention turned to the study of changing human behaviors. With the second revolution, the critical role of human behaviors in causing or preventing death, disease, and illness came to be more deeply appreciated. Research on health-related behaviors increased significantly after this time.

MID-1990s CONTEXT

To understand the mid-1990s context for the training and activities of public health professionals, it is helpful to turn to four national reports that have had a major influence in shaping the agenda for behavioral research in public health: *The Future of Public Health* (Institute Medicine [IOM], 1988), *The Public Health Faculty/ Agency Forum* (Sorenson & Bialek, n.d.), and two reports from the U.S. Surgeon General (1979, 1990), *Healthy People* and *Healthy People 2000*.

The Future of Public Health was a jeremiad in which the authors decried the state of public health then prevailing in the United States, finding that it had been allowed to "fall into disarray." For the purposes of this chapter, the report is important for two reasons: (1) It put forth a widely accepted definition of public health, and (2) it raised issues about a potential-mismatch between the types of training offered in most academic programs and the job skills needed in public health agencies.

After deploring how "the nation has lost sight of its public health goals" and "let down our public health guard," the IOM report set out a series of recommendations for rebuilding the public health infrastructure. These recommendations have been instrumental in redefining the core functions of public health. As a first step, the authors offered an original and authoritative definition of public health: "Public health is what we, as a society, do collectively to assure the conditions for people to be healthy." The reader will note that this definition is broad. Using this definition, social and behavioral sciences ranging from economics, management, and political science to anthropology, sociology, and psychology are intrinsic to the field. Indeed, all are drawn on liberally in academic training programs.

The second relevant point of the IOM report is its noting that "some schools have become somewhat isolated from public health practice." Following on *The Future of Public Health*, the Council on Education in Public Health (CEPH), the national public health accrediting body, revised its accreditation criteria. Schools of public health are now required to demonstrate that their curricula are strongly linked to the specific job skills needed in public health agencies. These skills and competencies are spelled out in detail in *The Public Health Faculty Agency Forum* (Sorenson & Bialek, n.d.).

The Faculty/Agency Forum specifies competencies in five areas: general or universal competencies expected of everyone in the field and competencies in each of the sub-disciplines of public health (epidemiology/biostatistics, health administration, environmental health sciences, and the behavioral sciences). Among the universal competencies, all public health professionals are expected to be competent in "identifying the role of cultural, social and behavioral factors in determining disease, disease prevention, health promoting behavior, and medical service organization and delivery." Thus, all public health professionals are expected to have a working knowledge of the behavioral sciences and their relevance to health outcomes.

The two U.S. Surgeon General reports, *Healthy People* and *Healthy People 2000*, complete this survey of the major influences that define the role of health behavior research in public health.

In 1979, the U.S. Surgeon General (1979) released a report titled *Healthy People*. This report was the first attempt by the U.S. Public Health Service to define public health goals for the nation. These goals were delineated in a companion report, *Promoting Health/Preventing Disease: Objectives for the Nation* (U.S. Department of Health and Human Services, 1980), that identified 243 objectives in 15 priority areas (e.g., immunizations, toxic controls, smoking, physical fitness). These objectives were to be achieved by the year 1990. Beyond identifying national objectives, the report is perhaps even more significant for having stated officially for the first time that "perhaps as much as half of U.S. mortality in 1976 was due to unhealthy behavior or lifestyle." Thus, the behavioral research agenda was set.

Based on the success and the model of the

Healthy People report, the U.S. Surgeon General (1990) issued *Healthy People 2000* a decade later. Like its predecessor, this report defined three overarching goals, broken down into 332 objectives organized into 22 priority areas. The three goals for the nation are to:

1. Increase the span of healthy life for Americans.
2. Reduce health disparities among Americans.
3. Achieve access to preventive services for all Americans.

In each priority area, objectives are categorized under five headings: improved health services, increased public and professional awareness, reduced risk factors, improved health status and surveillance. As explained by L. Green (L. Green, 1984; L. Green & Kreuter, 1991) (see Figure 2), these five categories provide the basic logic model for achieving the nation's goals and objectives. It is a simple linear framework. As shown in Figure 2, improved health services are expected to lead to increased public awareness, which in turn is expected to lead to reduced risk factors which finally will lead to improved health status.

In terms of the role of health behavior research in public health, it is important to point out that *Healthy People 2000* thus presented an explicit—albeit highly simplified—theory of human behavior: Knowledge causes action. Once people are made aware of the deleterious health effects of cigarette smoking, so the model suggests, they will stop smoking or not take it up.

In summary, with the largely effective control of infectious diseases (with the significant exception of HIV/AIDS) and the rise of chronic, or so-called "lifestyle," diseases, public health has come to pay increasing attention to the role of human behaviors in determining the health status of the nation. The etiology of the leading causes of morbidity and mortality now is largely social and behavioral, rather than biological. The significant exception is HIV/AIDS, but until such time as an effective vaccine or antiviral drugs are developed, HIV/AIDS prevention strategies will

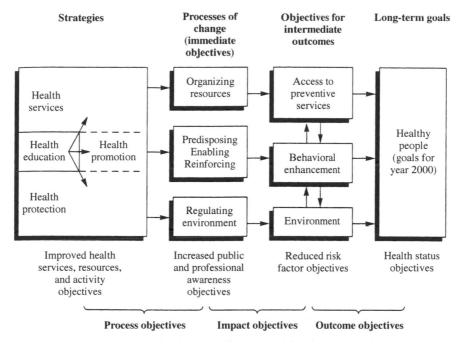

Figure 2. Approximate relationships among the objectives of interest and the objectives for the nation in disease prevention and health promotion. Reprinted with permission from L. Green and Kreuter (1991).

necessarily also focus on changing human behaviors.

Reflecting this shift in focus, a series of national reports in recent years have placed increasing importance on providing training and competencies in the behavioral sciences for all public health professionals. Moreover, a rudimentary model of human behavior is presented in the public health service's most prestigious planning document, *Healthy People 2000*. Before turning to the specific subdisciplines within public health to see how they are now utilizing health behavior research, a brief review of key controversies in the field brought on by the "second revolution" in public health will set the stage for the discussion in the subsequent sections.

CURRENT CONTROVERSIES

As described above, public health has always viewed health and disease as the product of the interaction of the agent, host, and environment. Historically, public health focused on changing the environment. With the first revolution and the rise of modern medicine, attention shifted to the role of bacterial agents in diseases processes. Many if not most people credit the development of vaccines and antibiotics for the virtual elimination of infectious diseases in developed countries, but this view has not gone unchallenged.

In a provocative analysis of the historical record, McKinlay and McKinlay (1977) found that the precipitous decline in infectious disease rates *preceded* the development of immunizations and antibiotics by several decades. For each of nine different infectious diseases, ranging from diphtheria to scarlet fever, the incidence rate plummeted long before the discovery of effective interventions to counteract the respective bacterial agent. Drawing on the work of McKeown (1976) and others, McKinlay and McKinlay attributed the declines to rising standards of living brought about by the industrial revolution—specifically, improved nutrition and reduced exposure to infection through improved hygiene—rather than the development of biological interventions. They concluded that at most, 3.5% of the total decline in mortality since 1900 could be ascribed to medical measures. Hence, they argued, the foundations of the first revolution in public health have been misattributed: Changes in environmental conditions, not in controlling disease-causing agents, were responsible for the dramatic improvements in the health of the public in the first half of this century.

The second revolution in public health has been marked by similar controversies (Neubrauer & Pratt, 1981). Here, the crux of the issue hinges on the relative contribution and independence of lifestyle behaviors in relation to socioeconomic status (e.g., see Antonovsky, 1967; Haan, Kaplan, & Camacho, 1987; M. Marmot, 1986; G. Marmot, Kogevinas, & Elston, 1987; Rose, 1985; Salmon, 1989). Critics argue that concentrating on changing individual lifestyle behaviors is yet another form of victim blaming (Becker, 1986; Marantz, 1990; Ryan, 1976).

The most compelling case against concentrating on the role of the host in health promotion and disease prevention was put forward in Great Britain in a report titled, *Inequalities in Health* (Department of Health and Social Security [DHSS], 1982). Released in 1982, *Inequalities in Health* is the British equivalent of the United States *Healthy People* (U.S. Surgeon General, 1979) report. Often referred to as the Black Report, it was prepared by the Working Group on Inequalities in Health which was commissioned by the British Secretary of State in 1977 and chaired by Sir Douglas Black, then Chair of the Royal College of Physicans.

Like *Healthy People*, the Black Report is a national public health planning document. Unlike the United States report, the Black Report examined four hypotheses regarding the distribution of health and illness in the general population. After a careful examination of the evidence, the Black Report rejected three alternative hypotheses: (1) that differences in health status were artifactual; (2) that differences in health status were due to downward drift, i.e., sick people become poor; and, significantly, (3) that differences in health status were due to differences in lifestyle. Instead, the report supported the fourth hypothesis, the materialist hypothesis, which states that differences in health status are attributable to differences in material conditions linked to socioeconomic status. Their recommendation: To improve the health status of the British people, it will be necessary to narrow the gap in income distribution in society (DHSS, 1982).

The controversy continues. More sophisticated analyses today find powerful correlations between lifestyle behaviors and socioeconomic status (SES), but even after taking these correlations into account, an independent contribution of SES to health status remains (MacIntyre, 1986) (for an elegant description of the interdependence of SES and lifestyle, see Graham, 1989). Whether lifestyle is independent of SES or not, questions persist about the potential effectiveness of attempts to encourage poor people with low levels of education to exercise, alter their diet, and give up smoking without significant improvements in their socioeconomic conditions. The most recent Canadian public health planning document, the Epp (1987) report, puts greater weight on changing socioenvironmental conditions than does the U.S. Surgeon General's *Healthy People 2000*.

Another more recent controversy concerns the ethical propriety of standard randomized experimental designs in the conduct of public health research. Most glaringly brought to light by the AIDS epidemic, the morality of withholding potentially effective medications from people otherwise doomed to die has been questioned by many people. On a less dramatic scale, many communities, particularly communities of color, are growing increasingly unwilling to be used as subjects to test disinterested researchers' hypotheses. They argue convincingly that they have a right to determine their own destiny.

In response to these concerns, many public health researchers are struggling to develop a more appropriate set of guidelines for conducting community research (Fawcett, 1989). This type of research is often grouped under labels such as "community action" or "participatory" research. The basic tenet of this type of research is that the subjects of inquiry should stand as equal partners with the researchers in determining the purposes of the research, the types of questions to be asked and the uses of the results (Brown & Tandor, 1983; Reason, 1995). Fawcett (1989) has identified a number of emerging standards for this type of research (see Table 1). These controversies play an important role in shaping the behavioral research agenda in public health today.

ORGANIZATION OF THE FIELD OF PUBLIC HEALTH

Academic training programs in public health are organized into five core disciplines: epidemiology, biostatistics, environmental health sciences, health administration, and the behavioral sciences. To become an accredited school of public health, a school must have a graduate training program that at a minimum offers all five core disciplines. As of 1995, there were 27 accredited schools of public health in the United States.

Epidemiology is the mother science of public health. It is concerned with studying the distribution and etiology of diseases in populations. Closely allied with epidemiology, biostatistics grounds all public health research in objective, quantifiable terms. The environmental health sciences concentrate on the health effects of air, water, and soil contaminants. Health administration is concerned with optimizing the trade-offs among cost, quality, and access in the provision of health care services. Finally, the behavioral sciences (or health education) are concerned with the role of human health behaviors in relation to disease prevention and health promotion.

In addition to core disciplines, there are a number of allied health sciences associated with the field of public health, including nutrition,

Table 1. Community Action Research Principles[a]

1. Community researchers should form collaborative relationships with the participants with whom they do the research.
2. Descriptive community research should provide information about relationships between environmental events, behaviors presumed relevant to community functioning, and related outcomes valued by communities.
3. Experimental community research should provide information on the effects of modifiable and sustainable environmental events on behaviors and outcomes of interest, on the generality and maintenance of the effects, and on the social importance and appropriateness of the research and action.
4. The chosen setting, participants, and research measures should be appropriate to the community problem under investigation.
5. The measurement of the dependent variables must be replicable by typically trained readers of community research reports, and chosen measures should attempt to capture the dynamic and transactional nature of the interaction between behavior and the environment.
6. Community interventions should be replicable by typically trained implementors and sustainable with local resources.
7. Community action should occur at the level of change and timing likely to optimize beneficial outcomes.
8. Researchers should develop a capacity to disseminate the effective social interventions they develop and provide training and technical assistance to change agents.
9. Results of community research and action must be communicated openly and effectively to clients, implementors, and purchasers of social interventions, decision makers, and, when appropriate, the broader public.
10. Community research and action projects should contribute to understanding and change, especially that which fosters prevention of problems in living and empowerment of people of marginal status.

[a]Reproduced with permission from Fawcett (1989).

exercise science, occupational health, maternal and child health, and international health. Each of these disciplines has its own well-defined content areas; each is related to the core disciplines in fairly self-evident ways.

Since health education and health administration are covered in Chapters 8 and 10 respectively, this chapter will focus on the remaining seven content areas: epidemiology and biostatistics, environmental health sciences, nutrition, exercise science, occupational health, maternal and child health, and international health.

Epidemiology and Biostatistics

As the mother science of public health, epidemiological research is at the foundation of each of the subdisciplines of public health. The relevance of the environmental health sciences, nutrition, exercise science, and so on to public health ultimately rests on epidemiological investigations into the relationship between specified content areas and their effects on human health status. In the discussion that follows, the examples cited are meant only to illustrate, not to exhaust the uses of behavioral research in public health.

On the basis of the successful model of the Framingham and Alameda County Population Laboratory studies, epidemiologists and biostatisticians have broadened the search for "risk factors" to include behavioral as well as biological risk factors. Much current epidemiological research focuses on discovering the behavioral analogues of cholesterol, hypertension, and smoking (Krantz, Glass, Contrada, & Miller, 1982; Raymond, 1989). What social and behavioral antecedents put people at higher risk for beginning to smoke, leading a sedentary lifestyle, eating a high-fat diet, or, of more recent concern, perpetrating violence (Prothrow-Stith, 1991; Rosenberg & Fenley, 1991) (see Figure 3). Studies of behavioral risk factors are now presented in a growing number of social epidemiology courses on campuses across the United States.

Because coronary heart disease is now the

Behavioral Risk Factors →	Risky Behaviors →	Poor Health Outcomes
[e.g., low self-esteem, family conflict, attitudes, perceived norms, social support, perceived susceptibility, etc.]	[e.g., smoking, violence, physical inactivity, obesity, precocious and promiscuous sexual behaviors, etc.]	[e.g., lung cancer, homicide, suicide, heart disease, strokes, etc.]

Figure 3. Flow chart of the presumed relationships among behavioral risk factors, risky behavior, and health outcomes.

leading cause of death in the United States, a number of large-scale public health intervention research trials have attempted to reduce its toll. On the basis of the results of the Framingham study, interventions have used theoretically based behavioral strategies to try to get people to change their smoking, dietary, and exercise behaviors. Using a highly intensive (and costly) individualized counseling model, the Multiple Risk Factor Intervention Trial (MRFIT) targeted smoking, cholesterol, and hypertension with state-of-the-art, one-on-one counseling techniques. The early results of the MRFIT program were disappointing (MRFIT Research Group, 1982), but follow-up studies demonstrated successful reductions in heart diseases linked to reductions in risk factors (MRFIT Research Group, 1990).

In contrast to the individualized MRFIT approach, the Stanford three- and five-community studies used population-based strategies to effect behavior changes to reduce known risk factors for heart disease (Farquhar, 1978; Farquhar et al., 1977, 1990). In the three-community study, three small matched towns were randomly assigned to a control condition (no intervention), media only group, or media plus community education condition. The behavioral interventions were based on an eclectic mix of behavioral theories, among them the health belief model, social learning theory, social marketing, and community organizing. The results of the Stanford three-community study, and the subsequent five-community study, provide modest support for the effectiveness of behavioral interventions in reducing mortality rates (Susser, 1995). The basic prototype of using population-based strategies to effect behavior change to reduce risk factors for heart disease has been replicated in several other large-scale studies with similar results (for a review of these studies, see Pancer & Nelson, 1989/1990).

Beyond the heart disease studies, the most advanced research program in identifying behavioral risk factors has focused on substance abuse. A number of reports have established near consensus in the field and have received the official endorsement of the federal Center for Substance Abuse Prevention. In these studies, a set of 17 risk factors, grouped into five major domains (community, school, peer, family, and individual), have been identified (Bry, McKeon, & Pandinam, 1982; Dupont, 1989; Goodstadt & Mitchell, 1992; Hawkins, Catalano, & Miller, 1992). These risk factors are shown in Table 2.

Like strategies to reduce the incidence of heart disease, the fundamental proposition of social epidemiology is that a reduction in behavioral risk factors will lead to a reduction in the physiological risk factors linked to the development of chronic diseases. To prevent heart disease, one needs to prevent smoking. To prevent smoking, one needs to identify, and then reduce or eliminate, the risk factors that increase the likelihood of people taking up smoking. Primary

Table 2. Risk Factors for Substance Abuse[a]

Laws and norms favorable toward behavior	Neighborhood disorganization
Extreme economic deprivation	Family alcohol and drug behavior and attitudes
Physiological factors	Family conflict
Poor and inconsistent family management practices	Early and persistent problem behaviors
Low bonding to family	Low degree of commitment to school
Academic failure	Association with drug-using peers
Peer rejection in elementary grades	Attitudes favorable to drug use
Alienation and rebelliousness	Availability
Early onset of drug use	

[a]Adapted from Hawkins, Catalano, and Miller (1992).

prevention is thus defined as the reduction or elimination of risk factors (Last, 1987).

In an important twist on the search for risk factors, there has also been a growing appreciation of the role of "protective" or "resiliency" factors in recent years in public health research. Resiliency factors are factors that protect people from or *decrease* their risk of taking up deleterious health behaviors. A warm, supportive family environment, religiosity, and social support (see below) are examples of resiliency factors that lower the odds of initiating unhealthy behaviors.

Evidence demonstrating the power of the behavioral risk factor model with respect to substance abuse is mixed. The most convincing case showing the relationship between primary risk factors and the initiation of unhealthy behaviors has been made in the case of smoking prevention. Drawing on Bandura's social learning theory (Bandura, 1977, 1986), researchers hypothesized that "peer pressure" is a major risk factor leading to teenage smoking. To counteract this risk factor, innumerable smoking prevention programs have implemented "resistance skills" programs utilizing the concepts of modeling and behavioral rehearsal, also from social learning theory (for a comprehensive review of school-based prevention programs, see Hansen, 1992). Harking back to an earlier public health model, McGuire (1964) named these strategies "inoculations." Although interventions demonstrating the effectiveness of this model for smoking prevention have been relatively consistent, the results have not generalized to other areas of substance abuse prevention.

One finds a similar picture if one examines the effects of resiliency factors. The most convincing evidence for the beneficial effects of resiliency factors has been uncovered for social support (House, Umberson, & Landis, 1988). One of the first demonstrations of the positive, protective effects of social support was carried out by Berkman in a re-analysis of the data collected in the Alameda County Population Laboratory study. Where the initial analyses had focused on health habits (e.g., smoking, drinking, physical activity), Berkman constructed a rudimentary measure of social support based on four items: marriage, church attendance, participation in social organizations, and time spent visiting friends (Berkman & Breslow, 1983). Even with this simple measure, her results were surprisingly robust. The impact of social support was of the same order of magnitude as the effects of health habits. The results held up even after controlling for health habits and social class. On the basis of Berkman's work and extensive other studies, it thus appears that seeing one's friends frequently may be as beneficial for one's health as regular exercise.

In seeking to explain the beneficial effects of social support, researchers have focused on the interaction of social support with stress and coping ability (Israel & Schurman, 1990). Two major alternative hypotheses have emerged: (1) Social support has a *direct* effect in reducing the health impact of stress, or (2) social support has an *indirect*, or buffering effect. In support of the direct effects model, there is some evidence that social support per se produces soothing biophysiological responses such as decreased heart rates and lowered blood pressure. In the indirect model, social support is seen as providing buffers to help people cope with stressors. These indirect mechanisms include providing people with information, instrumental support (e.g., money), emotional support, and feedback (Israel & Schurman, 1990).

Despite the logic and appeal of the behavioral risk and resiliency factor model, the amount of variability in human behaviors accounted for by this model has been low, especially when compared to biological risk factors, such as cholesterol or hypertension. The behavioral risk factors that increase the odds that people will take up smoking have not proven to be as robust as the relationship between biological risk factors (such as smoking) and heart disease. Cautious questions have been raised about whether the search for behavioral equivalents of biological risk factors will ultimately prove fruitful (Bucha-

nan, 1992, 1994; Kelly, 1989; McQueen & Noack, 1988; Research Unit, 1989).

Environmental Health Sciences

A new and rapidly growing area of research bringing together the behavioral sciences with the environmental health sciences is the topic of risk appraisal. For environmental health scientists, a major problem is presenting information about the health risks of exposures to different substances in ways that will engender appropriate public responses (see Figure 4). Their concern is that findings that establish very low risks, even infinitesmal risks, with regard to a suspected carcinogen often generate seemingly irrational overreactions on the part of the public. Conversely, other exposures fail to generate any response at all. What determines how people will perceive and react to the health risks inherent in exposures to different environmental health hazards?

Research into subjective risk appraisal has discovered several interesting and critical distinctions that people make in responding to potential hazards. One major difference that explains people's different reactions is whether the risk is voluntary (e.g., cigarette smoke) or nonvoluntary (e.g., asbestos) (National Research Council, 1989). When people feel they have control over their exposure to an identified carcinogen, they are willing to tolerate high levels of exposure. On the other hand, when people feel they do not have control over their level of exposure, they are unwilling to tolerate even minimal, inconsequential exposures. Hence, the public may demand extremely costly removals and cleanups of substances like asbestos (Abelson, 1990), while at the same time continuing to smoke, even though the chemicals in cigarette smoke pose an objectively much higher level of risk. Environmental health scientists are thus now teaming up with behavioral scientists to discover ways of framing information that will produce responses more consistent with objective levels of risks.

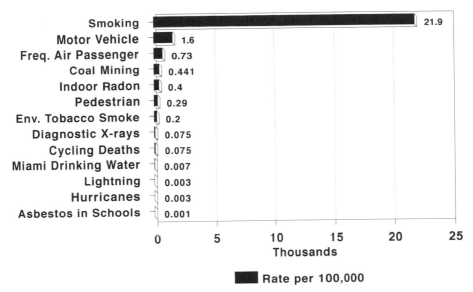

Figure 4. Relative risk to one's health due to exposure to different environmental contaminants and select behaviors.

Nutrition

Diet has a major influence on people's risk for heart disease, cancer, and stroke, the three leading causes of mortality in the United States today. Changes in people's patterns of food consumption, for better or worse, will have a major impact on the health status of the nation as a whole. *Healthy People 2000* therefore lists 21 objectives for improving dietary practices—from reducing fat intake to breast-feeding to food labels. Reflecting one of the controversies discussed earlier, there is continuing debate over whether strategies that target individual behavior change should take priority over strategies that focus on environmental change (e.g., regulations that mandate reduced salt content in canned foods).

As one of the allied health sciences, nutrition employs both clinical and public health approaches to understanding and altering people's dietary behaviors. On the clinical side, registered dieticians are trained in individual counseling techniques—frequently used in hospital settings—

as they seek to improve an individual's eating habits.

From a public health perspective, behavioral techniques of greater consequence are population-based approaches. As exemplified in the heart disease intervention programs, a large number of studies have attempted to modify a targeted population's eating habits—e.g., to reduce cholesterol levels, obesity, salt intake—to achieve national health goals. Another approach cited in *Healthy People 2000* is that of increasing the percentage of schoolchildren who receive nutrition education to at least 75% by the year 2000. Thus, Parcel et al. (1995) developed a school-based curriculum based on social learning theory to encourage more healthful eating habits starting at an early age. The preliminary evaluations of their research show promising results.

A pressing challenge facing the field of public health nutrition is overcoming public apathy and confusion that may result from inconsistent or seemingly contradictory messages. As nutritional science has progressed, the results of more recent studies have overturned, or made much more complex, findings from prior studies that demonstrated a relationship between a particular dietary factor and poor health outcomes. From cholesterol to bran to complex carbohydrates, health claims are put forward, only to be refuted by newer evidence. As a result, the general public has grown increasingly skeptical. The gap between the nutritional sciences and the behavioral sciences (communication theory, in particular) will need to be closed in the near future if public health nutrition is to achieve its goals.

Exercise Science

Like nutrition, physical activity and fitness are integrally related to people's overall physical and mental well-being. Accordingly, the Public Health Service has set out 12 objectives for the nation to achieve by the year 2000. The global goal is to improve physical fitness and decrease the toll of cardiovascular disease on society.

Like nutrition, changes in the population's level of physical activity—increases or decreases—will have significant implications for the nation's health bill. On the basis of the pioneering epidemiological studies by Paffenberger, being overweight and leading a sedentary lifestyle are now known to be major risk factors for coronary heart disease (Paffenberger, Hyde, Wing, & Hsieh, 1986; Paffenberger, Wing, & Hyde, 1978). Conversely, regular physical exercise is now recognized as one of the most powerful resiliency or protective factors known for warding off heart disease and a host of other ailments. Thus, programs are being developed for worksites and other locations to promote physical activity (Hooper & Veneziano, 1995).

Occupational Health

According to the U.S. Surgeon General (1990, p. 296): "Although the number of fatal occupational injuries has gradually declined in recent years, work-related illnesses and nonfatal injuries appear to be increasing. During 1987 alone, permanent impairments suffered on the job grew from 60,000 to 70,000, total disabling injuries number 1.8 million, and combined occupational illnesses and injuries in the manufacturing industries increased by 13.5 percent." Other studies have estimated that probably one half of all cancer cases are complicated by occupational exposures (Ashford, 1976).

A promising area of behavioral research in occupational health examines the relationship between job stress and job control (K. Green, 1988; Israel & Schurman, 1990; Wallerstein, 1992). Many studies have found that stress levels are inversely related to the amount of job control (autonomous decision-making authority), especially in high-demand positions. The implication of these studies is that stress, and hence associated health problems, could be reduced through increasing employees' control over their working conditions. The impetus to embrace a more participatory, inclusive decision-making process has been widely disseminated through programs like total quality management seminars.

More so than other areas of public health concern, the field of occupational health has been riven by contentions over the most appropriate target of change, the host or the environment. Here, the debate has become deeply political, taking on all the overtones of labor–management struggles. On its own behalf, management tends to blame work-related illnesses and injuries on an irresponsible work force, the solution to which is to set up counseling programs, such as employee assistance programs, for individual remediation. Labor, on the other hand, tends to see such problems as due to hazardous working conditions and fights for regulations to change the work environment, such as safer equipment, less stressful production demands, and less exposure to hazardous materials. As a result, the types of interventions that are implemented often have more to do with the particular federal administration in power than with any evidence about the respective merits of the interventions.

Maternal and Child Health

The United States has one of the worst infant mortality rates among all industrialized nations, ranking 21st in the world in 1994. There are also gaping disparities in infant mortality rates among the races in the United States. Because of these challenges, *Healthy People 2000* lists ten subobjectives to address infant mortality alone. Explanations for the dismal United States record commonly point to lifestyle factors such as illicit drug use and a high rate of unintended pregnancies.

Like smoking and other drug abuse prevention efforts, a number of programs have grown up around the idea of teaching young people "resistance skills" to give them the ability to withstand pressures to initiate sexual relations prematurely. Also like substance abuse prevention, the results of such abstinence-promoting programs are mixed.

Infant mortality is potentially preventable if a better understanding of the causes of risky behaviors could be formulated. For example, through comparisons with other countries, it is now clear that the provision of contraceptive devices (e.g., condoms) per se does not appear to encourage higher levels of sexual activity (Jones, 1986; Jones, Forrest, Henshaw, Silverman, & Torres, 1988).

International Health

Training public health professionals for positions in international settings is a two-way street. Many Americans are interested in working overseas, usually in the developing world, although events in Eastern Europe and the former Soviet Union in the 1990s point to the need for basic public health measures in these countries too. In the other direction, many health professionals from developing countries seek advanced training in the United States to prepare themselves for leadership positions in their native lands. About half of the schools of public health in the United States offer concentrations in international health.

Most of the public health problems in the developing world lie in the area of infectious diseases. Hence, the bulk of public health interventions there focus on basic environmental improvements, such as sanitation and water supplies. One of the most remarkable public health successes in this area is the worldwide elimination of smallpox.

Aside from environmental improvements, the area to receive the greatest attention of public health specialists in developing countries is maternal and child health, specifically childhood immunization campaigns and family planning. While not without its critics, the foundation of a major behavioral change strategy in immunization and family planning campaigns in the developing world is social marketing.

Social Marketing. Social marketing is based on principles and tenets employed in business marketing and advertising campaigns (Hastings & Haywood, 1991; Kotler & Roberto, 1989). To increase market "penetration" (i.e., to boost sales or, in the case of social marketing, to achieve social goals such as increasing levels of immunizations or numbers of contraceptors), social marketing targets four key variables: price, product, place, and promotion. "Price" refers to both the actual costs (e.g., for purchasing a condom) and the perceived psychological costs. Lowering the price, in both senses, will increase the number of adopters. "Product" refers to responding both to market demands (usually less relevant to social marketing campaigns) and to the relative advantages of one product over another (e.g., Norplant versus birth control pills). "Place" refers to making one's product readily accessible to the target population. "Promotion" refers to the deployment of a full range of mass media advertising techniques. It is important to note that social marketing is more than simply the use of the mass media. Price, product, and place are essential elements in any social marketing campaign.

The results of social marketing campaigns to boost immunization levels or promote contraceptive practices in international settings are un-even (Bloom & Novelli, 1981; Brieger & Rama-krishna, 1987). Media campaigns are frequently implemented without full attention to the other variables, with the result that problems such as accessiblility (place) are not overcome. As with other subspecialities in public health, critics charge that social marketing campaigns are the ultimate in "victim-blaming" approaches in seeking to improve the lives of poor, illiterate peasants. In their stead, proponents of environmental strate-gies point to the efficacy of other approaches, such as improving the status of women in society (e.g., through increasing literacy levels of women).

SUMMARY AND CONCLUSION: RESEARCH ISSUES

The relevance and application of health be-havior research to the field of public health should by now be apparent. There is one final point, however, that deserves further discussion.

Perhaps the most significant dividing line between public health and the behavioral sci-ences concerns the fundamental aims of research. The primary goal of research in the social and behavioral sciences is theory development. But the primary goal of epidemiological research is the discovery of risk and resiliency factors. Thus, researchers in the Research Unit in Health and Behavioural Change (1989) in England note (pp. 6-7):

> The role that epidemiology has taken on in becoming the underlying discipline of public health is a mixed blessing.... In the last analysis, epidemiology is only a method, it has no underlying theoretical, conceptual basis other than a belief in the current scientific para-digm. Lacking a theory, it has no guidelines as to where to place human behavior as a "factor"; it may be a determinant, it may be an outcome, but only rhetoric serves as a guide.

As noted, the basic paradigm of epidemiological research is rigidly empirical and atheoretical. Epi-demiological research indiscriminately incorpo-rates any factors that correlate significantly with

the health issue under investigation. Genetic, be-havioral, social, environmental, economic, and geographic factors—all are acceptable in trying to explain a disease process, no matter how eclectic, incongruous, or illogical. It is a "kitchen sink" approach that runs against the grain of principles prized in the behavioral sciences, principles such as parsimony, coherence, and meaningfulness.

The Ecological Model.   As an example, one model gaining increasing currency in public health these days is the ecological model de-scribed by McLeroy, Bibeau, Steckler, and Glanz (1988). McLeroy credits Bronfenbrenner (1979) and his "systems" analysis for inspiring the eco-logical model. In the ecological model, variables are seen as being located on different levels (or systems) corresponding to different levels of analysis. These different levels may be pictured as concentric circles, starting with the most micro-cosmic analysis in the center and expanding through outer circles of increasingly more macro-analyses.

The ecological model posits five system levels: intrapersonal, interpersonal, organiza-tional, community, and public policy. Intraperso-nal factors are individual psychological variables, such as self-efficacy, self-esteem, perceived sus-ceptibility, and the like. Interpersonal factors are social–psychological variables, such as norms and social support. Organizational factors mark the shift to more macroinstitutional levels of analysis.

Here, the model draws on theories of organi-zational development to identify factors (e.g., different management styles: authoritarian, dem-ocratic) that promote or impede more effective or efficient goal attainment. On the level of com-munity, the model draws on theories of commu-nity organization and community development with variables such as values, cultural norms and practices, anomie, and social bonding. Finally, on the level of public policy, the model looks at the impact of public policy on the distribution of socioeconomic goods, poverty, rights, and ac-cess to means of recourse to correct injustices.

In sum, the ecological model offers an enormous array of independent variables, all of which have been found separately to have some effect on human behavior. With the ecological model, the eclectic, multifactorial nature of epidemiological research finds its quintessential expression. It can accommodate virtually any social scientific variable ever identified, and as a perusal of the model suggests, it incorporates these variables without regard for the integrity of the theories of origin.

The basic paradigm of epidemiological research thus poses a major challenge to the aims and conduct of behavioral research. In epidemiological research, brute empirical relationships become the sole criterion for determining relevance, displacing research programs guided by deductive reasoning from theoretical premises. Theories developed in the behavioral sciences, such as those used in health behavior research, may therefore be used and useful in public health only in identifying new sets of variables for potential incorporation into one ever-growing larger model. In the end, the methods of epidemiological research threaten to supplant the development of theories that seek coherence, meaning, integrity, and parsimony with the simple accumulation of masses of distinct, unconnected factors.

REFERENCES

Abelson, P. (1990). The asbestos removal fiasco. *Science, 247,* 1017.

Antonovsky, A. (1967). Social class, life expectancy and overall mortality. *Milbank Memorial Fund Quarterly, 45,* 31-73.

Ashford, N. (1976). *Crisis in the workplace: Occupational disease and injury*. Cambridge, MA: MIT Press.

Bandura, A. (1977). *Social learning theory*. Englewood Cliffs, NJ: Prentice-Hall.

Bandura, A. (1986). *Social foundations of thought and action: A social cognitive theory*. Englewood Cliffs, NJ: Prentice-Hall.

Becker, M. (1986). The tyranny of health promotion. *Public Health Reviews, 14,* 15-25.

Belloc, N., & Breslow, L. (1972). Relationship of physical health status and health practices. *Preventive Medicine, 1,* 409-421.

Berkman, L., & Breslow, L. (1983). *Health and ways of living: The Alameda County Study*. New York: Oxford University Press.

Bloom, P., & Novelli, W. (1981). Problems and challenges in social marketing. *Journal of Marketing, 45,* 79-85.

Brieger, W., & Ramakrishna, J. (1987) Health education: Social marketing does not have all of the answers. *World Health Forum, 8,* 384-386.

Brofenbrenner, U. (1979). *The ecology of human development*. Cambridge, MA: Harvard University Press.

Brown, L., & Tandor, R. (1983). Ideology and political economy in inquiry: Action research and participatory research. *Journal of Applied Behavioral Sciences, 19,* 277-294.

Bry, B., McKeon, P., & Pandinam, K. (1982). Extent of drug use as a function of the number of risk factors. *Journal of Abnormal Psychology, 91,* 273-279.

Buchanan, D. (1992). An uneasy alliance: Combining quantitative and qualitative research methods. *Health Education Quarterly, 19,* 117-135.

Buchanan, D. (1994). Reflections on the relationship between theory and practice. *Health Education Research, 9,* 273-283.

Dawber, T., Meadors, G., & Moore, F. (1951). Epidemiologcal approaches to heart disease: The Framingham Study. *American Journal of Public Health, 41,* 279-286.

Department of Health and Social Security. (1982). *Inequalities in health (Black Report): Report of a research working group*. National Health Service. London: Pelican.

Dupont, R. (Ed.). (1989). *Stopping alcohol and other drug use before it starts: The future of prevention*. OSAP Prevention Monograph No. 1, U.S. Department of Health and Human Services. DHHS Publication No. (ADM) 89-1645. Washington, DC: U.S. Government Printing Office.

Epp, J. (1987). Achieving health for all: A framework for health promotion [The Ottawa Charter]. *Health Promotion, 1,* 419-428.

Farquhar, J. (1978). The community-based model of lifestyle intervention trials. *American Journal of Epidemiology, 108,* 103-111.

Farquhar, J., Fortmann, S., Flora, J., Taylor, B., Haskell, W., Williams, P., Maccoby, N., & Wood, P. (1990). Effects of communitywide education on cardiovascular disease risk factors: The Stanford Five-City Project. *Journal of the American Medical Association, 264,* 359-365.

Farquhar, J., Wood, P., Breitrose, H., Haskell, W., Meyer, A., Maccoby, N., Alexander, J., Brown, B., McAlister, A., Nash, J., & Stern, M. (1977). Community education for cardiovascular health. *Lancet, 1,* 1192-1195.

Fawcett, S. (1989). Some emerging standards for community research and action. In P. Tolan, C. Keys, F. Chertok, & L. Jason (Eds.), *Researching community psychology: Issues of theory and methods* (pp. 64-57). Washington, DC: American Psychological Association.

Goodstadt, M., & Mitchell, E. (1992). Prevention theory and research related to high-risk youth. OSAP Technical Report. *Breaking new ground for youth at risk: Program summaries*. Washington, DC: U.S. Department of Health and Human Services.

Graham, H. (1989). Women and smoking in the United Kingdom: The implications for health promotion. *Health Promotion, 3*, 371-382.

Green, K. (1988). Issues of control and responsibility in workers' health. *Health Education Quarterly, 15*, 473-486.

Green, L. (1984). Modifying and developing health behavior. *Annual Review of Public Health, 5*, 215-236.

Green, L., & Kreuter, M. (1991). *Health promotion planning: An educational and environmental approach*, (2nd ed). Mountain View, CA: Mayfield.

Haan, M., Kaplan, G., & Camacho, T. (1987). Poverty and health: Prospective evidence from the Alameda County Study. *American Journal of Epidemiology, 125*, 989-998.

Hansen, W. (1992). School-based substance abuse prevention: A review of the state of the art in curriculum, 1980-1990. *Health Education Research, 7*, 403-430.

Hastings, G., & Haywood, A. (1991) Social marketing and communication in health promotion. *Health Promotion International, 6*, 135-145.

Hawkins, J., Catalano, R., & Miller, J. (1992). Risk and protective factors for alcohol and other drug problems in adolescence and early adulthood: Implications for substance abuse prevention. *Psychological Bulletin, 112*, 64-105.

Hooper, J., & Veneziano, L. (1995). Distinguishing starters from non-starters in an employee physical activity incentive program. *Health Education Quarterly, 22*, 49-60.

House, J., Umberson, D., & Landis, K. (1988). Structures and processes of social support. *Annual Review of Sociology, 14*, 293-318.

Institute of Medicine. (1988). *The future of public health*. Washington, DC: National Academy Press.

Israel, B., & Schurman, S. (1990). Social support, control and the stress process. In K. Glanz, F. Lewis, & B. Rimer (Eds.), *Health behavior and health education: Theory, research and practice* (pp. 187-215). San Francisco: Jossey-Bass.

Jones, E. (1986). *Teenage pregnancy in industrialized countries*. New Haven, CT: Yale University Press.

Jones, E., Forrest, J., Henshaw, S., Silverman, J., & Torres, A. (1988). Unintended pregnancy, contraceptive practices, and family planning services in developed countries. *Family Planning Perspectives, 20*, 53-67.

Kannel, W., Dawber, T., Kagan, A., Revotskie, N., & Stokes, J. (1961). Factors of risk in the development of coronary heart disease—Six-year follow-up experience: The Framingham Study. *Annals of Internal Medicine, 55*, 33-49.

Kelly, M. (1989). Some problems in health promotion research. *Health Promotion International, 4*, 317-330.

Kotler, P., & Roberto, E. (1989). *Social marketing: Strategies for changing public behavior*. New York: Free Press.

Krantz, D., Glass, D., Contrada, R., & Miller, N. (1982). Behavior and health: The biobehavioral paradigm. In R. Adams, N. Smelser, & D. Treiman (Eds.), *Behavioral and social science research: A national resource: Part II* (pp. 76-145). Washington, DC: National Academy Press.

Last, J. (1987). *Public health and human ecology*. East Norwalk, CT: Appleton & Lange.

MacIntyre, S. (1986). The patterning of health by social position in contemporary Britain: Directions for sociological research. *Social Science and Medicine, 23*, 393-415.

Marantz, P. (1990). Blaming the victim: The negative consequences of preventive medicine. *American Journal of Public Health, 80*, 1186-1187.

Marmot, G., Kogevinas, M., & Elston, M. (1987). Social/economic status and disease. *Annual Review of Public Health, 8*, 111-135.

Marmot, M. (1986). Social inequalities in mortality: The social environment. In R. Wilkinson (Ed.), *Class and health* (pp. 21-33). London: Tavistock.

McGuire, W. (1964). Inducing resistance to persuasion. In L. Berkowitz (Ed.), *Advances in experimental and social psychology: Vol. 1*, (pp. 191-229). New York: Academic Press.

McKeown, T. (1976). *The role of medicine: Dream, mirage or nemesis*. London: Nuffield Provincial Hospitals Trust.

McKinlay, J., & McKinlay, S. (1977). The questionable contribution of medical measures to the decline of mortality in the United States in the twentieth century. *Milbank Memorial Fund Quarterly, 55*, 405-428.

McLeroy, K., Bibeau, D., Steckler, A. & Glanz, K. (1988). An ecological perspective on health promotion programs. *Health Education Quarterly, 15*, 351-377.

McQueen, D., & Noack, H. (1988). Health promotion indicators: Current status, issues and problems. *Health Promotion, 3*, 117-125.

MRFIT Research Group. (1982). Multiple risk factor research trial: Risk factor changes and mortality results. *Journal of the American Medical Association, 248*, 1465-1477.

MRFIT Research Group. (1990). Mortality rates after 10.5 years for participants in the Multiple Risk Factor Intervention Trial. *Journal of the American Medical Association, 263*, 1795-1801.

National Research Council. (1989). *Improving risk communication*. Washington, DC: National Academy Press.

Neubrauer, D., & Pratt, R. (1981). The second public health revolution: A critical appraisal. *Journal of Health Politics Policy and Law, 6*, 205-228.

Paffenberger, R., Hyde, R., Wing, A., & Hsieh, C. (1986). Physical activity, all-cause mortality, and longevity of college alumni. *New England Journal of Medicine, 314*, 605-613.

Paffenberger, R., Wing, A., Hyde, R. (1978). Physical activity as an index of heart attack risk in college alumni. *American Journal of Epidemiology, 108*, 161-175.

Pancer, M., & Nelson, G. (1989-1990). Community-based approaches to health promotion: Guidelines for community mobilization. *International Quarterly of Community Health Education, 10,* 91–112.

Parcel, G., Edmundson, E., Perry, C., Feldman, H., O'Hara-Tompkins, N., Nader, P., Johnson, C., & Stone, E. (1995). Measurement of self-efficacy for diet-related behaviors among elementary school children. *Journal of School Health, 65,* 23–27.

Prothrow-Stith, D. (1991) *Deadly consequences.* New York: HarperCollins.

Raymond, J. (1989). Behavioral epidemiology: The science of health promotion. *Health Promotion International, 4,* 281–286.

Reason, P. (Ed.). (1995). *Participation in human inquiry,* Thousand Oaks, CA: Sage.

Research Unit in Health and Behavioural Change. (1989). *Changing the public health.* Chichester, England: Wiley.

Rose, G. (1985). Sick individuals and sick populations. *International Journal of Epidemiology, 14,* 32–38.

Rosen, G. (1958). *A history of public health.* New York: MD Publications.

Rosenberg, M., & Fenley, M. (Eds.). (1991). *Violence in America: A public health approach.* New York: Oxford University Press.

Ryan, W. (1976). *Blaming the victim.* New York: Vintage Books.

Salmon, J. (1989). Dilemmas in studying social change versus individual change: Considerations from political economy. *Health Promotion International, 4,* 43–49.

Sorenson, A., & Bialek, R. (Eds.). (n.d.) *The public health faculty/agency forum: Linking graduate education and practice.* Bureau of Health Professions, Health Resources and Services Administration. Gainesville, FL: University Press of Florida.

Susser, M. (1995). Editorial: The tribulations of trials—Interventions in communities. *Journal of the American Public Health Association, 85,* 156–158.

U.S. Department of Health and Human Services. (1980). *Promoting health/preventing disease: Objectives for the nation.* Washington, DC: U.S. Government Printing Office.

U.S. Surgeon General. (1979). *Healthy people: The Surgeon General's report on health promotion and disease prevention.* DHEW (PHS) Publication No. 79-55071. Washington, DC: U.S. Department of Health, Education and Welfare.

U.S. Surgeon General. (1990). *Healthy people 2000: National health promotion and disease prevention objectives.* DHHS Publication No. 91-50212. Washington, DC: U.S. Department of Health and Human Services.

Wallerstein, N. (1992). Powerlessness, empowerment and health: Implications for health promotion programming. *American Journal of Health Promotion, 6,* 197–205.

II

HEALTH MANAGEMENT AND HEALTH POLICY

Although health behavior research has considerable *potential* value for the management or administration of health services and for health policies, virtually no such research relevant to management has been conducted. The process of developing policy, moreover, has far too often neglected an appreciable body of health behavior research findings.

HEALTH MANAGEMENT

Some data exist on the differential use of managed care and fee-for-service by Medicaid patients and nonmedicaid patients. For example, Krieger, Connell, and LoGerfo (1992) reported that Medicaid patients made less use of managed care services than did non-Medicaid patients; that Medicaid patients used services in a different way than non-Medicaid patients, in particular, that they used prenatal services less frequently and in a less timely manner. While such studies present problems in rigor and control, they reveal personal and social behavior factors that underlie care seeking, above and beyond the ability to pay. They also reveal issues to be resolved by health service managers in the future in order to increase the productivity and profitability (and possibly even the effectiveness) of managed care. In Chapter 10, Daugherty presents an agenda for

health behavior research directly relevant to management of health services, and especially directed toward the increases in managed care that began in the mid-1980s and can be expected to continue through the early 21st century.

HEALTH POLICY

Appropriate contexts for discussions of the relevance of health behavior research to health policy are considerations of what is meant by health policy, the behavioral factors that drive policy development, the role of government, and specific behaviors and risks toward which policy has been directed.

Health Policy: Toward a Definition

On the basis of extensive literature review of English language materials in medicine, nursing, hospital administration, and the policy sciences, Rodgers (1989) reported that policy was seldom referred to as a generic concept, but was most often defined in terms of specific policy formulation: "Rarely was an actual definition of the term 'health policy' provided" (p. 697). Rodgers provides four attributes of policy as a concept: reflections of a particular attitude toward significant health issues that imply values about some aspect of health care; expressions of a desire to move in a certain direction in relation to these values; involvement of some type of activity or behavior in relation to health care; and reference to a specific domain of health care, such as expenditures, organization of services, or health care personnel.

Often, terms such as "program," "legislation," "regulation," and "decision" are substituted for "policy," but policy need not be limited to legislation or regulations. It encompasses a wider array of values, decisions, and behaviors. Health policy, like all policy, needs to be considered as a product of human activity, preceded by a question or problem, and by the influence of various agencies, either persons or groups with specific interests or policy analysts or researchers (Rodgers, 1989).

Behavioral Factors That Drive Policy Formulation

As a reflection of human activity, the development and implementation of health policy need to be examined in terms of personal, social, and political factors. Somers (1986) provides a discussion of changes in demography and in public sentiment that appear to affect the demand for care and ultimately the development of health policy. Her discussion includes health behavior data that show increasing public skepticism of new drugs and therapies, increasing emphasis on patient autonomy and on laypersons assuming more responsibilities for their own health, and changing attitudes toward acute care conditions. The specific impact of these changes in health-related cognitions on demand for care and on health policy remains uncertain.

Kinston (1983), observing the British use of research on health services, suggests that the process of policy development is at risk for being co-opted by political factors and that what might appear to be a neutral "scientific" process is often a social construction. Kinston warns against the domination of the health services research process by a single, monolithic model, yet notes that

professional prestige, career openings, institutional reward systems, and social values all operate to influence the production of knowledge and to move it in particular directions. Ultimately, these influences affect the formulation of health policy.

Particularly insidious examples of how economic and political factors affect health policy are provided in Nestle's (1994) account of how United States Department of Health and Human Services/Department of Agriculture *Dietary Guidelines for Americans*, the federal policy statement on diet and disease prevention, has been watered down, as a result of food lobbyist activities, to suit the economic interests of the food industry. Although basic nutritional guidelines themselves had not changed, the substitution of words such as "choose" for "avoid" lead to public misperceptions and increase the likelihood of inappropriate food purchasing and poorer nutritional behaviors.

In contrast, evidence of positive benefits of alcohol consumption, e.g., on coronary heart disease—remain excluded from policy formulations, and the position that drinking in moderation should be encouraged and taught to youngsters has been "expunged from the American scene" (Peele, 1993, p. 805). Peele claims the temperance movement in the United States—in reality, an abstinence movement—has a disproportionate influence on public attitudes toward, and thus policies related to, alcohol consumption. Comparisons of temperance with nontemperance cultures suggest that alcohol policies reflect a society's reliance more on historical, cultural, and religious attitudes toward beverage alcohol than on supposedly scientific and medical evidence (Levine, 1992, cited in Peele, 1993).

With violence increasingly being defined as a public health issue, appropriate measures should be taken to reduce it and the injuries it causes. Yet Kellermann (1994) identifies major gaps in statistics relevant to policy formulation, noting that guns are specifically excluded from the jurisdiction of the Consumer Product Safety Commission, that the domestic gun industry is exempt from regulations establishing design and performance, and that questions about firearms-related injuries were omitted from the National Health Interview Survey after 1972. Gun lobby interests have successfully prevented the establishment of an appropriate database for intelligent policy development. Kellermann recognizes that these injuries and the societal ignorance about them are not accidental and urges collection of relevant health behavior data to help address this issue.

Role of Government

The role of government and its agencies in regulating health behavior remains undefined. In the United States, federal or state policies or both regulate a range of health behaviors, including (but not limited to) the purchase and use of alcohol, tobacco, and firearms; driving and vehicular safety; food and drug consumption; as well as environmental factors related to pollution; smoke and fire protection; and transportation and occupational safety. States also regulate the training and performance of many health professionals.

Levy (1986) provides an insightful analysis of the linkage between governmental policy, the 1976 National Health Information and Health Promotion Act, and worksite health promotion programs. She notes the dramatic increase of such programs and the relationship between several of them, those dealing with stress, smoking, fitness, nutrition, and hypertension, and the federal government's health objectives.

At the mid-1990s, the role of government in underwriting, guaranteeing, or facilitating payment for health services and in structuring or organizing or coordinating the delivery of health services and the activities of health professionals remains a focus of fierce political debate, as it has been for decades. A quarter of a century earlier, Kalimo (1971) demonstrated how health behavior data could be used to evaluate the impact of a government health insurance program in Finland. Such data showed that the introduction of

insurance had a positive impact in diminishing the effect of financial resources on care seeking and on reducing the ratio of care needed to care obtained.

High estimates or perceptions of costs—in contrast to actual costs—appear to be a barrier to seeking mammography among samples of United States women (Urban, Anderson, & Peacock, 1994); women who did not participate in screenings made higher estimates of their costs than women who did participate. Although providing insurance reimbursement for mammograms might not itself improve the rate of participation, if it influenced physicians' perceptions of patients' ability to pay, it might increase the likelihood that physicians would recommend a mammogram, which itself is a major determinant of participation (Urban et al., 1994). The question that logically emerges from such findings is: Does government have a role to play in providing such reimbursement?

At the same time, questions arise about who decides what is necessary care, who has what rights to experimental treatments, and whether there are there rights to care for non-necessary and nonestablished treatments (Mariner, 1994). Health behavior research has shown considerable variation in individual perceptions of treatment effectiveness and appropriateness, and Mariner notes the lack of consensus in the medical profession about what is standard, medically necessary treatment. This ambiguity raises the question of whether the physician, the insurer, the government, or the patient is to make the decision about appropriate and necessary treatment.

The absence in the United States of any policy, or coordination of policies, leads to major problems in maintaining appropriate levels of immunization for measles (e.g., Bernier, 1994), which should ordinarily be a simple thing. It also leads to confusion about who is responsible for what areas of public health. Pless (1994) relates this lack of a system to the underreporting of adolescent work injuries, with different governmental levels trying to place the burden of responsibility on the injured youngsters and their families, assuming that simply providing them with information about what to do will result in their reporting such injuries. Accumulated health behavior research testifies to the inadequacy and inappropriateness of such assumptions. Pless raises the question of whether state health departments should be given the authority to ensure improved reporting in place of the assumption that injured persons will do so.

Questions arise continually about the limits of the governmental role, about how far health policy should go in relation to individual behavior. AIDS provides a case in which the public health interest is juxtaposed with human rights interests. Scheper-Hughes (1994) observes that in the United States, AIDS was viewed as a human rights crisis with some public health connotations rather than a public health crisis with some human rights connotations (as it was elsewhere, e.g., in Cuba), with the results that mandatory testing and mandatory notification of partners have never been implemented. Legitimate questions arise about the effectiveness of such policies and about whether mandatory notification of partners would be a barrier to persons seeking HIV testing. Potterat, Spencer, Woodhouse, and Muth (1989) provide a model for evaluating the benefits and costs of such notification and indicate that the nature of the condition nonetheless warrants notification, even in the absence of much data on the impact and acceptability of notification.

Wikler (1978), for example, examined the moral basis for an increased governmental role in lifestyle behavior and raised ethical questions about the limits to which health education programs might go before they become coercive. In considering principles such as beneficence and paternalism, he cautions against overly simple moral justifications for intrusive, coercive governmental actions on behalf of health. Häyry, Häyry, and Karjalainen (1989) examined the Finnish policy toward smoking and, since it protected others from harm, found major parts of it not paternalistic. Nor did they find most of it to

be that coercive or restrictive, only the banning of "strong" tobacco products, i.e., those with the highest levels of tar, nicotine, and carbon monoxide. In Chapter 11, Nilstun provides a philosophical analysis of paternalism in relation to health policy and health behavior.

Specific Behaviors and Risks

The general question of how far policy should reach points to other more specific issues. Should governmental policy relate to the control of reproductive behavior, including regulation of the menstrual cycle? Such questions arise in the face of a technology, RU 486 (Misoprostal), that facilitates the interruption of pregnancy shortly after conception. "The desire to have access to a drug that inhibits or interrupts pregnancy is universal" (Banwell & Paxman, 1992, p. 1400). Knowledge of human behavior in this area indicates that any policy that restricts access to such a drug will lead to a black market for that drug. Health behavior research suggests that definitions of pregnancy and implantation will be problematic for any policy related to its use, as will the cultural definitions of when life begins. Moreover, the label it is given, i.e., "contraceptive" or "abortifacient" or "death pill," will have an impact on its availability (Banwell & Paxton, 1992).

Health policies generally tend to mandate individuals to change their behaviors rather than to mandate change in organizational, corporate, societal, political, or institutional structures. Even when institutions are subject to health policy, they often fail to adhere to it. Berliner (1988) observes that hospitals engaged in patient dumping even though it clearly violated anti–patient dumping legislation and COBRA (Combined Omnibus Budget Reconciliation Action of 1985). Berliner also suggested that even if economic dumping were eliminated, there would probably still be social dumping based on race, ethnicity, the nature of the insurance provider, and disease status.

In a view of several governmental goal statements for health and health promotion, including the United States Surgeon General's *Healthy People* (1979), and *Healthy People 2000* (1990), Lalonde's *A New Perspective on the Health of Canadians* (1974), the United Kingdom's *Prevention & Health: Everybody's Business* (1976), the American Public Health Association's *Model Standards* (1979), and the World Health Organization's *Global Strategy for Health for All by the Year 2000* (1977), McBeath (1991) makes clear the overemphasis in *Healthy People 2000* on individual responsibility and comments that LaLonde's reference to "lifestyle" factors in health risks may have resulted in reinforcing and compounding the erroneous assumption that personal behavior is largely voluntary and a result of individual choice. There is a simultaneous failure to recognize that lifestyle is influenced by life situations and that health status is a function of people's political, social, cultural, economic, and physical contexts. McBeath further observes the retreat of the United States government from support of the public health infrastructure necessary for attaining the objectives identified in its own documents, at the same time that other governments and agencies in Canada, Great Britain, and Scandinavia are "repenting of exaggerated stress on individual life-style, and embracing an expanded concept of health promotion" (McBeath, 1991, p. 1564).

In relation to injuries resulting from violence, traditional criminal justice policies based on deterrence, incapacitation, and rehabilitation target individual offenders and are ineffective. These policies should be broadened to include modification of high-risk situations and settings, and gun-control policy (Kellermann, 1994).

In addition to alcohol consumption, which the United States attempted to eliminate entirely through a constitutional amendment, with disastrous results, major health policy efforts have been directed at injury control and tobacco use. Mortality rates show the impact of increasing the speed limits on United States interstate highways on injuries and presumably on the behaviors that lead to them (e.g., Baum, Lund, & Wells, 1989). Other data fail to show the anticipated impact of

high school driver education programs or delayed licensure on fatal crash involvement, and in fact indicate that increasing enrollment in driver education simply increases the number of unseasoned drivers on the road and thus increases the absolute number of crashes (e.g., Robertson & Zador, 1978).

In Chapter 12, Robertson examines policies directed at automotive injury control that mistakenly focus almost solely on individual driving behaviors and desired injury control outcomes. Such policies fail to make appropriate use of available health behavior knowledge indicating that individual driving behavior is responsible for less of the variance in vehicular injuries than are poor automotive design and highway policies. In Chapter 13, Cummings similarly shows that attempts at reducing tobacco usage through health policies that affect taxes and advertising are more effective than programs designed around individual behavior change, since persistent tobacco use is not an informed choice but an addictive behavior.

REFERENCES

Banwell, S. S., & Paxman, J. M. (1992). The search for meaning: RU 486 and the law of abortion. *American Journal of Public Health, 82,* 1399–1406.

Baum, H. M., Lund, A. K., & Wells, J. K. (1989). The mortality consequences of raising the speed limit to 65 MPH on rural interstates. *American Journal of Public Health, 79,* 1392–1395.

Berliner, H. S. (1988). Patient dumping—No one wins and we all lose. *American Journal of Public Health, 78,* 1279–1280.

Bernier, R. H. (1994). Toward a more population-based approach to immunization: Fostering private- and public-sector collaboration. *American Journal of Public Health, 84,* 1567–1568.

Häyry, H., Häyry, M., & Karjalainen, S. (1989). Paternalism and Finnish anti-smoking policy. *Social Science and Medicine, 28,* 293–297.

Kalimo, E. (1971). Medical care research in the planning of social security in Finland. *Medical Care, 9,* 304–310.

Kellermann, A. L. (1994). Annotation: Firearm-related violence—What we don't know is killing us. *American Journal of Public Health, 84,* 541–542.

Kinston, W. (1983). Pluralism in the organisation of health services research. *Social Science and Medicine, 17*, 299–313.

Krieger, J. W., Connell, F. A., & LoGerfo, J. P. (1992). Medicaid prenatal care: A comparison of use and outcomes in fee-for-service and managed care. *American Journal of Public Health, 82*, 185–190.

Levine, H. G. (1992). Temperance cultures: Alcohol as a problem in Nordic and English-speaking cultures. In M. Lader, G. Edwards, & C. Drummond (Eds.), *The nature of alcohol and drug-related problems.* New York: Oxford University Press. [Cited in Peele, 1993]

Levy, S. R. (1986). Work site health promotion. *Family and Community Health, 9*(3), 51–62.

Mariner, W. K. (1994). Patients' rights after health care reform: Who decides what is medically necessary. *American Journal of Public Health, 84*, 1515–1520.

McBeath, W. H. (1991). Health for all: A public health vision. *American Journal of Public Health, 81*, 1560–1565.

Nestle, M. (1994). Editorial: The politics of dietary guidance— A new opportunity. *American Journal of Public Health, 84*, 713–715.

Peele, S. (1993). The conflict between public health goals and the temperance mentality. *American Journal of Public Health, 83*, 805–810.

Pless, I. B. (1994). Editorial: Unintentional childhood injury— Where the buck should stop. *American Journal of Public Health, 84*, 537–539.

Potterat, J. J., Spencer, N. E., Woodhouse, D. E., & Muth, J. B. (1989). Partner notification in the control of human immunodeficiency virus infection. *American Journal of Public Health, 79*, 874–876.

Robertson, L. S., & Zador, P. L. (1978). Driver education and fatal crash involvement of teenaged drivers. *American Journal of Public Health, 68*, 959–965.

Rodgers, B. L. (1989). Exploring health policy as a concept. *Western Journal of Nursing Research, 11*, 694–702.

Scheper-Hughes, N. (1994). An essay: AIDS and the social body. *Social Science and Medicine, 39*, 991–1003.

Somers, A. R. (1986). The changing demand for health services: A historical perspective and some thoughts for the future. *Inquiry, 23*(Winter), 395–402.

Urban, N., Anderson, G. L., & Peacock, S. (1994). Mammography screening: How important is cost as a barrier to use? *American Journal of Public Health, 84*, 50–55.

Wikler, D. L. (1978). Persuasion and coercion for health: Ethical issues in government efforts to change life-styles. *Health and Society/Millbank Memorial Fund Quarterly, 56*, 303–338.

10

Health Services Management and Health Behavior

Robert H. Daugherty

INTRODUCTION AND OVERVIEW

This chapter will address the influence on and interplay of health behavior research in the management of health care organizations. It will discuss the conceptual relationship between health behavior and health care management, assess the degree to which this relationship has been empirically researched, and suggest fruitful avenues of inquiry for the future.

The term *management* will be used throughout this chapter to denote the tasks of planning, organizing, directing, communicating, coordinating, and monitoring organizational functions by persons specifically designated and empowered to do so. The generic term *manager* will be used to refer an administrator, executive, director, chief—whoever has, or shares in, the legal authority and responsibility for an organization's functions, direction, and achievements. By the same token, management refers to the execution of the management tasks through an orderly institutional process carried out by those designated as managers, whatever their specific titles (Drucker, 1973).

The field of management in health care has been little researched within a health behavior framework. Research has primarily focused upon the organizational aspects vis-à-vis provider and consumer behavior and has paid little attention to the managerial functions, behavior, or perspective (Flood & Fennell, 1995; Greenley & Davidson, 1988). Almost all of the research has centered either on acute care episodes or on prevention and promotion as the settings for scientific study (Glanz, Lewis, & Rimer, 1990; Gochman, 1988), with little attention given to the chronic illness conditions that are now the leading causes of morbidity and mortality in Western developed countries (Cockerham, 1995; Gallagher, 1988; Strauss & Corbin, 1988). As a result, research in health behavior has a fragmented, disjointed character that has minimized the impact both of managerial roles and of behavior in the nexus of health care delivery and has tended to skew the perspective of health behavior research toward a functionalist social psychological focus that emphasizes interaction within the

Robert H. Daugherty • 4403 Lynnbrook Drive, Louisville, Kentucky 40220.

Handbook of Health Behavior Research IV: Relevance for Professionals and Issues for the Future, edited by David S. Gochman. Plenum Press, New York, 1997.

sick role framework posited by Parsons (1951, 1976). While this approach has clearly been valuable and fruitful in furthering understanding of the role and function of health and illness as they relate to human behavior, the rather disjointed nature of the studies conducted has served to obscure some important organizational and social systems perspectives (Flood & Fennell, 1995). It is this lack of perspective that would seem to have contributed to the dearth of research on the interplay of health care management and health behavior.

Health care management is not a new field in the health services professions, just as management in general is not new to the organizations in American society. It has evolved concurrently with both the ascendance and the professionalization of scientific medicine since the early 1900s and the development of the modern hospital in the late 19th and early 20th centuries (Hudak, 1993; Stevens, 1989). Its focus, emphasis, and underpinnings have changed significantly during this time, however, with the most dramatic changes occurring since 1980. These changes have been congruent with, and influenced by, four distinct but interrelated trends: (1) the development of the field of management in general and of health care management in particular (Filerman, 1994); (2) the coalescing of medical practice into one dominated by allopathic practitioners having the sole and legal prerogative to diagnose and treat, and the specialization of physician practices since the 1950s (Nuland, 1988; Starr, 1982); (3) the development of hospitals as the primary institution for health care research and delivery in communities, and the subsequent proliferation of medical technology since the 1970s (Rosenberg, 1987; Stevens, 1989); and (4) the increasing focus in the last 30 years on patients as consumers, rather than passive recipients of health care, coupled with the shift in illness burden in the United States from acute to chronic illness (Starr, 1982; Strauss & Corbin, 1988). It is important that these four phenomena be understood, since it is the historically changing contextual relationship of administrators, physicians, consumers, and the institutions in which health care has been carried out that has influenced how the field of health care management has evolved.

Health Care Management Professionalization. Health care management has developed from the relatively uneducated and untrained superintendent administering a hospital at the turn of the century to today's manager with a master's degree. During its first 60 years of development in this century, health care management followed a public health–public administration model, reflecting the fact that the training was oriented toward producing administrators for the large public and nonprofit hospitals that predominated (Hudak, 1993; Stevens, 1989).

Since the mid-1960s, there has been an upsurge of business interest and activity in the health care field, resulting in an emergent ideological view of health care as a profit-making enterprise (Gray, 1991), and the education and training of health care managers since the mid-1970s has become more oriented toward the principles of business management, reflecting this emphasis on health care in a context of business, rather than of public service (Hudak, 1993).

Provider Dominance and Specialization. The Flexner Report in 1910 signaled the rise of physicians as the predominant socially and legally sanctioned medical practitioners (Wolinsky, 1988). This predominance was true not only for the practice of medicine, but also for its overall development and the education and training of physicians (Nuland, 1988).

The years since 1970 have witnessed a dramatic increase in the number of physician specialties together with a marked decrease in the number of persons being trained in primary care (Cockerham, 1995; Wolinsky, 1988). This trend, resulting from medical, technical, and knowledge developments, has thus been driven by physician practice, rather than by patient needs, and has intensified the overly individualistic approach of physician practice that is the hallmark of the American medical system (Starr, 1982).

Organizational and Technological Proliferation. Until the end of the 1970s, almost all extensive diagnostic- and treatment-oriented medical procedures were performed in hospitals due to the technological complexity and expense of the procedures (Stevens, 1989). As with electronic technology in computers, however, the expansion of health care technology has made the offering of such services practical and cost-effective in settings outside the hospital, including the patient's home. The years since 1980 have produced a burgeoning of new nonhospital health care delivery organizations: free-standing emergency centers, primary care centers in shopping malls, home health care and hospice agencies, ambulatory surgery and diagnostic centers, and physician clinics offering complete laboratory services.

Patients as Consumers. The rise of health care consumerism, spawned during the social upheaval of the 1960s has become increasingly sophisticated over the last 30 years. In doing so, it has documented the self-serving nature of the delivery system and fueled the erosion of public faith and trust in the almost absolute efficacy of medicine and its primary practitioners, physicians, and at the same time has placed pressure on this system to become more responsive to the needs of consumers (Starr, 1982).

Health behavior research, however, took little note of these trends, and their impact upon consumers, providers, managers and organizations, until the 1990s. As a result, there is little to inform managers—or anyone, for that matter—of the extent to which these trends have influenced health behavior and of their likely influence on future health behavior.

HEALTH CARE MANAGEMENT AND THE STATUS OF HEALTH BEHAVIOR RESEARCH

Greenley and Davidson (1988) identified the principal issues for organizations and health behavior as the interaction between patient behavior and organizational processes, the effect of organizational forms (as a result of health policy decisions and technological development) on health behavior, and the response of managers, practitioners, and clients to organizational factors. Alonzo (1993) has argued that the prevailing American ideology of individualism and risk taking, overlaid with value orientations of freedom of choice and medical care as an economic as well as a social venture, has moved health behavior away from a social and toward an individualistic context. The results of this ideology have thus tended to focus recent change efforts on episodic ameliorization of health problems, in large part because they are more easily identified and controlled. Its scope, however, has been limited to viewing such research in the context of the influence of the actors upon each other in health and medical encounters, on one hand, and social and policy influences upon the behavior of the actors in medical encounters, on the other (Alonzo, 1993).

Health Behavior and Health Management

Health care delivery takes place in and through organizations, and the conceptual basis of management assumes an organizational context through which to carry out its functions (Drucker, 1973). The presence of organizations and management is so ubiquitous in modern society that it has often become an assumption rather than a focus of inquiry.

On the basis of extensive in-depth comparative research in two different health care institutional areas—nursing homes and acute care hospitals—two research studies concluded that the most apparent influence upon the quality and efficaciousness of services was that of management (Bowker, 1982; Gerteis, Edgman-Levitan, Daley, & Delbanco, 1993). The studies, however, did not specify precisely how management influenced service delivery, and although the impressionistic evidence tended to support the notion that the way in which the facilities were managed dictated the service received, management was never operationally defined, nor were attempts made in either study to single out any definitive managerial variables as determinants of service. What is clear is that the influence exists, and very little in the way of research has been performed to link various aspects of health management behavior to effective organizational outcomes. The literature of health services management has tended to focus upon the standard functions of business management, planning and market strategy, financial management, and technological resource allocation (Hudak, 1993; Wallace, 1994).

A social anthropological study that attempted to address behavior compared the approaches of health care managers, physicians, politicians, and social scientists in the United States and France in the application of diagnostic related group (DRG) management methods in hospitals (Pouvourville, 1989). DRG, which was developed by Yale University, consists of 438 groupings of patient conditions and is the method by which the federal government has paid hospitals for Medicare patients since 1983. The Pouvourville (1989) study suggested a fruitful avenue for management research and, as well, pointed out the relationship between the rise in influence and power of the health care executive in hospitals in the 1980s and the implementation of DRGs by the federal government through Medicare in 1983. It also provided some insight into the problems that surround the role of the health care manager in decision making. Until the introduction of DRGs, health care managers in hospitals had few tools or methods to measure or control hospital resources. Resource use was under the purview of the physicians, who were in control of both the service delivery process and the information on which that process was based, and whose modus operandi was to provide to administrators only the information they wanted them to have, in order to secure for themselves the things they wanted. Payment for services was retrospective and was based upon reasonable and customary fees and charges, which meant that payment both to hospitals and to physicians was based simply on the amount of services pro-

vided, rather than on any rational notion of effective use of resources. As DRGs were implemented, hospital executives for the first time had a resource allocation measure independent of the hospital physician staff, at least for Medicare patients, whose fees often amounted to between 50% and 70% of hospital revenues. One could argue that the rise to prominence and influence of health care managers in the 1980s was predominantly based upon this new management knowledge (Pouvourville, 1989).

Prompted by concern about medical ethics in the wake of the sea changes in medicine, some studies attempted to explore the ethical behavior of health care managers (Callahan, 1990; Williamson & Jauch, 1995). These studies researched attitudes and choices in hypothetical situations; there has been no exploration of the actual ethical behavior of managers through field research.

There has been little if any health behavior research exploring or linking health care managerial behavior to the behavior of consumers, other providers, or efficacious health outcomes, or demonstrating the link between the recent technological advances, their influence on organizational delivery modes, and the subsequent impact on managerial behavior and behavior change.

Health Behavior and the Consumer

Research in health consumer behavior since the 1960s has focused upon the issues of patienthood; beliefs about and reactions to illness; health-seeking behavior; interactions with health care professionals, particularly physicians; how health care is perceived and used by the patient; and since the mid-1980s, the patient's satisfaction with (as well as willingness to carry out) the treatment prescribed (Aharony & Strasser, 1993; Andersen, 1995; Gochman, 1988; Lewis, 1994). During the 1980s, research emerged that focused upon the patient as customer in a competitive health market (Aharony & Strasser, 1993; Rudd & Glanz, 1990) and was influenced more by business interests as health services managers sought to determine factors that influence use and satisfaction with services in order to compete effectively with one another (Gray, 1991; Shortell, Morrison, & Friedman, 1990).

Because of the clinical bias implicit in the physician-medical model-hospital approach to health services delivery and use, behavioral research has tended to focus upon physician-patient interaction, patient health behavioral characteristics and compliance, role behavior of service providers, and, to some limited extent, the effect of organizational factors on health behavior—primarily of patients (Alonzo, 1993). Almost completely lacking are studies of patient behavior outside the physician encounter context. Even within the physician encounter context, only since the mid-1980s has the research begun to scratch the surface of understanding the encounter from the perspective of the receiver of service (Bursztajn, Feinbloom, Hamm, & Brodsky, 1990; Gerteis et al., 1993). More recent research has focused upon the issues of patient participation in care decisions, the influence of economic variables, and how patients do change or will need to change their behavior in order to participate fully and direct in the management of their health care (Rice & Morrison, 1994; Rice, Nelson, & Colby, 1992).

Thus, health care managers have very little guidance as to how best to structure and deliver health care services and what will promote the most efficacious of health service interactions. Further, to the extent that there is any guidance at all, it is tending to emanate from consumer behavior market studies rather than health behavior research (Shortell & Kalusny, 1994).

Health Behavior and Physicians

Physician practice is moving away from the independent practitioner model of service provision to a more organizational—some would say bureaucratic—form of practice either in groups or within the corporate structures of health provider institutions. At the same time, the shift in consumer behavior has posed a challenge to the supremacy of physicians and their almost absolute authority in health care delivery. While it is probably extreme to characterize this trend as presaging the deprofessionalization of physicians (Ritzer & Walczak, 1988), their accountability is coming increasingly under more organized scrutiny (Halverson, 1993; Starr, 1982).

Of primary concern for managers is how physicians accept accountability for their professional work. Colombotos and Kirchner (1986) argue that physicians, even though they are becoming more and more willing to accept review and oversight, are much more amenable to broad guidelines informally enforced, than to specific criteria and standards, which they view as "cookbook medicine." As professionals, they see themselves as trained to control the methods, timing, and application of their knowledge, skills, and abilities in their area of expertise. External imposition of standards and protocols for performance implies that there is little professional discretion, and discretion in the work of professionals is akin to the sorcerer's magic. Rationality aside, discretion is an almost mystical component of the professional's work that is crucial to maintaining professional autonomy. To acknowledge that this seeming discretion is illusory, and that most actions are guided by processes that can be defined, routinized, and codified, symbolically reduces the professional power that attends indefinable, and therefore unchallengeable, professional discretion. There should be no mystery about why physicians are slow to define protocols and reduce their diagnostic and treatment processes to writing. The demand for just this kind of accountability, however, is a constant theme that has resulted in the recent increase in interest in managed care approaches to American health care reform (Meyer & Silow-Carroll, 1993).

From a management point of view, one of the most frustrating aspects of working with physicians has been their behavior in the organizational setting (Freidson, 1963; Goldsmith, 1992; Smith, 1955; Starr, 1982). The transformation that has occurred in physician-hospital and physician-patient relations since the late 1970s has exacerbated the conflict between the physician and almost everyone else in the health delivery system and has highlighted the problems that health care managers have in the management of those systems (Goldsmith, 1992; Starr, 1982).

Since 1980, research in physician behavior widened from a focus on physician–patient interaction to include physician practice patterns during the end of the 1980s. Spawned by concern about resource utilization and cost containment, this research has uncovered substantial variations in physician practice patterns with varying resource use, all unrelated to patient outcomes. These studies found that there were wide variations in practice patterns by specialty, procedure, and protocols within practice activities. Other research on high-technology procedures such as carotid endarterectomies has found as many as 32% to be inappropriate and another 32% to be of questionable efficacy (Meyer & Silow-Carroll, 1993; Tillman & Sullivan, 1993). The implication of this emerging research is that while there are some standards, as yet largely unwritten, physicians generally adhere to their own idiosyncratic practice styles. One could hypothesize that this is in large measure the result of the independence in the individual practitioners of medicine so prevalent throughout the 20th century, and of their obdurate refusal to submit to any authority, or oversight, including that of their own profession (Goldsmith, 1992; Starr, 1992).

Research on nonphysician providers other than nurses has been limited. This limitation perhaps reflects the hegemony of physicians in health care delivery, but may also indicate that it is assumed that nonphysicians have little impact upon the efficacy or patient-perceived quality of and satisfaction with care. Managed care may change this situation, as it places more emphasis upon the health care team, rather than physicians, and increasingly recognizes that the other professions may have as much effect on quality and outcomes, if not the same level of input, as physicians (Pendergast, Kimberlin, Berardo, & McKenzie, 1995; Uili & Wood, 1995).

A recent study of pharmacy roles yields some preliminary findings on at least two areas in which pharmacists can have influence: (1) training and socialization, and (2) organizational setting (Pendergast et al., 1995). Training and socialization dimensions are of critical importance, since they involve the sustaining of the organization's values and vision. The pharmacist, like the physician, is a professional whose orientation has changed dramatically since the 1960s, from technical scientist to knowledge consultant. The advent of preproportioned, packaged drugs has diminished the need for pharmacists' technical ability in preparing and mixing drug compounds. At the same time, the proliferation in medical care of drugs, and of drug administration, has significantly increased the need for patient understanding of and compliance with drug treatment regimens (Pendergast et al., 1995). Thus, the knowledge consultation role of the pharmacist has become of major importance in managing health care for individual patients. Pendergast and her associates found that both role orientation in professional training and on-the-job socialization had significant effects upon whether or not pharmacists saw importance in the role of patient consultant. The salient points for health care executives are that role definition is of importance and that positive reinforcement for that role needs to be consciously attended to and designed into the patient–provider interactional framework of the health delivery system in order to maximize its effectiveness.

Health Behavior and Organizational Settings

Weber (1947) noted that organizational forms arise out of a historical social context and that these organizational forms drive the behavior of the actors—managers, professional practitioners, and consumers—who operate within those forms. Later theorists (Perrow, 1965; Scott, 1987) noted that while organizations may arise out of a seemingly normative social need that appears coherent and uniform in its goals, modern organizations are made up of people with many competing professional and cultural interests who use the organization as a means of attaining their own ends. Thus, the organization actually embodies a system of competing and contradictory goals, values, and activities of the various subgroups that it encompasses and becomes a political arena in which these competing interests play out their claims for dominance in defining the goals and direction for the organization (Scott, 1987).

This description is especially true of the health care field, in which the conflict over the differing perspectives of managers, physicians, other health professionals, and the consumer has intensified, ostensibly over the cost and value of health care (Goldsmith, 1992). On closer inspection, however, one could argue that the real conflict is over control of the goals, direction, and content of health care in the United States, as it has become clearer that the medical profession's claim to hegemony through its scientific base fails to stand up under increasing scrutiny (Meyer & Silow-Carroll, 1993; Starr, 1982).

There has been insufficient recognition of the demographic forces at work that pose problems for the way health care has been organized and managed. The aging of the population coupled with the shifting incidence of acute infectious conditions and diseases to chronic illness has yet to affect, to any appreciable degree, a delivery system primarily oriented to high-technology, short-stay acute treatment (Bopp, Brown, & Daugherty, 1994; Gallagher, 1988; Halverson, 1993; Strauss & Corbin, 1988). Research has reflected the dominance of the hospital setting as the locus of health care organizational activity, ignoring the larger interorganizational service delivery phenomenon that is implicit in the informal, unorganized network that characterizes the "health care delivery system" in the United States.

Thus, for example, while there are studies of physician–patient interaction, there is almost no research on the organization and management of the setting of the interaction incorporating factors that affect the behavior of both the physician and the patient—e.g., ease of obtaining appointments, waiting time, attitudes and behavior of office staff, billing process—and thereby influence the physician–patient interaction. Yet organizational and market research indicates that these factors do influence interaction behavior patterns in the delivery of services in general (Czepiel, Solomon, & Surprenant, 1985) and of health care services in particular (Shortell, Becker, & Neuhauser, 1976). To date, such research has been heavily organizational and marketing-oriented. This limited approach has virtually ignored one of the most fundamental of issues in American medicine that is a driving force behind much of health behavior—that the *disorganization* of health care services is itself a determinant of health behavior.

The impact of organizational modes and the management of health care delivery, and their effects upon the participants in the system, have been given scant attention, and such research has tended to be in the realm of organizational influences on patient behavior (Greenley & Davidson, 1988).

FUTURE DIRECTIONS IN HEALTH CARE MANAGEMENT

Until the early 1980s, the health care manager's role was seen as one of passive administrative caretaking (Shortell & Kaluzny, 1994). During the 1980s, the increasing influence of health care management, and its challenge to physicians over resource control and orientation of medicine, were largely ignored by behavioral research. This is not to say that health behavior research was of no value to health care executives. It is simply that health care managers had to reinterpret into organizational contexts what are essentially discrete and clinically oriented studies and information. Health care managers would benefit from systematic research that addressed the changing health service configuration and recognized the emergence of chronic illness and the continuum of care needs, managed care, and the new tasks of the health care manager.

Continuum of Care

The continuum concept of illness and care views illness not as a discrete series of bio-physiological threats to the body that must be rooted out through medical diagnosis and treatment, but as impairments of a person's ability to function in any or a combination of the biological, physiological, and psychosocial areas of life. Given the prevalence of chronic illnesses as chief health maladies, the continuum of care addresses the fact that chronic illness (e.g., long-term conditions such as hypertension, diabetes, heart disease, cancer, and multiple sclerosis) is seldom "cured," in the conventional sense in which this term has been applied to infectious illnesses of the past. Rather, chronic illness is a condition that must be managed, i.e., integrated, controlled, and monitored within a person's total pattern of living (Strauss & Corbin, 1988). Further, the continuum concept gives credence to the fact that much of this management of illness takes place outside health institutions in the course of an individual's normal activities of work, family life, and other aspects of living (Bopp et al., 1994).

Managed Care

Embodying the conceptual framework of the continuum of care, the emergence of managed care in the form of organizations that are fully integrated, though geographically limited, is beginning to take shape (Halverson, 1993, Meyer & Silow-Carroll, 1993). Managed care organizations can take many forms, but their main characteristic is the assumption of risk, as well as service, for the populations they serve. Managed care is an outgrowth of health maintenance organizations (HMOs) and most often resembles them in organizational form. HMOs, which have been established mainly in urban areas, are characterized by a redefinition from the conventional mission of producing successful health medical procedures and treatment (although no one would deny that these are necessary ingredients) to that of producing healthy, or at least healthier,

populations (Halverson, 1993). Doing so turns the previous medical care incentive system on its head: Instead of benefiting from illness by being paid for full hospital beds and for performing more and more high-tech and expensive procedures, the system benefits economically to the extent that it can keep its participants from needing expensive services by emphasizing illness prevention, healthy lifestyles, and effective management of chronic illness in its early stages to obviate expensive acute intervention.

Greenley and Davidson (1988) argued that the HMO approach produces unintended consequences of undertreating patients or of not providing care, since the service incentive is mitigated by a fixed sum allotted per patient in the system. This argument misses the point of the managed care outcomes approach. In managed care, the health delivery organization (i.e., the HMO) assumes total responsibility and financial risk for its participants' health. Certainly there is incentive *not* to provide service, but presumably the managed care service provider also recognizes the risk that not providing inexpensive prevention-oriented services will often lead to the necessity for costlier services in the future, the costs of which the organization would also be required to absorb.

New Focus for Management

The changes in the health care system place demands upon health care managers to exhibit new knowledge, skills, and abilities (Hudak, 1993; Leadership Center, 1992; Wallace, 1994). For the first time, health care management is in a position not only to clarify its roles, but also to articulate its fundamental cultural foundations in values and beliefs. Executive management is moving away from emphasis upon technical and organizational skills to focus on conceptual and human behavior skills (Zuckerman, 1989). These skills relate primarily to behavioral aspects of management: mastering and leading change, systems thinking, shared vision, continuous quality improvement, redefining health care, and creation of public–community linkage (Leadership Center, 1992).

It is one thing to call upon managers to retool to provide leadership in new health care design; it is quite another to ensure that they have the conceptual and managerial tools to do so. What is abundantly clear is that new skills and abilities will need to be articulated in new roles for health care managers and indeed for all providers of health services. The old roles, as noted earlier, required knowledge, skills, and abilities to administer within a predetermined framework, primarily that of the community or specialty hospital or clinic. The new roles will require an ability to create the institutional framework and to manage through an interorganizational network that responds equally to population-based as well as resource-based initiatives and change (Zuckerman, 1989). There are at present no studies that explore these changing roles.

HEALTH BEHAVIOR RESEARCH NEEDS OF HEALTH CARE MANAGERS

If health services managers are to play the leadership and professional management and coordination role that is being envisioned under the emerging service delivery systems, health behavior research will need to focus on the issues of chronic illness management and on the organizational and management behavioral structures, processes, and linkages necessary to articulate effective illness management outcomes (Gallagher, 1988; Greenley & Davidson, 1988; Scott, 1990). In most of the discussions, the behavior change is assumed, or at least the policy antecedents of this change are assumed, yet there is little in the way of behavior research to assist the manager in predicting, or even taking into account on any rational basis, the future behavioral components or actions that will coincide with the society-wide managed care concept presented in the previous section. What is needed in health behavior research is the validation of these proposed management concepts through care-

fully designed studies that link these roles to organizational outcomes.

Moving toward a more encompassing social–psychological systems conception of health will require health care managers to articulate a new vision for health care participants to which they can relate their efforts. This framework will need to address not only the vision of a health care future, but also the organizational contexts through which this vision can be, and is being, realized. It is clear from even the paucity of recent research that current traditional organizational structures inhibit the efficacious delivery of managed care, and future research will need to take into account the organizational and social setting to a greater degree than has been done in the past (Filerman, 1994).

Paradigm Components

To consider both the existing impact and the future direction of health behavior research in health care management, it is necessary to have a conceptual framework within which to view what is known and is not known. The behavioral paradigm suggested is a health systems network as a subsystem of society. This network is composed of the various health delivery units and actors and constitutes an ideal typology with the purpose of systemizing inquiry. The units of analysis of this typology are (1) health provider behavior, (2) health consumer behavior, and (3) health management behavior. The context, however, needs to be the process of health care delivery management as a service phenomenon.

The organizational frames of reference have been suggested by Scott (1982), who proposes three models of managing the work of health care professionals, which, he notes, have developed historically in the United States. The first is the autonomous professional organization that characterized most community hospitals until the end of the 1970s. The autonomous professional organization is characterized by accountability of the organization's core service operations to peer professional groups, rather than through the hierarchy of the organization to its policy and governance functions.

The second organizational form is the heteronomous professional organization, in which there is subordination of the professional functions of an organization to administrative controls and general supervision. This form has generally characterized the work of most nonphysician health care professionals in hospitals and increasingly since the 1980s has characterized physician–hospital relations. As noted earlier, the advent of the DRG payer system together with the ascendance of a profit-making ideology among professional health care managers exacerbated the organizational–physician conflicts of interest and contributed to an increasingly negative interactional pattern (Goldsmith, 1992).

The third form of management, the conjoint professional organization, describes a context not much in evidence, but one upon which the upsurge in managed care will increasingly depend. A conjoint professional organization is one in which the professionals and managers are balanced in their power and importance relationships and are functionally highly interdependent. Its relationships are also complex and dependent upon effectively designed and executed human communication patterns. But this complexity also provides improved flexibility and responsiveness to customer (patient) needs and requirements (Scott, 1982).

These three typologies can effectively form the background against which both to analyze the extent and impact of health behavior research from a health care management perspective and to suggest the framework in which future research might be fruitful. It might also be fruitful to invoke a cultural–subcultural context in analyzing these interactions in terms of their respective patterns of belief, values, roles, and relationship prescriptions. Managerial behavior is not simply a response to policy and organizational factors, but plays an increasingly important role in the formation of policy and organizational forms and behavior through the active application of its professional values and beliefs (Zucker-man, 1989). It has already been noted that changing consumer beliefs and values and the reaction of health care professionals to assaults upon their value and belief systems have influenced health behavior in increasingly significant ways.

While not necessarily articulated in those terms, more recent writings on health care management (Filerman, 1994; Shortell & Kaluzny, 1994; Zuckerman, 1989) have also noted the need to change organizational relationships and roles in order to provide for improved organizational and management approaches to the provision of health services.

Consumer/Patient Research

Studies of health consumer behavior have tended to focus on satisfaction with services, physician–patient interactions, and the attitudinal prerequisites of behavior with relation to health issues, although there is ample evidence that health is affected not only by biophysiology, but also by the environment, the organizational ecosystem, sociocultural factors, lifestyle, and economics (Alonzo, 1993). There has been but very little research on the effects of organizational and economic factors on the health behavior of consumers, and such research as there is has been subject to varying interpretation (Kronick, 1992; Rice & Morrison, 1994; Rice et al., 1992). Although much has been written about the medical and organizational deficiencies of a health care system that places science rather than the patient at the center of the process (e.g., Bursztajn et al., 1990; Cassell, 1991; Gerteis et al., 1993), such studies have been either case histories or anecdotally based, and few if any rigorous studies have been performed to verify the efficacy of patient-centered care. Such studies would have to go beyond the context of patient–physician (or other provider) interaction and investigate the setting, organizational, and managerial decision-making variables that are attendant to the concept of patient-centered care.

The concept of equity as a basis for both patient and physician satisfaction may have significant potential for health care managers, since it reframes the physician–patient relationship away from a win–lose struggle for power and focuses instead on a therapeutic communication process in which the end product is neither patient nor physician satisfaction, but rather an ongoing series of mutually enhancing interactions (Koehler, Fottler, & Swan, 1992). The outcome sought is quality care both as objectively defined by the physician and as judgmentally perceived by the patient. Equity occurs when each participant feels that the ratio of benefits received to effort and resources expended is equal or skewed in his or her favor. Both physicians and patients have satisfiers that are idiosyncratically determined by their expectations and level of satisfaction, and thus are not mutually exclusive. The physician–patient relationship is therefore not a zero-sum game such that if one is to be satisfied the other must be dissatisfied; rather, it is a mutually reinforcing interaction in which physicians, as professionals, can initiate the behavior change and thereby simultaneously enhance both their own and their patients' satisfaction within the encounter (Koehler et al., 1992).

Although the studies supporting the concept of equity are not conclusive, it would appear, on the basis of the research to date, to be a fruitful area of inquiry for health care executives. Further, the notion of equity is consistent with social–psychological research on customer and employee satisfaction that has been performed in the service industry since the mid-1970s. This research indicates that consumer satisfaction in the long run depends on the total service experience and that the quality of the service interactional process depends upon the dynamics of the service encounter in such a way that the satisfaction and interpersonal gains of both the provider and the consumer are enhanced (Czepiel et al., 1985; Norman, 1984).

If managing one's health is a lifelong issue, as has been argued, health behavior research will need to include how health care professionals influence health behavior outside the illness episode, how the illness management process works, and how the roles of the chronically ill person, the primary caregivers, and the health professionals interrelate and conflict (Strauss & Corbin, 1988). Within a multicultural context, such research will need to investigate the cultural barriers to increased involvement of consumers. Such barriers exist within the culture of the health provider groups as they prescribe the roles that consumers can legitimately take and the role of the physician provider as the one best equipped to make and influence decisions (Gerhardt, 1989). The provider cultural ideology generally does not recognize that many of the decisions that persons must make with regard to their health are also value decisions with respect to how they want to live.

Provider Behavior Research

Like consumer research, health behavior research from the provider perspective has tended to focus upon the physician–patient interaction and its relationship to patient compliance, the quality of care, and patient satisfaction. One glaring omission is the lack of studies of physician influence upon other physicians or of the influence of specialist and generalist physicians on each other.

Research on the variations in physician practice found that while physicians resist definitive protocols as "cookbook medicine," there is evidence that when confronted with scientific data on practice variation, they will voluntarily bring their patterns more in line with identified norms (Gerteis et al., 1993). Unfortunately, the data concerning what conditions predispose changes in physician practice pattern are inconclusive. Given the mandate for physician behavior change under managed care, this lack of information is particularly critical for health care managers. Future research can take some cues, however, from current findings. It would seem reasonable to hypothesize, for example, that a combination of information and a practice setting that reinforces equity norms of physician–patient satisfaction would be more conducive to physician behavior change than simply the provision of the information. This hypothesis would need further study under controlled conditions in order to test the role of the effectiveness-satisfaction nexus in managed care.

The health behavior research field needs comparative studies of differences in physician behavior, satisfaction, and communication under managed care and non-managed care conditions. Such inquiry would need to address three key issues: (1) How can managers most positively go about involving physicians in a teamwork approach to providing health care services? (2) How can physicians best be trained and motivated to work toward managing health care? (3) How can physicians' behavior be influenced to relate to patients on a consultant/partnership basis, rather than on an expert/advice-follower basis?

Research in Health Care Management

Research in managers' behavior will need to take on more prominence in the health behavior field. Most research has dealt with their attitudes. The role and effect of the health care manager on performance and behavior of organizations has been implied in organizational studies, but not explicitly identified or verified (Gerteis et al., 1993; Shortel & Kaluzny, 1994). Much of the work on management roles and behavior has centered around prescriptions for the future, which, however conceptually useful, provide little insight into how health care executives actually behave and their effect on the health care system (Hudak, 1993; Vladeck, 1986; Wallace, 1994; Williamson & Jauch, 1995).

Future research on health care management behavior will need to focus upon the mutual interaction and influence patterns between managers and practitioners, the role of information and decision making, and the effect of increasing structure on the roles, relationships, and well-being of patients, practitioners, and managers. The literature suggests that service quality in the future will be greatly determined by the degree to which managers can influence, balance, and synthesize the traditionally competing interests

of the actors in the health care arena (Shortell & Kaluzny, 1994).

There is a dearth of research on organizational impact on health behavior, with little having emerged since Greenley and Davidson (1988, p. 226) noted the need for further investigation based on the increasing corporatization and bureaucratization of health care. Perhaps one reason for the dearth is that the health care delivery system has continued to undergo dramatic change and that it is therefore difficult to identify the appropriate variables for study. The implications of the extent to which the focus in health care has shifted to chronic illness and managed care are still not well understood, nor is the notion of how patient outcomes are related to the changed economic incentives of managed care and its potential for changing behavior.

Rationality in personal and organizational decision making would suggest that organizations not behave in ways that would knowingly put them at greater financial risk in the future. The extent to which rationality actually exists in health care organizations, however, has not yet been empirically verified. There is some limited research on the functions and scope of managed care systems, but none comparing behavior of participants in managed care with that of participants in traditional health care programs. There is also anecdotal evidence relating organizational design and management functions to defined outcomes, but no systematic research in the health behavior field. Existing research focused upon comparisons of reduction of acute hospital stays and of inappropriate use of medical resources by HMO participants and by fee-for-service participants. Presumably, there is behavior change on the part of both providers and consumers of health services, but there is no indication of exactly what change has occurred. Thus, research on future health care organizational and management forms will need to take into account the impact of differing economic incentives, differing organizational designs, and the degree to which managers and other health care providers engage in rational decision-making behavior.

Koehler et al. (1992) and others (Halverson,

1993; Meyer & Silow-Carroll, 1993) noted how measures of service quality and efficacy have shifted in focus from structure and process of service to outcomes. This shift has followed the shift in economic incentives away from reimbursement for specific procedures and treatments toward prospective payment for health maintenance. A part of the same trend is the shift away from small single or group practice settings toward larger organizations or networks of organizations with the resources to take on the economic risk for groups of people. Thus, for health care managers, research such as that by Dutton, Gomby, and Fowles (1985) showing that patient satisfaction tends to be highest in solo practices must be examined for variables that will translate to larger settings.

In the final analysis, managed care has the potential to produce an organizational rationalization of health care practice that could qualitatively improve the health of the nation. Health behavior research needs to be in the forefront of this effort in view of the substantial evidence that the behavioral aspects of health services delivery are as important as the technical aspects (Halverson, 1994; Meyer & Silow-Carroll, 1993).

REFERENCES

Aharony, L., & Strasser, S. (1993). Patient satisfaction: What we know about and what we still need to explore. *Medical Care Review, 50,* 49–79.

Alexander, J., Morrisey, M., & Shortell, S. (1986). The effects of competition, regulation and corporatization on hospital–physician relationships. *Journal of Health and Social Behavior, 27,* 220–235.

Alonzo, A. (1993). Health behavior: Issues, contradictions and dilemmas. *Social Science and Medicine, 37*(8), 1019–1034.

Andersen, R. (1995). Revisiting the behavioral model and access to medical care: Does it matter? *Journal of Health and Social Behavior, 36,* 1–10.

Barr, J., & Steinberg, M. (1983). Professional participation in organizational decision-making: Physicians in HMOs. *Journal of Community Health, 8*(3), 160–173.

Bopp, K., Brown, G., & Daugherty, R. (1994). Continuum of care In R. Taylor & S. Taylor (Eds.), *The AUPHA manual of health services management* (pp. 623–640) Gaithersburg, MD: Aspen.

Bowker, L. (1982). *Humanizing institutions for the aged.* Lexington, MA: D. C. Heath.

Bursztajn, H., Feinbloom, R., Hamm, R., & Brodsky, A. (1990). *Medical choices, medical chances.* New York: Routledge.

Callahan, D. (1990). *What kind of life: The limits of medical progress.* New York: Simon & Schuster.

Cassell, E. (1991). *The nature of suffering and the goals of medicine.* New York: Oxford University Press.

Charles, C., & DeMaio, S. (1993). Lay participation in health care decision making: A conceptual framework. *Journal of Health Politics, Policy and Law, 18,* 881–904.

Cockerham, W. (1995). *Medical sociology* (6th ed.). Englewood Cliffs, NJ: Prentice-Hall.

Colombotos, J., & Kirchner, C. (1986). *Physicians and social change.* New York: Oxford University Press.

Czepiel, J., Solomon, M., & Surprenant, C. (1985). *The service encounter: Managing employee customer interaction in service businesses.* Lexington, MA: Lexington Books.

Drucker, P. (1973). *Management: Tasks—responsibilities—practices.* New York: Harper & Row.

Dutton, D., Gomby, D., & Fowles, J. (1985). Satisfaction with children's medical care in six different ambulatory settings. *Medical Care, 23*(7) 894–911.

Filerman, G. (1994). Health: The emerging context of management. In R. Taylor & S. Taylor (Eds.), *The AUPHA manual of health services management* (pp. 3–18). Gaithersburg, MD: Aspen.

Flood, A., & Fennell, M. (1995). Through the lenses of organizational sociology: The role of organizational theory and research in conceptualizing and examining our health care system. *Journal of Health and Social Behavior* (Extra Issue), pp. 154–169.

Freidson, E. (1963). *The hospital in modern society.* New York: Macmillan.

Gallagher, E. (1988). Chronic illness management: A focus for future research applications. In D. S. Gochman (Ed.), *Health behavior: Emerging research perspectives* (pp. 397–407). New York: Plenum Press.

Gerhardt, U. (1989). The sociological image of medicine and the patient. *Social Science and Medicine, 29,* 721–728.

Gerteis, M., Edgman-Levitan, S., Daley, J., & Delbanco, T. (1993). *Through the patient's eyes: Understanding and promoting patient-centered care.* San Francisco: Jossey-Bass.

Glanz, K., Lewis, F. M., & Rimer, B. K. (1990). *Health behavior and health education.* San Francisco: Jossey-Bass.

Gochman, D. (1988). *Health behavior: Emerging research perspectives.* New York: Plenum Press.

Goldsmith, J. (1992). The reshaping of health care. *Health Care Forum Journal, 35*(3), 19–27.

Goldsmith, J. (1993). Driving the nitroglycerin truck. *Health Care Forum Journal, 36*(2), 36–41.

Gray, B. (1991). *The profit motive and patient care.* Cambridge, MA: Harvard University Press.

Greenley, J., & Davidson, R. (1988). Organizational influences patient health behaviors. In D. S. Gochman (Ed.), *Health behavior: Emerging research perspectives* (pp. 215-229). New York: Plenum Press.

Halverson, G. (1993). *Strong medicine*. New York: Random House.

Hudak, R. (1993). Health care administrator in the year 2000: Practitioners' views of future issues and job requirements. *Hospital and Health Services Administration, 38*, 181-195.

Hurka, S. (1980). Need satisfaction among health care managers. *Hospital and Health Services Administration, 25*(3), 43-54.

Koehler, W., Fottler, M., & Swan, J. (1992). Physician-patient satisfaction: Equity in the health services encounter. *Medical Care Review, 49*, 455-484.

Kronick, R. (1992). Can consumer choice reward quality and economy? Towards a test of economic competition. *Journal of Health Politics, Policy and Law, 17*(1), 25-37.

Leadership Center. (1992). Bridging the leadership gap. *Health Care Forum Journal* (May/June), *35*(3), 43-47.

Lewis, J. (1994). Patient views on quality care in general practice: Literature review. *Social Science and Medicine, 39*, 655-670.

Meyer, J., & Silow-Carroll, S. (Eds.) (1993). *Building blocks for change: How health care reform affects our future*. Washington, DC: Economic and Social Research Institute.

Norman, R. (1984). *Service management: Strategy and leadership in service businesses*. New York: Wiley.

Nuland, S. (1988). *Doctors: The biography of medicine*. New York: Knopf.

Pappas, G. (1990). Some implications for the study of the doctor-patient interaction: Power, structure, and agency in the works of Howard Waitzkin and Arthur Kleinman. *Social Science in Medicine, 30*, 199-204.

Parsons, T. (1951). *The social system*. New York: Free Press.

Parsons, T. (1975). The sick role and the role of the physician reconsidered. *Milbank Memorial Fund Quarterly, 53*, 257-278.

Pendergast, J., Kimberlin, C., Berardo, D., & McKenzie, L. (1995). Role orientation and community pharmacists' participation in a project to improve patient care. *Social Science and Medicine, 40*, 557-565.

Perrow, C. (1963). Goals and power structures: A historical case study. In E. Freidson (Ed.), *The hospital in modern society*, (pp. 112-146). New York: Macmillan.

Perrow, C. (1965). Hospitals: Technology, structure, and goals. In J. March (Ed.), *Handbook of organizations* (pp. 910-971). Chicago: Rand McNally.

Pouvourville, G. (1989). Differences in the approaches of the doctor, manager, politician and social scientist in health care controversies—Hospital case-mix management methods: An illustration of the manager's approach in health care controversies. *Social Science and Medicine, 29*, 341-349.

Rice, T., & Morrison, K. (1994). Patient cost sharing for medical services: A review of the literature. *Medical Care Review, 51*, 235-287.

Rice, T., Nelson, L., & Colby, D. (1992). Will Medicare beneficiaries switch physicians? A test of economic competition. *Journal of Health Politics, Policy and Law, 17*, 3-24.

Ritzer, G., & Walczak, D. (1988). Rationalization and the deprofessionalization of physicians. *Social Forces, 67*, 1-22.

Rosenberg, C. (1987). *The care of strangers: The rise of America's hospital system*. New York. Basic Books.

Rudd, J., & Glanz, K. (1990). How individuals use information for health action: Consumer information processing. In K. Glanz, F. Lewis, & B. Rimer (Eds.), *Health behavior and health education: Theory, research and practice* (pp. 115-139). San Francisco: Jossey-Bass.

Scott W. (1982). Managing professional work: Three models of control for health organizations. *Health Services Research, 17*, 213-240.

Scott, W. (1987). *Organizations: Rational, natural and open systems*. Englewood Cliffs, NJ: Prentice-Hall.

Scott W. (1990). Innovation in medical care organizations: A synthetic review. *Medical Care Review, 47*, 165-192.

Shortell, S., Becker, S., & Neuhauser, D. (1976). The effects of management practices on hospital efficiency and quality of care. In S. Shortell & M. Brown (Eds.), *Organizational research and hospitals* (pp. 77-103). Chicago, IL: Blue Cross Association.

Shortell, S., & Kaluzny, A. (1994). *Health care management: Organizational design and behavior* (3rd ed.). Albany, NY: Delmar.

Shortell, S., Morrison, E., & Friedman, B. (1990). *Strategic choices for America's hospitals*. San Francisco: Jossey-Bass.

Smith, H. (1955). Two lines of authority: The hospital's dilemma. *Modern Hospital, 85*(3), 48-52.

Squier, R. (1990). A model of empathetic understanding and adherence to treatment regimens in practitioner-patient relationships. *Social Science and Medicine, 30*, 325-339.

Starr, P. (1982). *The social transformation of American medicine*. New York: Basic Books.

Stevens, R. (1989). *In sickness and in wealth: American hospitals in the twentieth century*. New York: Basic Books.

Strauss, A., & Corbin, J. (1988). *Shaping a new health care system*. San Francisco: Jossey-Bass.

Tillman, I., & Sullivan, S. (1993). Quality and the future of American health care. In J. Meyer & S. Silow-Carroll (Eds.), *Building blocks for change: How health care reform affects our future*. Washington, DC: Economic and Social Research Institute.

Uili, R., & Wood, R. (1995). The effect of third party payers on the clinical decision-making of physical therapists. *Social Science and Medicine, 40*(7), 873-879.

Vladeck, B. (1986). Health, health care executives, and their communities. *Hospital and Health Services Administration, 31*, 7-15.

Wallace, P. (1994). Hospital executives: Perceptions of skills and experiences desired in health care graduates. *Journal of Health Administration Education, 12*, 1-14.

Weber, M. (1947). *The theory of social and economic organizations.* New York: Free Press.

Weisman, C., & Nathanson, C. (1985). Professional satisfaction and client outcomes: A comparative organizational analysis. *Medical Care, 23*, 79-119.

Williamson, S., & Jauch, L. (1995). Research on hospital administrators' ethics: An agenda. *Medical Care Research and Review, 52*, 134-144.

Wolinsky, F. (1988). *Sociology of health: Principles, practitioners, and issues* (2nd ed.) Belmont, CA: Wadsworth.

Wright, A., & Morgan, W. (1990). On the creation of "problem" patients. *Social Science and Medicine, 30*, 951-959.

Zuckerman, H. S. (1989). Redefining the role of the CEO: Challenges and conflicts. *Hospital and Health Services, 34*, 25-38.

11

Paternalism and Health Behavior

Tore Nilstun

Smoking is a preventable health risk to smokers as well as to nonsmokers who are exposed to tobacco smoke (Eriksson, LaMaistre, & Newell, 1988; *Healthy People 2000*, 1991; Peto, 1994), and costs related to the use of tobacco are substantial (Hocking, Grain, & Gordon, 1994). It is therefore not surprising that far-reaching measures have been suggested to protect individuals against the dangers of smoking (Leppo & Verio, 1986; Roemer, 1993), frequently with strong opposition from the tobacco industry (Editorial, 1994; Stanton & Begay, 1994).

Attempts to modify smoking behavior raise the controversial issue of paternalism, and the purpose of this chapter is to discuss the ethics of paternalism in the context of health maintenance, health restoration, and health improvement. First, the concept of "paternalism" is defined; second, different types of paternalism are identified; third, the relevant value premises are formulated and applied in the analysis of paternalistic measures suggested to protect against the dangers of smoking.

Tore Nilstun • Department of Medical Ethics, University of Lund, S-222 22 Lund, Sweden.

Handbook of Health Behavior Research IV: Relevance for Professionals and Issues for the Future, edited by David S. Gochman. Plenum Press, New York, 1997.

DEFINITIONS OF PATERNALISM

In the *Compact Edition of the Oxford English Dictionary* (1971), *paternalism* is defined as follows:

> *Definition 1*: the claim or attempt to supply the needs and to control the life of a nation, a community, a group or an individual in a way like that of a father towards his children.

There have been several attempts in the literature on medical ethics to make this definition more precise. Though the basic idea is usually preserved, the meaning is somewhat changed, as illustrated by the following examples:

> *Definition 2*: Paternalism, then, is the intentional overriding of one person's known preferences or actions by another, where the person who overrides justifies the action by the goal of benefiting or avoiding harm to the person whose will is overridden (Beauchamp & Childress, 1994, p. 274).
>
> *Definition 3*: Paternalism [is] the use of (varying degrees of) coercion to impose another's vision—where the other might be the state, private institutions, or individuals—on a single individual or class of individuals (Agich, 1993, p. 3).
>
> *Definition 4*: Paternalism refers to behaviour that attempts to interfere with the autonomy of an individual without his/her consent (explicit or presumed) for the express purpose of benefiting that individual (Veatch & Spicer, 1994).
>
> *Definition 5*: Briefly, paternalism is the belief that it

can be right to order the lives of others for their own good, irrespective of their own wishes or judgments (Harris, 1985, p. 194).

Definition 6: Paternalism is the protection of individuals from self-inflicted harm, … Decisions are taken, choices made and freedom inhibited, all for the good of the patient. There is no element of consent (Downie & Calman, 1994, p. 163).

Definition 7: Paternalism characteristically involves making people's decisions for them or keeping certain information from them on the grounds that it would be better for them not to know (Shinebourne & Bush, 1994).

Definition 8: Paternalistic actions [means that] A is acting towards B for the purpose of benefiting B but without B's informed consent (Nikku, 1994).

Definition 9: P acts paternalistically towards Q if and only if (a) P acts with the intent of averting some harm or promoting some good for Q, (b) P acts contrary to the current preferences, desires or dispositions of Q, (c) P's act is a limitation of Q's autonomy (Dworkin, 1992).

On the population level, however, there are several problems with these definitions. First, most of the definitions (2, 4, 6, 8, and 9; possibly also 5 and 7) require that the beneficiary be identical with the one whose autonomy is limited. But in health behavior modification, the would-be paternalist is usually an authority that acts toward the whole population or a group with the purpose of benefiting some unidentified persons (Nikku, 1994). When health behavior modification is the issue, acts with the motive of benefiting a group or class of individuals (and not a particular individual) would not be paternalistic by these definitions.

Second, according to some of the definitions (2, 3, and 9), an act is paternalistic only if the act, *as a matter of fact*, contradicts the current preferences, desires, or dispositions of the individual or the group. According to the other definitions (1, 4, 5, 6, 7, and 8), this condition is not necessary; they require only that the person who acts paternalistically not know what these preferences, desires, or dispositions are. The first condition (that the act should contradict such preferences …) is, in the view of this chapter, too strong. But the second condition (that the paternalist not know what these preferences, desires,

or dispositions are) is too weak. This chapter proposes a somewhat modified version of the second requirement in the last definition (9). The condition "P acts contrary to the current preferences, desires or dispositions of Q" should be replaced with a somewhat weaker requirement: "P has no reason to believe that the act agrees with the current preferences, desires, or dispositions of Q."

The following definition incorporating this substitute second condition and a slight rewording of the third is suggested:

P acts paternalistically toward an individual or a group Q if and only if
(1) P acts with the intent of averting some harm or promoting some good for Q;
(2) P has no reason to believe that the act agrees with the current preferences, desires, or dispositions of Q; and
(3) P's act is a limitation of Q's right to self-determination.

DIFFERENT TYPES OF PATERNALISM

On the basis of these three conditions, six different types of paternalism may be identified. The requirement that P act with the intent of averting some harm or promoting some good for Q suggests the first distinction. If the would-be paternalist's only motive is to benefit an individual Q (in one way or another) the act may be called *individual paternalism*. It is also called *medical paternalism* (Giesen, 1988). But if the motive is to protect a group or class of individuals from harm, the act may be called *social paternalism* (Kjellin & Nilstun, 1993). The expressions "pure paternalism" and "impure paternalism" are sometimes used to indicate this distinction (Beauchamp & Childress, 1994, p. 275).

In the clinical setting, individual paternalism is more common than social paternalism: The motive is primarily to benefit a particular patient. Antismoking policies (which are based on the idea that individuals are not to be relied on in assessing the health risks of tobacco use), however, aim at the prevention of harm to the general public, both smokers and nonsmokers. Most such attempts to modify health behavior therefore exemplify social paternalism.

The second requirement in the definition relates to the current preferences, desires, or dispositions of Q. Since Q may prefer in some situations that P act and in other situations that P abstain from acting, a distinction is sometimes made between *active paternalism* and *passive paternalism*. Passive paternalism obtains when P refuses to execute the positive preferences of Q. Debates about paternalism typically focus on active paternalism, i.e., situations in which P acts on the grounds that it is to Q's benefits even though Q prefers nonintervention (Beauchamp & Childress, 1994, p. 288).

Many smokers prefer nonintervention. Attempts to modify their smoking behavior would therefore, as a rule, exemplify active paternalism. Passive paternalism is probably more frequent in other areas, e.g., in sports medicine, when a physician refuses to provide an athlete with anabolic steroids.

The third requirement in the definition relates to the concept of autonomy. Depending on the degree to which Q is an autonomous person, *weak paternalism* can be distinguished from

strong paternalism (Feinberg, 1971). In weak paternalism, the would-be paternalist intervenes to protect persons against their own nonautonomous actions; in strong paternalism, the purpose is to protect persons against their autonomous actions (Beauchamp & Childress, 1994, p. 277).

Unfortunately, there is no general agreement on where to draw the line between weak and strong paternalism. One attempt, which makes much sense, was made by Harris (1985, pp. 195–201). His point of departure was that perfect autonomy is, like any ideal, unattainable. The line should therefore be drawn where an individual is as autonomous as can reasonably be expected. This is the case when there are no apparent defects in the agent's control (such as mental illness or drug addiction), reasoning, or available information relevant to the decision at hand. Accordingly, most of the current attempts to modify health behavior related to smoking would be classified, if they were classified as paternalistic at all, as strong paternalism.

These six different types of paternalism are summarized in Table 1.

Other subclasses of paternalism have also been suggested. For instance, Häyry, Häyry, and Karjalainen (1989) distinguish three levels of paternalism: *paternalistic paternalism* (such as

**Table 1. Six Different Types of Paternalistic Acts[a]
by P toward Q, and Their Respective Frequency
in Smoking Behavior Modification at the Population Level**

Characteristics of the paternalistic act	Type of paternalism	Frequency in smoking behavior modification
P's intention is to:		
Benefit only an individual Q	Individual paternalism	Seldom
Benefit a group or class Q	Social paternalism	Often
Q prefers or desires:		
Interference	Passive paternalism	Seldom
Noninterference	Active paternalism	Often
Q is:		
Autonomous	Strong paternalism	Often
Nonautonomous	Weak paternalism	Seldom

[a]An act is paternalistic if and only if (1) P acts with the intent of averting some harm or promoting some good for Q; (2) P has no reason to believe that the act agrees with the current preferences, desires, or dispositions of Q; and (3) P's act is a limitation of Q's right to self-determination.

health education in schools, total ban on advertisements, and sale restrictions to minors), *weak paternalism* (such as health education in mass media, by health professionals, and by voluntary organizations), and *strong paternalism* (such as a ban on brands exceeding an upper limit of hazardous substances).

VALUE PREMISES

Justification of paternalism requires value premises. Such premises are often taken from or inspired by ethical theories. This chapter therefore provides a short summary of the three most discussed and applied theories in medical ethics: utilitarianism, libertarianism, and justice as fairness.

There are several forms of utilitarianism. According to *act utilitarianism*, an act is right if and only if it maximizes utility (Jeremy Bentham, 1789; John Stuart Mill, 1861)—or, in some versions, minimizes suffering (Popper, 1966). According to *rule utilitarianism*, an ethical rule is right if and only if general compliance with the rule maximizes utility, and a particular act is right if and only if it falls under such a rule. According to *classical utilitarianism*, the aim should be the maximization of aggregate utility, while *average utilitarianism* requires maximization of utility per capita. There is no general agreement on the definition of *utility*. Some define it as pleasure or happiness (and absence of pain or suffering); others, as satisfaction of preferences or needs.

The most influential modern exponent of the *libertarian* theory is Nozick (1974), but a similar theory was earlier formulated by John Locke (1690). The basic assumption of the theory is the liberty of all individuals to do what they please with themselves and their property, provided that they do not interfere with the like liberty of others. A further limitation on the right to liberty is given by the harm principle. This principle says that the liberty of one person should be restricted only to prevent harm to others (Feinberg, 1973; Mill, 1859). The right to property is fundamental to the libertarian theory, and it determines both the role of the state and the rules of individual conduct. When a person finds or "mixes labour with" an unowned item, there is initial acquisition of property. The owner of the property may sell it on the free market or give it away as the owner pleases.

Rawls (1952, 1972) is a defender of *justice as fairness*. This theory contains three principles: Each person is to have an equal right to liberty (greatest equal liberty), persons with similar abilities and skills are to have equal access to offices and positions (equality of fair opportunity), and social economic institutions are to be arranged so as to benefit maximally the least well off (fair differences).

Inspired by the ethical theories of utilitarianism, libertarianism, and justice as fairness, three value premises may be identified:

- *The principle of beneficence* states the moral obligation to benefit others, especially not to harm them (utilitarianism).
- *The principle of autonomy* states the moral obligation to respect each other's right to self-determination (libertarianism).
- *The principle of justice* states the moral obligation to act fairly in the distribution of burdens and benefits, especially not to discriminate against anyone (justice).

These principles, which are commonly accepted in medical ethics (Beauchamp & Childress, 1994; Gillon, 1994; *International Guidelines for Biomedical Research*, 1993; *International Guidelines for Ethical Review*, 1991; Stanley, 1989), are rather vague and do not themselves provide a method for balancing them against each other when making moral decisions. They do provide, however, a potentially international and intercultural basis for a common moral commitment that requires that transgression of any one of them can be justified only by pointing to the overriding application of one or more of the others (Gillon, 1993).

IDENTIFICATION AND ANALYSIS OF ETHICAL CONFLICTS

An ethical conflict is a situation where there is at the same time, a moral obligation to adopt each of two alternatives, and the agent cannot adopt both alternatives together (Gowan, 1987; Sinnott-Armstrong, 1988). When paternalism and smoking behavior modification is the issue, the ethical conflicts often (but not always) arise because principle of beneficence and the principle of autonomy cannot be satisfied at the same time.

Examples of measures suggested (and often implemented) to change smoking behavior are (1) health education in schools, via the mass media, for people using health services, and by voluntary organizations (Flynn et al., 1992, 1994; Gregorio, 1994); (2) price policy, such as regular price revisions and differential taxation (Townsend, Roderick & Cooper, 1994; Yach, 1994); (3) premarket licensing, such as quality control, health warning on packages, ban on brands exceeding the upper limits of hazardous substances, and classification of products as "harmful" and "very harmful" (Benhamou, Benhamou, Auquier, & Flamant, 1994); (4) total ban on advertisement and sales promotion—so far only on the national level (British Airways' response, 1994; Fulop, & Mckee, 1994)—or at least on campaigns with special appeal to teenagers (Hastings, Ryan, Teer, & MacKintosh, 1994); (5) sale restriction (Leppo & Verio, 1986); (6) restriction on smoking in schools, nurseries, public transport, and other public locales (Moore, Wolfe, Lindes, & Douglas, 1994); (7) restriction on portrayal in films and television of smokers as successful and attractive (Hazan, Lipton, & Glantz, 1994); and (8) research, planning, and evaluation of consumption levels and trends and their distribution and of the health effects of smoking (Gritz, 1994; Wynder & Hoffmann, 1994). It has also been suggested that smokers (as a group) should be held accountable. Revenues from cigarette taxation should be placed in a specific trust to pay for heart disease costs (Kaesemeyer, 1994).

A model that combines ideas from Hermerén (1986) and Francoeur (1983) facilitates the identification and analysis of ethical conflicts raised by such measures. The model—which is more fully discussed in Nilstrun (1990), Haglund, Nilstun, Westrin, and Smedby (1991), Westrin, Nilstun, Smedby, and Haglund (1992), and Nilstun and Westrin (1994)—has two dimensions. The first dimension specifies the relevant ethical principles (in this chapter, the three principles of beneficence, autonomy, and justice are used) and the second dimension specifies the different groups of individuals involved in or affected by the attempts to modify smoking behavior.

Each group should consist of persons who, in relation to antismoking policies, have similar interests. The groups should be exhaustive; i.e., all those who are involved in or affected by the policy should belong to at least one group. But the groups are not necessarily exclusive; i.e., one individual may belong to more than one group. The groups involved in or affected by antismoking policies are:

- Smokers (many of whom want to go on using tobacco).
- Adult nonsmokers (most of whom don't want to be exposed to tobacco smoke).
- Children (who should be protected from passive smoking and prevented from using tobacco).
- Fetuses (all of whom should be protected from maternal smoking).
- Pets (which should be protected from being exposed to tobacco smoke).
- Tobacco industries and trades (which want to manufacture and sell their products).
- Employees in tobacco industries and trade (who don't want to lose their jobs).
- Employers (who want to reduce their costs due to smoking).
- The state (which gets revenue by taxing tobacco products but pays for health care).
- Health care professionals (who want to reduce the use of tobacco).

The task, when applying the model to assess attempts to modify health behavior, is to identify ethical costs and benefits to those involved or affected. Since the words "costs" and "benefits" here are used in a rather wide sense, some clarification is needed. To identify and assess the rightness or wrongness of attempts to modify health behavior with reference to the principle of beneficence is to determine their tendency to produce good or bad consequences. Within the utilitarian tradition, it is natural to call fulfillments of the principle of beneficence (i.e., the good consequences) ethical benefits and violations of the principle (i.e. the bad consequences) ethical costs.

In the literature on medical ethics, the words "costs" and "benefits" are not used in connection with the principle of autonomy. To assess a health behavior modification policy with reference to this principle is not to determine any good consequences. The rightness or wrongness of the policy is assessed by reference to the obligation to respect the right to self-determination of the persons involved (no matter what its consequences might be). Though less common, in order to facilitate comparison, the expression "ethical costs" is used to denote violations of the principle of autonomy and the expression "ethical benefits" to denote fulfillments.

In the same way, violations of the principle of justice are called "ethical costs" and fulfillments "ethical benefits."

The official smoking policy in the 1960s (in this chapter called the "liberal smoking policy") is used as a baseline, which means that this policy is treated as though it has no ethical costs and no ethical benefits. Given this simplifying assumption, the question to be answered is: What are the differences, in terms of ethical costs and ethical benefits, to the groups involved in or affected by an antismoking policy (as suggested by the different measures identified to reduce smoking) compared to a liberal smoking policy?

Ethical benefits related to the principle of beneficence consist of prevention of harm to smokers (who are induced to quit smoking or

reduce their consumption), adult nonsmokers (who don't start smoking or are less exposed to tobacco smoke), children, fetuses, and pets. Reduced tobacco-related health care costs and absence due to illness are ethical benefits to the state and employers, respectively. The joy felt by many health care professionals when smoking is reduced might also be considered an ethical benefit. Not only ethical benefits, however, but also ethical costs fall upon smokers. Most of them really enjoy smoking and many are not harmed. Nevertheless, they are forced to abstain, e.g., at work, due to antismoking policies. (Many health care workers seem to take for granted that the benefits always outweigh the costs to smokers. But is this assumption correct?) In addition, there are costs to the tobacco industry, both employers and employees. The costs and benefits related to the principle of beneficence are indicated in the first column of Table 2.

Ethical costs related to the principle of autonomy consist of interferences with the right to self-determination. Smokers' freedom to act on their desire to smoke is limited by the antismoking policy. There are also autonomy costs to the tobacco industry and the employees in these industries. As to autonomy benefits, the prohibition of smoking in public premises favors the freedom of those individuals who want to avoid health risks posed by exposure to tobacco smoke. The costs and benefits related to the principle of autonomy are indicated in the second column of Table 2.

There are also ethical benefits and costs related to the principle of justice. A liberal smoking policy is to the advantage of smokers at the expense of non-smokers. But antismoking policies reverse the situation. Smokers, at least in Sweden, are now frequently treated in ways that can only be described as discrimination. A change from liberal to antismoking policy implies justice costs to smokers and justice benefits to nonsmokers. The costs and benefits related to the principle of justice are indicated in the third column of Table 2.

To make a complete ethical analysis of anti-

**Table 2. Ethical Benefits and Ethical Costs
of an Antismoking Policy Compared to a Liberal Smoking Policy[a]**

Persons involved or affected	Ethical principles		
	Beneficence	Autonomy	Justice
Smokers	Benefits	Costs	Costs
Nonsmokers			
Adults	Benefits	Benefits	Benefits
Children	Benefits	—	Benefits
Fetuses	Benefits	—	Benefits
Pets	Benefits	—	—
Tobacco industries and trades	Costs	Costs	—
Employees in tobacco industries	Costs	Costs	—
Employers	Benefits	—	—
The state	Benefits	—	—
Health care professionals	Benefits	—	—

[a]The liberal smoking policy (premised on the principle of autonomy) is the baseline for comparison.

smoking policies (compared to a liberal smoking policy), all the costs and benefits in Table 2 should be taken into consideration. In this chapter, however, the purpose is only to discuss the two ethical conflicts raised by paternalism. For both of these conflicts, the requirement of the principle of beneficence (in relation to smokers and nonsmokers) comes into conflict with the requirement of the principle of autonomy (in relation to smokers).

Antismoking measures, the purpose of which is to benefit not only smokers but also nonsmokers, give rise to the first ethical conflict. This conflict arises because it is not always possible to satisfy both the obligation to respect smokers' right to self-determination and the obligation to prevent them from harming others (social paternalism). Antismoking measures that aim at benefiting smokers give rise to the second conflict because it is always possible to satisfy both the obligation to respect smokers' right to self-determination and the obligation to prevent them from harming themselves (individual paternalism). The two most important benefits and the most important cost relevant to the assessment of paternalism that accrue to smokers and nonsmokers are indicated in Table 3.

BALANCING ETHICAL COSTS AND BENEFITS

So far, this approach has been descriptive and analytical and the objective has been to meet a minimal standard of intersubjectivity; i.e., competent persons, asking the same questions and using similar methods, should also reach similar conclusions (Hermerén, 1972, p. 121). The choice of value premises and the identification of ethical costs and benefits to those involved and affected are intersubjective in this sense. But when the ethical costs and ethical benefits are to be bal-

**Table 3. Most Important Ethical Cost and Two
Most Important Benefits Relevant to the
Assessment of Paternalism of an Antismoking
Policy Compared to a Liberal Smoking Policy[a]**

Persons involved or affected	Ethical principle	
	Beneficence	Autonomy
Smokers	Benefits	Costs
Nonsmokers	Benefits	—

[a]The liberal smoking policy (premised on the principle of autonomy) is the baseline for comparison.

anced, it is difficult to satisfy the requirement of intersubjectivity.

The harm principle, as formulated by Mill (1859), justifies different solutions to the two ethical conflicts raised by paternalism:

> ... the sole end for which mankind are warranted, individually or collectively, in interfering with the liberty of action of any of their number, is self-protection. That the only purpose for which power can be rightfully exercised over any member of a civilized community, against his will, is to prevent harm to others. His own good, either physical or moral, is not a sufficient warrant.

According to Mill, individual paternalism should be avoided; i.e., priority should in this situation be given to the principle of autonomy at the expense of the principle of beneficence. But social paternalism is sometimes ethically justified; i.e., priority should in such situations sometimes be given to the principle of beneficence at the expense of the principle of autonomy.

A similar position is defended by VanDeVeer (1986) and Feinberg (1986). According to VanDeVeer, individual paternalism is never justified when it is incompatible with respecting competent persons' right to direct their own lives within the sphere of acts that do not wrong others. According to Feinberg, the right to self-determination always takes precedence in the rare cases in which there is a conflict between promoting a person's good and respecting the personal right of self-determination.

If the harm principle is accepted, antismoking policies are justified only when they are aimed at protecting nonsmokers from being exposed to tobacco smoke. Consistent application of the harm principle implies that all public premises (including restaurants and other eating places) should have nonsmoking areas even if their having them may be inconvenient to smokers.

But antismoking policies cannot be justified by reference to the good of the person being coerced. At least some of the many restrictions placed on adult smoking in the workplace and in hospitals are hard to justify with reference to the harm principle. Pleasant smoking rooms, conve-

niently located and with adequate ventilation, would protect nonsmokers from the danger of passive smoking.

There are several problems, however, with the harm principle. The most important is that few if any find the principle acceptable without exceptions. Also, there is no consensus as to what particular antismoking policies should be considered as such exceptions. This lack of agreement makes the harm principle lose much of its force when ethical conflicts are to be solved. It also explains the popularity of "commonsense morality." According to this morality, to solve an ethical conflict raised by paternalism requires a determination, *in any particular case*, of which principle—beneficence or autonomy—is more important (Brock, 1994):

> The cost to the subject's well-being from respecting a particular choice of the subject can vary greatly in degree—from the loss of the subject's life at one end of a continuum to the most trivial of adverse effects at the other end. Likewise, the importance of respecting the individual's autonomy can vary substantially from case to case depending on such factors as how central and far-reaching the choice is within the particular individual's plan of life, how strongly the individual wants to make the choice in question for him- or herself, and so forth.

Ross (1940), an important source of inspiration for the theory of bioethics that emanated from the Kennedy Center in Georgetown in the late 1970s (Beauchamp & Childress, 1994), makes this problem with ethical conflicts explicit. According to Ross's theory, one enters into a decision-making situation equipped with a set of basic ethical principles that are used to identify and examine the problems at hand (Ross, 1940, p. 41):

> ... right acts can be distinguished from wrong acts only as being those which, of all those possible for the agent in the circumstances, have the greatest balance of *prima facie* rightness ... over their *prima facie* wrongness,... For the estimation of the comparative stringency of these *prima facie* obligations no general rules can, as far as I can see, be laid down.

By "prima facie rightness or obligation" is meant that the act is right or obligatory unless it conflicts with an equal or stronger right or obligation. A prima facie right is binding unless overridden or outweighed by competing moral rights (Ross, 1940, pp. 18–22; cf. also Beauchamp & Childress, 1994, p. 33).

One can agree with Ross that no such general rules can be laid down. That they cannot be does not imply, however, that ethical principles are useless. On the contrary, the effort to formulate such principles and identify the ethical costs and benefits to those involved or affected not only improves knowledge about the alternatives and their probable consequences, but also counteracts the human tendency to "forget" ethical costs and benefits. When it is believed that the right solution to an ethical conflict has been found, the capacity for unbiased assessment of counterargument is easily lost.

The use of principles to identify ethical costs and ethical benefits is therefore essential to ethical analysis. But when one has to decide how to solve an ethical conflict, the use of analogy is often more convincing (Winkler, 1993, 1994). That it is can be illustrated by comparing the ethics of data utilization in epidemiology and in journalism (Westrin & Nilstun, 1994).

Much of the available knowledge about the harmful effects of smoking derives from epidemiology, often using case registers and record linkage. The purpose of such studies is to prevent harm to unidentified individuals. But the large number of individuals investigated often makes it practically impossible to obtain individually informed consent, and without such consent there is infringement on personal autonomy. This means that epidemiology is almost inconceivable without some element of social paternalism.

In the European countries, there is at present a strong antipaternalistic trend. Legal controls over data collection have adversely affected the prospects for epidemiology, especially in countries with previously favorable conditions for epidemiological research, such as Sweden. Far greater damage to environmental epidemiology is likely if a recent proposal by the European Commission is implemented. Its key paragraph states that "member states shall prohibit the automatic processing of sensitive data—for example, regarding health—without the expressed and written consent freely given of the data subjects." This restriction reflects a desire to give priority to respect for individual autonomy at the expense of benefits to the whole population. According to this paragraph, paternalism is not justified in epidemiology.

By contrast, journalists have been allowed far greater freedoms. One reason is that the aims and tasks of journalism—with its emphasis on an open society—are not compatible with strict adherence to the principles of respect for individual autonomy and of doing no harm. Hence, infringements on both the principle of beneficence and the principle of autonomy by journalism are unavoidable ethical costs in an open society. This means that paternalistic acts sometimes are justified with reference to journalism.

But is this difference between journalism and epidemiology justifiable? One can argue that it is not. In epidemiology, which also aims at benefits to the open society, there is no need to harm research subjects. But it is not possible to carry out case register research and record linkage without some infringement on individual autonomy. Compared with the ethical costs of journalism, however, the ethical costs of epidemiology are very modest. So if social paternalism is justified with reference to journalism (and in my opinion it is), it should also be accepted with reference to epidemiology.

CONCLUDING REMARKS

Any attempt to resolve the ethical conflicts related to paternalism in the context of health maintenance, health restoration, and health improvement is dependent not only on personal values and factual assumptions but also on the choice of analogy. Since people differ over values, many assumptions about health behavior modification are questionable; further, since the force of reasoning by analogy is highly dependent on cultural affiliation, different conclusions as to paternalism may be equally rational or irrational. Competent persons, facing the same ethical conflicts and using similar methods, do not always reach similar conclusions; i.e., the requirement of intersubjectivity is not always satisfied.

If the authority of science ends where intersubjectivity ends (which seems reasonable), medical ethicists do not have any special mandate to solve these ethical conflicts. Thus, the task of setting limits on the use of paternalism in health behavior modification falls outside the scope of medical ethics and into the realm of politics.

REFERENCES

Agich, G. J. (1993). *Autonomy and long-term care*. New York: Oxford University Press.

Beauchamp, T. L., & Childress, J. F. (1994). *Principles of biomedical ethics* (4th ed.). New York: Oxford University Press (originally published in 1979).

Benhamou, S., Benhamou, E., Auquier, A., & Flamant, R. (1994). Differential effects of tar content, type of tobacco and use of a filter on lung cancer risk in male cigarette smokers. *International Journal of Epidemiology, 23*(3), 437–443.

Bentham, J. (1789). *An introduction to the principles of morals and legislation*. London (originally printed in 1780).

British Airways' response. (1994). Airline's magazine promotes production of tobacco products. *British Medical Journal, 309*(6953), 544.

Brock, D. W. (1994). Paternalism and autonomy. *Ethics, 98*(3), 550–565.

The compact edition of the Oxford English dictionary. (1971). Oxford: Clarendon Press.

Downie, R. S., & Calman, K. C. (1994). *Healthy respect: Ethics in health care* (2nd ed.). New York: Oxford University Press.

Dworkin, G. (1992). Paternalism. In L. C. Becker & C. B. Becker (Eds.), *Encyclopedia of ethics* (pp. 939–942). London: St James Press.

Editorial. (1994). Revealing the link between campaign financing and deaths caused by tobacco. *Journal of the American Medical Association, 272*(15), 1217–1218.

Eriksson, M.P., LaMaistre, C. A., & Newell, G. R. (1988). Health hazards of passive smoking. *American Review of Public Health, 9*, 7–70.

Feinberg, J. (1971). Legal paternalism. *Canadian Journal of Philosophy, 1*, 105–124.

Feinberg, J. (1973). *Social philosophy*. Englewood Cliffs, NJ: Prentice-Hall.

Feinberg, J. (1986). *Harm to self*. New York: Oxford University Press.

Flynn, B. S., Worden, J. K., Secker-Walker, R. H., Bchir, M. B., Badger, G. J., Geller, B. M., & Costanza, M. C. (1992). Prevention of cigarette smoking through mass media interventions and school programs. *American Journal of Health, 82*(6), 827–834.

Flynn, B. S., Worden, J. K., Secker-Walker, R. H., Pirie, P. L., Badger, G. J., Carpenter, J. H., & Geller. B. M. (1994). Mass media and school interventions for cigarette smoking prevention: Effects 2 years after completion. *American Journal of Health, 84*(7), 1148–1150.

Francoeur, R. T. (1983). *Biomedical ethics: A guide to decision making*. New York: Oxford University Press.

Fulop, N. J., & Mckee, M. (1994). Airline's magazine promotes production of tobacco products. *British Medical Journal, 309*(6953), 544.

Giesen, D. (1988). *International medical malpractice law: A comparative study of civil liability arising from medical care*. Tübingen: J. C. B. Mohr; Dordrecht, Boston, & London: Martinus Nijhoff.

Gillon, R. (1993). Ethical review procedures: A developed countries' perspective. In *International guidelines for biomedical research involving human subjects*, (pp. 70–87). Geneva: CIOMS.

Gillon, R. (Ed.). (1994). *Principles of health care ethics*. New York: Wiley.

Gowan, C. W. (Ed.). (1987). *Moral dilemmas*. New York: Oxford University Press.

Gregorio, D. I. (1994). Counselling adolescents for smoking prevention: A survey of primary care physicians and dentists. *American Journal of Health, 84*(7), 1151–1153.

Gritz, E. R. (1994). Reaching toward and beyond the year 2000 goal for cigarette smoking: Research and public health priorities. *Cancer, 74*(4)(Supplement), 1423–1432.

Haglund, B., Nilstun, T., Westrin, C.-G., & Smedby, B. (1991). Longitudinal studies on environmental factors and disease. *Scandinavian Journal of Social Medicine, 19*(2), 81–85.

Harris, J. (1985) *The value of life*. London: Routledge.

Hastings, G. B., Ryan, H., Teer, P., & MacKintosh, A. M. (1994). Cigarette advertising and children's smoking: Why Reg was withdrawn. *British Medical Journal, 309*(6959), 933–937.

Häyry, H., Häyry, M., & Karjalainen, S. (1989). Paternalism and Finnish antismoking policy. *Social Science and Medicine, 28*, 293–297.

Hazan, A. R., Lipton, H. L., & Glantz, S. A. (1994). Popular films do not reflect current tobacco use. *American Journal of Public Health, 84*(6), 998–1000.

Healthy people 2000: National health promotion and disease prevention objectives. (1994). DHHS Publication No. PHS 91-50212. Washington, DC: U.S. Department of Health and Human Services.

Hermerén, G. (1972). *Värdering och objektivitet [Valuation and objectivity]*. Lund: Studentlitteratur [in Swedish].

Hermerén, G. (1986). *Kunskapens pris [The price of knowledge]*. Stockholm: Forskningsrådsnämndens Förlagstjänst [in Swedish].

Hocking, B., Grain, H., & Gordon, I. (1994). Cost to industry of illness related to alcohol and smoking: A study of Telecom Australia employees. *Medical Journal of Australia, 161*(7), 407–412.

International guidelines for biomedical research involving human subjects. (1993). Geneva: CIOMS.

International guidelines for ethical review of epidemiological studies. (1991). Geneva: CIOMS.

Kaesemeyer, W. H. (1994). Holding smokers accountable for heart disease costs. *Circulation, 90*(2), 1029–1032.

Kjellin, L., & Nilstun, T. (1993). Medical and social paternalism: Regulation of and attitudes towards compulsory psychiatric care. *Acta Psychiatria Scandinavica. 88*, 415–419

Leppo, K., & Verio, H. (1986). Smoking control in Finland: A case study in policy formulation and implementation. *Health Promotion, 1*, 5–16.

Locke, J. (1670). *Two treatises on government.* London.

Mill, J. S. (1859). *On liberty.* London.

Mill, J. S. (1861). *Utilitarianism.* London.

Moore, S., Wolfe, S.M., Lindes, D., & Douglas, C.E. (1994). Epidemiology of failed tobacco control legislation. *Journal of the American Medical Association, 272*(15), 1171–1175.

Nikku, N. (1994). Paternalism and autonomy in health promotion. In, P. E. Liss & N. Nikku (Eds.), *Health promotion and prevention: Theoretical and ethical aspects* (pp. 110–116). Stockholm: Swedish Council for Planning and Coordination of Research.

Nilstun, T. (1990). Public health measures with HIV infection: A model for identification and analysis of ethical conflicts. In B. Janson, & P. Allebeck (Eds.), *Ethics in medicine: Individual integrity versus demands of society* (pp. 203–213). New York: Raven Press.

Nilstun, T., & Westrin, C.-G. (1994). The use of numbers in ethical analysis. *Health Care Analysis, 2*(1), 43–46.

Nozick, R. (1974). *Anarchy, state and Utopia.* New York: Basic Books.

Peto, R. (1994). Smoking and death: The past 40 years and the next 40. *British Medical Journal, 309*(6959), 937–939.

Popper, K. R. (1966). *The open society and its enemies.* London: Routledge & Kegan Paul (originally published in 1945).

Rawls, J. (1952). Justice as fairness. *Philosophical Review, 67*, 164–194.

Rawls, J. (1972). *A theory of justice.* New York: Oxford University Press.

Roemer, R. (1993). *Legislative action to combat the tobacco epidemic* (2nd ed.). Geneva. World Health Organization.

Ross, W. D. (1940). *The right and the good.* Oxford: Oxford University Press.

Shinebourne, E. A., & Bush, A. (1994). For paternalism in the doctor-patient relationship. In R. Gillon (Ed.), *Principles of health care ethics* (pp. 399–408). New York: Wiley.

Sinnott-Armstrong, W. (1988). *Moral dilemmas.* New York: Basil Blackwell.

Stanley, J. M. (Ed.). (1989). The Appleton consensus: Suggested international guidelines for decisions to forgo medical treatment. *Journal of Medical Ethics, 14*, 128–136.

Stanton, A. G., & Begay, M. E. (1994). Tobacco industry campaign contributions are affecting tobacco control policymaking in California. *Journal of the American Medical Association, 272*(1), 1176–1182.

Townsend, J., Roderick, P., & Cooper, J. (1994). Cigarette smoking by socioeconomic group, sex and age: Effects of price, income, and health publicity. *British Medical Journal, 309*(6959), 923–927.

VanDeVeer, D. (1986). *Paternalistic intervention.* Princeton NJ: Princeton University Press.

Veatch, R. M., & Spicer, C. M. (1994). Against paternalism in the patient-physician relationship. In R. Gillon (Ed.), *Principles of health care ethics* (pp. 409–419). New York: Wiley.

Westrin, C. G., & Nilstun, T. (1994). The ethics of data utilization: A comparison between epidemiology and journalism. *British Medical Journal, 308*, 522–523.

Westrin, C. G., Nilstun, T., Smedby, B., & Haglund, B. (1992). Epidemiology and moral philosophy. *Journal of Medical Ethics. 18*(4), 193–196.

Winkler, E. R. (1993). From Kantianism to contextualism: The rise and fall of the paradigm theory in bioethics. In E. R. Winkler & J. R. Coombs (Eds.), *Applied ethics: A reader* (pp. 343–365). Oxford: Blackwell.

Winkler, E. R. (1994). *Reflections on the relevance of the Georgetown paradigm for the ethics of environmental epidemiology.* Working paper EHAZ 14/WS01/10. Rome: WHO Regional Office for Europe.

Wynder, E. L., & Hoffmann, D. (1994). Smoking and lung cancer: Scientific challenges and opportunities. *Cancer Research, 54*, 5284–5295.

Yach, D. (1994). Tobacco excise tax and children. *South African Medical Journal, 84*(8), 507.

12

Health Policy, Health Behavior, and Injury Control

Leon S. Robertson

INTRODUCTION

The United States has two policies that contribute substantially to its excessive health care costs: (1) neglect of application of cost-effective injury reduction programs and (2) required medical treatment of the injured on demand. The neglect of effective prevention programs is partly due to a non sequitur espoused since the early days of the automobile by its manufacturers (Eastman, 1984) and in recent decades by some professionals in public health, medicine, and engineering: Behavior is a major factor in injury causation; therefore, behavior must be changed to reduce injury. This false bromide is often applied as well to other major health problems, such as cancer and heart disease (e.g., American Public Health Association, 1994).

If health problems are framed as mainly behavioral in origin, and behavior is difficult to

Leon S. Robertson • Yale University and Nanlee Research, Branford, Connecticut 06405-5115.

Handbook of Health Behavior Research IV: Relevance for Professionals and Issues for the Future, edited by David S. Gochman. Plenum Press, New York, 1997.

change because of its complexity as well as constitutional and ethical constraints, then the health problems will persist. If treatment cannot be denied once an individual develops the health problem, then the cost to the individual, or more likely to all of us through insurance and governmental payment programs, will be high.

This chapter focuses on behaviors in various sectors of United States society that contribute to the incidence, severity, and costs of injuries in the United States and the policy alternatives to reduce them. Because injury is, by definition, an instantaneous event, the potential for immediate cost savings from prevention is huge. For example, a seat belt law reduces deaths and injuries as soon as it is enforced. Efforts to reduce heart disease and cancer, while desirable, have lower cost savings in the short run because of the lag, often decades, between exposure to risk factors and manifestation of the disease. The median age at death from cardiovascular disease is 76 and that from cancer is 68, compared to a median age at death from motor vehicle crashes of 28. Because of such differences, injury results in more lost years of life than do cardiovascular disease and cancer combined (Rice & MacKenzie, 1989).

INDIVIDUAL BEHAVIOR

Is it necessary to change behaviors of individuals at risk to reduce injury or other diseases related to those behaviors? Numerous studies have illustrated the efficacy of interventions that did not directly address behavioral risk factors.

In New York City, child deaths in falls from high-rise buildings were reduced about 80% by programs and regulations requiring window barrier that could not be breached by children in such buildings (Bergner, 1982). Had the programs been directed at myriad behaviors, such as leaving children unattended, parents or guardians becoming intoxicated, and interruptions of supervision by causes such as demands from other children or telephone calls, it is unlikely that much if any reduction in falls would have resulted.

In White River, Arizona, during a 2-year period, injury control specialists of the Indian Health Service (IHS) identified a 2-mile section of road in which numerous pedestrians had sustained serious injuries, mainly in nighttime collisions. The White Mountain Apache Tribe and the IHS collaborated in a project to install streetlights along the road. In the subsequent 4 years, only 2 pedestrians were struck at night (Robertson, 1992). Again, it has proved difficult to change numerous known behavioral risk factors for pedestrian injury—e.g., alcohol intoxication, unsupervised children, children darting into the road—and attempting to do so would not have been nearly as successful as lighting the road.

Both federal safety standards and nonrequired changes in car crashworthiness by manufacturers have greatly reduced death and severe injury in crashes. The federal safety standards initiated in 1968 prevented about 15,000 deaths per year by the early 1980s, when most vehicles that did not meet the standards had been scrapped (Robertson, 1984). Crashworthiness of front ends was improved by manufacturers in response to 35-mile-per-hour frontal barrier crash tests by the National Highway Traffic Safety Administration (NHTSA) (Kahane, 1994). Further

reductions will occur as cars without air bags are junked in this decade and the next. Vehicle crashworthiness protects both those whose behavior contributes to the crash and others who might otherwise have also been injured.

The point in this argument is not to exclude individual behavior change as an option for improving public health. The point is to indicate that (1) the widespread assumption that behavior causes the problem and must therefore be changed to reduce the problem is not true, and (2) a variety of options should be considered and the most cost-effective one(s) should be applied.

Attempts at individual behavior change include: (1) persuasion through education, media advertising, incentives, and disincentives; and (2) requiring or prohibiting behaviors that reduce or increase risk, respectively, by law or administrative directive. Regulation is generally more effective than persuasion, but the effects of either approach depend on several contingencies (Robertson, 1983).

Persuasion

Two types of individual behavior are important in considering behavior as a risk factor for disease or injury: (1) behavior that exposes the person or others in proximity to hazardous pathogens and (2) behavior intended to protect the individual from hazardous agents. The former and occasionally the absence of the latter is sometimes called "risk-taking" behavior. This label is unfortunate in view of the evidence that the opposite, i.e., misunderstanding or denial of risk, is prevalent. People do not gather information on risks and choose to act on the basis of that information, as the descriptor "risk-taking" implies; rather, they have vague and inconsistent perceptions of risk (Slovic, Fischoff & Lichtenstein, 1987) and often deny that the perceived risk applies to them personally (Robertson, 1992).

While denial has been demonstrated, the effect it has on self-protective behavior has not been investigated adequately. Are risk-deniers less likely to take precautions than others? If so, are there ways to confront or reverse the denial in such a way as to increase protective behavior?

Principles for efficient and effective behavior change have been established, but are often ignored in practice. For example, it is well known that changing a one-time or infrequent decision to reduce risk, such as installing a smoke detector or buying a more crashworthy vehicle, is easier than changing a frequently required behavior, such as child supervision or seat belt use (Robertson, 1975). Indeed, the risk reduction, given the behavior change, can sometimes be larger for the one-time decision compared to the frequent decision. Nonuse of seat belts increases risk of death in a crash by about 40%, while purchase of certain "sport utility" vehicles, pickup trucks, and the least crashworthy cars can increase risk to 3–20 times that of the safest vehicles (Robertson, 1989, 1992). Yet enormous resources have been expended on seat belt use campaigns, while little is done to influence choice in vehicle purchases based on risk.

Despite evidence that advertising campaigns alone have little or no effect on behaviors such as seat belt use, alcohol use, and driving behavior (Robertson, 1983), not only are such campaigns frequently launched, but also those who produce them claim credit for reduced risk that occurred for other reasons. A recent ad campaign in South Carolina was claimed to reduce motor vehicle fatalities 38% from the beginning of the campaign in 1988 through 1992. During those years, however, the death rate in South Carolina was higher than expected compared to its historic relation to the United States rate and the rate of other states in the region. The death rate was in decline nationwide because of such factors as junking of less crashworthy older vehicles, increase in seat belt use because of laws and belts that automatically encircle occupants, more vehicles with air bags, and greater police and court attention to alcohol-influenced driving. Actually, South Carolina was not keeping pace, and the ad campaign had no apparent effect (Robertson, 1994).

The South Carolina campaign was preceded by focus group discussions and public opinion polls that formed the basis for the campaign. Unfortunately, these methods are insufficient to assess the potential effectiveness of a campaign in changing actual behavior. There are cable television systems that are divided so that the researcher can do a controlled experiment, showing ads on one cable and using the households on the second cable as a control (Robertson et al., 1974). Proponents of "public service" advertising seldom make use of such research before launching their campaigns.

Furthermore, persuasion is not only often ineffective, but also can be harmful. If education results in greater participation in a hazardous activity without reducing the risk per participation, the problem is increased. Such was the case with high school driver education. Introduced with no experimentation to establish efficacy historically, it was eventually claimed to be effective by its advocates because those who took the course had lower crash rates than those who did not. A controlled experiment in England indicated that individual risk of a crash was not reduced by the course when self-selection into the course was eliminated. In the aggregate, however, the risk per population was increased because of increased licensure and driving by those who had taken the course (Shaoul, 1975).

In the United States, the states with larger proportions of 16- to 17-year-olds taking driver education in high school had more such persons licensed per population, but no fewer fatal crashes per number licensed. The net result was greater fatal crash involvement per population of 16- to 17-year-old drivers in states with more drivers educated per population (Robertson & Zador, 1978). A study of communities that dropped driver education from school curricula, compared with communities of similar size that retained the course, indicated a reduction in licensure and crash involvement per 16- to 17-year-old population in the communities that dropped the course (Robertson, 1980).

An attempt by the federal government to devise an improved high school driver education course proved futile. The course was designed by educators and psychologists using principles thought to be effective in changing behavior. In a controlled experiment, the students who had the new "safe performance curriculum" had no better subsequent crash records than the control group licensed without formal training (Lund, Williams, & Zador, 1986).

The demonstration of effectiveness of educational efforts has been shown in certain instances. Pedestrian injuries to children who dart out in front of vehicles were reduced by a combination of public service advertising on television and instruction in public schools in four cities. The campaign was focused on a cartoon character, "Willy Whistle," portrayed in film and television in interaction with children in traffic situations. The basic message is that the child should stop and look at any curb or at any cars parked along the roadside before entering the street (Blomberg, Preusser, & Hale, 1983). This gives approaching drivers the opportunity to slow down even if the child subsequently darts out.

Combinations of information, education, and incentives have been found to increase bicycle helmet use. In Australia and Seattle, campaigns that included promotion of helmet use in the schools and by community groups, discounts on helmets offered by merchants, and prizes for children wearing helmets at bicycling events increased use (DiGuiseppi, Rivara, Koepsell, & Polissar, 1990; Wood & Milne, 1988). In the Seattle study, bicycle helmet use was also surveyed in Portland, Oregon, before and during the Seattle campaign to be sure that any general increase in bicycle helmet use in the region that might occur would not be falsely attributed to the campaign. The use in Portland changed only slightly, increasing confidence that the increased helmet use in Seattle was a result of the campaign.

Incentives alone have substantial effect. Studies of lottery-like incentives to use seat belts have increased use, at least during the period of the incentives. For example, in work settings, employees' use of seat belts observed as they leave parking lots, is increased substantially during periods that belt use is the qualifier to receive cash or other prizes in periodic drawings. When the incentives are no longer offered, however, belt use soon declines (Geller, 1988).

Several controlled experiments in which clinicians or health educators in clinical settings have attempted to influence injury-related behavior or the use of protective equipment have produced mixed results. Brochures regarding household hazards (Dershewitz & Williamson, 1977) and brochures plus counseling by a health educator regarding use of child restraints (Reisinger & Williams, 1978) had no effect in controlled experiments. Counseling by physicians regarding use of child restraints had a small effect (Reisinger et al., 1981), and such counseling regarding use of smoke detectors (Miller et al., 1982) and infant falls (Kravitz, 1973) had a larger effect.

Several generalizations regarding the potential effectiveness of individual behavior change efforts can be stated tentatively on the basis of the research cited. Obviously, it is easier and more effective to influence a behavior that, once accomplished, will reduce risk for a sustained period of time (e.g., purchase of a lower-risk motor vehicle, smoke detector) than to influence a frequently required behavior (e.g., use of seat belts and child restraints). Concentrating on a single behavior (e.g., darting into traffic) is usually more effective than a more diffuse effort (e.g., warning against various household hazards). Personal counseling, particularly by an authority figure such as a physician, seems to have more effect than less personal television ads or counseling by persons who, however knowledgeable, may not be perceived as authoritative by the average person. Reduction of costs by discounts or possibility of short-term tangible reward, as in a lottery, has some effect.

One should note that demonstrated effectiveness or lack of effectiveness of a particular effort will not necessarily result in its use or nonuse. The "Willy Whistle" materials were provided to schools and television stations throughout the country by the NHTSA, but this author could find only one city (Miami, Florida) in which they had been used in any sustained effort. Yet high school driver education, despite its harmful result, remains a ubiquitous and costly program in many communities.

There is no governmental or other system to monitor or control the selection of injury control efforts at the local level or in clinical settings, nor is one likely to be developed. Such efforts will remain ad hoc and only occasionally based on scientific demonstration of effectiveness.

Law

Coalitions of injury researchers and groups interested in reducing particular injuries have influenced the enactment of injury control laws in selected states and local communities. These laws have included those concerning seat belt use, child restraint use, motorcycle helmet use, increased penalties for driving while intoxicated, taxes on cigarettes and alcohol, cigarette burn rates, tap water temperature, and some aspects of gun control (Bergman, 1992). These efforts tend to be ad hoc, dependent on the enthusiasm and influence of advocates with interest in a particular injury. When such legislation is publicized, however, law-making bodies in other jurisdictions will often adopt similar laws.

Classic experimental–control design is seldom used in the study of effects of laws. Legislators and the judiciary have resisted randomly assigning offenders to various treatments or applying various laws to different jurisdictions. Occasionally, police agencies have agreed to random assignment of patrol or other enforcement modalities (Kelling et al., 1974). The more convincing design, given no random assignment, is a quasi-experimental design in which the function of control is served by one or more comparable jurisdictions in which the legal intervention is not implemented.

The involvement of alcohol in motor vehicle crashes has periodically received major attention, although not always in ways that led to effective public policy. As with "crime" generally, the emphasis is usually on severe punishment for offenders without consideration of the research

evidence that severity of punishment is the least effective policy for prevention (Ross, 1992).

Policies directed at those with convictions for driving under the influence (DUI)—whether license suspension, jail, detoxification, or education—cannot have any major effect on the total problem because 5 of every 6 drivers with illegal blood alcohol concentrations in crashes have no prior conviction for DUI (Ross, 1992).

The effect of laws governing drinking and driving in deterring people in general from driving under the influence of alcohol, not just those caught doing so, is difficult to measure. Self-reports of drinking and driving (as well as of seat belt use and other behaviors) is not correlated with objective measures of the phenomenon, e.g., blood alcohol of fatally injured drivers (Robertson, 1992). Quasi-experimental studies of injury incidence occasionally find some small effects of increments in anti-alcohol legislation on crash rates (Zador, Lund, Fields, & Weinberg, 1988).

Programs aimed at reducing drunk driving without reducing drinking (e.g., designated drivers, provision of rides by volunteers or taxi subsidies) ignore the fact that alcohol is involved more in assaults than in motor vehicle crashes and is a factor in other forms of injury. Apparently, no one has studied the net effects on alcohol-related injuries of such policies. If people drink as much or more when there is a designated driver and proceed to become involved in violence or to take a fall on the stairs at home, the overall injury rates and accompanying costs may not be reduced.

Policies that attempt to reduce alcohol consumption generally, such as increasing the minimum legal drinking age, have had an effect on injury reduction generally in the targeted age groups (Jones, Pieper, & Robertson, 1992). Consumption of alcohol and its consequences (cirrhosis as well as injury) are substantially reduced as the price of alcohol increases. Increments in alcohol taxes have a substantial effect on consumption and alcohol-related problems (Cook, 1981; Cook & Tauchen, 1982; Saffer & Grossman,

1987). Since taxes are often not adjusted for inflation, however, the effect erodes in time. Despite increases in the federal excise taxes on alcohol in 1985 and 1990, the real tax, adjusted for inflation, was less after the 1990 increase than it was in the 1950s (Ross, 1992).

Because the energy inherent in motion increases in direct proportion to the square of the speed of motion, control of speed on roads is an important factor in injury control. Maximum speed limits were lowered to save fuel, not to reduce injuries, after the Arab oil boycott in 1973. Nevertheless, analyses of the effects of the speed limit separate from the changes in driving patterns indicate a reduction of about 5000 deaths a year attributable to the reduced speed limit (Kemper & Byington, 1977). When the limit was raised back to 65 mph on rural interstate highways, the death rate on these roads increased (Insurance Institute for Highway Safety, 1994).

Traditional criminology and popular culture emphasize risk of arrest and punishment as primary factors in the effect of law. Perhaps more important, however, are factors such as observability of the behavior and augumentation of police enforcement by others in the community (Robertson, 1983). A law regarding an observable behavior such as helmet or belt use may be obeyed more readily, not because it is more often enforced, but because the wearer knows that a police officer can easily detect a violation. Laws that can be enforced by the community, such as age of purchase of alcohol and curfews for teenagers, are probably enforced by the members of the community (proprietors of retail outlets and parents, respectively) more often than by the police.

CORPORATE BEHAVIOR

Most of the severe injury in industrialized societies is the result of modifications of materials and energy by corporations (e.g., motor vehicles, guns, stairs, cigarettes that ignite house fires). People do not necessarily behave in corporate settings as they would in other contexts. Corporate decisions are usually made in groups and approved by higher-ranking groups. In such situations, the group may make a decision that no one individual in the group would make or endorse. This phenomenon has been called *pluralistic ignorance*. Individual persons think that they have much to lose and nothing to gain by opposing or advocating a position that will affect the "bottom line," i.e., profits. At least that seems the only explanation for corporate behavior that knowingly leads to unnecessary death and disability when the decision makers would not, as individuals, kill or maim anyone.

For example, in the late 1960s, Eaton, Yale and Towne—a major supplier of components to automobile assembly companies—developed a practical application of a device that was patented in the 1940s. The device detects crash forces in the front end of a vehicle and, if the forces are above a preset level, inflates a cushion in front of the driver or front seat passengers. This device, which came to be known as an "air bag," set in motion more than two decades of delay and deception by the motor vehicle manufacturers.

When the government attempted to impose regulations that would put air bags in every new car by the mid-1970s, the manufacturers opposed it on various grounds. One or another of the companies did promise, on several occasions, to install air bags on large numbers of vehicles to test their effectiveness, but most such promises were broken. Because of poor marketing efforts, only about 12,000 were sold in the 1970s (Karr, 1976).

One of the false arguments used in opposition to air bags was that if people would wear the seat belts already in the vehicles, air bags would not be necessary. Actually, there is only partial overlap in the injuries reduced by air bags and those reduced by seat belts. Air bags spread the force of a crash over a much larger area of the anatomy than seat belts, and thus there is less force at any given point. Seat belts reduce ejections, which are unaffected by air bags. Nevertheless, the governmental standard was revised to allow, as an alterative to air bags, so-called "automatic" seat belts that wrap around a driver or front seat passenger when the door is closed.

The whole standard was then rescinded by the Reagan administration and was reinstated only after protracted litigation ending in a court decision that the government's recission of the standard was illegal. If the original standard had been adopted, air bags would have been installed on the vast majority of cars on the road by the mid-1980s. Given the time necessary for older vehicles to be scrapped, that goal will not be reached until after the turn of the century.

The motor vehicle industry continues to mislead the public in its advertising on vehicle design and safety. On April 3, 1994, *The New York Times* (1994) published a supplement on cars that included a feature-like article, "Safety Smart," with "Advertisement" at the top of the article, but no advertiser or author identified. The article said that lap–shoulder belts would "reduce traffic fatalities by 50 percent if all drivers and passengers would wear them, compared to the 20 to 40 percent reduction possible with airbags. Since many foolish Americans still refuse to buckle up, the automobile industry is spending billions of dollars to engineer ever more clever passive safety devices to protect us from ourselves." The article went on to describe an air bag that would increase protection in side crashes. It ended with an old falsehood once used to support the claim that "safety doesn't sell": "In 1957, Ford offered seat belts, but no one would buy them."

In fact, the belt use in air-bag-equipped vehicles is similar to that in vehicles without air bags. If taken seriously, the article's implication that the protection is redundant could lead to less belt use in air-bag-equipped vehicles.

As to side air bags in side crashes, contrary to the quoted passage, there would be virtually no overlap in the injuries reduced relative to seat belts. Such side air bags would protect heads and shoulders from impact with side glass or pillars, and to some degree from penetrating vehicles or other objects, neither of which is affected much by belts. The major function of belts in side crashes is to prevent ejection, which side air bags will not do.

Notice the resentment in the article at having to provide increased protection for "foolish Americans" at increased expense. In fact, when Ford offered seat belts in 1957, the demand from wise Americans was so large that the company could not produce enough to keep up with demand. Nevertheless, because the models in which belts were offered did not sell as well as the competing Chevrolet, the "safety doesn't sell" myth was born (Eastman, 1984). Most manufacturers did not provide lap seat belts even as an option until 14 states required them as standard equipment in 1964.

In addition to the malfeasance of a corporation that would perpetuate such misinformation, there is the newspaper's culpability. The corporate officers of *The New York Times* apparently take little responsibility for the content of its pages if the section is labeled as "advertisement."

Another tragic example of manufacturers placing profits ahead of the health of their customers is the design and aggressive marketing of "sport utility vehicles"—a cross between a truck and a station wagon. In the 1980s, despite knowledge of the vehicles' propensity to roll over easily at moderate speeds, many manufacturers developed such vehicles to compete with the Jeep CJ (CJ denotes "Civilian Jeep," but it is similar to the military vehicle).

In 1961, a General Motors engineer noted that rollover of automobiles was greatly reduced by lowering the center of gravity (Stonex, 1961). In 1980, a study of Jeep CJs and other "utility vehicles" indicated that rollover rates were several times those of cars and that the vehicles were too narrow relative to the height of their center of gravity (Snyder et al., 1980). Tests of Jeep CJs, operated by remote control, found that they could overturn in turns taken as slow as 22 miles per hour. These tests were shown on the popular television program "60 Minutes." Other studies showed the same problem with some pickup trucks (Reinfurt et al., 1981).

The manufacturers' response was to ignore the simple physics and develop more and more such vehicles—e.g., Ford BroncoII, Toyota 4Runner, Nissan Pathfinder, General Motors small Blazer and Jimmy, Suzuki Samurai, Isuzu Trooper—as well as narrower pickup trucks. Study after study has indicated that these vehicles have 3–20 times the rollover rate per vehicle in use compared to the average of passenger cars. The correlation of rollover rates to static stability of the vehicles (the ratio of the distance between center of the tires to the height of the center of gravity) is extraordinary. From 55% to 90% of the variation among rollover rates of the noted vehicles is explained by static stability, and controls for other risk factors do not reduce the correlation (Harwin & Brewer, 1990; Mengert et al., 1989; Robertson, 1989).

By 1992, almost 1 of every 10 motor vehicle fatalities—some 3800 people per year—died in rollovers of utility vehicles and small pickup trucks. At least 1000 per year and probably more would have lived had the manufacturers made the vehicles 1–9 inches wider or lowered the center of gravity by half that amount. The only difference between the motor vehicle manufacturers who market these unstable vehicles and serial killers is that the corporations do not choose their victims.

The typical response of manufacturers when their vehicles are found defective is to blame the drivers. For example, General Motors Corporation (GM) chose to place fuel tanks in its C/K-series pickup trucks outside the frame of the vehicle next to the sheet metal "skin" to increase fuel capacity relative to competitive trucks in its 1973–1987 models. Other manufacturers placed the tank within the frame. The issue of risk of fire in GM pickups received widespread public attention in 1992 when a family whose son died in a GM truck fire sued GM and demanded a trial rather than accept a private settlement from the company (Applebone, 1993).

The Center for Auto Safety petitioned the NHTSA to recall the vehicles, partly on the basis of data indicating higher fatal fire rates in GM compared to similar-sized Ford pickups during 1981–1986. GM hired a consulting firm that claimed the GM trucks posed no unreasonable risk because some small cars and trucks had a higher fire risk, although its data clearly indicated a higher fatal fire rate in GM compared to similar-sized pickups (Lange, Ray, & McCarthy, 1992). Imputed overall fire rates, based on crash rates from a few states, were said to be no different among GM and other vehicles. GM retracted the claim that its pickups had a lower overall fatality rate than Ford's pickups—admitting that the total occupant fatality rate in GM C/K pickups was actually higher than that of Fords of similar size (Meier, 1992). More recently, GM has attempted to turn that argument on its head. In a submission to the NHTSA, GM argued that its trucks have higher fatal fire rates because they are driven by "more aggressive" drivers (General Motors, 1993).

In 1988, GM introduced a redesigned pickup truck with the gasoline tank inside the frame. The fatal fire rates in C/K pickup trucks made by General Motors and the F-series pickups made by Ford Motor Company were examined by this author to assess the reduction in such rates associated with placement of fuel tanks within the frame. GM and Ford trucks were chosen for comparison because they had sufficient sales for statistical reliability, were of similar size and weight, and were major competitors in the market for pickup trucks of the size examined.

Data on all 1981–1991 model year GM C/K and Ford F-series pickups involved in fatal crashes were extracted from the 1981–1992 Fatal Accident Reporting System (FARS) computer tapes. Only vehicles that had identification numbers indicative of this group were included. The data on each vehicle included whether or not a fire occurred, whether the fire was considered the most harmful event (the event that did the most harm to the occupants), number of occupant deaths, principal point of impact on the vehicle, vehicle identification number, and model year.

The number of vehicles in use during each of the calendar years 1981–1992 was estimated from sales data and a scrappage rate from previous studies (*Ward's Automotive Yearbook*, 1982–1992). The original sales of a given model year were multiplied by the proportion remaining in use at a given vehicle age in a given calendar year after the first year of use (Oak Ridge National Laboratory, 1984). The use in the first fractional year of sale was calculated by summing months remaining in the year from month of sale for a given set of vehicle sales and dividing the total by 12. The sum of each of these calculations for each manufacturer's trucks sold before and after October 1, 1987, indicates years of use by model and fuel tank location.

Fatal fire and nonfire crash involvement rates and occupant fatality rates per million vehicle-years of use were calculated and compared by manufacturer and location of fuel tanks. If the placement of fuel tanks outside the frame increased the risk of a fire-related fatality, the GM trucks should have had higher fatal fire rates in the pre-1988 models compared to Ford trucks of the same vintage. Also, after GM placed the tank inside the frame in 1988 and subsequent models, the fatal fire rate of GM and Ford trucks should have been comparable in 1988 and subsequent model years.

Fuel tanks could be on either side of a GM vehicle (dual tanks were optional). If a fuel tank outside the frame posed a greater risk, there should have been a markedly higher rate of fire-related deaths, particularly when the impact was to the side of the pickups (at clock positions 2–4 and 8–10). If GM trucks are driven more aggressively, the GM trucks should have been involved in total fatal crashes at a higher rate than Ford trucks. The latter comparison included, in addition to fatalities of truck occupants, death of one or more occupants in vehicles in collisions with the pickup trucks when no occupant in the truck died, as well as deaths of pedestrians and bicyclists struck by the trucks. To the extent that "aggressive driving" is a factor in fatal crash rates, it should have contributed proportionately to the total death rate in all such crashes, not just to those in which an occupant of the driver's vehicle died.

The fatal fire and nonfire rates of GM and Ford trucks during 1981–1992 are presented in Table 1. The 1981–1987 GM trucks, which have "side-saddle" tanks, had higher fire rates than 1981–1987 Ford trucks with the tanks inside the frame. The occupant death rate in crashes in

Table 1. Fatal Crash Rates per Million Vehicle-Years of 1981–1991 GM and Ford Pickup Trucks in Calendar Years 1981–1992[a]

	Model years							
	1981–1987				1988–1991			
	GM		Ford		GM		Ford	
Crashes	*N*	Rate	*N*	Rate	*N*	Rate	*N*	Rate
Fire most harm[b]								
Vehicles	140	5.1	85	3.4	23	3.2	26	4.2
Occupant deaths	165	6.0	104	4.2	29	4.1	32	5.2
All fires[b]								
Vehicles	391	14.3	265	10.6	66	9.3	66	10.8
Occupant deaths	401	14.6	245	9.8	71	10.0	76	12.4
Nonfire								
Vehicles	9231	336.8	8376	336.0	2843	400.4	2241	365.8
Occupant deaths	4709	171.8	3595	144.2	1473	207.5	892	145.6

[a]The estimated vehicle-years of use (see the text) are: 1981–1987 models: GM, 27.41 million; Ford, 24.93 million; 1988–1991 models: GM, 7.10 million; Ford, 6.13 million.
[b]Crashes classified as "Fire most harm" are also included in "All fires."

which fire was considered the most harmful event was 1.43 times higher for GM trucks than Ford trucks, and the occupant death rate in all crashes in which fires occurred was 1.49 higher for GM trucks than for Ford trucks.

Although the nonfire occupant death rate for GM trucks was higher than that for Ford trucks, the total nonfire fatal crash involvement rate was virtually the same in the 1981–1987 GM and Ford trucks. In the 1988–1991 model years, when both manufacturers placed the fuel tanks inside the frame, the fatal fire rates for GM trucks were somewhat less than those for Ford trucks, even though the nonfire fatal crash rate and the occupant death rate for GM trucks were each higher than the corresponding rate for Ford trucks.

Fatal fire rates in side crashes (principal impact at clock positions 2–4 and 8–10) are presented in Table 2. For the 1981–1987 model GM trucks, the total fatal fire rates in side impacts were more than 3 times higher than the rates for Ford trucks of the same model years. In the 1988–1991 models, in which the gasoline tanks are inside the frame, there was essentially no difference between the fire rates in side impacts for the trucks of the two manufacturers.

The data clearly indicate that 1981–1987 GM trucks posed higher risks of fire-related deaths than Ford trucks. The largest difference was found in side impacts in the area of the gasoline tanks. Since sheet metal can be crushed into the side of the vehicle and puncture side tanks when the primary impact is frontal or rearward, the risk is not exclusively in side crashes. This writer has examined photographs of the underside of a burned GM truck involved in a frontal collision in which the side tank was clearly punctured by deformation that would not have reached a tank located inside the frame.

GM's argument that more aggressive driving explains the difference in fire death rates between GM and Ford trucks is not supported by the data. GM and Ford trucks had virtually the same nonfire fatal crash involvement rates in the pre-1988 models (see Table 1). The changes in nonfire fatal crash involvement rates before and after the change in placement of tanks in GM trucks are not consistent with the changes in fire death rates. The fire death rate in GM trucks declined as the overall occupant death rate and the total fatal crash involvement rate increased. GM considered only occupant death rates in pre-1988 trucks in its argument that its customers are more aggressive.

GM also constructed an "Aggressive Driver Demographic Factors Index" by adding the percentages of 21 factors available in the FARS, some

Table 2. Fatal Fire Rates in Side Impacts per Million Vehicle-Years of 1981–1991 GM and Ford Pickup Trucks in Calendar Years 1981–1992

Crashes	1981–1987 GM N	1981–1987 GM Rate	1981–1987 Ford N	1981–1987 Ford Rate	1988–1991 GM N	1988–1991 GM Rate	1988–1991 Ford N	1988–1991 Ford Rate
Fire most harm								
Vehicles	36	1.3	11	0.4	2	0.3	2	0.3
Occupant deaths	41	1.5	11	0.4	3	0.4	2	0.3
All fires								
Vehicles	72	2.6	30	1.1	7	1.0	6	1.0
Occupant deaths	84	3.1	31	1.1	9	1.3	8	1.3

of which were driver characteristics and some of which were other factors, e.g., number of vehicles in the crash, ran off the road, and posted speed 55 mph or greater (General Motors, 1993). Several of the factors are known to be correlated (age 29 years or younger, police indicate "driving too fast," one or more speeding convictions, vehicle speed 55 mph or greater). Posted speed is obviously not indicative of aggressive driving, and the speed-related factors are obviously not additive. The summation of several indicators of the same phenomenon is methodologically indefensible. Also, data on actual vehicle speeds in the crashes are missing on more than half the cases.

The philosophy of appropriate and inappropriate risk comparisons raised in the GM truck fire case is also of interest to risk analysts more generally. GM's consultants from Failure Analysis Associates seem to believe that if one can find a worse risk to compare to whatever risk is at issue, then the risk at issue is reasonable. By that philosophy, only the highest risk would be unreasonable and subject to correction. The false claim that the total occupant fatality risk in GM trucks was the same as or less than in similar-sized Ford trucks, even if true, would not justify the introduction of an unnecessary higher risk of fire by placement of the fuel tanks outside the frame. The primary objective of risk analysis should be to find means of reducing specific risks, not to justify a risk by the presence or absence of another (Robertson, 1992).

GOVERNMENT BEHAVIOR

Several federal regulatory agencies have been authorized to set standards for injurious products. In addition, at the federal level, injury control research and some state and local programs are funded by several agencies. Motor vehicle safety standards are promulgated by the NHTSA in the U.S. Department of Transportation (DOT), which also supports some research and state programs. Also within DOT, the Coast Guard has the authority to issue standards for boats and their operation, the Federal Aviation Administration can do so for aircraft and their operation, and the Federal Railway Administration can do so for trains.

Standards for injury reduction in most workplaces are promulgated by the Occupational Safety and Health Administration in the Department of Labor, which maintains an inspectorate in states that do not have workplace inspection programs that meet federal criteria. Mine safety standards and inspections are under the jurisdiction of a separate agency, the Mine Safety and Health Administration. The vast majority of consumer products, excepting (by statute) motor vehicles, cigarettes, and guns, can be regulated by the Consumer Product Safety Commission, a small agency with commissioners appointed by the President and approved by the Congress.

A few types of machine guns, assault weapons, cheap handguns, and ammunition are banned for sale to the public by the federal government, and the Bureau of Alcohol, Tobacco and Firearms has jurisdiction for licensure of gun dealers and enforcement of prevailing laws. Most guns are unregulated regarding important characteristics such as usability by children, lethality of muzzle speed and ammunition (e.g., size, shape), and defects in design and manufacture.

The priorities of the federal agencies are determined largely by the Congress and the executive branch, sometimes through specific statutes to pursue an issue, but more often by budget allocations (or denial) to specific agencies and the ideology of political appointees. Occasionally, the White House intervenes in agency actions, such as the noted rescinding of the air bag standard or in the implementation of a federal rule or law. Ideology, testimony in hearings by agency personnel and others, lobbying by interest groups, and the personal interest of legislators and executives—not necessarily in that order—determine the budgets and direction (or lack thereof) of agency actions.

In some instances, the logic invoked by government officials to avoid action is bizarre. In

1987, the NHTSA refused to adopt a minimum stability standard to reduce rollover in utility vehicles and pickup trucks (National Highway Traffic Safety Administration, 1987). This refusal was not surprising in an administration that adopted deregulation as a major theme. After the change in administrations, and accumulation of much more data by government and private researchers, the agency again refused to set such a standard (National Highway Traffic Safety Administration, 1994). The arguments against a standard, bipartisan yet deceptive, are apparent attempts to protect the motor vehicle industry from its folly in producing unstable vehicles.

Consider a few of the statements made by the agency in the aforecited document to justify the more recent decision: "The agency believes that no single type of rulemaking or other agency action could solve all, or even a majority of, the problems associated with rollover." With few exceptions, that is true of every Federal Motor Vehicle Safety Standard issued in the past and is no excuse for not issuing a standard. Air bags, for example, do not reduce occupant fatalities by 100%, but by about 30%, but that is no reason not to provide them. The evidence on rollover of low-stability vehicles indicates that a minimum standard for stability would substantially reduce the total rollover and rollover fatality rates of those vehicles.

The government emphasized belt use and alcohol and implied that these factors are disproportionately involved in most of the rollover problems. The document itself, however, contradicts that implication when it later notes that the majority of variation in rollovers among vehicles is explained by stability of the vehicle as measured by tilt-table angle (the angle at which a vehicle's upper wheels lose contact when a test table on which it is sitting is tilted).

In its "Estimates of the Benefits of a Standard," "the agency assumed that the severity of the accidents would be reduced but that the accidents would not be prevented.... This assumption is somewhat pessimistic because an unknown number of crashes would most likely

be avoided." Actually, the most common rollover scenario for unstable vehicles involves a driver who perceives that one or both right tires are off the pavement, or about to leave the pavement, and turns the steering wheel sharply to stay on or get back on the pavement. This creates a roll motion that would not occur if the vehicle had a lower center of gravity, a wider track, or both. In a study of utility vehicle rollovers, 9 of 10 vehicles had fatal rollover rates per vehicle in use that were 3–20 times those of passenger cars, but 8 of the 10 had fatal *nonrollover rates* similar to or less than those of passenger cars (Robertson, 1989). The drivers of these vehicles are no more likely to crash than anyone else except that their vehicles roll unnecessarily under circumstances easily foreseeable by the vehicle's manufacturers.

The NHTSA said: "Net reductions of 3 to 61 serious injuries and 4 to 63 fatalities would be expected for a minimum tilt table angle standard in the range of 42.8 to 46.4 degrees. Net reductions of 3 to 68 serious injuries and 2 to 68 fatalities would be expected for a minimum critical sliding velocity in the range studied, i.e., 14.68 to 16.73 kph.... A minimum tilt table angle of 45 degrees, which is higher than the tilt table angle of 69 percent of present compact sport utility vehicles, would save 23 lives.... An increase in track width, derived from frame or suspension alterations, or a decrease in center of gravity height are the only methods of improving stability without potential safety liabilities. Such changes would require large initial costs related to the design and development of major vehicle components, if not the entire vehicle.... Based on these estimates of the benefits and costs of a minimum stability standard, NHTSA believes that the benefits would not be sufficient to justify the expected costs."

This exceedingly bizarre cost-benefit statement is grotesquely deceptive. The upper limit of the analysis is set at 46.4° when the high rollover rates are found in vehicles with tilt angles up to 47.7°. The numbers of deaths and injuries that would be prevented are so obviously wrong based on the numbers that occur in low-stability vehicles (about 3800 per year in the early 1990s), combined with the correlation of death and injury rates to stability, that it is difficult to see how anyone with any sense of arithmetic would not say, "That can't be right." Even if the numbers were correct, it is outrageously misleading to state the reductions in injury and death on the basis of one year's use of a cohort of vehicles, not on the lifetime of the vehicle cohort, and at the same time to state the costs in terms of initial design-change costs, when designs of this class of vehicles remain essentially the same for many model years, spreading the design costs over large numbers of vehicles and many years, resulting in minimum unit costs. The Jeep Wrangler's rollover rate is little more than half that of the vehicle it replaced, the CJ-7 (the nonrollover crash rates of the two are virtually identical), yet its base price in 1989, $9430 according to Ward's Automotive Yearbook, was among the lowest of the vehicles in the "light duty truck" market segment. Making the Jeep more stable certainly did not put it into a different vehicle class or render it unaffordable, and making it even more stable would not do so.

The NHSTA mentioned that the estimates of death and injury reductions were based on a "hypothetical" population of vehicles, but did not mention that the hypothetical population (1882) was less than half the 3800 fatalities in rollovers that occurred in light trucks, utility vehicles, and vans in 1991. Also, the assumption that vehicles in 1991 were representative of vehicles that will be sold in the future was unfounded. Without a minimum stability standard, there is nothing to prevent one or more manufacturers from producing vehicles as bad as or worse than, say, the CJ5, or BroncoII.

The situation in state governments seems no better. In 1993, I gave a talk at a seminar presented by the federal government for state legislators and health department officials. About 20 states were represented at the meeting. I asked for a show of hands by participants from states that have an office in the legislature or administrative branch that systematically assesses the health needs of the state and reviews the alternative means of reducing the priority problems in terms of effectiveness and costs. Not one hand was raised. There is a lack of focus at the state or federal level on the relative importance of specific injuries in loss of life, morbidity, and costs, and a lack of rational allocation of resources toward injury control strategies of known effectiveness.

The need for a more data-driven effort and coordination among the various agencies was recognized in the report *Injury in America* (Committee on Trauma Research, 1986), and the Centers for Disease Control and Prevention (CDC) was subsequently designated as the lead agency for coordination. In addition, the CDC supports research and "capacity building" for injury surveillance and control programs among state and local health departments. While some significant research has been done under CDC sponsorship, the agency has no power to allocate funds among the regulatory agencies. The states are developing better data systems, but the injury control programs that most have adopted are of dubious or untested effectiveness.

A review of the intentions of state and local health departments supported by the CDC's "capacity-building" grants is not encouraging (CDC, 1991). While the data systems may be improved by many of the proposed efforts, the announced injury control projects are mainly oriented to the very difficult aim of changing behaviors, to the neglect of the principles noted in the discussion of behavior change in this chapter. Even the New York City Health Department, which years earlier accomplished the noted reduction in children's falls by requiring window barriers, still emphasizes unproven approaches (educational campaigns, conflict resolution) to solving other problems and promotes the demonstrably harmful driver education in public schools. It seems that many health departments have no acquaintance with the research literature, and some have no institutional memory. The CDC may be supporting "capacity building" for failure.

CONCLUSION

This chapter has illustrated the extent to which public policy to reduce injuries is often misguided and unfocused. Behavioral factors can be changed to reduce injury, given certain conditions, but it is possible to control injuries substantially by changing environment and products irrespective of behavior. Too often, the correlation of injury to behavioral factors is used an excuse for doing nothing.

On the basis of research evidence, several principles for policy formation regarding injuries can be stated. Calculation of years of expected life lost and inpatient hospital days from particular subsets of injuries and diseases may help policy makers avoid concentration of resources on more frequent but relatively trivial subsets. If an environmental modification is available to reduce a particular subset, that modification is likely to be more effective than an attempt to modify behavior. Numerous behavioral and environmental approaches and their effects have been identified (Rice & MacKenzie, 1989), and the new ones are being studied and reported in the research literature. Where behavior change is the only recourse, motivating a single action that will have a sustained effect (e.g., purchase of a safer vehicle, smoke detector) will likely be more effective than attempting to modify more frequently required behaviors. Behavioral approaches shown to be effective by good research must be implementable and sustained in the population at risk. The policy maker who feels unqualified to judge what constitutes "good" research may wish to contact the Centers for Disease Control and Prevention for a list of injury prevention research centers that have experts on the research literature.

On a positive note, there are numerous injury control researchers who are not afraid to engage in the policy debate. At the risk of losing academic standing among colleagues who look down on "advocacy" and the loss of research grants from government agencies, they continue to produce data on the importance of the problem and the means of reducing it. They are putting the "public" back into public health.

REFERENCES

American Public Health Association. (1994). Behavior kills more in U.S. than anything. *Nation's Health*, January.

Applebone, P. (1993). GM is held liable over fuel tanks in pickup trucks. *The New York Times*, April 5, p. 1.

Bergman, A. B. (Ed.). (1992). *Political approaches to injury control at the state level.* Seattle: University of Washington Press.

Bergner, L. (1982). Environmental factors in injury control: Preventing falls from heights. In A. B. Bergman (Ed.), *Preventing childhood injuries* (pp. 57–60). Columbus, OH: Ross Laboratories.

Blomberg, R. D., Preusser, D. F., & Hale, A. (1983). *Experimental field test of proposed pedestrian safety messages: Vol. 2. Child messages.* Washington, DC: U.S. Department of Transportation.

Centers for Disease Control. (1991). Summaries: State and community-based injury control projects, applied methods for injury surveillance projects, incentive grants for injury control intervention projects. Atlanta, GA: U.S. Department of Health and Human Services.

Committee on Trauma Research. (1986). *Injury in America.* Washington, DC: National Academy Press.

Cook, P.H. (1981). The effect of liquor taxes on drinking, cirrhosis, and auto accidents. In M. Moore & D. Gerstein, (Eds.), *Alcohol and public policy: Beyond the shadow of prohibition* (pp. 255–285). Washington, DC: National Academy Press.

Cook, P. H., & Tauchen, G. (1982). The effect of liquor taxes on heavy drinking. *Bell Journal of Economics, 13,* 379–390.

Dershewitz, R. A. & Williamson, J. W. (1977). Prevention of childhood household injuries: A controlled clinical trial. *American Journal of Public Health, 67,* 1148–1153.

DiGiuseppi, C. G., Rivara, F. P., Koepsell, T. D., & Polissar, L. (1990). Bicycle helmet use by children: Evaluation of a community-wide helmet campaign. *Journal of the American Medical Association, 262,* 2256–2261.

Eastman, J. W. (1984). *Styling vs. safety.* New York: University Press of America.

Geller, E. S. (1988). A behavioral approach to transportation safety. *Bulletin of the New York Academy of Medicine, 64,* 632–661.

General Motors Corporation. (1993). Evaluation of GM 1973–87 C/K pickup trucks. Part III. Analysis of FARS fire rates in side collisions for fullsize pickups and supplemental statistical presentations. Submission to the National Highway Traffic Safety Administration, August 10.

Harwin, E. A., & Brewer, H. K. (1990). Analysis of the relationship between vehicle rollover stability and rollover risk using the NHTSA CARDfile Accident Database. *Journal of Traffic Medicine, 18*, 109-122.

Insurance Institute for Highway Safety. (1994, Sept. 10). Seven straight years: Deaths higher after 65 MPH speed limits than before. *Status Report, 29*, 2.

Jones, N. E., Pieper, C. F., & Robertson, L. S. (1992). The effect of legal drinking age on fatal injuries of adolescents and young adults. *American Journal of Public Health, 82*, 112-115.

Kahane, C. J. (1994). *Correlation of NCAP performance with fatality risk in actual head-on collisions*. Washington, DC: National Highway Traffic Safety Administration.

Karr, A. R. (1976, Nov. 11). Saga of the air bag, or the slow deflation of a car-safety idea. *Wall Street Journal*, p. 1.

Kelling, G. L., et al. (1974). *The Kansas City preventive patrol experiment*. Washington, DC: The Police Foundation.

Kemper, W. J., & Byington, S. R. (1977). Safety aspects of the 55 MPH speed limit. *Public Roads, 41*, 58-67.

Kravitz, H. (1973). Prevention of falls in infancy by counseling mothers. *Illinois Medical Journal, 144*, 570-573.

Lange, R. C., Ray, R. M., & McCarthy, R. M. (1992). Analysis of light-duty motor vehicle collision-fire rates. Menlo Park, CA: Failure Analysis Associates.

Lund, A. K., Williams, A. F., & Zador, P. F. (1986). High school driver education: Further analysis of the DeKalb County study. *Accident Analysis and Prevention, 18*, 349.

Meier, B. (1992, Dec. 2). GM retreats on claims about fatal truck fires. *The New York Times*, p. A20.

Mengert, P., Salvatore, S., DiSario, R., & Walter, R. (1989). *Statistical estimation of rollover risk*. Washington, DC: National Highway Traffic Safety Administration.

Miller, R. E., Reisinger, K. S., Blatter, M. M., & Wucher, F. (1982). Pediatric counseling and subsequent use of smoke detectors. *American Journal of Public Health, 72*, 392-393.

National Highway Traffic Safety Administration. (1987). Federal Motor Vehicle Safety Standards; denial of petition for rulemaking: vehicle rollover resistance. *Federal Register, 52*, 49,033-49,038.

National Highway Traffic Safety Administration. (1994). Consumer information regulations; Federal Motor Vehicle Safety Standards; rollover prevention. *Federal Register, 59*, 33,254-33,272.

Oak Ridge National Laboratory. (1984). Scrappage and survival rates of passenger cars and trucks in 1970-82. *Ward's Automotive Yearbook*. Detroit, MI: Ward's Communications.

Reinfurt, D. W., Li, L. K., Popkin, C. L., O'Neill, B., Burchman, P. F., & Wells, J. A. K. (1981). *A comparison of the crash experience of utility vehicles, pickup trucks and pas-* senger cars. Chapel Hill: Highway Safety Research Center, University of North Carolina.

Reisinger, K. S. & Williams, A. F. (1978). Evaluation of programs designed to increase protection of infants in cars. *Pediatrics, 62*, 280-287.

Reisinger, K. S., Williams, A. F., Wells, J. A. K., John, C. E., Roberts, T. R., & Podgainy, H. J. (1981). The effect of pediatricians counseling on infant restraint use. *Pediatrics, 67*, 201-206.

Rice, D. P., & MacKenzie, E. J. (Eds.) (1989). *Cost of injury in the U.S.: A report to Congress, 1989*. San Francisco: Institute for Health and Aging, University of California.

Robertson, L. S. (1975). Behavioral research and strategies in public health: A demur. *Social Science and Medicine, 9*, 165.

Robertson, L. S. (1980). Crash involvement of teenaged drivers when driver education is eliminated from high school. *American Journal of Public Health, 70*, 599-603.

Robertson, L. S. (1983). *Injuries: Causes, control strategies and public policy*. Lexington, MA: D. C. Heath.

Robertson, L. S. (1984). Automobile safety regulations: Rebuttal and new data. *American Journal of Public Health, 74*, 1390-1394.

Robertson, L. S. (1989). Risk of rollover in utility vehicles relative to static stability. *American Journal of Public Health, 79*, 300-303.

Robertson, L. S. (1992). *Injury epidemiology*. New York: Oxford University Press.

Robertson, L. S. (1994). Highway deaths: False PR on the effects of PR. *Journal of Public Health Policy, 86*, 437-442.

Robertson, L. S., Kelley, A. B., O'Neill, B., Wixom, C. W., Eiswirth, R. S., & Haddon, W., Jr. (1974). A controlled study of the effect of television messages on safety belt use. *American Journal of Public Health, 64*, 1071-1080.

Robertson, L. S., & Zador, P. (1978). Driver education and crash involvement of teenaged drivers. *American Journal of Public Health, 68*, 959-965.

Ross, H. L. (1992). *Confronting drunk driving: Social policy for saving lives*. New Haven, CT: Yale University Press.

Safety smart. (1994, April 3). *The New York Times*, "Auto Show" supplement, p. 36.

Saffer, H., & Grossman, M. (1987). Beer taxes, the legal drinking age, and motor vehicle fatalities. *Journal of Legal Studies, 16*, 351-374.

Shaoul, J. (1975). *The use of accidents and traffic offenses as criteria for evaluating courses in driver education*. Salford, England: University of Salford.

Slovic, P., Fischhoff, B., & Lichtenstein, S. (1987). Behavioral decision theory perspectives on protective behavior. In N. D. Weinstein (Ed.), *Taking care: Understanding and encouraging self-protective behavior* (pp. 14-41). New York: Cambridge University Press.

Snyder, R. G., McDole, T. L., Ladd, W. M., & Minahan, D. J.

(1980). *On-road crash experience of utility vehicles*. Ann Arbor: Highway Safety Research Institute, University of Michigan.

Stonex, K. A. (1961). Road design for safety. *Traffic Safety Research Review, 5*, 18–30.

Ward's Automotive Yearbook. (1982–1992). U.S. new truck sales by line by month. Detroit, MI: Ward's Communications.

Wood, T. & Milne, P. (1988). Head injuries to pedal cyclists and the promotion of helmet use in Victoria, Australia. *Accident Analysis and Prevention, 20*, 177.

Zador, P. L., Lund, A. K., Fields, M., & Weinberg, K. (1988). Fatal crash involvement and laws against alcohol-impaired driving. Washington. DC: Insurance Institute for Highway Safety.

13

Health Policy and Smoking and Tobacco Use

K. Michael Cummings

OVERVIEW

In the 1990s, public and governmental attitudes toward tobacco use are dramatically different in comparison to the attitudes of the 1950s and before. Smoking then was widely perceived as a mark of sophistication and a natural accompaniment of work and play. In the 1990s, smoking is seen as an unhealthful behavior that is increasingly unacceptable in social settings (U.S. Department of Health and Human Services [DHHS], 1989). The evidence that smoking poses a serious health risk is relatively recent in origin. Although studies demonstrating health risks associated with smoking date back to the 1920s, tobacco use was not widely accepted as dangerous until publication of the 1964 Surgeon General's Report on Smoking and Health (DHHS, 1989). That report stated in unequivocal terms that "cigarette smoking is a health hazard of sufficient importance in the United States to warrant appropriate remedial action" (U.S. Public Health Service, 1964).

With the widespread publicity of the findings in the 1964 report, tobacco use was added, virtually overnight, to the political agenda (DHHS, 1989; Rabin & Sugarman, 1993; Simonich, 1991). Since the mid-1960s, public attitudes about smoking have changed dramatically, and political activity addressing the conduct of smokers and the tobacco industry has increased correspondingly. This chapter reviews the rationale and success of different public and private policies to reduce tobacco use since 1964.

The Tobacco Problem

Cigarette smoking has been identified as the single most important source of preventable morbidity and mortality in the United States (DHHS, 1989). During the decade of the 1990s, an estimated 4.5 million Americans will die from smoking-caused diseases (Peto, Lopez, Boreham, Thun, & Heath, 1992). The worldwide death toll from tobacco is about 3 million each year (Connolly, 1992). In the United States, cigarette smoking is the main cause of 87% of deaths from lung cancer, 30% of all cancer deaths, 82% of deaths

K. Michael Cummings • Department of Cancer Control and Epidemiology, Roswell Park Cancer Institute, Buffalo, New York 14263.

Handbook of Health Behavior Research IV: Relevance for Professionals and Issues for the Future, edited by David S. Gochman. Plenum Press, New York, 1997.

from pulmonary disease, and 21% of deaths from chronic heart disease (DHHS, 1989). In 1993, the medical care costs associated with the treatment of smoking-related illnesses were estimated to be $50 billion (Centers for Disease Control and Prevention [CDC], 1994a). Although less commonly used, other forms of tobacco such as chewing tobacco, snuff, cigars, and pipe tobacco also are important causes of morbidity and mortality in this country (National Cancer Institute [NCI], 1992).

Exposure of nonsmokers to environmental tobacco smoke (ETS) has increasingly become recognized as a health problem. The 1986 Surgeon General's Report on Smoking and Health brought to public attention the findings that "sidestream" smoke is at least as rich in carcinogens as inhaled tobacco smoke (DHHS, 1986). Since 1980, scientific studies have linked ETS exposure to higher rates of lung cancer and other cancers and heart disease and to a wide range of respiratory illnesses (DHHS, 1989). In 1992, the U.S. Environmental Protection Agency (EPA) confirmed the link between ETS and cancer by classifying secondhand smoke as a Group A carcinogen (EPA, 1992). This category includes only the most potent cancer-causing agents, such as benzene, vinyl chloride, asbestos, and arsenic. The EPA study estimated that ETS exposure is responsible for approximately 3000 lung cancer deaths, 37,000 cardiovascular disease–related deaths, and between 150,000 and 300,000 lower respiratory ailments in young children each year (EPA, 1992).

Who Smokes?

At the mid-1990s, the cigarette-smoking population of the United States consisted of roughly equal numbers of males and females, totaling roughly 25% of the adult population (CDC, 1994b). The appearance of parity between the sexes, however, masks important differences in the smoking habits of men and women over the past century. Prior to World War II, social taboos against smoking by women limited cigarette use primarily to men (Warner, 1986). In the

immediate post–World War II period, smoking rates among women increased dramatically, as smoking became socially acceptable for women. In 1955, 24% of women and 53% of men were smoking (Giovino et al., 1994). One decade later, the smoking rate had risen to 34% among women but had remained essentially unchanged among men (52%) (Giovino et al., 1994).

Since the mid-1960s, the overall prevalence of smoking has declined at a rate of about 0.62% per year. The decline in smoking, however, has not been equal among the sexes. Among women, the prevalence of smoking has declined at a rate of about 0.41% per year, from 34% in 1965 to 23% in 1993 (Giovino et al., 1994). For men, the rate of decline has been faster than for women. Smoking prevalence among men declined at a rate of 0.86% per year, from 52% in 1965 to 28% in 1993 (Giovino et al., 1994).

Data on smoking habits also reveal marked differences in use patterns by age, race, and education (DHHS, 1989; Giovino et al., 1994). For example, while cigarette smoking has declined steadily among adults, the prevalence of smoking among teenagers has remained stubbornly constant between 1984 and 1994, and may even be increasing (DHHS, 1994; Giovino et al., 1994). Also, the use of smokeless tobacco by adolescent males increased dramatically during the 1980s (Giovino et al., 1994).

During the first part of the 20th century, cigarette smoking was associated with wealth and social standing. In the United States at the century's end, tobacco use is increasingly seen as behavior of the lower classes (DHHS, 1989). For example, recent analyses of smoking prevalence found that educational status is the demographic variable most predictive of cigarette smoking status (Giovino et al., 1994; Pierce, Fiore, Novotny, Hatziandrev, & Davis, 1989). A predictable result of this shift in the demographic pattern of smoking is that the gap in the health status between the affluent and poor segments of society is likely to widen in the next few decades.

Currently, 46 million American adults and an additional 3 million teenagers smoke (CDC,

1994b). Changes in cigarette consumption in the United States seem to mirror shifts in public attitudes about smoking, with increasing consumption between 1900 and 1950 related to newly developed techniques for advertising and marketing cigarettes and the impact of World Wars I and II; declining cigarette consumption since the 1960s is associated with increased public awareness of the dangers of tobacco use and governmental actions to regulate the use, sale, and advertising of tobacco products (Warner, 1986).

WHY DO PEOPLE SMOKE?

According to Simonich (1991), theories concerning why people smoke can be divided into two broad categories: cognitive and noncognitive. Cognitive theories are based on the assumption that a person's behavior is influenced by what the person knows and believes. Noncognitive theories assume that a person's decision to smoke is outside the person's direct control.

Cognitive Theories of Smoking Behavior

Cognitive theories operate on the assumption that people weigh the likely costs and benefits of their actions to attain valued outcomes and choose to act in ways that maximize benefits and reduce costs (Wright, 1984). In cognitive theory, what is important is not what may be true, but rather what the person believes to be true. The importance of subjective thought in explaining smoking behavior is reflected in an ironic anecdote reported by Blum (1989): A pregnant smoker stated in all seriousness that she used the cigarette warning labels to help her avoid harming her unborn child. She reported that she never smoked the cigarettes that had the "fetal injury" warning label, only the ones with the "carbon monoxide" warning label. According to a cognitive model of smoking behavior, the key to behavior change is the ability to alter a person's subjective thought processes. For exam-

ple, if a person could be convinced that cigarettes have many more bad effects than good effects, that person would be less likely to smoke.

Cognitive theories of smoking behavior predict that smoking will be discouraged by interventions that increase people's awareness of the negative attributes of smoking (e.g., the dangers of smoking, higher cigarette prices, restrictions on when and where smoking is allowed) or promote the positive attributes of not smoking (e.g., better health, money saved) or do both. Support for a cognitive theory of smoking behavior can be found in ecological studies that show a strong association between public and private sector activities to reduce smoking, increase public awareness of the dangers of smoking, and change attitudes about tobacco, on one hand, and declining cigarette consumption during the past 25 years, on the other (Warner, 1989).

In the same way that antitobacco interventions might discourage smoking, messages that extol the benefits of smoking via direct advertising or other means (e.g., role modeling) could be expected to encourage smoking behavior (Institute of Medicine [IOM], 1994). The importance of the perceived benefits of smoking as a predictor of smoking was examined in a study of teen smokers in California (Pierce, Evans, et al., 1994). In surveys conducted in 1990 and 1992, adolescents were asked if they believed that smoking helps people when they are bored, helps them relax, helps people feel more comfortable at parties and in other social situations, and helps them keep their weight down. One quarter of adolescents expressed belief in one of these benefits of smoking; 30%, in two or three; and 12%, in four or five. In cross-sectional analyses, a measure of the risk of engaging in smoking behavior was directly related to the number of benefits associated with using tobacco. The impact of cigarette advertising on smoking behavior was further demonstrated in a study by Pierce, Lara, and Gilpin (1994), that showed a strong association between trends in smoking initiation by adolescent females and expenditures for cigarette advertising promoting the sale of brands targeting women.

Noncognitive Theories of Smoking Behavior

Noncognitive theories of smoking behavior see cigarette smokers as victims needing help. Smoking is not seen as a voluntary behavior, but is attributed to conditions not under the victim's direct control. A popular noncognitive theory of smoking is one that attributes smoking to nicotine addiction (Henningfeld, Cohen, & Pickworth, 1993). Those who see smoking as an addiction argue that smokers do not have the ability to exercise personal choice to quit smoking. In short, smokers have been duped. They are lured into smoking and are then stuck with a behavior they cannot easily control. Smoking is considered an irrational choice and one that nearly all smokers regret. The results of the NCI's Community Intervention Trial for Smoking Cessation (COMMIT) provide evidence to support the concept that for many smokers, smoking is not a volitional behavior but an addiction (COMMIT Research Group, 1995). COMMIT found that an intensive 4-year educational campaign directed at smokers was inadequate to substantially increase cessation rates in heavy smokers exposed to the campaign. The study concluded that more must be done to prevent people from beginning to smoke in the first place.

The 1988 Surgeon General's Report provides voluminous evidence to support the view that nicotine in tobacco can cause addiction (DHHS, 1988). Further support for the addiction claim is found in the following facts regarding tobacco use (CDC, 1994b):

- Seventy percent of adults who smoke say they wish they could quit smoking completely.
- Seventeen million try to quit each year, but fewer than one out of ten succeed. For every smoker who quits, nine try and fail.
- Heavy smokers (>25 cigarettes per day) are much less successful in stopping smoking compared to lighter smokers.
- Three out of four adult smokers say that they are addicted.

- Eight out of ten smokers say they wish they had never started smoking.

Nicotine is believed to be the prime addictive substance in tobacco. Nicotine is a central nervous system stimulant that produces effects in the brain that are reinforcing. The consumer becomes addicted as he or she seeks the sensations nicotine provides, gradually requiring an increasing dose to obtain the desired effects. Sudden stopping of nicotine use often produces withdrawal symptoms characterized by central nervous system effects such as irritability, difficulty concentrating, trouble sleeping, feelings of anxiety, and depression (DHHS, 1988; Henningfeld et al., 1993). These symptoms may persist for weeks unless nicotine ingestion is begun again.

Despite public denials from the tobacco industry that tobacco is not addictive, evidence from internal industry research reports, memoranda, and product patents suggests otherwise (Hilts, 1994a; Kessler, 1994a,b). For example, a 1973 Philip Morris internal research report described the cigarette in the following way (Dunn, 1972):

> The cigarette should be conceived not as a product, but as a package. The product is nicotine. The cigarette is but one of many package layers. There is the carton, which contains the pack, which contains the cigarette, which contains the smoke. The smoke is the final package. The smoker must strip off all these package layers to get to that which he seeks. Think of the cigarette pack as a storage container for a day's supply of nicotine. Think of the cigarette as a dispenser for a dose unit of nicotine. Think of a puff of smoke as the vehicle of nicotine. Smoke is beyond question the most optimized vehicle of nicotine and the cigarette the most optimized dispenser of smoke.

CHOICE VERSUS ADDICTION: IMPLICATIONS FOR POLICY

While the debate about whether smoking is a choice or an addiction is often presented in the popular media as an either/or proposition, most serious researchers in the field view smoking behavior as a blend of both cognitive and noncognitive elements (Orleans & Slade, 1993; Simonich, 1991). To date, however, public and private policies regarding tobacco have largely ignored the concept of smoking behavior as an addiction, and the data supporting this concept. Instead, the focus of public policy efforts to reduce tobacco use have relied mainly on an informed consumer orientation (DHHS, 1989; Rabin & Sugarman, 1993; Simonich, 1991). This focus has been maintained despite the substantial body of scientific evidence from health behavior research that has repeatedly demonstrated that educational campaigns typically have little impact on changing health-related behaviors (COMMIT Research Group, 1995; Wallack, 1981).

Informed Choice

An informed-choice perspective is based on the notion that individuals should decide for themselves whether or not to smoke. The government's role is to ensure truly informed individual decision making. The informed-choice perspective is consistent with the laws requiring warning labels on tobacco products and with efforts to regulate or counter tobacco advertising that interferes with the consumer's ability to make an informed choice about smoking.

Government efforts to prevent the sale of tobacco products to minors are also consistent with an informed-choice perspective, except that for children the assumption is that their immaturity prevents them from making the sort of informed choice adults can make. Hence, public policies targeting children tend to be more restrictive than those for adults and include laws prohibiting tobacco sales to minors, bans on smoking in public schools, and restrictions on advertising and promotions thought to be attractive to youth (i.e., federal ban on broadcast advertising of cigarettes, the Food and Drug Administration's regulations on the distribution and advertising of tobacco products, state and local laws regulating the free distribution of tobacco samples, and point-of-sale and billboard advertising).

Smoking as an Addiction

Those who adhere to the perspective of smoking as an addiction perceive the tobacco industry as the primary cause of the tobacco problem. The concept of smoking as an addiction offers a number of interesting, although little used, policy options, including (1) government regulation of tobacco products, (2) tort damage claims by smokers and states against the tobacco companies, and (3) the provision of free or low-cost smoking cessation programs funded by tobacco companies, taxes on tobacco products, or a requirement that such services be included in ordinary health insurance (Schauffler, 1993). Policies protecting smokers from discrimination in employment, or requiring that smokers be assured of a place to smoke during the workday, also fit within the perspective of smokers as victims (Sugarman, 1993).

Protection of Nonsmokers

A third perspective on regulating tobacco ignores the reasons that someone might smoke and instead focuses attention on the harm to others from smoking. The nonsmoker's rights model views smokers as polluters and nonsmokers as victims. In this perspective, the goal is not to help smokers, but rather to protect the health of nonsmokers. Since the mid-1980s, scientific evidence regarding the health risks of passive smoking has grown rapidly. This evidence has undercut social support for smoking and contributed to increased public demand for limits on indoor smoking. Since the 1970s, hundreds of laws have been enacted limiting smoking on airplanes, and in workplaces, shopping malls, government buildings, hospitals, restaurants, and elsewhere (NCI, 1993).

HISTORY OF TOBACCO CONTROL POLICIES

In the 40 years before publication of the 1964 Surgeon General's report on Smoking and

Health, the government did virtually nothing to discourage tobacco use (Rabin & Sugarman, 1993). To the contrary, before 1964, government policies promoted smoking by offering subsidies to tobacco growers and by giving out free cigarettes to soldiers during wartime. The government's involvement in tobacco control changed following the publication of the 1964 Surgeon General's Report. Within a year of the report, Congress enacted the Federal Cigarette Labeling and Advertising Act requiring health warnings on cigarette packages (DHHS, 1989). A few years later, Congress passed legislation banning the advertising of cigarettes on television and radio.

Since the mid-1960s, a wide array of public and private policy initiatives aimed at reducing use of tobacco have been enacted. Table 1 includes a summary of different types of policy actions adapted from the 1989 Surgeon General's Report (DHHS, 1989). This summary includes policies directed toward (1) informing and educating consumers, (2) increasing the cost of tobacco use through the use of economic incentives, and (3) limiting opportunities to use, manufacture, and/or sell tobacco products.

The next section of this chapter briefly describes and evaluates tobacco control policy measures in each of these three categories. For a more comprehensive review and evaluation of tobacco control policies, the reader is referred to other sources (DHHS, 1989; IOM, 1994; Rabin & Sugarman, 1993; Simonich, 1991).

Information and Education

As a general rule, society does not impose bans on dangerous and deleterious products. Instead, the goal of government regulation with regard to product safety is to ensure that consumers are informed about the inherent dangers of products. Government activities regarding tobacco have generally followed this approach, establishing policies to require the provision of information and education about the dangers of tobacco use so that individuals can make an informed choice whether to smoke or not (DHHS, 1989).

Government efforts to warn the public about the dangers of tobacco use have included (1) requiring information about the health risks of tobacco on advertising and packages of cigarettes and smokeless tobacco products; (2) mandating the broadcast of antismoking messages on the electronic media in the late 1960s under the Federal Communication Commission's Fairness Doctrine; (3) state-financed counter–tobacco advertising campaigns designed to reverse the appeal of pro-tobacco messages; and (4) requiring the government to issue reports summarizing information on the health risks of using tobacco and disclosing the levels of certain tobacco smoke constituents.

Warning Labels.   Since 1964, Congress has enacted a series of laws specifying that warning labels be placed on cigarette packages. The first

Table 1. Tobacco Control Policies[a]

Information dissemination	Economic incentives	Restraints on tobacco use and marketing
Warning labels	Tobacco taxes	Restrictions on smoking in certain places (e.g., public places, workplaces, schools)
Counteradvertising	Tobacco product litigation	Restrictions on tobacco sales to minors
Government reports	Life and health insurance premium differentials for smokers and nonsmokers	Restrictions on tobacco advertising and promotions
		Product regulation

[a]Adapted from DHHS (1989).

of these laws was enacted in 1965, updated in 1969, and revised again in 1984 (USDHHS, 1989). Also, in 1986, Congress enacted warning requirements for smokeless tobacco products (USDHHS, 1989).

Eleven days after the 1964 Surgeon General's Report on Smoking and Health was released, the Federal Trade Commission (FTC) proposed rules requiring cigarette manufacturers to disclose on all cigarette packages and advertising that "cigarette smoking is dangerous to health" and "may cause death from cancer and other diseases" (FTC, 1964). Before the FTC rule could take effect, Congress passed the Cigarette Labeling and Advertising Act of 1965 (DHHS, 1989). This law preempted the FTC warning label and in its place required that the following health warning be placed on all cigarette packages: "Caution: Cigarette smoking may be dangerous to your health." Unlike the proposed FTC regulation, Congress did not require the warnings on product advertisements. The 1965 act also preempted federal agencies and state and local governments from issuing their own health warnings and prohibited the FTC from requiring health warnings on cigarette advertising until July 1, 1969.

In 1969, the FTC again proposed regulations requiring manufacturers to print a stronger health warning on cigarette packages and on cigarette advertisements (FTC, 1969). In response to the regulations proposed by the FTC, Congress passed the Public Health Cigarette Smoking Act of 1969, which amended the 1965 labeling act to require a slightly strengthened health warning: "Warning: The Surgeon General Has Determined That Cigarette Smoking Is Dangerous to Your Health" (DHHS, 1989). Again, the Congressionally mandated warning was milder than that recommended by the FTC and omitted reference to death and to other specific diseases. The 1969 act also prohibited the FTC from requiring health warnings on cigarette advertisements until July 1, 1971. The 1969 act also preempted state and local governments from regulating cigarette advertising on the basis of smoking and health concerns. In March 1972, FTC rules went into effect requir-

ing manufacturers to display on all cigarette advertising the same health warning mandated on cigarette packages.

In 1981, the FTC (1981a) issued a report on the effectiveness of federally mandated cigarette warning labels. The report concluded that the warning label was "worn out" and had little impact on the public's level of knowledge about smoking (FTC, 1981a). This report helped create Congressional support for new, stronger health warnings on cigarette packages and advertisements. In 1984, Congress enacted the Comprehensive Smoking Education Act, which required four rotating health warnings on all cigarette packages and advertisements (DHHS, 1989):

- SURGEON GENERAL'S WARNING: Smoking Causes Lung Cancer, Heart Disease, Emphysema, and May Complicate Pregnancy.
- SURGEON GENERAL'S WARNING: Quitting Smoking Now Greatly Reduces Serious Risks to Your Health.
- SURGEON GENERAL'S WARNING: Smoking by Pregnant Women May Result in Fetal Injury, Premature Birth, and Low Birth Weight.
- SURGEON GENERAL'S WARNING: Cigarette Smoke Contains Carbon Monoxide.

Despite an FTC recommendation that the size of the health warning label be increased and that the shape be changed to a circle-and-arrow format to make it more noticeable, Congress retained the size and rectangular format of the previous health warnings.

In 1986, Congress passed the Comprehensive Smokeless Tobacco Health Education Act, which for the first time mandated warning labels on smokeless tobacco products and advertisements (DHHS, 1989). Under the act, three rotating warning labels are required to be printed on smokeless tobacco packaging and advertisements in the circle-and-arrow format originally recommended for cigarettes by the FTC. The three required health warnings are:

- WARNING: This product may cause mouth cancer.

- WARNING: This product may cause gum disease and tooth loss.
- WARNING: This product is not a safe alternative to cigarettes.

The 1986 law also preempted federal agencies and state and local governments from imposing additional health warnings on smokeless tobacco packages and advertisements.

Even though government-mandated health warning labels are an important area of government intervention against tobacco use, few studies have actually evaluated the impact of warning labels on knowledge, beliefs, attitudes, or tobacco use behaviors (DHHS, 1989; Simonich, 1991). The body of research that does exist suggests that warning labels on cigarettes and smokeless tobacco products and advertisements are ineffective in reducing consumption (Simonich, 1991). Several studies suggest that current health warnings on tobacco products and advertisements are too small and inconspicuous in relationship to the imagery in tobacco advertising to be noticed (Bhalla & Lastovicka, 1984; FTC, 1981a; Fischer, Krugman, Fletcher, Fox, & Ras, 1993; Fischer, Richards, Berman, & Krugman, 1989). In one study using a sophisticated eye-tracking device, 44% of adolescents asked to view cigarette advertisements did not even look at the warning label displayed on the ad (Fischer et al., 1989). Research also suggests that the warnings on tobacco products are too lengthy to be read. A study of roadside billboards found that under typical driving conditions, observers could read the entire warning message on only 5% of cigarette advertisements (Davis & Kendrick, 1989). Observers were able, however, to identify the brand name and advertising message on the billboards. The 1981 FTC study on cigarette warning labels concluded that the 1966 and 1970 warnings were ineffective because they had become worn out and stale, were too abstract, and lacked personal relevance (FTC, 1981a). The FTC study recommended using rotating warnings that were short, concrete, and personalized. They

also suggested that the format for the warnings be changed in shape and increased in size.

To increase the noticeability of health warnings, Canada and Australia mandated that warnings on cigarette packages be increased in size (Hill, 1993; Kaiserman, 1993). In Canada, the law requires that all sides of tobacco packaging display one of eight rotating warnings that occupy from 30% to 40% of the main display area of the package. Information regarding the toxic constituents present in cigarette smoke must also be displayed. The Canadian law also stipulated that tobacco billboards erected after January 1, 1991, carry a health warning equal to 20% of the size of the billboard. Interestingly, tobacco billboards began disappearing in Canada shortly after this law took effect.

In 1992, Australia strengthened its regulations for tobacco warning labels and packaging by requiring a series of 12 rotating health warnings to appear on the top front of cigarette packages (Hill, 1993). In addition to the warning message, information on the tar, nicotine, and carbon monoxide yields must appear on the side of the pack, along with a detailed message about the hazards of smoking and a quitline telephone number displayed on the back of the package.

While the stronger and more prominently displayed health warnings on tobacco products and advertisements in Canada and Australia would appear to have a greater chance of discouraging consumption than the health warnings mandated on tobacco products sold in the United States, studies have not yet confirmed this prediction (Slade et al., 1992).

In a comprehensive analysis of different government anti-smoking policies in the United States, Simonich (1991) argued that the apparent ineffectiveness of mandated warning labels is the result of the future-oriented health messages that are not relevant to the majority of consumers. Simonich (1991) suggested that most people are influenced by information that is relevant to their present concerns. For example, warning labels deal only with health risks, a future concern. On the other hand, cigarette advertising promotes smoking satisfaction and social acceptance, present-oriented concerns. Since most people are present-oriented, they are susceptible to messages relevant to the present and discount messages about the future (i.e., health risks). Simonich recommended that warning labels be changed to include messages that are more present-oriented, such as "A pack a day costs you over $700 per year" or "Your smoking hurts those closest to you."

Simonich (1991) also suggested that warning labels on cigarettes may be ineffective in reducing consumption because smokers do not have close substitutes to use in place of cigarettes. He noted that a number of studies have found that labeling of food products substantially alters consumption so long as close substitutes exist (i.e., shifting from high-fat to lower-fat foods). Since cigarette warning labels provide exactly the same information for every brand, they cannot stimulate brand switching. As a group, however, cigarettes now have a close substitute that can be used to provide the nicotine that most smokers crave. In the United States, nicotine gum and nicotine skin patches, once available only by prescription, have been made available over the counter and for some smokers may serve as substitutes for cigarettes or as an aid to smoking cessation. Cigarette companies are also developing nicotine delivery devices that look and taste like regular cigarettes, but do not burn tobacco, thus potentially eliminating many of the harmful chemicals found in tobacco smoke (Hilts, 1994c) These alternative nicotine delivery devices are being designed to appeal to the health concerns of smokers and may represent substitutes for cigarettes. Nicotine itself, however, is not entirely harmless (DHHS, 1988). At high exposure levels, nicotine is a potentially lethal poison. At lower exposure levels, long-term nicotine use may contribute to cardiovascular disease and peptic ulcer disease. It is not clear whether these alternative nicotine delivery devices should be required to carry the same health warning found on regular cigarettes.

The Fairness Doctrine. The first and to date the only large-scale national counteradvertising campaign to educate the public about the health risks of tobacco use occurred between 1967 and 1970, when the Federal Communications Commission (FCC) required licensees who broadcast cigarette commercials to provide free media time for antismoking public service announcements (PSAs) under the Fairness Doctrine (DHHS, 1989). The Fairness Doctrine, which was repealed by the FCC in 1988, obligated licensed broadcasters to "encourage and implement the broadcast of all sides of controversial public issues over their facilities, over and beyond their obligation to make available on demand opportunities for the expression of opposing views" (FCC, 1987).

In January 1967, John Banzhaf, an attorney, petitioned the FCC to apply the Fairness Doctrine to cigarette advertising (DHHS, 1989). In June 1967, the FCC accepted Banzhaf's petition and ruled that licensed broadcasters were required to air roughly one antismoking message for every three cigarette commercials. In July 1967, antismoking PSAs developed by voluntary health agencies and the government began to air. Unlike most public service advertising campaigns, many of the antismoking ads aired during prime time. The time donated for the antismoking messages amounted to approximately $276 million per year (in 1993 dollars). The Fairness Doctrine campaign ended in January 1971, as a result of a federal law that banned cigarette advertising on television and radio. After 1970, the number of antismoking PSAs declined markedly as antismoking messages were forced to compete for donated air time.

Between 1967 and 1970, cigarette consumption in the United States dropped at a much faster rate than during the period immediately before or after the time when the Fairness Doctrine antismoking campaign was operational (DHHS, 1989). While it is impossible to rule out the effects of other influences that may have contributed to the decline in cigarette consumption between

1967 and 1970, several studies have concluded that the antismoking messages mandated by the Fairness Doctrine were responsible for much of the reduction in smoking during that period (Hamilton, 1972; O'Keefe, 1971; Simonich, 1991, Warner, 1989). Support for this conclusion is found in the study published by O'Keefe (1971), which found high levels of recall for the antismoking PSAs aired as part of the campaign among both adults and youth. Analysis of trends in national survey data also suggests that the Fairness Doctrine PSAs contributed to increases in public knowledge of the health hazards of smoking (DHHS, 1989).

State-Financed Counter-Tobacco Advertising Campaigns. The experience with the Fairness Doctrine antismoking messages between 1967 and 1970 prompted some public health advocates to call on the-government to implement paid antitobacco advertising campaigns to counteract the impact of cigarette advertising. The main problem with a counteradvertising approach is funding it. Several states, including California, Massachusetts, and Minnesota, have implemented paid antitobacco counteradvertising campaigns financed from cigarette excise tax collections. The impact of these counteradvertising campaigns on changing public knowledge, attitudes, and behavior related to tobacco is still unclear. A recent analysis of the Proposition 99–funded California antitobacco program found, however, that among the many diverse elements of the program, the paid media campaign was one of the most important in contributing to an overall decline in cigarette consumption between 1988 and 1992 (Pierce, Evans, et al., 1994).

Government Reports. Since 1964, government agencies have issued hundreds of reports summarizing the scientific evidence about the health risks of tobacco use (DHHS, 1989). Many of these reports are required under legislative mandate. Because these reports frequently receive extensive media coverage and are widely disseminated, they have helped educate the public about the health risks of tobacco.

The Federal Cigarette Labeling Act of 1965 and the Public Health Cigarette Smoking Act of 1969 require that the Secretary of Health and Human Services produce an annual report for Congress updating information on the health consequences of smoking. These reports are referred to as Surgeon General's Reports. Including the 1964 Surgeon General's Report (which was *not* mandated by Congress), there have been 23 Surgeon General's Reports on smoking.

The impact of these reports on smoking behavior is difficult to assess, although several studies suggest that the first Surgeon General's Report in 1964 contributed to a drop in cigarette consumption (Hamilton, 1992; Simonich, 1991; Warner, 1989). Reports have helped influence policy development on such issues as passive smoking (DHHS, 1986), nicotine addiction (DHHS, 1988), and youth tobacco use (DHHS, 1994).

Federal law also requires the FTC to produce an annual report for Congress on cigarettes sales and advertising (DHHS, 1989). These reports generally include data on per capita cigarette sales, market share for filtered and unfiltered cigarettes, market share for cigarettes of varying tar and nicotine yields, and cigarette advertising and promotional expenditures. Over the years, the FTC has proposed rules that would require cigarette manufacturers to list yields of tar, nicotine, and other hazardous components on their packages and in their advertising.

In 1967, the FTC opened its own laboratory to analyze the tar and nicotine content of cigarette smoke. In 1981, the FTC published a list showing the tar, nicotine, and carbon monoxide yields of domestic cigarette brands based on its own laboratory tests (FTC, 1981b). The FTC has also acknowledged, however, that its testing procedures are flawed and probably underestimate the amount of tar, nicotine, and carbon monoxide that smokers receive from smoking (Hilts, 1994b).

In 1987, the FTC closed its laboratory and

has since relied on nicotine, tar, and carbon monoxide ratings provided by the cigarette industry under a voluntary reporting agreement (USDHHS, 1989). Today, cigarette companies are not required to disclose information about the tar and nicotine content of cigarettes. Tar and nicotine levels are frequently seen, however, on packaging and in advertising. Such disclosure is done voluntarily and usually appears on cigarette brands with 8 mg or less of tar, but rarely on brands with higher tar content. Some researchers have speculated that the FTC effort to inform people about tar and nicotine yields of cigarettes may have inadvertently increased cigarette demand by suggesting that some cigarette brands are less dangerous (Warner & Slade, 1992).

The Comprehensive Smoking Education Act of 1984 and the Comprehensive Smokeless Tobacco Health Education Act of 1986 require manufacturers of tobacco products to annually provide to the Secretary of Health and Human Services a list of additives used in manufacturing (DHHS, 1989). The government is required, however, to treat the lists as "trade secrets." Under these laws, Congress can be informed about research activities on health risks of these additives and may call attention to ingredients that pose a health risk to smokers. Otherwise, the lists of additives must be treated confidentially and not divulged to the public. These laws also did *not* give the government authority to regulate the use of additives in tobacco products, even if a health hazard is identified.

Many government reports are issued without a specific legislative mandate. For example, in 1992, the EPA issued an important scientific report on the health risks of environmental tobacco smoke (EPA, 1992). This report received extensive media coverage and helped reinforce public concern about the dangers of ETS and served as a springboard for both public and private regulatory initiatives to protect nonsmokers from tobacco smoke.

The publication and dissemination of scientific information on the health consequences of tobacco use represents the least coercive of government interventions to combat tobacco (Samet, Lewit, & Warner, 1994). The impact of this effort on tobacco use behavior is impossible to measure precisely. Information dissemination is essential, however, to the formulation of all other policy initiatives. Without appropriate information, it is difficult to form the popular consensus necessary to create and enforce more restrictive policies.

Economic Incentives

It is well recognized in economic theory, as well as in everyday life, that purchasing decisions are influenced by the affordability of a product (Watson, 1972). The affordability of a good is influenced both by the price of the good and by the consumer's income. The price of tobacco products is determined by the manufacturer's price, wholesale and retail markups, and tobacco taxes.

Numerous studies, using a variety of methodologies, have shown that overall cigarette consumption is responsive to price changes (DHHS, 1989; IOM, 1994; Lewit, 1989). Estimates of the price effect vary, but generally speaking a 10% increase in the retail price reduces consumption by about 4% (Lewit, 1989). Consumption is reduced both because some people choose not to smoke (either by not starting to smoke or by quitting smoking) and because some smokers choose to smoke fewer cigarettes. Approximately two thirds of the decreased consumption is the result of people choosing not to smoke at all (Lewit, 1989). Conversely, a decline in the retail price of tobacco leads to increased consumption.

Tobacco Taxes. One of the most straightforward ways to influence the price of tobacco products is through taxation. Studies indicate that taxes on tobacco products, usually in the form of an excise tax, are passed directly on to the consumer. In the United States, tobacco is taxed by federal, state, and local governments (Lewit, 1989).

Historically, governments have levied tobacco taxes to generate revenues. Increasingly, however, taxation of tobacco products is being recognized as an effective strategy to discourage tobacco use (IOM, 1994). For example, it has been estimated that if Congress were to raise the federal cigarette tax on cigarettes by $2 per pack and maintain this tax in real terms, cigarette consumption would decrease by 23% (i.e., by approximately 7 million fewer smokers) (Coalition on Smoking or Health, 1993). The politics of tobacco, however, has hindered the use of tax policy as a means to discourage tobacco use in the United States (Kagan & Vogel, 1993).

While the actual total tax amount on cigarettes increased nearly 5-fold from 1955 to 1993 (from 11¢ per pack to 53¢ per pack), the real value of the tax was less in the mid-1990s than it was during the mid-1950s due to inflation (IOM, 1994). Interestingly, the inflation-adjusted price of cigarettes was about 45% higher in the mid-1990s, than in 1955 as a result of tobacco manufacturers' price increases, not taxes. Increases in the standard of living (i.e., more money to spend on goods) helped make cigarettes more affordable in the 1990s than they were 30 years earlier (IOM, 1994).

Thus, while increasing tobacco taxes is one of the most direct and effective means of discouraging tobacco use, the federal government and most state governments have made little use of taxation policy as a way of controlling tobacco consumption. The IOM (1994) report on preventing nicotine addiction in children recommended that "tobacco tax policies at the federal and state levels should be linked directly to the national objectives for reducing tobacco use." In other words, the IOM report recommended that government policy makers should use tobacco taxes as an intervention to reduce tobacco consumption, not merely to raise government revenues. The IOM (1994) report further recommended that Congress increase the federal excise tax on cigarettes to $2 a pack by 1995 and tax all tobacco

products on an equivalent basis so that increases in the price of one type of tobacco product (e.g., cigarettes) will not result in increased consumption of other types of tobacco products (e.g., smokeless tobacco); the report also recommended that tax policy take into account the affordability of tobacco products to prevent tobacco from becoming more affordable in the future.

Indirect Economic Incentives. While tobacco taxes represent a fairly direct means of influencing consumption, other types of policies can influence the price of tobacco products indirectly. For example, the federal policy of tobacco price supports and the allotment system, which were designed to aid tobacco farmers, have helped keep the price of domestically produced tobacco artificially elevated (Northup, 1993). Also, product liability suits against tobacco manufacturers have the potential of significantly increasing the price of tobacco products (Daynard, 1988). In 1994, attorneys general in over a dozen states have initiated product liability actions against cigarette manufacturers to recover costs associated with public-financed insurance for treatment of tobacco-caused illnesses (Tobacco Product Liability Project, 1995). For each of these states, the estimated annual expenditure for treatment of tobacco-caused illnesses is in the hundreds of millions of dollars. Although product liability suits are not policies per se, legislation pertaining to them could influence the impact of legal actions against tobacco manufacturers. For example, in California, legislation specifically exempts tobacco manufacturers from product liability actions.

Life and Health Insurance. In 1964, whether or not a person smoked was not a consideration in the premiums paid for insurance. Today, premium differentials based on whether a person smokes or does not smoke are nearly universal for life insurance and increasingly common for health insurance. Smoker/nonsmoker premium differentials were first introduced by the life insurance industry in the mid-1960s when actuarial studies demonstrated the higher mortality of smokers compared to nonsmokers (DHHS, 1989; Schauffler, 1993). Because life insurance is usually sold on an individual basis, it is possible to adjust prices according to the applicant's mortality risk status. Health insurance, on the other hand, is typically purchased on a group basis, usually as an employment benefit. As a result, health insurance policies are seldom tailored to individual health risks. As a result, smoker/nonsmoker premium differentials are much less commonly offered by health insurers, although, as noted, this situation is changing (DHHS, 1989; Parkinson et al., 1992).

For example, the Contra Costa County California health plan and the King County Washington Medical Blue Shield plan began offering group policy discounts based on the smoking status of their enrollees (Parkinson et al., 1992). In Contra Costa County, if a company bans smoking in the workplace, and is shown to have a 90% prevalence of nonsmoking employees, a 15% group insurance premium discount is given. In the King County plan, employees who smoke can take advantage of a $500 lifetime benefit for any smoking cessation intervention offered in the community, with a 25% copayment required. Currently, publicly funded health insurance such as Medicaid includes coverage for nicotine replacement therapy in about 20 states, although eligibility requirements vary widely among states. In the past, Congress has considered legislation that would mandate that publicly funded insurance include smoking cessation treatments (DHHS, 1989).

There are no studies that have evaluated the impact of smoking-related insurance premium differentials and their effect on smoking behavior (Parkinson et al., 1992). Premium differentials would not be expected to influence smoking initiation, since most individuals make decisions about smoking during adolescence. Among adult smokers, however, premium differentials may have both an economic and an educational effect in discouraging smoking (DHHS, 1989). In addition to increasing the cost of smoking, higher premiums charged to smokers help to reinforce knowledge of the harm caused by smoking. Health insurers who cover the cost of smoking cessation programs and aids reduce the cost of quitting for the smoker and provide an economic incentive to cessation providers to offer more services.

Restrictions on Tobacco

Public policies intended to inform consumers about the health hazards of tobacco or to make tobacco products more costly discourage tobacco use indirectly. A third category of policies affect tobacco use more directly by limiting locations in which tobacco can be used and by restricting the sale and advertising of tobacco products.

Restrictions on Where Tobacco Is Used.   In 1964, the health risks of smoking were a concern for smokers only. There were no laws regulating smoking in public locations. Scientific studies documenting the health risk of passive smoking published during the 1980s made smoking a health issue for nonsmokers. Organizations that monitor smoking laws and policies have documented increasing numbers of laws and policies restricting the locations in which people can smoke (NCI, 1993). In 1993, nearly all states and over 500 local communities had laws restricting smoking in public places and workplaces (NCI, 1993). Thousands of businesses, including a majority of large corporations and several fast food restaurant chains, have instituted "smoke free" policies. Federal laws prohibit smoking on buses, trains, and domestic airline flights (DHHS, 1989). In 1994, Congress outlawed smoking in most of the nation's public schools and in federally funded programs that serve children, including Head Start centers, day care centers, and community health centers. The United States military prohibits smoking in common work areas. Smoking has even been restricted in many outdoor sports arenas. As Brandt (1990) pointed out, "... cigarette smoking has become the most rigorously defined of all public behaviors." Kagan and Skolnick (1993) also suggested that laws restricting smoking in public locations have also influenced attitudes about smoking in settings in which there are as yet no such formal rules. For example, a 1992–1993 national survey found that 67% of households had rules that prohibited smoking indoors (Census Bureau, 1992).

Policies restricting where people can smoke have made smoking less socially acceptable and have almost certainly contributed to reductions in smoking behavior, although the precise impact on smoking behavior is difficult to quantify. Pierce, Lara, and Gilpin (1994) found that smoking prevalence declined between 1990 and 1992 at a faster pace in companies in California that were 100% smoke free compared to those that merely segregated smokers and nonsmokers. Separately conducted econometric studies by Simonich (1991), Wassermann, Manning, Newhouse, and Winkler (1991), and Emont, Lhoi, and Novotny (1993) each found that the restrictiveness of state-level smoking rules was an important predictor of reduced aggregate cigarette consumption, even after controlling for other types of government policies (e.g., higher taxes). Thus, while rules limiting the locations in which people can smoke are intended to protect the health of nonsmokers, these rules have helped redefine smoking behavior in American society, making it less acceptable, more inconvenient, and less pleasurable, thereby encouraging cessation and discouraging uptake of smoking.

Restrictions on Tobacco Sales. With approximately 46 million adult cigarette smokers, a total prohibition on tobacco sales is not practical (Coalition on Smoking or Health, 1995). In the United States, however, there is a tradition of limiting minors' access to tobacco products. The argument for limiting tobacco sales to minors is based on the idea that children and adolescents may not be mature enough to appreciate adequately the long-term consequences of their use of tobacco. Abundant evidence illustrates that many youths who begin to use tobacco do not fully comprehend the nature of addiction and

therefore believe that they will be able to avoid the harmful consequences of smoking by stopping smoking after a few years (DHHS, 1994; IOM, 1994). Like their adult counterparts, however, many adolescent smokers would like to quit smoking, but feel that they cannot do so easily. The 1989 national survey of teenagers 12–18 years of age found that over 60% of adolescent smokers had thought seriously about stopping smoking and that nearly half had tried unsuccessfully to quit (Allen, Moss, Giovino, Shopland, & Pierce, 1993).

Laws intended to curtail tobacco sales to minors date back to the turn of the 20th century (DHHS, 1994; IOM, 1994). In 1964, all but two states had laws that prohibited selling or giving tobacco to children. After 1964, several states repealed their tobacco access laws because they were not being enforced. In recent years, however, governments at all levels have begun to address the problem of youth access to tobacco. Today, all states have enacted laws that prohibit the sale of tobacco products to persons under the age of 18 years (IOM, 1994). In 1992, Congress amended the Public Health Service Act to include section 1926, known as the Synar Amendment, which linked ongoing program funding to control of youth access to tobacco (DHHS, 1994). In addition, several states and hundreds of localities have taken meaningful steps to enforce youth access laws. For example, California, New York, Florida, and Vermont have implemented a retailer licensing system that enables health departments or other law enforcement officials to identify and monitor retailer compliance with youth access laws (IOM, 1994). As of July 1993, 170 communities had adopted ordinances eliminating or severely restricting cigarette vending machines (NCI, 1993). Many communities have banned self-service displays of tobacco on the grounds that they promote experimentation, impulse buying, and shoplifting by teenagers (NCI, 1993; IOM, 1994). Finally, several states and communities have enacted ordinances banning or restricting the distribution of free tobacco product samples (NCI, 1993).

The effects of youth access laws on deterring tobacco use by minors are still unclear. Studies indicate that compliance with laws prohibiting tobacco sales to minors remains low (Office of the Inspector General, 1992). Thus, in most localities, minors are able to obtain tobacco products with relative ease. Evidence from several studies indicates that when tobacco age-restriction laws are actively enforced, tobacco sales to minors can be sharply reduced (IOM, 1994). Two studies found that active enforcement of local age-restriction laws on tobacco sales was associated with a decline in teenage smoking (DiFranza, Carlson, & Caissc, 1992; Jason, Ji, Ames, & Birhead, 1991). Neither study included a no-enforcement comparison condition, but as stated in the IOM (1994) report on nicotine addition and youth: "In the long run, the real public health benefit of a reinvigorated youth access policy lies not in its effect on consumer choices, but rather in its declarative effects—that is, in its capacity to symbolize and reinforce the emerging social norm that disapproves of tobacco use." The report goes on to state that "… failure to implement the youth access restrictions actually undermines the tobacco-free norm; an unenforced restriction is probably worse than no restriction at all" (IOM, 1994). As the public's attitudes toward a tobacco-free norm have evolved, so has support for stronger measures to limit youth access to tobacco products, even though doing so means further inconveniencing adult tobacco users.

Restrictions on Tobacco Advertising and Promotions. In the United States, the FTC has the authority under the Federal Trade Commission Act to regulate the advertising of consumer products to prevent "unfair or deceptive acts or practices in commerce" (FTC, 1964). Over the years, the FTC has used its regulatory authority to challenge the advertising practices of cigarette manufacturers. For example, in 1950, the FTC prohibited the R.J. Reynolds company from claiming in its advertising that Camel cigarettes aided digestion, did not impair the wind or physi-

cal condition of athletes, would never harm or irritate the throat or leave an aftertaste, were soothing, restful, and comforting to the nerves, and contained less nicotine than any of the four highest-selling brands (Wagner, 1971). In 1983, the FTC blocked the advertising of Brown and Williamson's Barclay cigarettes for incorrectly stating the tar yield. In 1986, the FTC successfully challenged an R.J. Reynold's advertisement that misrepresented the results of a study on heart disease and smoking (USDHHS, 1989).

In 1964, the FTC proposed rules for regulating the imagery and copy of cigarette ads to prohibit unsubstantiated health claims (FTC, 1964). The FTC rules were never adopted, however, due to passage of the 1965 Federal Cigarette Labeling and Advertising Act. Public pressure to regulate tobacco advertising was widespread and strong in the mid-1960s, especially because of concerns regarding youth smoking. In 1963, the average teenager viewed 100 cigarette commercials a month (Pollay, 1994a). In response to mounting pressure to limit cigarette advertising, the tobacco industry in 1964 adopted a voluntary code of conduct (Pollay, 1994b). The tobacco industry's self-regulatory code, which is still in use today, covered four areas: (1) advertising appealing to the young, (2) advertising containing health representations, (3) the provision of free tobacco samples, and (4) the distribution of promotional items to the young (Pollay, 1994b). For example, a specific stipulation of the voluntary code is that models used in ads should not appear to be younger than 25 years of age. Over the years, public health groups have argued that the voluntary code is inadequate and largely ignored by the tobacco industry (Blum & Myers, 1993; IOM, 1994).

In 1969, the FTC recommended in a report to Congress that a ban on cigarette advertising on television and radio be enacted (FTC, 1969). In 1969, Congress passed the Public Health Cigarette Smoking Act, which prohibited cigarette advertising in the broadcast media effective beginning in 1971 (DHHS, 1989). Congress extended the ban on broadcast advertising to small cigars in 1973 and to smokeless tobacco products in 1986 (DHHS, 1989). The federal law banning cigarette advertising on television and radio also included a clause preempting states and localities from regulating or prohibiting cigarette advertising or promotions for health reasons. The purpose of the preemption was to avoid chaos created by different, potentially conflicting regulations. The effect of the federal preemption, however, has been that few states and localities have attempted to regulate advertising of tobacco products (DHHS, 1989). A number of cities and states have acted to restrict transit advertising, the free distribution of tobacco product samples, and point-of-sale advertising. Whether these actions are lawful remains unclear. In Massachusetts, a local law prohibiting point-of-sale advertising was recently challenged on the basis that it violates the federal preemption on cigarette advertising. The IOM (1994) report recommended that Congress repeal the federal law preempting state regulation of tobacco promotion and advertising that occurs entirely with the states' borders.

There has been little formal evaluation of the impact of government actions concerning tobacco advertising and promotion. The impact of the broadcast advertising ban on consumption is difficult to determine, since the ban also eliminated the airing of the Fairness Doctrine PSAs that were associated with a drop in cigarette consumption (Simonich, 1991). Also, the savings from reduced advertising may have allowed the cigarette companies to hold down the price of cigarettes temporarily, which in turn may have affected sales. Cigarette advertising expenditures actually increased following the 1971 broadcast ad ban and were redirected into print ads, billboards, and promotions.

A number of studies have attempted to estimate the impact of the federal broadcast advertising ban on consumption. Hamilton (1972), Schneider, Klein, and Murphy (1981), and Warner (1989) all concluded that the net effect of the ad ban was to increase cigarette consumption in the short term.

Cigarettes remain among the most heavily advertised consumer products on the market. In 1991, the tobacco industry spent $4.6 billion on advertising and promotion of cigarettes and over $100 million on advertising and promotion of smokeless tobacco products (IOM, 1994). Between 1975 and 1991, cigarette advertising and promotional expenditures in the United States more than quadrupled. Published studies offer substantial evidence to support the argument that advertising and promotion influence tobacco consumption, although the precise mechanisms by which they operate are not fully understood. Advertising may influence tobacco use in a number of ways. For example, advertising could encourage current smokers to smoke more, reduce the resolve of current smokers to stop or to consider stopping, encourage ex-smokers to take up smoking again, and seduce nonsmokers, especially children, to use tobacco (Warner, 1986). Critics of the cigarette industry have argued that a share of cigarette advertising is intended to encourage young people to smoke (Blum & Myers, 1993). For example, surveys conducted between 1976 and 1990 among high school students suggested an association between the use of Camel cigarettes and the 1988 introduction of the cartoon character "Joe Camel" advertising campaign (DiFranza et al., 1991; Pierce et al., 1991).

A study that examined trends in smoking behavior by adolescents and young adults between 1984 and 1989 found that initiation of smoking by teenagers increased at about the same time that spending on cigarette advertising and promotions increased. Smoking initiation rates among young adults did not follow the same pattern as observed among teenagers (CDC, 1995) (see Figure 1).

Concerns about the effects of advertising on adolescent tobacco use have prompted a number of public health groups to call for stronger regulations on tobacco advertising. For example the IOM (1994) report called for legislation to either ban tobacco advertising and promotion altogether or restrict such messages to a "tombstone" format.

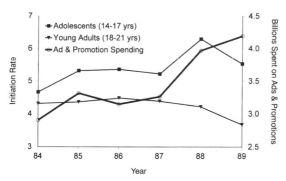

Figure 1. Trends in smoking initiation rates for adolescents (age 14–17 years) and young adults (age 18–21 years) and total advertising and promotional expenditures for cigarettes by year in the United States, 1984–1989. Smoking initiation rates were computed as follows: Using the age of respondents at the time of the interview and the age they reported starting smoking, the age of respondents and their smoking status was calculated for each year between 1984 and 1989. The denominator of the initiation rate for a given year was the number of respondents at risk for starting smoking during the year (i.e., persons already smoking were eliminated from the denominator that year). The numerator was the number of respondents who reported initiating smoking during that year.

Product Regulation. In the United States, nearly all consumer products are subject to a variety of federal regulatory statutes designed to ensure that the products are safe and that consumers are informed about possible risks. Tobacco products, however, are an exception (IOM, 1994; Kessler, 1994a). With the exception of warning labels, Congress has explicitly excluded tobacco products from regulatory control for both political and practical reasons. The only federal agency with any jurisdiction over tobacco products is the Food and Drug Administration (FDA). The Food, Drug, and Cosmetic Act (FDCA) gives the FDA authority to regulate drugs "intended to affect the structure or any function of the body of man" (Kessler, 1994a). The act does not exclude tobacco products, although until recently, the FDA had taken the position that tobacco products are intended for "smoking pleasure" and not to affect the structure or function of the body. On February 25, 1994, however, FDA Commissioner David Kessler indicated that

he was reconsidering the view that tobacco products are not drugs under the FDCA (IOM, 1994). In raising this issue, Dr. Kessler presented evidence that cigarette manufacturers deliberately manipulate nicotine levels in tobacco products to satisfy an addiction on the part of some of their customers. He also acknowledged in testimony to Congress that if nicotine-containing cigarettes were regulated as drugs, strict application of the FDCA could result in the removal from the market of all tobacco products, an option that he admitted is not practically feasible. In essence, Dr. Kessler asked Congress for direction about how to develop a regulatory response for tobacco products under a scheme whereby these products would remain lawfully available for adult consumption.

Barring a complete ban on tobacco products, Congress could instruct the FDA, or some other agency of the government, to regulate the content, marketing, and sale of tobacco products. For example, Benowitz and Henningfield (1994) suggested that it might be possible to establish threshold limits on the amount of tar and nicotine allowed in cigarettes to reduce addiction. Under the current regulatory system, however, there is little incentive for the tobacco industry to design its products to be less dependence-producing and safer. It is likely that at least in the near future, tobacco products will remain lawfully available for adults and accessible to minors (IOM, 1994). For this reason, efforts aimed at regulating the design and content of tobacco products to promote the marketing of safer products seem logical, and may represent the single best policy option for lowering the disease burden caused by tobacco use (IOM, 1994).

METHODOLOGICAL ISSUES RELEVANT TO TOBACCO POLICY RESEARCH

It is evident from this review of research on tobacco policies that it is nearly impossible to precisely quantify the impact of different policy measures on behavior. Econometricians have dominated the research on tobacco policy, often employing complex statistical models to quantify the impact of different policies on tobacco use. Econometric methods are intrinsically limited, however, in their ability to adequately isolate the impact of specific policies independent of other influences on tobacco use (Chapman, 1989). The development of valid measures that capture the essential features of tobacco policies is another problem plaguing econometric studies. For example, with the exception of cigarette prices, most tobacco policy measures are not easily quantified. How does one meaningfully equate or assign a numerical value to different health education approaches or to weak compared to robust health warnings? Recently, researchers have begun to advocate the use of qualitative approaches, in addition to quantitative methods, to judge the impact of tobacco policies on behavior (Chapman, 1989).

CONCLUSIONS: RESEARCH AND POLICY ISSUES

The years since the mid-1950s have witnessed a dramatic change in attitudes toward and use of tobacco by Americans. Most public health scholars believe that this change has been accelerated by public policy interventions to reduce tobacco use (IOM, 1994; Simonich, 1991; Warner, 1989). Simonich's (1991) analysis of government antismoking policies enacted between 1964 and 1987 concluded that among the most potent demand-reducing tobacco policies were higher tobacco taxes, restrictions on smoking in public locations, and paid counteradvertising. Other policies, such as the requirement of warning labels on tobacco products and limits on advertising, appear to have had less direct impact on discouraging tobacco use, although these policies may have contributed to altering cultural norms concerning tobacco.

This chapter has attempted to chronicle policy approaches to curb tobacco use, describe their rationale, and review evidence of efficacy.

Ultimately, this review leads one to ask about the need for continuing activity in the public policy sphere for tobacco control.

This question is the subject of ongoing debate and controversy, because the answer depends on one's view of why people smoke and the government's authority to regulate behavior (Rabin & Sugarman, 1993). To a large extent, tobacco control policies enacted to date have been based on the concept of informed consumer choice. This theory is based on the premise that consumers are capable of making a rational and voluntary choice to use tobacco. Under an informed-choice theory, the government's role in tobacco control is limited to ensuring truly informed individual decision making.

Empirical support for an informed-choice theory of tobacco use is weak. The conclusions of most behavioral studies of tobacco users suggest that for many smokers, tobacco use is not a voluntary behavior, but an addiction (DHHS, 1988). Thus, there appears to be little real world connection between what behavioral research says about the factors that motivate tobacco use and the development of tobacco control policy. Up to now, tobacco control policies have been determined mainly by political and economic forces. This situation is unfortunate, since health behavior research has the capacity to inform policy development as well as to provide relevant feedback on existing policies.

REFERENCES

Allen, K., Moss, A., Giovino, G. A., Shopland, D. R., & Pierce, J. P. (1993). Teenage tobacco use data: Estimates from the teenage attitudes and practices survey, United States, 1989. *Advance Data*, No. 224.
Benowitz, N. L., Henningfeld, J. E. (1994). Establishing a nicotine threshold for addiction. *New England Journal of Medicine, 331*, 123–125.
Bhalla, G., Lastovicka, J. L. (1984). The impact of changing cigarette warning message content and format. *Advertising and Consumer Research, 11*, 305–310.
Blum, A. (1989). Warnings: Smokers opt for the new, prefer carbon monoxide poisoning to fatal injury. *Journal of the American Medical Association, 261*, 44–45.

Blum A., & Myers, M. (1993). Tobacco marketing and promotion. In T. P. Houston (Ed.), *Tobacco use: An American crisis* (pp. 63-71). Chicago: American Medical Association.

Brandt, A. (1990). The cigarette, risk, and American culture. *Daedalus, 119*, 155-176.

Centers for Disease Control and Prevention. (1994a). Medical-care expenditures attributable to cigarette smoking—United States. *Morbidity and Mortality Weekly Report, 43*(26), 469-472.

Centers for Disease Control and Prevention (1994b). Cigarette smoking among adults—United States, 1993. *Morbidity and Mortality Weekly Report, 43*(50), 925-930.

Centers for Disease Control and Prevention. (1995). Trends in smoking initiation among adolescents and young adults—United States, 1980-1989. *Morbidity and Mortality Weekly Report, 44*(28), 521-525.

Chapman, S. (1989). The limitations of econometric analysis in cigarette advertising studies. *British Journal of Addiction, 84*, 1267-1274.

Coalition on Smoking or Health. (1993). *Saving lives and raising revenues: The case for major increases in state and federal tobacco taxes.* Washington DC: Coalition on Smoking or Health.

Coalition on Smoking or Health. (1995). *Protecting our families and children from tobacco: Public policy activities of the Coalition on Smoking or Health 1995 and 1996.* Washington DC: Coalition on Smoking or Health.

COMMIT Research Group (1995). Community intervention trial for smoking cessation (COMMIT). I. Cohort results from a four year community intervention. *American Journal of Public Health, 85*(2), 183-192.

Connolly, G. N. (1992). Worldwide expansion of transnational tobacco industry. *Journal of the National Cancer Institute Monograph, 12*, 29-35.

Davis, R. M., & Kendrick, J. S. (1989). The Surgeon General's warnings in outdoor cigarette advertising: Are they readable? *Journal of the American Medical Association, 261*, 90-94.

Daynard, R. A. (1988). Tobacco litigation as a cancer control strategy. *Journal of the National Cancer Institute, 80*, 9-12.

DiFranza, J. R., Carlson, R. P., Caisse, R. E. (1992). Reducing youth access to tobacco. *Tobacco Control, 1*, 58.

DiFranza, J. R., Richards, J. W., Paulman, P. M., Wol, F., Gillespie, N., Fletcher, C., Jaffe, R. D., Murray, D. (1991). RJR Nabisco's cartoon camel promotes camel cigarettes to children. *Journal of the American Medical Association, 266*, 3149-3153.

Dunn, W. L., Jr. (1972). *Motives and incentives in cigarettes.* Richmond, VA: Philip Morris Research Center.

Emont, S. L., Lhoi, W. S., Novotny, T. E. (1993). Clean indoor air legislation, taxation, and smoking behavior in the United States: An ecological analysis. *Tobacco Control, 2*, 13-17.

Federal Communications Commission. (1987). Inquiry into section 73.1910 of the Commission's rules and regulations concerning alternatives to the general Fairness Doctrine obligations of broadcast licensees. *Federal Communications Commission Record, 2*, 5272.

Federal Trade Commission. (1964). Advertising and labeling of cigarettes: Notice of rulemaking proceedings for establishment of trade regulation roles. *Federal Register, 29*, 530-532.

Federal Trade Commission. (1969). Cigarettes in relation to the health hazards of smoking: Unfair or deceptive advertising and labeling. *Federal Registry, 34*, 7917-7918.

Federal Trade Commission. (1981a). Federal Trade Commission staff report on the cigarette advertising investigation. *Federal Trade Commission.*

Federal Trade Commission. (1981b). Report of tar, nicotine and carbon monoxide of the smoke of 187 varieties of cigarettes. *Federal Trade Commission.*

Fischer, P. M., Krugman, D. M., Fletcher, J. E., Fox, R. J., Ras, T. H. (1993). An evaluation of health warnings in cigarette advertisements using standard market research methods: What does it mean to warn? *Tobacco Control, 2*, 279-285.

Fischer, P.M., Richards, J. W., Berman, E. F., & Krugman, D. M. (1989). Recall and eye tracking study of adolescents viewing tobacco advertisements. *Journal of the American Medical Association, 261*, 84-89.

Giovino, G. A., Schooley, M. W., Zhu, B. P., Chrisman, J. H., Tomar, S. L., Peddicord, J. P., Merritt, R. K., Husten, C. G., & Eriksen, M. P. (1994, Nov. 18). Surveillance for selected tobacco-use behaviors—United States, 1900-1994 *CDC Surveillance Summaries, 43* (SS-3), 1-43.

Hamilton, J. L. (1972). The demand for cigarettes: Advertising, health scare, and the cigarette advertising ban. *Review of Economics and Statistics, 54*, 401-411.

Henningfeld, J. E., Cohen, C., & Pickworth, W. D. (1993). Psychopharmacology of nicotine. In C. T. Orleans & J. Slade (Eds.), *Nicotine addiction: Principles and management.* (pp. 24-45). New York: Oxford University Press.

Hill, D. (1993). Australia's new health warnings on cigarette packaging. *Tobacco Control, 2*, 92-94.

Hilts, P. J. (1994a, April 29). Scientists say cigarette company suppressed findings on nicotine. *The New York Times*, p. A1.

Hilts, P. J. (1994b, May 2). Major flaw cited in cigarette data: Testing for tar and nicotine under reports amounts. *The New York Times*, p. A1.

Hilts, P. J. (1994c, Nov. 27). Little smoke, little tar, but still lots of nicotine. *The New York Times*, p. A1.

Institute of Medicine. (1994). *Growing up tobacco free: Preventing nicotine addiction in children and youths.* Washington, DC: National Academy Press.

Jason, L. A., Ji, P. Y., Ames, M. D., & Birhead, S. H. (1991). Active enforcement of cigarette control laws in the prevention of cigarette sales to minors. *Journal of the American Medical Association, 166*, 3159-3161.

Kagan, R. A., & Skolnick, J. H. (1993). Banning smoking:

Compliance without enforcement. In R. L. Rabin & S. D. Sugarman (Eds.), *Smoking policy: Law, politics and culture,* (pp. 69–94). New York: Oxford University Press.

Kagan, R. A., & Vogel, D. (1993). The politics of smoking regulation: Canada, France, the United States. In R. L. Rabin & S. D. Sugarman (Eds.), *Smoking policy: Law, politics, and culture* (pp. 22–48). New York: Oxford University Press.

Kaiserman, M. J. (1993). The effectiveness of health warning messages. *Tobacco Control, 2,* 267–269.

Kessler, D. A. (1994a, March 25). *Statement on nicotine-containing cigarettes.* Testimony before the House Subcommittee on Health and the Environment.

Kessler, D. A. (1994b, June 21). *The control and manipulation of nicotine in cigarettes.* Testimony before the House Subcommittee on Health and the Environment.

Lewit, E. M. (1989). U.S. tobacco taxes: Behavioral effects and policy implications. *British Journal of Addiction, 84,* 1217–1234.

National Cancer Institute. (1992). *Smokeless tobacco or health: An international perspective.* NIH Publication No. 92-3461. Washington, DC: National Institutes of Health, Public Health Service, U.S. Department of Health and Human Services.

National Cancer Institute. (1993). *Major local tobacco control ordinances in the United States.* NIH Publication No. 93-3532. National Institutes of Health, Public Health Service, U.S. Department of Health and Human Services.

Northup, A. M. (1993). U.S. agricultural policy on tobacco. In T. P. Houston (Ed.), *Tobacco use: an American crisis,* Chicago: American Medical Association.

Office of the Inspector General. (1992). Youth access to tobacco. OEI-02-92-00880. Washington DC: U.S. Department of Health and Human Services.

O'Keefe, M. T. (1971). The anti-smoking commercials: A study of television's impact on behavior. *Public Opinion Quarterly, 35,* 242–248.

Orleans, C. T., Slade, J. (1993). *Nicotine addiction: Principles and management.* New York: Oxford University Press.

Parkinson, M. D., Schauffler, H. H., Kottke, T. E., Curry, S. J., Sulberg, L. I., Arnold, C. B., Butz, R. H., Taylor, R., Halloway, J. B., & Meltzer, C. (1992). Report of the tobacco policy research study group on reimbursement and insurance in the United States. *Tobacco Control 1* (Supplement), 552–556.

Peto, R., Lopez, A. D., Boreham, J., Thun, M., & Heath, C., Jr. (1992). Mortality from tobacco in developed countries: Indirect estimates from national vital statistics. *Lancet, 339,* 1268–1278.

Pierce, J. P., Evans, N., Farkas, A. J., Cavin, S. W., Berly, C., Kramer, M., Konley, S., Rosbrook, B., Choi, W., & Kaplan R. M. (1994). *Tobacco use in California: An evaluation of the tobacco control program, 1989–1993.* La Jolla: University of California, San Diego.

Pierce, J. P., Fiore M. C., Novotny, T. E., Hatziandrev, E. J., &

Davis, R. M. (1989). Trends in cigarette smoking in the United States: Educational differences are increasing. *Journal of the American Medical Association, 261,* 56–60.

Pierce, J. P., Gilpin, E., Burns, D. M., Whalen, E., Rosbrook, B., Shopland, D., & Johnson, M. (1991). Does tobacco advertising target young people to start smoking? *Journal of the American Medical Association, 266,* 3154–3158.

Pierce, J. P., Lara, L., & Gilpin, E. (1994). Smoking initiation by adolescent girls, 1944 through 1988. *Journal of the American Medical Association, 271*(8), 608–611.

Pollay, R. W. (1994a). Exposure of U.S. youth to cigarette television advertising in the 1960's. *Tobacco Control, 3,* 130–133.

Pollay, R. W. (1994b). Promises, promises: Self-regulation of U.S. cigarette broadcast advertising in the 1960's. *Tobacco Control, 3,* 134–144.

Rabin, R. L., Sugarman, S. D. (Eds.). (1993). *Smoking policy: Law, politics and culture.* New York: Oxford University Press.

Samet, J. M., Lewit, E. M., & Warner K. E. (1994). Involuntary smoking and children's health. *The Future of Children: Critical Health Issues for Children and Youth, 4,* 94–114.

Schauffler, H. H. (1993). Health insurance policy and the politics of tobacco. In R. L. Rabin & S. D. Sugarman (Eds.), *Smoking policy: Law, politics, and culture* (pp. 184–207). New York: Oxford University Press.

Schneider, L., Klein, B., & Murphy K. M. (1981). Government regulation of cigarette health information. *Journal of Law and Economics, 24,* 575–612.

Simonich, W. L. (1991). *Government anti-smoking policies.* New York: Peter Lang.

Slade, J., Connolly, G. N., Davis, R. M., Douglas, C. E., Henningfeld, J. E., Hughes, J. R., Kozlowski, L. T. & Myers, M. L. (1992). Report of the policy research study group on tobacco products. *Tobacco Control 1*(Supplement), 54–59.

Sugarman, S. D. (1993). Disparate treatment of smokers on employment and insurance. In R. L. Rabin & S. D. Sugarman (Eds.), *Smoking policy: Law, politics, and culture* (pp. 161–183). New York: Oxford University Press.

Tobacco Product Liability Protect (1995). 1994 Year in Review. *Tobacco on Trial 1,* 1–44.

U.S. Census Bureau Current Population Survey. (1992, September). Washington, DC: Bureau of the Census, U.S. Department of Commerce.

U.S. Department of Health and Human Services. (1986). *The health consequences of involuntary smoking: A report of the Surgeon General.* DHHS Publication No. (CDC) 87-8398. Washington, DC: Centers for Disease Control, U.S. Public Health Service, U.S. Department of Health and Human Services.

U.S. Department of Health and Human Services. (1988). *The health consequences of smoking: Nicotine addiction—A report of the Surgeon General, 1988.* DHHS Publication No. (CDC) 88-8406. Washington, DC: Office on Smoking and Health. Center for Health Promotion and Education,

Centers for Disease Control, U.S. Public Health Service, U.S. Department of Health and Human Services.

U.S. Department of Health and Human Services. (1989). *Reducing the health consequences of smoking: 25 Years of progress—A report of the Surgeon General*. DHHS Publication No. (CDC) 89-8411. Washington, DC: Office on Smoking and Health, Center for Chronic Disease Prevention and Health Promotion, Centers for Disease Control, U.S. Public Health Service, U.S. Department of Health and Human Services.

U.S. Department of Health and Human Services. (1994). *Preventing tobacco use among young people: A report of the Surgeon General*. Atlanta, GA: Office on Smoking and Health, Center for Chronic Disease Prevention and Health Promotion, Centers for Disease Control and Prevention, U.S. Public Health Service, U.S. Department of Health and Human Services.

U.S. Environmental Protection Agency. (1992). *Respiratory health effects of passive smoking: Lung cancer and other disorders*. EPA 600/6-90/006F. Washington, DC: Office of Health and Environmental Assessment, Office of Research and Development.

U.S. Public Health Service. (1964). *Smoking and health: Report of the Advisory Committee to the Surgeon General of the Public Health Service*. PHS Publication No. 1103. Washington, DC: Centers for Disease Control, U.S. Department of Health, Education and Welfare.

Wagner, S. (1971). *The Federal Trade Commission*. New York: Praeger.

Wallack, L. M. (1981). Mass media campaigns: The odds against finding behavior change. *Health Education Quarterly, 8*, 209-260.

Warner, K. E. (1986). *Selling smoking: Cigarette advertising and public health*. Washington, DC: American Public Health Association.

Warner, K. (1989). Effects of the anti-smoking campaign: An update. *American Journal of Public Health, 79*, 144-151.

Warner, K. E., Slade, J. (1992). Low tar, high toll. *American Journal of Public Health, 82*, 17-18.

Wasserman, J., Manning, W. E., Newhouse, J. P., & Winkler, J. D. (1991). The effects of excise taxes and regulations on cigarette smoking. *Journal of Health Economics, 10*, 43-64.

Watson, D. S. (1972). *Price theory and its uses*. Boston: Houghton Mifflin.

Wright, G. (1984). *Behavioral decision theory: An introduction*. Beverly Hills, CA: Sage.

III

PLANNED APPLICATIONS

A number of deliberately planned efforts to induce behavioral change to enhance health and safety were presented in Volume II of this *Handbook*, particularly in the chapters on adhering to regimens for weight loss and nutrition (Chrisler, Chapter 17), smoking cessation (Glasgow & Orleans, Chapter 19), exercise (Marcus, Bock, & Pinto, Chapter 18), and occupational safety (Cohen & Colligan, Chapter 20). Planned efforts to reduce smoking, drug and alcohol usage, and risky sexual behaviors were described in Volume III, particularly in the chapters on health behavior in children (O'Brien & Bush, Chapter 3), and adolescents (Cowell & Marks, Chapter 4). These planned applications often involve three highly interdependent processes: health promotion, health education, and communication campaigns.

HEALTH PROMOTION
AND HEALTH EDUCATION

The relevance of health behavior knowledge for health promotion and health education (HP/HE) has long been acknowledged. Graham (1973), using health behavior research data, identified cultural barriers to acceptance of innovations in relation to engaging in new, preventive behaviors and urged that campaigns designed to change behaviors, or to elicit innovative behaviors, be sensitive to the cultural meanings of the new behavior. Richards (1975) noted the particular relevance of knowledge about the cultural symbolic value of healing and medicine and the need for Eurocentric health professionals to understand the belief systems of non-Eurocentric cultures and the cultural norms for gender-appropriate behavior.

Knowledge generated by health behavior research was the basis for England's (1978) conclusion that it was necessary to cast off myths about the ease of establishing successful prevention programs in underdeveloped countries. Other myths, as well as untested assumptions, about health promotion and health education programs were identified by Johnson (1981) through knowledge generated by health behavior research. Johnson used knowledge of *real* data on the age of onset of smoking to urge that antismoking programs begin at an appropriate age, an age that is not *so* early that the program effects would boomerang. Johnson also used health behavior research data to argue against erroneous assumptions about the long-term effects of health as a value compared with the effects of social approval.

West, Graham, Swanson, and Wilkinson (1977) urged the need for follow-up health behavior data on smoking cessation. Nearly a decade later, Shumaker and Grunberg (1986) provided an account of the factors involved in smoking relapse. Although the systemic effects of nicotine themselves require greater understanding, they operate in conjunction with a variety of behavioral cues (e.g., Pomerlau, 1986), and improving the success of interventions requires understanding of personal motivation, social support, and family determinants of health behavior (e.g., Brownell et al., 1986).

Eardley and Elkind (1990) demonstrated how concepts from the health services utilization model, such as predisposing and enabling factors, together with an understanding of factors that reinforce health behavior affected participation in breast-screening programs in the United Kingdom. Their findings have implications for the organization of screenings to reduce barriers to participation.

Simonds (1984) acknowledged the increasing emphasis in health education on the determinants of human behavior and on health behavior research. Green (1984) similarly noted that effective models for health education require greater knowledge of (1) the personal determinants of health behavior, including individual cognitive factors such as interests, attitudes, perceptions, beliefs, values, motives, and the skills necessary to estimate risks or vulnerabilities and to recognize symptoms; and (2) the social determinants such as peer influences. Stanton, Black, Engle, and Pelto (1992) demonstrated the broad implications of a range of health behavior theories for identifying motivational issues that underlie behavioral change in developing countries, particularly in relation to control of diarrheal diseases.

A major work by Glanz, Lewis, and Rimer (1990) demonstrated how a number of health behavior conceptual models and data are used in individual, interpersonal, and group interventions to change health behaviors. Despite the demonstrated value of health behavior knowledge and perspectives, however, HP/HE interventions do not universally incorporate such knowledge in their planning or implementation.

Discussions of the relevance of health behavior for HP/HE can be considered within a context of definitions, conceptualizations, critical views, evaluation models, and specific contents and targets.

Definitions

Health Promotion. In addition to the definitions presented by Glanz and Oldenburg in Chapter 8 of this volume, Dines and Cribb (1993) draw from both a business and marketing perspective—in which "promotion" emphasizes placing a product at the forefront of consumer attention to encourage consumption—and a workplace perspective—in which "promotion" connotes moving to a higher level—and define health promotion as "placing the absence of disease, foundations for achievement and well being in the forefront of attention. Alternatively it becomes raising well-being and strengthening foundations so achievement may be at a higher level, or eliminating more disease so that the human state remaining exists at a higher level" (Dines & Cribb, 1993, p. 21). Furthermore, health promotion as a concept is independent of disease prevention and includes advocacy of values together with effective and concrete public participation in order to give a population the internal and external resources necessary "to increase control over, and to improve, their health" (WHO, 1986a, cited in Dines & Cribb, 1993) and to make more healthful lifestyles easier to lead (Dines & Cribb, 1993, p. 30). Health promotion thus involves strategies to change public policy, create supportive environments, strengthen community action, develop personal skills, and reorient health services.

Health Education. Health education denotes the imparting of information and knowledge and is a vital component of health promotion. "Health education has been defined by the World Health Organization as any combination of planned activities leading to a situation where people want to be healthy; know how to attain health; do what they can individually and collectively; and seek help when needed (WHO, 1981a,b, cited in Kolbe, 1988). Milio (1976) views health education as a way of developing options rather than as a strategy for restricting choice.

"From time immemorial there has clearly

existed some form of Health Education which has become esconced in the social and cultural milieu" (Richards, 1975, p. 141). Health education exists as the crossroads of social science and medicine and translates social science findings into action programs designed to improve health knowledge and behaviors (Richards, 1975). Health education is a much older term than health promotion, but the terms are increasingly used together.

Conceptualization

Questions arise about the conceptualization of HP/HE, i.e., about their domain and their objectives. What types of behaviors should be their focus? What levels of personal and social systems should be their targets? Dines and Cribb (1993), for example, recognize as an extreme that all of life's activities can be seen as health promoting and that such a broad definition reduces the value of the concept immeasurably.

More specifically, although many HP/HE campaigns have been largely directed at specific diseases and the behavioral risk factors that underlie them, e.g., smoking, cholesterol intake, and the like, this may be an inappropriate direction for HP/HE. It has been argued that overidentification with risk factors and disease is an inappropriate, ineffective approach to health promotion campaigns. Fielding (1977) points out the problems that result when health promotion is co-opted as the preventive part of specific medical regimens, e.g., when exercise programs or smoking reduction programs are perceived as part of regimens for heart disease, rather than as general health-promotion behaviors. Health promotion has thus acquired a disease-specific orientation and connotation. Fielding urged health promotion programs to emphasize the nondisease factors that determine health behavior—e.g., patterns of reinforcement that increase the likelihood of such behaviors occurring; tax structures and insurance policy premiums that reward health-promoting behavior—which can be potent factors in moving health promotion away from risk

reduction, disease-specific models. Knowledge generated by health behavior research can identify the nondisease factors that generate and support preventive behaviors. Dines and Cribb (1993) also argued that health promotion needs to be considered as separate from disease prevention, which is largely a medical issue.

In evaluating several large-scale health promotion interventions, Fincham (1992) not only notes the relevance of a number of health behavior models and knowledge for understanding the factors that influence individual decisions to adopt healthy behaviors, but also stresses the inadequacy of the traditional public health approach to health promotion and risk reduction of simply providing education and information. Fincham endorses introducing a wide range of psychological and social factors into the intervention process.

Love and Kalnins (1984) used knowledge generated by health behavior research to support "structuralist" approaches to health promotion programs, rather than the more traditional approaches that attempt to change individuals. In nutrition education, for example, structuralist programs would focus on the community, on the food industry, and on television advertising as ways of changing dietary patterns.

Similar in perspective are de Leeuw's (1989) views, which emphasize the need for health promotion to focus on policy development and change in combination with efforts at individual behavior change. De Leeuw particularly stresses the importance of understanding the policy-making process, the "policy-making-environment-analysis," and of the multiple and special interests that control this process. Using the acronyms HE/SHE to reflect two extreme points of view—respectively, "Hyper-Expansionist," a business-as-usual, analytical, uncritical perspective of health education with "masculine" values related to technocracy, formal organizations, and increased medicalization, and "Sane, Humane, and Ecological," a more "feminine" perspective stressing decentralization, reintegration of work with other aspects of life, self-help, and mutual aid—

de Leeuw suggests that health promotion efforts need to integrate these two positions.

Similarly, and congruent with knowledge generated by health behavior research, Milio (1976) argued that health education becomes more effective if it is group-focused rather than focused on individuals, particularly when the group serves as a social network to support norms that endorse health-generating behaviors. Frazier (1978), basing her arguments on health behavior research data demonstrating the great difficulty of changing motives and of overcoming the social and cultural barriers to care, urged health education programs to move away from traditional attempts to change individual motives through typical dental health education programs for school-age children. Instead, she favored changing community policies through the skillful use of group and community planning processes.

On the basis of health behavior research data, Jenny (1976) urged that dental health promotion campaigns become more ecologically focused and deal with the family as a whole, and with the community as well, rather than attempt to change individual diet and other behaviors that place dental health at risk. Community values encourage families to use refined carbohydrates. School health materials are ineffective in this context. Furthermore, Jenny identified barriers to care that reduce the effectiveness of health education programs and urged that services and facilities be brought closer to the population to be served.

Knowledge generated by health behavior research can determine how social networks and other social and community factors support or impede preventive, health-promoting behaviors. Fielding (1977) argued for the greater involvement of community groups in the planning of health promotion programs. Greater involvement of community agencies in the early stages of planning an intervention was found to increase levels of community participation (Davis & Iverson, 1984).

Critical Views

In addition to suggesting the need to expand the domain of HP/HE, critical questions arise about their legitimacy and value. Becker (1993) urges a critical look at enthusiasm for health promotion in relation to disease prevention. Underlying his criticism are the dubiousness of many findings, the reversals of "what is known to be good," the minimal calculated benefits of lifestyle changes, together with (Becker, 1993, p. 5)

... the devotion of high resources (and often low scholarship) to a relentless search for "risk factors"; premature exhortation of the public to adopt numerous health-related behaviors, with great lack of success, frequent reversals of advice, and unfulfilled promises concerning what such behaviors would achieve for the adopters; a public generally confused and skeptical with regard to public health advice; a scientific community that rushes tentative findings into print; a mass media community that worsens the problem; and an introspective approach to health that fosters victim-blaming and stigmatization, ignores critical social, economic and environmental issues that have major impacts on health, and further encourages an already unhealthy level in our society of concern for person, rather than societal, well-being.

Evans (1988) similarly cautions against over-acceptance of the concept and technology of prevention. Goodman and Goodman (1986) note not only the minimal or nonexistent gains in mortality rates for coronary heart disease associated with interventions to reduce its risk, but also the increased risk attributable to hypertensive drug therapy. Goodman and Goodman further observe that prevention campaigns are often driven by economic and market interests. Brownell (1991) admonishes health professionals to recognize that biological realities have a far greater impact on risk than do individual behaviors, yet profits are made from the public's search for absolute answers, as exemplified by the commercial success of books on diet, exercise, bodies, and health in general. The media and marketing interests are well served by continual news and emphasis on new scientific findings. Brownell further points out the vested corporate and managerial interests in stress management programs that absolve the organization of responsibility for a noxious work environment. Finally, Levy (1986), recognizing the ineffectiveness of many interventions and programs, together with the gains to be made from marketing them, raises questions about the ethics of encouraging participation.

Evaluation Models

Evaluation of HP/HE interventions is often complex and difficult, and historically many interventions have been inadequately evaluated. D. G. Altman and his colleagues (e.g., D. G. Altman, 1986; Jackson, Altman, Howard-Pitney, & Farquhar, 1989) propose an evaluation framework that recognizes the transactional nature of community programs. This framework transcends tight evaluation designs in order to reflect aspects of the settings and context, understanding of the phenomenological perspectives of the participants, and appreciation of the role of the evaluator.

Cheadle and his colleagues (e.g., Cheadle et al., 1992–1993; Cheadle, Wagner, Koepsell, Kristal, & Patrick, 1992) propose an alternative evaluation model for community programs that emphasizes the degree to which the community becomes increasingly "activated," i.e., the degree to which major community institutions become involved in the process of increasing community initiatives and resources for health promotion and of improving awareness of health issues (Cheadle et al., 1992). Wickizer et al. (1993) further stress the importance of observing community activation as a process (in addition to outcomes), emphasizing that health promotion strategies should include organized efforts to increase community awareness and consensus about health problems, coordinated planning of prevention and environmental change programs, interorganizational allocation of resources, and citizen involvement in these processes. Wickizer et al. (1993) draw upon network analysis to measure coordination of community efforts.

Community participation is considered to be part of a broad process of community development. Cook et al. (1988) identify some processes critical to both development of and participation in health interventions. These processes include defining a community, reaching a community, considering cultural differences in a community, involving community residents, and recognizing tensions among those providing health care services, those conducting experiments and research, and those promoting community participation.

Specific Targets and Levels of Intervention

HP/HE interventions have been targeted at a wide range of health behaviors, and several levels are available for such interventions. In addition to long-standing traditional efforts to influence diet, exercise, smoking, worksite safety, smoking, drug and alcohol use, and risky sexual behaviors (described in the chapters in Volumes II and III of this *Handbook* identified earlier in this discussion), HP/HE efforts are also being directed at injury and violence reduction. Large-scale programs involve schools, communities, families, and worksites, as well as efforts to affect minority and marginalized populations.

Injury Reduction. The traditional educational programs aimed at highway safety have not proven to be effective (Robertson, Chapter 12 in this volume; Nichols, 1994). Information by itself hasn't proven successful in changing patterns of drunk driving or of the use of child safety seats, seat belts, and motorcycle helmets. Information can sometimes lead, however, to changes in community attitudes, which have an impact on legislation, which then may have a greater chance of changing behavior (Nichols, 1994). A review of the literature (Pless & Arsenault, 1987) does suggest that combining information and education with a behavioral or social learning component and other forms of persuasion with changes in the larger system, such as legislation, have had an impact on certain aspects of child safety, such as home injuries, burns, and scalds and use of seat restraints.

A particular need for health promotion efforts is manifested by the number of injuries sustained in home driveway accidents. Brison, Wicklund, and Mueller (1988) note that parents' backing up of vehicles is a major cause of injuries and fatalities to their children, particularly as use of vans and larger family vehicles has increased. They suggest the need to develop new strategies such as safeguarding driveways and reassessing the ways in which their vehicles may obstruct vision, since the conventional wisdom of discouraging children from "darting out" into traffic is clearly irrelevant in these instances.

Playground and street safety for children was successfully increased through the Safe Kids/ Healthy Neighborhoods Program in Harlem, in New York City. This program created safe playground areas; involved children and adolescents in safe, supervised activity to teach them useful skills; provided injury and violence prevention education; and made safety equipment (e.g., helmets) available at reasonable cost (Davidson et al., 1994).

Violence Reduction and Empowerment. Violence and violent behaviors are suggested as appropriate targets for HP/HE (e.g., Christoffel, 1994), and violence reduction is urged as an addition to the more traditional objectives. Another object for HP/HE is the empowerment of children as health consumers (Igoe, 1991).

School Programs. Schools have been the historic locus of health education programs, and typically most such programs have imparted knowledge and information, guided by the assumption that such information will in itself lead to appropriate behavior or to behavioral change. Health behavior research has demonstrated the error of this assumption. School-based programs increasingly make use of knowledge about the development of beliefs about health and illness

and about the role of peer, family, and environmental factors in health beliefs and actions. Simons-Morton, Parcel, Baranowski, Forthofer, and O'Hara (1991) provide an account of a school based program that modified environmental characteristics, i.e., the school lunches served, together with a physical education program to improve diet and levels of physical activity. They note that, of course, schools do not change readily. In Chapter 14, Kelder, Edmundson, and Lytle provide a comprehensive discussion of how health behavior research findings inform school-based programs, how the effectiveness of such programs is increased when they are made part of a community-based approach, and how the results of such interventions in turn add to knowledge about health behavior.

Community Programs. McAlister, Puska, Salonen, Tuomilehto, and Koskela (1982) based their comprehensive community and regional approach to health promotion in the North Karelia Project on knowledge generated by health behavior research. Knowledge about the difficulty of changing individual preventive behaviors, including use of preventive services, together with data on the existing beliefs in their target population, led them to develop a program aimed at changing larger system variables. Their project in Finland, which has been recognized globally, mobilized a variety of community resources in a successful attempt at changing risk factors for cardiovascular disease. Wherever possible, families were involved by including them in cooking demonstrations or by encouraging spousal support for adherence to regimens. Among the environmental changes included were implementation of restaurant policies on smoking and successful encouragement of the development of a sausage with lower fat content. Significant reductions in risk estimates based on smoking, serum cholesterol, and blood pressure were obtained over a 5-year period. Moreover, long-term differences in patterns of smoking were attributed more to this overall community program than to specific school-based smoking prevention programs for adolescents (Vartiainen, Fallonen, McAlister, & Puska, 1990). In Chapter 15, Schooler and Flora discuss community-based programs, including their effect on the structure and functioning of the communities themselves.

Family Programs. Several major intervention programs to change dietary behaviors have focused on the family as a social unit. Atkins et al. (1990), Baranowski et al. (1990), and Perry et al. (1988) provide insights into the mixed success of these programs in changing family eating behaviors. Many family interventions unfortunately do not draw widely upon any body of health behavior research *findings*, but are derived instead from general social learning theories or cognitive learning theories or both.

In Chapter 16, Baranowski and Hearn acknowledge the lack of success of many such programs and provide a developmental perspective for discussing them.

Worksite Programs. The relevance of health behavior research to worksite interventions is affirmed in the context of a demonstration of the value of the Pender health promotion model, based on social cognitive theory: The "design of workplace health promotion programs must be based on knowledge of factors influencing the adoption of healthy lifestyle by employees" (Pender, Walker, Sechrist, & Frank-Stromborg, 1990, p 331). The major variables in this model are the importance of health, perceived control over health, and perceived self-efficacy. The effectiveness of worksite programs is seen to hinge on skill building, use of coworker support systems, provision of current information on the controllability of health, and employee involvement in planning lifestyle modifications, as well as supportive change in the work environment. Pender et al. (1990) suggest the need to reconceptualize workplace health as multidimensional well-being—not just as the absence of injury or illness or a reduction in risk behaviors.

Numerous workplace interventions drawing upon health behavior knowledge have been implemented, with varying degrees of design rigor and success (e.g., Glasgow, Terborg, Hollis, Severson, & Boles, et al., 1993). Klesges et al. (1988) characterize many such programs as having low participation, high attrition, and modest outcomes. Sorensen et al. (1992) describe a multisite nutrition intervention to reduce cancer risks involving classes and food demonstrations targeted at individuals, point-of-choice labeling of cafeteria items to provide environmental support, and an employee advisory board at each site. One of the few interventions to employ a randomized design, it resulted in some reduction of fat intake.

Workplace programs raise the questions of whose interests are served by health promotion interventions and whether such interests are congruent. Eakin (Volume I, Chapter 16) observes that workers often believe they will be penalized for engaging in safe behavior. Political, social, and economic changes may sharpen any already existing differences between workers, employers, and health professionals. In the context of the economic transitions taking place in Poland in the early 1990s, for example, health was recognized as having different meanings for workers and employers. Health was treated as a commodity; workers were less interested in health than employers or government officials charged with workplace safety, and were willing to accept unhealthful conditions for extra pay (Ratajczak, 1993).

The use of narrative paradigms for instruction to increase worker safety reflects an abstraction from a wide range of health behavior research findings. In Chapter 17, Cole describes how narratives based on real worksite experiences increase the effectiveness of industrial safety programs.

Marginalized and Minority Populations. Eardley et al. (1985), studying attendance at British cervical screenings, showed that those women most in need of the services were least likely to take the initiative in making the appointments and might be most threatened by the screening procedure and its potential findings. Their data showed that such programs would be more successful if the providers took initiative both in identifying participants and in the appointment-setting process and that information about the screening should be directed more at the needs and fears of the target population.

Botvin et al. (1992) demonstrated how health behavior research findings, particularly relating to personal factors and peer and media influences, were incorporated in the design of interventions for a predominantly Hispanic population. Davidson et al. (1994) demonstrated how health behavior research could be used to improve the safety of minority youngsters in Harlem. Thomas, Quinn, Billingsley, and Caldwell (1994) provided important data on characteristics that relate to black churches' likelihood of participating in community health outreach programs. They found, for example, that churches more likely to participate were medium to large in size, rather than small, and had clergy with a graduate degree.

COMMUNICATION CAMPAIGNS

British data point to the inappropriate and stereotyped interpretations made by health professionals about working-class beliefs and note how such misinterpretations impede effective HP/HE programs (Pill & Stott, 1987). Steuart (1993) cautioned against similar stereotyping and inappropriate assumptions about the health beliefs of the elderly.

In relation to health-screening campaigns, Kirscht, Haefner, and Eveland (1975) stressed the importance of coordinating types of appeals with characteristics of the target population. Stahl, Lawrie, Neill, and Kelley (1977) similarly endorsed adapting specific techniques to the characteristics of their target areas in a community hypertension screening program. Health behavior research has an important contribution to

make in generating knowledge of such target population characteristics.

The importance of readability of health promotion materials was underscored by Meade and Byrd's (1989) analysis of smoking education materials. Patients in the primary care units in which the materials were distributed often had difficulty comprehending them. Skinner, Strecher, and Hospers (1994), using a stages of change model, found that tailoring messages from physicians about mammography to make them appropriate to the woman's stage of readiness of change increased the likelihood that the message would be read more thoroughly and remembered. Further, among black and poorer women who were initially precontemplators and contemplators, such tailoring was more likely to move them to have a mammogram.

In Chapter 18, on communication campaigns, Swinehart demonstrates the interaction between media programs and health behavior research data. The chapter identifies a number of instances in which such knowledge appropriately sharpened or redirected the focus of a media campaign.

REFERENCES

Altman, D. G. (1986). A framework for evaluating community-based heart disease prevention programs. *Social Science and Medicine, 22,* 479–487.

Atkins, C. J., Senn, K., Rupp, J., Kaplan, R. M., Patterson, T. L., Sallis, J. F., Jr., & Nader, P. R. (1990). Attendance at health promotion programs: Baseline predictors and program outcomes. *Health Education Quarterly, 17,* 417–428.

Baranowski, T., Simons-Morton, B., Hooks, P., Henske, J., Tiernan, K., Dunn, J. K., Burkhalter, H., Harper, J., & Palmer, J. (1990). A center-based program for exercise change among black-American families. *Health Education Quarterly, 17,* 179–196.

Becker, M. H. (1993). A medical sociologist looks at health promotion. *Journal of Health and Social Behavior, 34,* 1–6.

Botvin, G. J., Dusenbury, L., Baker, E., James-Ortiz, S., Botvin, E. M., & Kerner, J. (1992). Smoking prevention among urban minority youth: Assessing effects on outcome and mediating variables. *Health Psychology, 11,* 290–299.

Brison, R. J., Wicklund, K., & Mueller, B. A. (1988). Fatal

pedestrian injuries to young children: A different pattern of injury. *American Journal of Public Health, 78,* 793-795.

Brownell, K. D. (1991). Personal responsibility and control over our bodies: When expectation exceeds reality. *Health Psychology, 10,* 303-310.

Brownell, K. D., Glynn, T. J., Glasgow, R., Lando, H., Rand, C., Gottlieb, A., & Pinney, J. M. (1986). Task Force 5: Interventions to prevent relapse. In S. A. Shumaker & N. E. Grunberg (Eds.), *Proceedings of the National Working Conference on Smoking Relapse. Health Psychology, 5*(Supplement), 53-68.

Cheadle, A., Psaty, B. M., Diehr, P., Koepsell, T., Wagner, E., Wickizer, T., & Curry, S. (1992-1993). An empirical exploration of a conceptual model for community-based health promotion. *International Quarterly of Community Health Education, 13,* 329-363.

Cheadle, A., Wagner, E., Koepsell, T., Kristal, A., & Patrick, D. (1992). Environmental indicators: A tool for evaluating community-based health-promotion programs. *American Journal of Preventive Medicine, 8,* 345-350.

Christoffel, K. K. (1994). Editorial: Reducing violence—How do we proceed? *American Journal of Public Health, 84,* 539-541.

Cook, H. L., Goeppinger, J., Brunk, S. E., Price, L. J., Whitehead, T. L., & Sauter, S. V. H. (1988). A reexamination of community participation in health: Lessons from three community health projects. *Family and Community Health, 11*(2), 1-13.

Davidson, L. L., Durkin, M. S., Kuhn, L., O'Connor, P., Barlow, B., & Heagarty, M. C. (1994). The impact of the Safe Kids/Healthy Neighborhoods injury prevention program in Harlem, 1988 through 1991. *American Journal of Public Health, 84,* 580-586.

Davis, M. F., & Iverson, D. C. (1984). An overview and analysis of the health style campaign. *Health Education Quarterly, 11,* 253-272.

de Leeuw, E. (1989). Concepts in health promotion: The notion of relativism. *Social Science and Medicine, 29,* 1281-1288.

Dines, A., & Cribb, A. (Eds.). (1993). *Health promotion concepts and practice.* Oxford, England: Blackwell.

Eardley, A., & Elkind, A. (1990). A pilot study of attendance for breast cancer screening. *Social Science and Medicine, 30,* 693-699.

Eardley, A., Elkind, A. K., Spencer, B., Hobbs, P., Pendleton, L. L., & Haran, D. (1985). Attendance for cervical screening—Whose problem? *Social Science and Medicine, 20,* 955-962.

England, R. (1978). More myths in international health planning. *American Journal of Public Health, 68,* 153-159.

Evans, R. I. (1988). Health promotion—Science or ideology? *Health Psychology, 7,* 203-219.

Fielding, J. E. (1977). Health promotion—Some notions in search of a constituency. *American Journal of Public Health, 67,* 1082-1085.

Fincham, S. (1992). Community health promotion programs. *Social Science and Medicine, 35,* 239-249.

Frazier, P. J. (1978). A new look at dental health education in community programs. *Dental Hygiene, 52,* 176-186.

Glanz, K., Lewis, F. M., & Rimer, B. K. (Eds.). (1990). *Health behavior and health education: Theory, research and practice.* San Francisco: Jossey-Bass.

Glasgow, R. E., Terborg, J. R., Hollis, J. F., Severson, H. H., & Boles, S. M. (1995). Take heart: Results from the initial phase of a work-site wellness program. *American Journal of Public Health, 85,* 209-216.

Goodman, L. E., & Goodman, M. J. (1986). Prevention—How misuse of a concept undercuts its worth. *Hastings Center Report, April,* 26-38.

Graham, S. (1973). Studies of behavior change to enhance public health. *American Journal of Public Health, 63,* 327-334.

Green, L. W. (1984). Health education models. In J. D. Matarazzo, S. M. Weiss, J. A. Herd, N. E. Miller, & S. M. Weiss (Eds.), *Behavioral health: A handbook of health enhancement and disease prevention* (pp. 181-198). New York: Wiley.

Igoe, J. B. (1991). Empowerment of children and youth for consumer self-care. *American Journal of Health Promotion, 6*(1), 55-65.

Jackson, C., Altman, D. G., Howard-Pitney, B., & Farquhar, J. W. (1989). Evaluating community-level health promotion and disease prevention interventions. In M. T. Braverman (Ed.), *Evaluating health promotion programs. New directions for program evaluation: Vol. 43* (pp. 19-32). San Francisco: Jossey-Bass.

Jeffrey, R. W., Forster, J. L., French, S. A., Kelder, S. H., Lando, H. A., McGovern, P. G., Jacobs, D. R., Jr., & Baxter, J. E. (1993). The Health Worker Project: A work-site intervention for weight control and smoking cessation. *American Journal of Public Health, 83,* 395-401.

Jenny, J. (1976). Promoting dental health—An ecological approach. *Dental Assistant, 45,* 14-19, 48-49.

Johnson, C. A. (1981). Untested and erroneous assumptions underlying antismoking programs. In *Promoting adolescent health: A dialog on research and practice* (pp. 149-165). New York: Academic Press.

Kirscht, J. P., Haefner, D. P., & Eveland, J. D. (1975). Public response to various written appeals to participate in health screening. *Public Health Reports, 90,* 539-543.

Klesges, R. C., Brown, K., Pascale, R. W., Murphy, M., Williams, E., & Cigrang, J. A. (1988). Factors associated with participation, attrition, and outcome in a smoking cessation program at the workplace. *Health Psychology, 7,* 575-589.

Kolbe, L. J. (1988). The application of health behavior research: Health education and health promotion. In D. S. Gochman (Ed.), *Health behavior: Emerging research perspectives* (pp. 381-396). New York: Plenum Press.

Levy, S. R. (1986). Work site health promotion. *Family and Community Health, 9*(3), 51-62.

Love, R., & Kalnins, I. (1984). Individualist and structuralist perspectives on nutrition education for Canadian children. *Social Science and Medicine, 18*, 199-204.

McCalister, A., Puska, P., Salonen, J. T., Tuomilehto, J., & Koskela, K. (1982). Theory and action for health promotion: Illustrations from the North Karelia Project. *American Journal of Public Health, 72*, 43-50.

Meade, C. D., & Byrd, J. C. (1989). Patient literacy and the readability of smoking education literature. *American Journal of Public Health, 79*, 204-206.

Milio, N. (1976). A framework for prevention: Changing health-damaging to health-generating life patterns. *American Journal of Public Health, 66*, 435-439.

Nichols, J. L. (1994). Changing public behavior for better health: Is education enough? *American Journal of Preventive Medicine, 10*, 19-22.

Pender, N. J., Walker, S. N., Sechrist, K. R., & Frank-Stromborg, M. (1990). Predicting health-promoting lifestyles in the workplace. *Nursing Research, 39*, 326-332.

Perry, C. L., Luepker, R. V., Murray, D. M., Kurth, C., Mullis, R., Crockett, S., & Jacobs, D. R. J. (1988). Parent involvement with children's health promotion: The Minnesota home team. *American Journal of Public Health, 78*, 1156-1160.

Pill, R. M., & Stott, N. C. H. (1987). The stereotype of "working-class fatalism" and the challenge for primary care health promotion. *Health Education Research: Theory and Practice, 2*, 105-114.

Pless, I. B., & Arsenault, L. (1987). The role of health education in the prevention of injuries to children. *Journal of Social Issues, 43*, 87-103.

Pomerlau, O. F. (1986). Neuroregulators and the reinforcement of smoking. In S. A. Shumaker & N. E. Grunberg (Eds.), Proceedings of the National Working Conference on Smoking Relapse, *Health Psychology, 5*(Supplement), 85-86.

Ratajczak, Z. (1993). Conflicting perspective (sic) on health promotion in the workplace. *Polish Psychological Bulletin, 24*(1), 75-81.

Richards, N. D. (1975). Methods and effectiveness of health education: The past, present and future of social scientific involvement. *Social Science and Medicine, 9*, 141-156.

Shumaker, S. A., & Grunberg, N. E. (Eds.). (1986). Proceedings of the National Working Conference on Smoking Relapse. *Health Psychology, 5*(Supplement) (entire issue).

Simonds, S. K. (1984). Health education. In J. D. Matarazzo, S. M. Weiss, J. A. Herd, N. E. Miller, & S. M. Weiss (Eds.), *Behavioral health: A handbook of health enhancement and disease prevention* (pp. 1223-1229). New York: Wiley.

Simons-Morton, B. G., Parcel, G. S., Baranowski, T., Forthofer, R., & O'Hara, N. M. (1991). Promoting physical activity and a healthful diet among children: Results of a school-based intervention study. *American Journal of Public Health, 81*, 986-991.

Skinner, C. S., Strecher, V. J., & Hospers, H. (1994). Physicians' recommendations for mammography: Do tailored messages make a difference? *American Journal of Public Health, 84*, 43-49.

Sorensen, G., Morris, D. M., Hunt, M. K., Hebert, J. R., Harris, D. R., Stoddard, A., & Ockene, J. K. (1992). Work-site nutrition intervention and employees' dietary habits: The Treatwell program. *American Journal of Public Health, 82*, 877-880.

Stahl, S. M., Lawrie, T., Neill, P., & Kelley, C. (1977). Motivational interventions in community hypertension screening. *American Journal of Public Health, 67*, 345-352.

Stanton, B., Black, R., Engle, P., & Pelto, G. (1992). Theory-driven behavioral intervention research for the control of diarrheal diseases. *Social Science and Medicine, 35*, 1405-1420.

Steuart, G. W. (1993). Social and behavioral change strategies. *Health Education Quarterly, 1993*(Supplement), S113-S135.

Thomas, S. B., Quinn, S. C., Billingsley, A., & Caldwell, C. (1994). The characteristics of northern black churches with community health outreach programs. *American Journal of Public Health, 84*, 575-579.

Vartiainen, E., Fallonen, U., McAlister, A. L., & Puska, P. (1990). Eight-year follow-up results of an adolescent smoking prevention program: The North Karelia Youth Project. *American Journal of Public Health, 80*, 78-79.

West, D. W., Graham, S., Swanson, M., & Wilkinson, G. (1977). Five year follow-up of a smoking withdrawal clinic population. *American Journal of Public Health, 67*, 536-544.

WHO. (1981a). Global strategy of health for all by the year 2000. *Health for all series* (No. 3). Geneva: Author. (Cited by Kolbe, 1988.)

WHO. (1986b). A discussion document on the concept and principles of health promotion. *Health Promotion, 1*(1), 73-76 [Cited by Dines and Cribb, 1993].

Wickizer, T. M., Von Korff, M., Cheadle, A., Maeser, J., Wagner, E. H., Pearson, D., Beery, W., & Psaty, B. M. (1993). Activating communities for health promotion: A process evaluation method. *American Journal of Public Health, 83*, 561-567.

14

Health Behavior Research and School and Youth Health Promotion

Steven H. Kelder, Elizabeth W. Edmundson, and Leslie A. Lytle

INTRODUCTION

Adolescents are frequently considered among the healthiest of all Americans, with nearly the lowest mortality rate of all age groups (Coira, Zill, & Bloom, 1994). They also have morbidity rates for chronic medical and psychiatric disorders that are low in comparison to those in the adult population (Gans, 1990). A closer look reveals that morbidity and mortality rates do not adequately portray the health status of most adolescents. A far greater number of American adolescents are threatened by what has been called "social morbidities," which include unintended pregnancy, sexually transmitted diseases, homicide, suicide, injuries related to violence, and substance abuse. Adolescents also may develop

unhealthful and persistent behavior patterns such as poor dietary intake, low levels of physical activity, and tobacco use. These social morbidities and unhealthful behavior patterns not only threaten adolescents' current physical health status, but also are linked throughout the life span to adult chronic diseases and ultimately to adult mortality.

The task of improving the health status of youth is complex and difficult. Great strides in medical treatments have alleviated many acute and chronic conditions, yet in 1991 it was reported that 46% of black, 40% of Hispanic, and 16% of white children were living in poverty, most with limited access to health care services (U.S. Bureau of the Census, 1992). The task is made more difficult by concurrent problems in educational performance, interrupted family relationships, poor living conditions, and a culture that supports and reinforces many unhealthful behaviors (U.S. Department of Education, 1993). Dramatic improvements in adolescent health are unlikely without global changes in health care provision, improvements in economic conditions, and wide-scale health promotion efforts. While health care provision and economic reform are beyond the scope of this chapter, sev-

Steven H. Kelder • School of Public Health, University of Texas Health Science Center at Houston, Houston, Texas 77225. Elizabeth W. Edmundson • Department of Kinesiology and Health Education, University of Texas at Austin, Austin, Texas 78712. Leslie A. Lytle • Division of Epidemiology, School of Public Health, University of Minnesota, Minneapolis, Minnesota 55454-1015.

Handbook of Health Behavior Research IV: Relevance for Professionals and Issues for the Future, edited by David S. Gochman. Plenum Press, New York, 1997.

eral innovative health promotion strategies have shown promise. This chapter will provide an overview of the rationale for youth health promotion, present a theoretical model for health promotion, and review the youth health promotion literature.

RATIONALE FOR YOUTH HEALTH PROMOTION

For adolescents, health promotion interventions are most often concerned with the modifiable risk factors that are closely related to current or future health outcomes. The Centers for Disease Control and Prevention (CDC) have identi-

fied six behaviors that place adolescents at higher risk for chronic and acute conditions: intentional and unintentional injuries, substance use, early and unprotected sexual activity, tobacco use, poor nutrition, and low levels of physical activity (Kolbe, 1990). Table 1 provides data from the 1993 Youth Risk Behavior Survey, a national representative sample of high school students conducted by the CDC. These data indicate that many youths are engaging in behaviors that place them at risk for health problems.

Although acute risk due to unhealthful behaviors clearly warrants immediate intervention, a great deal of research has been conducted on means of altering future chronic disease risk. Efforts directed toward the early prevention of

Table 1. Percentage of High School Students Who Reported Each Risk Behavior by Gender. United States, Youth Risk Behavior Survey, 1993

Risk behavior	Females (%)	Males (%)
Rarely or never used safety belts	14.3	23.8
Rarely or never used motorcycle helmets[a]	39.0	40.4
Rarely or never used bicycle helmets[b]	93.6	92.2
Rode with a driver who had been drinking alcohol[c]	34.5	36.3
Carried a weapon[c]	9.2	34.3
In a physical fight[d]	31.7	51.2
Made a suicide plan[d]	22.9	15.3
Attempted suicide[d]	12.5	5.0
Current cigarette use[c]	31.2	29.8
Smokeless tobacco use[c]	2.0	20.4
Current alcohol use[c]	45.9	50.1
Five or more drinks of alcohol on one occasion[c]	26.0	33.7
Current marijuana use[c]	14.6	20.6
Current cocaine use[c]	1.4	2.3
Ever had sexual intercourse	50.2	55.6
Four or more sex partners during lifetime	15.0	22.3
Currently sexually active (sex in past 3 months)	37.5	37.5
Condom use during last sexual intercourse[e]	46.0	59.2
Birth control pill use during last sexual intercourse[e]	22.3	14.7
Ate two or more fruits and vegetables[f]	13.0	17.6
Ate two or fewer servings of high-fat food[f]	75.6	57.6
Engaged in vigorous physical activity on 3 or more of past 7 days	56.2	74.7

[a]Among students who rode a motorcycle at least once during the 12 months preceding the survey.
[b]Among students who rode a bicycle at least once during the 12 months preceding the survey.
[c]One or more times during the 30 days preceding the survey.
[d]One or more times during the 12 months preceding the survey.
[e]Among students who have had sex during the 3 months preceding the survey.
[f]During the day preceding the survey.
Source: Kann et al. (1995).

adult chronic diseases have typically focused on the modification of health behaviors such as physical activity, dietary intake, and cigarette smoking. The rationale behind this type of youth health promotion is that (1) a certain proportion of children and adolescents are at excess physiological and behavioral risk; (2) the development of physiological risk factors begins early in life and tracks from childhood into adulthood; (3) the development of physiological risk depends largely upon the initiation of health-compromising behaviors that also track into adulthood; and (4) primary prevention can be achieved through the modification of behaviors related to physiological risk factors, before behavior patterns are more fully established and resistant to change (Perry, Kelder, & Klepp, 1994a,b).

SOCIAL COGNITIVE THEORY: A MODEL OF YOUTH HEALTH PROMOTION

Many models developed to explain or predict health behaviors provide useful constructs with which to design interventions (Petraits, Flay, & Miller, 1995). While it is beyond the scope of this chapter to review these theories in great detail, it is worth noting that social cognitive theory (SCT) is often cited in the youth health promotion literature as the predominant model used in the design of successful health promotion programs (Bandura, 1986; Baranowski, Perry, & Parcel, 1997). SCT addresses both the psychosocial dynamics that underlie health behavior and the methods of promoting behavior change while emphasizing cognitive processes and their effect on behavior. Human behavior is explained by SCT in terms of a triadic, dynamic, and reciprocal model in which behavior, social–environmental influences, and personal factors (such as personality and affect) all interact. An individual's behavior is uniquely determined by these factors.

The determinants of behavior have been further elucidated as (1) *social–environmental* factors, which are aspects of the environment that support, permit, or discourage engagement in a particular behavior, including influential role models (including peers), situational contexts, social norms for behavior, social support from family and friends, and specific opportunities; (2) *behavioral factors*, such as existing behavioral repertoire, and behavioral intentions, capabilities, or coping skills; and (3) *personal factors*, which are particular personal dispositions and cognitive processes that increase or decrease the likelihood of a person's engaging in a given behavior, including level of knowledge, personal values, attitudes, beliefs, and self-efficacy (Perry, Stone, et al., 1990). Among the crucial personal factors are the individual's capabilities to symbolize the meanings of behavior, to foresee the outcomes of given behaviors, to learn by observing others, to self-determine or self-regulate behavior, and to reflect and analyze experience. These ideas have been particularly valuable in designing effective health education programs.

In the development of school health promotion programs, great emphasis is currently placed on multicomponent interventions. Approaches include interventions that address not only behavioral change at the individual level, but also changes within the environment designed to support behavioral change (Parcel, Simons-Morton, & Kolbe, 1988). In the translation from theory to programmatic components, several intervention strategies for youth health promotion are being developed and studied. Classroom curriculum, school environment, parental education, and community reinforcement are examples of strategies currently under evaluation or being implemented.

Curriculum

Most traditional programs are based on the assumption that if students clearly understand the negative consequences of certain health behaviors, they will make the rational decision not to engage in them. During the 1980s, it became clearer from health behavior research that adolescents' decisions to engage in high-risk behaviors also involve social influences and normative expectations, not just knowledge. It has been hypothesized that resistance to the social pressures to engage in health-compromising behaviors such as tobacco use will be greater if the student has been "inoculated" or has developed specific behavioral skills in advance to counter such pressures. Likewise, students with specific healthful eating, physical activity, or conflict resolution skills would be expected to eat better, exercise more often, and resolve conflict peaceably.

The new generation of health promotion programs have successfully incorporated developmentally appropriate strategies such as the importance of peers in adolescent life, particularly the extent to which adolescents are affected by the perceived norms and behaviors of their peers (Klepp, Halper, & Perry, 1986). This body of research has demonstrated that teenagers tend to respond more favorably to their peers' encouragement to avoid drug use, delay intercourse, or use condoms than to the same messages delivered by teachers or other adults.

Changes in the school organization offer powerful means of modifying the school environment and culture to support health promotion goals. Research has identified organizational factors such as policy and practices, organizational mission, and human resource development as important instruments for institutional change (Parcel et al., 1988). Examples of policy actions include school-wide smoking bans, nutritional content standards of school food service (in both purchasing and food preparation), parental fines for their children's fighting, and athletic eligibility criteria.

Policy-level intervention calls for the creation of local coalitions and planning councils to define, coordinate, and implement health promotion programs. Ideally, teachers, administrators, parents, and other interested citizens would participate in discussions to increase their awareness of the importance of school health promo-

tion and be given guidance on how to establish a policy in their schools. This process includes the following steps: (1) obtain commitment, (2) form an advisory committee, (3) gather information, (4) develop the policy, (5) plan the implementation strategy, (6) communicate the policy, (7) implement the new policy, and (8) evaluate policy effectiveness (Kelder, Parcel, & Perry, 1995). These activities are theoretically consistent; i.e., the school environment reinforces the norms, skills, and behaviors emphasized by the health curriculum.

Parent Education

Parents are perhaps the most potent and significant health role models for their children (Coleman, 1991; Nader et al., 1989). They also provide specific opportunities for or barriers to adolescent health behaviors such as determining the foods that are purchased, access to physical activity, selection of school and neighborhood, and alcohol use at home. Health behavior research in youth health promotion supports the inclusion of parents through home learning to increase program efficacy (Perry, Kelder, & Komro, 1992). In these programs, parents are given activities to complete with their children that typically include parenting tip sheets, games, or parent interviews. These activities are designed to increase communication between parents and children and to reinforce at home the messages learned at school.

In addition, several studies have demonstrated the importance of parents in adolescent life. Children's attitudes about risk behaviors such as sexual initiation (Treboux & Busch-Rossnagel, 1990), condom use (Schaalma, Kok, & Peters, 1993), and drug experimentation (Jurich, Polson, Jurich, & Bates, 1985) have been found to be positively related to their parents' attitudes about these behaviors. Parents are important role models prior to substance use onset and can be useful allies in drug prevention programs. After students begin to use alcohol and drugs, however, peers appear to exert greater influence (Kandel & Andrews, 1987). Parents maintain their influence if they exercise some control in the determination of their child's peer group, given that group norms often dominate health choices (Brown, Mounts, Lamborn, & Steinberg, 1993). In this sense, parents can directly and indirectly influence their child's health behaviors.

Community Reinforcement

Although schools are efficient and appropriate organizations for implementing prevention programs, outside support and reinforcement for these programs appears to be necessary for sustained change. There are several reasons for considering health promotion efforts that are community-wide (Perry, Kelder, & Komro, 1992). First, high-risk students, those most likely to use substances or engage in early sexual activity, are also most likely to drop out of school prior to graduation, and therefore might be missed with a school-based program. These same high-risk students may also be more alienated from messages that are delivered at school.

Second, the social influences that affect high-risk behaviors hold sway predominantly outside schools. The direct modeling of healthful or unhealthful behaviors and the support for or against these behaviors come from family members, other peers, adults in the community, and mass media images. A consistent preventive message from these various sources would arguably be optimal.

Third, community policies that regulate the opportunities and barriers for health behaviors, as well as the normative climate of a community, all appear to affect adolescents.

Finally, in some communities, the school is the safest place for children to go, and many do not want to leave school and go home. For these children, an expansion of health promotion efforts into the local housing project, community center, or parks and recreation areas is warranted.

EFFECTIVENESS OF INTERVENTIONS

Substance Use Prevention

The earliest drug prevention programs were founded on the premise that increased knowledge would deter adolescent drug use (Goodstadt, 1978). This model typically made use of fear arousal or "scare tactics" as well as messages with moral overtones. The exaggerated claims about the negative and immoral effects of drugs (e.g., films such as "Reefer Madness") frequently did more to undermine the credibility of adults and authority than to deter drug use. Subsequent programs, commonly called "affective education," focused on individual deficiencies such as a lack of self-esteem or undeveloped values. These programs attempted to remediate psychological factors that place adolescents at risk for drug use. Research over more than a dozen years evaluating knowledge- and affective-based approaches suggested that these approaches produced little effect on substance use behaviors and may even have encouraged experimentation (Bruvold, 1993; Hansen, 1992; Tobler, 1992).

During the 1970s, it became increasingly understood from health behavior research that social factors in favor of experimenting with tobacco are of greater importance to adolescents than the well-known consequences. Evans and Raines (1982) utilized social psychological principles to explain the etiology of substance use and focused prevention efforts on the social causes of these behaviors, rather than on personal attitudes and knowledge. Evans and Raines's program was based on social inoculation theory (McGuire, 1968), which hypothesized that resistance to the social pressures to use tobacco and other drugs would be greater if the person had been inoculated or had developed arguments in advance to counter such pressures. The work of Evans and Raines provided an important foundation and shift in direction for current prevention programs and is frequently referred to as the "social influences" type of prevention.

School-Based Smoking Prevention. Most of the studies that have applied the social influences model to smoking prevention have done so with 6th through 8th grade students and have demonstrated a significant impact on smoking onset rates. Several comprehensive reviews of the smoking prevention literature, including several meta-analyses, have reported positive intervention group findings in smoking onset when compared with an equivalent or randomly assigned control group (Bruvold, 1993; Pentz et al., 1989; Tobler, 1992). In these studies, the interventions were found to produce reductions in regular (i.e., weekly) smoking ranging from 43% to 60%, with maintenance of these effects generally 1–3 years postintervention. Unfortunately, the effects of the social influences programs appear to diminish over time, suggesting that additional booster education programs are needed during middle adolescence (Botvin, Baker, Dusenbury, Tortu, & Botvin, 1990; Flay et al., 1989). This need is particularly evident in the context of a multibillion-dollar advertising and promotion effort by the tobacco and alcohol industries.

In 1987, a National Cancer Institute advisory panel of expert smoking prevention researchers attempted to achieve consensus on the essential elements for school-based smoking prevention programs (Glynn, 1989). The panel concluded that sufficient data and experience existed to make the following eight recommendations considered necessary for successful school-based smoking prevention programs: (1) Give smoking prevention at least five classroom sessions in each of two years of junior high school and booster sessions in senior high school; (2) include information about the social influences of tobacco onset, short-term effects, and refusal skills; (3) fit the program into existing curricula; (4) start the program during the transition from elementary to middle school or junior high; (5) involve students in presenting the program; (6) encourage parent participation; (7) train teachers thoroughly—ideally for a full day; and (8) use a prevention program that fits with established community norms and needs so that it will be adopted readily.

School-Based Alcohol and Drug Use Prevention. Literature reviewing the impact of educational programs designed to delay the onset of alcohol and marijuana use among adolescents has often concluded that there is little evidence or contradictory evidence regarding the effectiveness of primary prevention programs. Hansen (1992) reviewed substance use prevention programs published between 1980 and 1990 and classified them according to curriculum content. He concluded that comprehensive and social influences programs were most successful in preventing the onset of substance use compared to other intervention techniques such as information/values clarification, affective, and alternative programs. Comprehensive programs go beyond the usual spectrum of prevention activities and include decision-making and life skills training.

The reported impact of the social influences model on adolescent marijuana use has been mixed, and continued intervention improvement and replication is necessary (Hansen, 1992). Alcohol use onset has proved difficult to delay, although modest reductions in the prevalence of alcohol use due to preventive efforts have been demonstrated (Botvin, 1990; Tobler, 1992). The overall implication of these studies is that students who are equipped with skills to resist the social influences to consume alcohol may still choose to use given the widespread social acceptance of alcohol.

One program, Drug Abuse Resistance Education (DARE), is noteworthy because it is one of the most widely used drug education programs in the country, having been implemented in 49 states, and is endorsed by the U.S. Department of Justice. DARE is a 17-session social influences and affective education curriculum in which law enforcement officers teach the program at school. Although early results were positive (Dejong, 1987), a large-scale study found no significant behavioral effects, although positive impact was demonstrated on several mediating variables (health consequences, media knowledge, assertiveness, attitudes toward drugs) (Ringwalt, Ennett, & Holt, 1991).

Community-Level Substance Use Prevention. Several smoking and drug use prevention programs have gone beyond the classroom into the larger school and community environments. The Minnesota Heart Health Program (Perry, Kelder, Murray, & Klepp, 1992), Finland North Karelia Project (Vartiainen, Pallonen, McAlister, & Puska, 1990), and Vermont School and Mass Media Project (Flynn et al., 1994) provide further support for the importance of community-level interventions. The first two studies included smoking prevention programs embedded within a larger heart health program that emphasized smoking cessation, healthy eating, and physical fitness for all community members. The Vermont study compared school plus mass media programs to school alone. Long-term results indicate that smoking rates throughout the follow-up period were substantially lower in the intervention communities. The risk of being a smoker in all of these intervention communities was slightly less than half that in the reference communities.

Project Northland (Perry et al., 1993) and the Midwestern Prevention Project (Pentz et al., 1989) are two community-wide substance use prevention programs that include (1) school-based education (using a peer-led social influences model), (2) parental education and organization, (3) mass media, (4) organized community efforts, and (5) changes in school and local government policy. By involving the community, both programs attempt to create environmental support for the changes made within the school-based component, thus changing the social norm of drug use. Results from both of these studies indicate that onset rates for alcohol and marijuana are significantly lower in the intervention communities (Johnson et al., 1990; Perry et al., 1996).

Nutrition and Physical Education

As in the case of smoking and substance use prevention, a multitude of educational programs have been developed to change the diet and physical activity patterns of children. The rationale behind programs of this type includes the substantial prevalence and burden of disease in adults and mass exposure to elevated risk factors beginning early in life (Strong & Kelder, 1996; Webber et al., 1995). A substantial portion of current and future physiological risk can be found in heath behaviors and hence is modifiable. Hyperlipidemia, sedentary lifestyle, obesity, and hypertension all appear in children, and all are associated with consumption of high-fat and sodium-rich diets, overconsumption of calories, and lack of physical activity.

School-Based Nutrition Education. Adolescence, more than any other time of life, requires greater caloric intake to accommodate the rapid pubertal growth spurt. For this reason, many parents and pediatricians have been more concerned with under- than with overconsumption of foods. Despite this emphasis, however, population rates of adolescent obesity have been increasing (Gortmaker, Dietz, & Sobol, 1987), and most school-age children consume a diet similar to that of adults, characterized by high intakes of sodium, refined carbohydrates, and animal protein and fat, and low intakes of potassium, complex carbohydrates, and vegetable protein and fat (Webber et al., 1995). Because dietary habits are formed during childhood and unhealthful dietary habits pose significant risk for acute and chronic diseases, research efforts have been directed toward modifying young people's unhealthful eating habits (Kelder, Perry, Klepp, & Lytle, 1994).

Much of the early research in this area has been focused on knowledge-based school programs. These programs have covered a variety of topics, such as the role of nutrients in the body, food sources of nutrients, food production and processing, and healthful eating in general. Early studies reported positive changes in student knowledge and attitudes regarding healthful eating, but generally failed to demonstrate improvement in adolescent eating behavior or positive changes in physiological risk patterns (Contento, Manning, & Shannon, 1992).

Neglected in the knowledge-based studies was consideration of the multiple factors in the etiology of eating behaviors. Food habits appear to be influenced by the interaction between individuals and their social and physical environment, not simply on knowledge of the healthfulness of foods. Although health behavior research on the development of food preferences is not conclusive, some evidence suggests that mere exposure to a wide variety of foods tends to increase preference and consumption (Rozin, 1984). In addition, a child's family and immediate cultural environment define the foods that a young person is exposed to as well as the skills in food selection and preparation that are established. At home, at school, and in the larger environment, adult role models instruct children through their own behaviors that food choices are based on habits learned or reinforcements received, not on nutrition knowledge, or are used as a method of coping with negative affective states. Finally, the mass media permeate communities with messages about food and eating patterns through both print and electronic channels, and specifically target youth as consumers and as influential members in food-related decisions. The amount of time children attend to the media has been relatively constant for the past three decades, yet the number of food advertisements has steadily increased, most promoting high-fat or calorie-laden foods (Sylvester, Achterberg, & Williams, 1995).

Several articles detailed the research efforts during the 1980s, sponsored by the National Heart, Lung, and Blood Institute and the National Cancer Institute, which tested components of the social cognitive theory model of intervention (Contento et al., 1992; Stone, Perry, & Luepker, 1989). These programs focused on the knowledge, skills, and behaviors needed to improve food quality or nutrient intake and maintain a healthful diet. The interventions ranged from 4 to 20 sessions involving a variety of grades, peer leaders, and parental involvement and reported favorable results for knowledge, attitudes, and skills, with modest improvements on behavior

and physiological measures. In addition, positive behavioral and physiological results have been achieved with the Know Your Body program. A comprehensive school health promotion program for kindergarten through 6th grade with intervention components incorporating several SCT concepts, Know Your Body is notable for its intervention effects with inner city minority children (Resnicow, Cross, & Wynder, 1993).

Several community-level health promotion interventions took the SCT model a step further and reported modest but encouraging results. In the Oslo Youth Study, significantly lower blood cholesterol levels were observed among both genders (Tell & Vellar, 1988). In the North Karelia Youth Study, fat consumption was reduced for both genders, and total cholesterol was reduced for females (Puska et al., 1982). Finally, results from the Class of 1989 study of the Minnesota Heart Health Program suggested that multicomponent interventions such as behavioral education in schools coupled with community-wide health promotion strategies can produce modest but lasting improvement in adolescent knowledge and choices of heart-healthy foods and less frequent food-salting practices (Kelder, Perry, Lytle, & Klepp, 1995).

School Food Service.   School food service also plays an important part in overall nutrition, directly affecting the nutrition of children through the daily provision of an estimated 27 million lunches and 3 million breakfasts. Lytle, Kelder, and Snyder (1993) reviewed the school food service research and found that most research focused on attempts to reduce total fat, saturated fat, cholesterol, or sodium in school cafeterias. These studies showed a trend toward being able to reduce fat and sodium without incurring resistance from students or prohibitive cost increases, but the reductions most often failed to meet recommended food intake guidelines.

A report reviewing the literature on school-based nutrition programs identified six elements of successful programs. Such programs (1) are behaviorally based and theory driven; (2) incorporate family involvement in programs for elementary children; (3) include self-assessment of eating patterns in programs for middle and senior high school children; (4) include behavior change programs that intervene in the school environment; (5) include behavior change programs that intervene in the larger community; and (6) provide more in-class instruction time to increase program impact (Lytle & Achterburg, 1995). The authors also recommended five broad-reaching objectives to improve the diet of American children: (1) School, school districts, and local, state, and federal governments need to commit to comprehensive, school-based nutrition education; (2) multiple instructional techniques should be included in nutrition education; (3) diet change for children should be viewed from an environmental perspective including the family, the community, the media, and the food industry; (4) federal and state governments must develop and promote a system to disseminate effective nutrition education materials; and (5) there must be evaluation of the effectiveness of national and statewide nutrition education and other behavior change programs for children. Similar recommendations can be found in a joint position by the Society for Nutrition Education, American Dietetic Association, and School Food Service Associations (Olson, 1995).

Physical Activity. Physical activity is important for the current and future health of youth. Among adults, physical activity is inversely related to coronary artery disease, hypertension, non-insulin-dependent diabetes mellitus, depression, colon and reproductive cancers, osteoporotic fractures, and total mortality (Baranowski et al., 1992). Physical activity is related to childhood obesity, and several studies have suggested that children and adolescents are not engaging in physical activity of sufficient length and intensity to improve their cardiovascular fitness. Ross (1994) reported data from the National Children and Youth Fitness Studies (conducted in 1984 and 1986) indicating that 59% of 5th–12th graders engaged in "appropriate physical activ-

ity" (defined as activity involving large muscle groups requiring 60% of cardiovascular capacity at least 3 times per week for at least 20 minutes). The same study reported that nearly all 5th- and 6th-grade students are enrolled in physical education (PE). Rates of enrollment decline with each successive grade, however, so that by 12th grade, only 56% of boys and 49% of girls take PE. Unfortunately, even when students are enrolled in PE, enrollment is no guarantee that they will be engaging in physical conditioning activities. Parcel et al. (1987) observed 3rd- and 4th-grade children during PE and reported that 32.8% of the available time was devoted to management and organization, 41% to games, sports, free play, and skills, and 17% to fitness activities, of which 6% was activities that were potentially aerobic.

Simons-Morton, Parcel, O'Hara, Blair, and Pate (1988) reviewed the physical education literature. While nearly all studies had only limited follow-up duration, they reported a variety of positive outcomes, including improvements in maximum physical working capacity, performance on distance runs, and increases in minutes of elevated heart rates during PE and during the total day. Typically, the activities of these programs included warm-up, running that was progressively longer over the school year, and a variety of aerobic activities. The studies in this review largely measured fitness variables and are unable to answer questions about physical activity outside school or after the completion of intervention.

More recent physical education programs have moved beyond sports-oriented or mandatory physical training and have incorporated new concepts made available through health behavior research. The newer behavior-oriented programs are designed to increase the amount of moderate to vigorous physical activity that children obtain during PE (Perry, Stone, et al., 1990). These programs often include (1) introductory/warm-up activities, (2) lesson focus, (3) fitness development, and (4) cool-down activities. The goal is to provide students with the opportunity to experience and practice physical activity that may be carried over into other times of the day and maintained later in life (Parcel, Simons-Morton, O'Hara, Baranowski, & Wilson, 1989).

Sallis and McKenzie (1992) also reviewed the literature on physical education and concluded that physical education programs have produced short-term improvements in physiological and behavioral outcomes, while classroom-based programs have not. Generally, a variety of learning activities are conducted in classroom programs, including modeling, monitoring, goal setting, contracting, skills training, and reinforcement. National Heart, Lung and Blood youth prevention interventions have indicated little long-term impact on physical activity behavior and modest positive short-term knowledge and physical activity outcomes (Stone et al., 1989). In addition, the Class of 1989 study reported modest improvements in physical activity using a classroom-based SCT approach (Kelder, Perry, & Klepp, 1993).

Sallis and Patrick (1994) issued two general population guidelines to improve youth physical activity. First, all adolescents should be physically active daily, or nearly every day, as part of play, games, transportation, physical education, or planned exercise, in the context of family, school, and community activities. Adolescents are encouraged to incorporate physical activity into their lifestyles by doing such things as walking upstairs and walking or riding a bicycle for errands. Second, adolescents should engage in 3 or more sessions per week of activities lasting 20 minutes that require moderate to vigorous levels of exertion.

Ross and Hohn (1994) issued a similar, but more specific, set of youth physical activity recommendations, among which are: The promotion of lifelong physical activity and fitness should be the primary goal of physical education, and PE curricula should be balanced so as to function effectively in the psychomotor, cognitive, and affective domains. Additionally, professional preparation programs should prepare future teachers of physical education to develop balanced curricula and to deliver instruction that

is effective in all three educational domains. Finally, PE programs should meet the needs of all youngsters, in particular those who have special needs and are "low-fit."

The culmination of the research investigations on nutrition and physical activity conducted during the 1980s was the Child and Adolescent Trial for Cardiovascular Health (CATCH) (Perry, Stone, et al., 1990). CATCH was a randomized, multicentered trial funded by The National Heart, Lung and Blood Institute and designed to assess the effects of a school- and family-based intervention for promoting healthful behaviors in elementary-school children to reduce their risk of cardiovascular disease (1987–1994). The interventions comprehensively applied the SCT model, including classroom curricula and school environmental modifications related to food consumption, physical activity, and tobacco use, as well as family- and home-based programs to complement the school-based activities. Main outcomes indicated that the CATCH project was able to safely modify and to maintain the health content of school lunches, increase moderate to vigorous physical activity in physical education classes, and improve nutrient intakes in healthy and ethnically diverse schoolchildren over a 3-year period (Luepker et al., 1996).

Sexuality Education

Sexuality education is unequivocally the most controversial of adolescent health promotion programs. The empirical evidence on adolescent reproductive health problems is undisputed by scientists and health professionals; in fact, these concerns have garnered political and community support for a call to action. Why have these programs generated an outpouring of social debate and political opposition? The disagreement and controversy center on exactly how to go about improving the disconcerting statistics on adolescent sexual health and sexual behavior.

In the United States, the average age of menarche is 12.5 years, and the development of secondary sex characteristics occurs within a corresponding window of time, usually during early to middle adolescence. Male fertility and sexual development also occur during adolescence. Essentially, between the ages of 11 and 16 years, adolescents experience a cascade of sexual development dominated by biological changes that must be interpreted within a cultural context (Alan Guttmacher Institute, 1994). That cultural context is infused with the psychosocial influences of parents and parental figures, peers, technology, increasing juvenile violence, and media-popularized role models. Sexuality education programs, grounded in health behavior research models, face the unique challenge of recognizing the diversity of sexual experiences among adolescents. Commonly included objectives are learning respectful and loving ways of experiencing intimacy without intercourse and awareness with acceptance of responsibility for the outcomes of sexual intimacy.

At the end of the 20th century, many parents and sexuality education programs (especially abstinence-only programs) indirectly advise adolescents to delay the onset of intercourse by about 12 years after they reach biological capacity for reproduction (Alan Guttmacher Institute, 1994). In 1890, the average time between puberty and marriage for women was 7.2 years; three to four generations later, in 1988, it was 11.8 years. Men have also delayed marriage in the last part of the 20th century; the time between first ejaculation and marriage was 12.5 years in 1988. Such a delay is unprecedented in American society, and the scientific evidence suggests that many adolescents do not wait for marriage to have intercourse. Indeed, not only are the majority of teens refusing to delay the onset of intercourse, but also many of them engage in unprotected intercourse. One million teenage women become pregnant every year, and 3 million teenagers each year contract a sexually transmitted disease (STD) (Alan Guttmacher Institute, 1994).

In direct contrast to sexual development information grounded in scientific integrity, school board members and legislators at the national, state, and local levels are the targets of intensive misinformation campaigns sponsored by various groups that oppose sexuality education (Kantor, 1992/1993; SIECUS, 1993). This misinformation is published by ultraconservative groups that describe the years between childhood and late adolescence as a "latency period," a time when youth are not concerned with sexual issues (Kantor & Haffner, 1995). Regardless, the biological, behavioral, and psychological evidence overwhelmingly supports the acknowledgement of teens as sexual beings (Alan Guttmacher Institute, 1994; Department of Health and Human Services [DHHS]/CDC, 1995; Dryfoos, 1990).

The process of collecting valid data on such a sensitive and private topic as sexual behavior has faced political challenges that most other areas of health promotion never encounter. In fact, since 1980, the obstacle faced by researchers trying to obtain valid estimates of sexual behavior among adolescents has been federal and state opposition—the result, again, of intense political lobbying by conservative and far-right groups opposed to making reproductive health information available to adolescents (Yarber, 1992).

The benchmark measures of adolescent sexual health are ever having had intercourse, pregnancy rates, and incidence/prevalence of STDs. Many teens are sexually active before they graduate from high school. Nationally, more than 53% of high school students report having had sexual intercourse (Surveillance United States, 1993). Not surprisingly, the likelihood of first intercourse increases with age. According to the CDC, pregnancy rates among adolescents age 15–19 remained about the same between 1980 and 1990 (approximately 11% annually). While pregnancy rates have remained stable, however, live birth rates have increased between 1980 and 1990, with the greatest increase among 15- to 17-year-old females (Spitz, 1993).

Sexual expression by adolescents generates alarm among health professionals because of the potential negative outcomes associated with the risks of unprotected sexual intercourse, such as

STDs, including AIDS, and premature or unintended pregnancy. The most prevalent STD among adolescents is chlamydia, which is a major cause of pelvic inflammatory disease and infertility (DHHS/CDC, 1995). AIDS is the sixth leading cause of death among young people ages 15–24 (DHHS/PHS, 1995). Moreover, the percentage of AIDS cases among women increased dramatically in the first five years of the 1990s, due in part to changes in the clinical definition and chronic underreporting during the 1980s. According to the CDC, the percentage of cases from heterosexual contact rose by 21% from 1990 to 1991 (CDC, 1994b). The CDC cautions that women, especially women of color, and adolescents are the groups experiencing the fastest increases in AIDS cases.

School-Based Sexuality Education. School-based sexuality education programs, most of which are designed to help teens avoid early pregnancy and STDs, have been under vicious attack by conservative political groups during the past decade (Yarber, 1992). As a result, adolescents receive, on average, no more than 5 hours of instruction on birth control and 6 hours of instruction on STDs between grades 7 and 12 (Alan Guttmacher Institute, 1994). Undoubtedly, this scant exposure to crucial information and skills training is reflected in the unchanging pregnancy rates, increasing STD rates, and research results indicating that adolescents do not perceive themselves as being at risk for STDs, including AIDS (Walter, Vaughan, Ragin, Cohall, & Kasen, 1994).

Holtzman et al. (1992) conducted a national survey of public school districts and discovered that the teaching of HIV prevention skills, when the district required that they be taught, was usually implemented in the upper grades. Of primary concern to Holtzman et al. (1992) was that delay of instruction in HIV prevention skills until after many teens have become sexually active forfeits the immediate benefit of instruction on condom use and, even more, the benefit of methods of sexual expression other than inter-

course (i.e., how to express feelings yet avoid intercourse). The results indicate that the median number of hours of annual HIV instruction provided to students ranged between 2 and 4 for all public school districts that participated in this national study. This amount of instruction falls short of the amount of instructional time allocated to other health behavior programs, such as smoking and substance use prevention.

Klein, Goodson, Serrins, Edmundson, and Evans (1994) conducted a content analysis of ten nationally available curricula/curricula guidelines and reported similar deficits. Instruction on topics and skills related to sexuality within society and culture as well as to sexual behaviors was essentially absent from all curricula save one. Gender and sexual orientation bias were quite prevalent; indeed, none of the materials reviewed provided any instruction regarding disease prevention in reference to homosexuality. The evaluation did detect an emphasis on personal skill development among the curricula. Unfortunately, most of the instruction was limited to "saying no." Topic-specific curricula, curricula that intentionally target one or two sexual behaviors (e.g., pregnancy prevention or HIV prevention), tended to provide realistic strategies and adequate depth of instruction for skill development.

Part of the answer to this overall lack of improvement in adolescent sexual health and health-related behaviors is the content, quality, and quantity of sexuality education provided. Kirby and colleagues have done yeoman service for the entire field of adolescent health by pioneering research on the effects and effectiveness of sexuality education (Kirby, Barth, Leland, & Fetro, 1991; Kirby et al., 1994). This body of work represents the results of health behavior research on many sexuality education programs, with several informative narratives on the recent history of sex education, as well as recommendations for the structure, content, and evaluation of programs. In particular, Kirby describes the primary features of each generation of curricula and highlights the features of more recently implemented programs that have been based upon health behavior research. These programs have successfully reduced sexual risk behavior among teens.

Although many programs, including those that comprise the recent fourth generation of curricula, have emphasized skill building in areas such as communications and assertiveness, Kirby's extensive review of the effects of such programs revealed that very little information is being collected about the quality of many of these interventions. In fact, there is such a diverse range in the quality and type of programs being implemented that the results measuring the impact on sexual behavior are mixed.

Nevertheless, several features of effective programs were identified in these reviews. First, effective programs were more likely to have a narrow focus, specifically on the reduction of sexual risk taking, with a small number of behavioral goals such as delaying the initiation of intercourse. These programs did not explore other sexuality issues such as parenting or gender identity. Second, programs were more effective when strategies and content were based on health behavior research generated by social cognitive theories. Third, experiential activities were used to demonstrate basic accurate information about the risks of unprotected intercourse and how to avoid engaging in unprotected sex. The instruction emphasized active learning methods and utilized peer educational techniques rater than teacher lectures. Fourth, effective programs directly addressed the interaction of social influences and the media upon sexual decisions. Fifth, reinforcement of social norms against unprotected sex, in conjunction with modeling and practice of communication and negotiating skills, were significant components of the effective programs. These strategies are consistent with those mentioned in other domains of effective health behavior research. The overwhelming evidence is that sexuality education does not increase sexual activity. The programs either delayed the onset of sexual intercourse or had no effect at all on intercourse but did increase contraceptive use among students who were sexually active at the onset of the intervention.

Violence Prevention

Violence among America's youth has emerged as a significant public health problem for which few effective prevention methods have been found. Young people are disproportionately represented among both perpetrators and victims of violence (Earls, Cairns, & Mercy, 1993; Mercy, Rosenberg, Powell, Broome, & Roper, 1993), with the average age of both groups growing younger in recent years. Arrest rates for homicide, rape, robbery, and aggravated assault in the United States peak among older adolescents and young adults. Homicide is the second leading cause of death for Americans of ages 15–34 and is the leading cause of death for young African-Americans. In addition, persons of ages 12–24 face the highest risk of nonfatal assault in our society.

The high rates of violence and aggression during adolescence are associated with behavior patterns and risk factors that are common to adolescent development (Pepler & Slaby, 1994). Although minority youth are particularly vulnerable to violence, the gross disparities observed between black and white mortality rates in the United States generally disappear once the equally gross disparities of socioeconomic status are accounted for (Centerwall, 1995). Other factors include gender, previous delinquent behavior, alcohol and drug use, conflict with parents, patterns of parental supervision, extended exposure to mass media, racial and ethnic discrimination, and pubertal development (Hill, Soriana, Chen, & LaFromboise, 1994). In addition, the school context may create a milieu conducive to aggression. Large classes, overcrowded schools, underskilled instructors, and poor discipline management all contribute to aggression and anger. Finally, although schools contribute to aggressive behavior, school is the safest place for many inner city students to be, since they have to dodge drug peddlers and gang conflicts on their way to and from school. Attention to these developmental and contextual factors is necessary in order to implement effective interventions.

A difficulty of interpreting the effectiveness literature is the broad range of violence definitions that demand similar and different programmatic responses. A conference for school counseling practitioners identified six ways in which violence is affecting youth today: (1) domestic violence, (2) dating violence, (3) sexual harassment, (4) childhood sexual abuse, (5) family alcoholism, and (6) television violence (Harvard University, 1993). Because the various forms of violence are diverse, prevention programs are abundant, vary widely in their theoretical perspective, and are created and carried out by sometimes mutually exclusive professional and academic disciplines. Although many efforts have been made to address violent injury, relatively few careful evaluations have been conducted, and few of those have demonstrated effectiveness. Tolan and Guerra (1994) conducted an exhaustive review of the literature and concluded (p. 46): "There has been relatively limited sound empirical program evaluation that permits judgment of effects. There is also a considerable gap between the most commonly used programs and the most frequently evaluated ones.... most approaches have not been well evaluated and the effects shown must be qualified and enthusiasm for given approaches tempered." In many cases, informal records of teacher or student enthusiasm about a program, individual success stories, or program longevity have been the only basis on which to judge program effects.

Program Components. Tolan and Guerra (1994) offered a practical perspective on the strong points of psychotherapy, behavior modification, cognitive–behavioral interventions, and social skills training as educational methods that may be used to address components of violent behavior at the individual level, as well as insight into other contextual dynamics of intervention. Similarly, other experts have discussed

the nature of an effective intervention as comprehensive or ecological in its orientation, consisting of prevention/intervention efforts across settings, individuals, and developmental levels (Larson, 1994). Applications of these strategies are incorporated in educational and social agency violence prevention programs, often as both peer mediation and conflict resolution curricula.

Peer Mediation. Enlisting adolescent peer models in lieu of adult authority figures to change youth norms is a widely used approach to curbing violence and is often adopted in conjunction with conflict resolution curricula and life and social skills training (Center for the Study & Prevention of Violence, 1995; National Center for Injury Prevention and Control, 1993; U.S. Department of Justice, 1994). Recognizing that children in alienating school environments may reject authority figures and instead ally themselves with other children for moral support, peer mediation programs are designed to empower children to help each other. Mediators may be called on directly by school administrators or teachers to negotiate conflicts among their classmates, they may assist younger age groups on or off campus as mentors, or they may simply be information carriers who, trained in prosocial behavior, change the norm among their own peer groups through modeling. The inclusion of peer role models is a significant component of current violence intervention programs.

Conflict Resolution Curricula. Conflict resolution curricula, which vary in length and number of lessons, often operate to improve behavioral indicators that are predictive of adult antisocial behavior. These behaviors translate into skills deficits that typically include a lack of empathy, impulse control, and problem-solving, assertiveness, and anger management skills. Most curricula include lessons on conflict identification and anticipation, anger management, ownership of emotions and behaviors, recognition of impulsive actions, and identification of choices and consequences of actions. Popular classroom techniques include video production and viewing, role playing, didactic presentations, and puppetry, which are often used to provide a basis for self-reflective discussion and antisocial behavior recognition and analysis. These activities are designed to teach adolescents about their risks of being injured or killed by violence, how to recognize and cope with anger, and how negative consequences of fighting usually outweigh any positives. Students are usually encouraged to find ways to deal with their anger and interpersonal conflicts other than with physical force and are provided opportunities to role play hypothetical conflict situations.

School Policy. Among the latest violence prevention policies are increases in on-campus police presence, random drug screening for athletes, community service, and municipal fines for fighting in amounts of hundreds of dollars. These school policies complement the more traditional policies of detention, in or out of school suspension, and expulsion. Locked doors and teachers and administrators equipped with walkie-talkies typify the prisonlike security systems of many urban schools. School priorities have necessarily shifted away from education and toward discipline and control. Pallas (1988) revealed that increased lack of control in the classroom and over school policy as well as poor student behavior are positively associated with increased proportions of students of low socioeconomic status and minority students. The Zero Tolerance drug and weapon policy, a nationwide campaign among inner city schools, may reflect not only a violence prevention policy but also perhaps the mind frame of school teachers and administrators who are subjected to unprecedented levels of cyclical adolescent failure, frustration, and hostility.

Law Enforcement Programs. Because the risk factors associated with perpetration of and victimization by violence have proven to be so diverse and are strongly linked to economic, physical, environmental, community, and human development, effective implementation and enforcement of legislation that influences any and all of these areas is promising. Legislative and criminal justice violence prevention activities that are currently employed include regulated use of and access to weapons (weaponless schools, control of concealed weapons, restrictive licensing, appropriate sale of guns), regulated use of and access to alcohol (appropriate sale of, prohibition or control of alcohol sales at events, training of servers), and punishment at schools and dress codes for school (National Center for Injury Prevention and Control, 1993). North Carolina Governor James B. Hunt's Task Force on Violence recommended similar efforts: tougher disciplinary measures for dealing with violent behavior and possession of weapons, parental responsibility laws, school suspension carryover policies so that winter and summer vacations do not exempt a student from the disciplinary action, statewide school violence reporting systems, increasing funding for alternative learning centers, and changes in the juvenile justice system to increase the penalties for juvenile violence (Easley, Ethridge, & Hampton, 1993).

Webster (1993) provided additional recommendations to prevent adolescent violence: (1) Fund long-term evaluations with sufficient sample size and follow-up to detect changes in perpetration and victimization rates; (2) restructure program content to include a behavioral focus, address known risk factors consistent with the developmental stage of the target audience, include training on how to handle put-downs and deescalate volatile situations, and include training in street survival skills; (3) focus on broader solutions to improve the environments in which underprivileged youth live, enhancing opportunities for them to live productive lives, and improve the social institutions that affect the quality of life; and (4) reduce the availability of guns. These recommendations are further developed in several reports that provide specific youth violence prevention activities at the individual, school, community, and government levels (Center for the Study and Prevention of Violence, 1995; National Center for Injury Prevention and Control, 1993; U.S. Department of Justice, 1994).

Finally, Slaby, Barham, Eron, and Wilcox (1994), as part of the American Psychological Association's Commission on Violence and Youth, distilled the conclusions of the commission: (1) Early childhood interventions can help children learn to deal with social conflict effectively and nonviolently; (2) schools can become a leading force in providing the safety and the effective educational programs by which children can learn to reduce and prevent violence; (3) all programmatic efforts to reduce and prevent violence will benefit from heightened awareness of cultural diversity; (4) television and other media can contribute to the solutions rather than to the problems of youth violence; (5) major reductions in the most damaging forms of youth violence can be achieved by limiting youth access to firearms and by teaching children and youth how to prevent firearm violence; (6) reductions of youth involvement with alcohol and other drugs can reduce violent behavior; (7) psychological health services for young perpetrators, victims, and witnesses of violence can ameliorate the damaging effects of violence and reduce further violence; (8) education programs can reduce the prejudice and hostility that lead to hate crimes and violence against social groups; (9) when groups become mobs, violence feeds on itself; (10) psychologists can act individually and in their professional organizations to reduce violence among youth.

While any of these efforts independently may have limited impact, the latest recommendations suggest that interagency collaboration is essential to successfully addressing this multifaceted problem. Moreover, in anticipation of federal funding cuts for social programs, it is clear that previously underfunded agencies facing additional budget cuts will be forced to share resources and responsibilities as well as to clarify goals in streamlining their programs.

RECOMMENDATIONS FOR FUTURE RESEARCH

Several avenues for refining and enhancing school-based health promotion remain to be explored. Best (1989) described the challenges as the following: (1) When should professionals intervene? All interventions must take into consideration the appropriate level of cognitive and behavioral development. (2) For how long should professionals intervene? Should interventions include booster sessions that span multiple age groups or just the age when the behavior is becoming established? (3) What mediates intervention effects? What are the effects of family- or community-based interventions that supplement school health promotion? (4) What are the intervention targets? Should the focus be on individual motivation or on social norms and policies that regulate behavior? Are social influence models that focus on specific substance use behaviors more appropriate than models that focus on generic life skills? Should abstinence or responsible use be the goal?

Others have noted the white middle-class homogeneity of research populations that have received most substance use prevention programs (Rotheram-Borus & Tsemberis, 1989). Prevention policy makers and researchers need to modify and evaluate the existing prevention interventions in a culturally sensitive manner. The extent to which the current social influences and life skills models generalize to low-income and minority populations deserves additional research.

Methodological Issues

Finally, even though dissemination of the current models of social influences and life skills curricula has been recommended, methodological flaws of the studies upon which judgment is based prohibit taking a conclusive position. Several articles (Cook, Anson, & Walchli, 1993; Murray et al., 1994; Pentz, 1994) reviewed shortcomings of health promotion research and offered recommendations calling for improvements in (1) reducing subject attrition and improved long-term tracking; (2) controlling for possible Hawthorne effects (i.e., novelty); (3) biochemical validation, where appropriate, to increase honesty of reporting; (4) ensuring that the unit of statistical analysis is the same as the unit of assignment; (5) standardizing dependent measures across studies; and (6) enhancing implementation integrity and training quality.

RECOMMENDATIONS FOR HEALTH PRACTITIONERS

Since the mid-1970s, researchers and health education specialists have searched for methods to enhance and sustain school-based intervention effects. Within the school, the several innovative strategies have included (1) delivering multiple years of behavioral interventions; (2) expanding the interventions to include other types of social skills, such as interpersonal skills, critical thinking, or assertiveness; (3) including same-age peer leaders as potent sources of social information; and (4) altering school policies, such as changing cafeteria menus to provide healthier foods and physical education.

In addition, recent advances in software have made interactive computer technology more accessible to educators, thus easing their burden of covering all areas of academic and health concerns. Interactive computer technology has many of the same attention-getting features as the mass media, but offers greater educational opportunities because learners can control the pace of learning, adjust the instruction to their existing level of knowledge, receive direct feedback for their responses, and have fun at the same time (Lytle & Achterberg, 1995).

There has been growing recognition, however, that instruction at school in behavioral skills to promote health and to resist the social influences to behave in unhealthy ways may have limited impact if most of the students' other sources of socialization (i.e., parents, siblings,

or the larger community culture) are delivering a contradictory message (Biglan, Glasgow, & Singer, 1990). Several of the studies reviewed herein support the use of mass media and other community-level interventions to achieve lasting effects.

Schools have the potential to have substantial impact on youth health behaviors. Unfortunately, effective programs and strategies are not being used by a majority of this nation's schools because there is a large gap between research and practice in school health. The existence of this gap has been recognized in a number of areas, including sexuality education and smoking. A recent analysis of state sexuality curricula guidelines concluded that most of the guidelines promote an emphasis on providing technical information about HIV infection and transmission and do not emphasize skill-building approaches (SIECUS, 1991). A comparison of practice and state of the art on smoking education revealed that the smoking curricula in use by middle schools do not emphasize social influences despite an accumulation of health behavior research data demonstrating their importance, but rather focus on providing information about the consequences of smoking (Silvestri & Flay, 1989).

Guidelines are increasingly perceived as a way to bridge the gap between research and practice and to transfer the successful characteristics of effective programs to more widespread use. The Division of School Health at the CDC has published guidelines for school health programs to prevent HIV/AIDS (CDC, 1988), tobacco use and addiction (CDC, 1994a), nutrition (CDC, 1997a), physical activity (CDC, 1997b), and comprehensive school health education (Kolbe, 1993).

Finally, health professionals must be aware of the social and economic conditions under which many target populations live. Social risk factors such as unemployment, high population density, poverty, drug use, historical and structural inequity, racism, and discrimination, among others, place some groups at higher risk than others (Hill et al., 1994; McLoyd, 1990). When parents have no telephone or permanent address, when children are not attending school or are living in extreme poverty with no adult supervision, when teachers with large class sizes and outdated instructional materials are facing children with little self-control, it is unrealistic to expect health promotion interventions to have any effect before there are changes in the social and economic conditions under which these young people live. To bring about any meaningful and lasting improvements in health, it may be necessary to bring economically and educationally disadvantaged children and their families up to a higher level of readiness for interventions to be effective.

ACKNOWLEDGMENTS. The authors wish to recognize and thank the following individuals for their assistance and important contributions: Jennifer Conroy, Andrew Fourney, K. K. Harris, Colleen Kelder, Laura McCormick, Nancy Murray, and Sema Spigner.

REFERENCES

Alan Guttmacher Institute. (1994). *Sex and America's teenagers*. New York: Author.

Bandura, A. (1986). *Social foundations of thought and action*. Englewood Cliffs, NJ: Prentice-Hall.

Baranowski, T., Bouchard, C., Bar-Or, O., Bricker, T., Health, G., Kinn, S. Y. E., Maline, R., Obarzanek, E., Pate, R., Strong, W. B., Truman, B., & Washington, R. (1992). Assessment, prevalence, and cardiovascular benefits of physical activity and fitness in youth. *Medicine and Science in Sports and Exercise*, (24), S237–S247.

Baranowski, T., Perry, C. L., & Parcel, G. S. (1997). How individuals, environments, and health behavior interact: Social learning theory. In K. Glantz, F. M. Lewis, & B. Rimer (Eds.), *Health behavior and health education* (2nd ed.) (pp. 161–186). San Francisco: Jossey-Bass.

Best, J. A. (1989). Intervention perspectives on school health promotion research. *Health Education Quarterly*, 16, 299–306.

Biglan, A., Glasgow, R. E., & Singer, G. (1990). The need for a science of larger social units: A contextual approach. *Behavior Therapy*, 21, 195–215.

Botvin, G. J. (1990). Substance abuse prevention: Theory, practice, and effectiveness. *Crime and Justice*, 13, 461–519.

Botvin, G. J., Baker, E., Dusenbury, L., Tortu, S., & Botvin, E. M. (1990). Preventing adolescent drug abuse through a multimodal cognitive–behavioral approach: Results of a 3-year study. *Journal of Consulting and Clinical Psychology*, 58(4), 437–446.

Brown, B. B., Mounts, N., Lamborn, S. D., & Steinberg, L. (1993). Parenting practices and peer group affiliation in adolescence. *Child Development*, 64, 467–482.

Bruvold, W. H. (1993). A meta-analysis of adolescent smoking prevention programs. *American Journal of Public Health*, 83(6), 872–880.

Center for the Study and Prevention of Violence. (1995). *Violence and conflict resolution for youth: Curriculum and videos*. Boulder, CO: CSPV.

Centers for Disease Control. (1988). Guidelines for effective school health education to prevent the spread of AIDS. *Morbidity and Mortality Weekly Report*, 37(S-2), 1–3.

Centers for Disease Control and Prevention. (1994a). Guidelines for school health programs to prevent tobacco use and addiction. *Morbidity and Mortality Weekly Report*, 43(RR-2), 1–18.

Centers for Disease Control and Prevention. (1994b). AIDS information: Cumulative cases. *HIV AIDS Surveillance Report*, year ended.

Centers for Disease Control and Prevention. (1997a). Guidelines for school health programs to promote healthy eating. *Journal of School Health*, 67, 9–26.

Centers for Disease Control and Prevention. (1997b). Guidelines for school and community programs to promote lifelong physical activity among young people. *Morbidity and Mortality Weekly Report*, 46(RR-6), 1–36.

Centerwall, B. S. (1995). Race, socioeconomic status, and domestic homicide. *Journal of the American Medical Association*, 273(22), 1755–1758.

Coira, M. J., Zill, N., & Bloom, B. (1994). Health of our nation's children. National Center for Health Statistics. *Vital Health Statistics*, 10(191).

Coleman, J. (1991). *Parental involvement in education*. PIP 91-983. Office of Educational Research and Improvement. U. S. Department of Education. Washington, DC: U.S. Government Printing Office.

Contento, I. R., Manning, A. D., & Shannon, B. (1992). Research perspective on school-based nutrition education. *Journal of Nutrition Education*, 24, 247–260.

Cook, T. D., Anson, A. R., & Walchli, S. B. (1993). From causal description to causal explanation: Improving three already good evaluations of adolescent health programs. In S. G. Millstien, A. C. Petersen, & E. O. Nightingale (Eds.), *Promoting the health of adolescents: New directions for the twenty-first century* (pp. 339–374). New York: Oxford University Press.

DeJong, W. (1987). A short-term evaluation of Project DARE (Drug Abuse Resistance Education). *Journal of Drug Education*, 17, 279–294.

Department of Health and Human Services/Centers for Disease Control and Prevention. (1995). Pregnancy, sexually transmitted diseases, and related risk behaviors among U.S. adolescents. *Adolescent Health: State of the Nation, Monograph Series No. 2.*

Department of Health and Human Services/Public Health Service. (1995). Update: AIDS among women, United States, 1994. *Morbidity and Mortality Weekly Report, 44*(5), 81–99.

Dryfoos, J. G. (1990). Adolescents at risk: Prevalence and prevention. New York: Oxford University Press.

Earls, F., Cairns, R. B., & Mercy, J. A. (1993). The control of violence and the promotion of nonviolence. In S. G. Mill-stien, A. C. Petersen, & E. O. Nightingale (Eds.), *Promoting the health of adolescents: New directions for the twenty-first century* (pp 285–304). New York: Oxford University Press.

Easley, M., Ethridge, B., & Hampton, S. (1993). *Executive summary report of the task force on school violence.* Raleigh, NC: Office of the Attorney General.

Evans, R. I., & Raines, B. E. (1982). Control and prevention of smoking in adolescents: A psychosocial perspective. In T. J. Coates, A. C. Petersen, & C. Perry (Eds.), *Promoting adolescent health: A dialog on research and practice* (pp. 101–136). New York: Academic Press.

Flay, B. R., Koepke, D., Thompson, S. J., Santi, S., Best, J. A., & Brown, K. S. (1989). Six-year follow-up of the first Waterloo School Smoking Prevention Trial. *American Journal of Public Health, 79,* 1371–1375.

Flynn, B. S., Wordon, J. K., Sacker-Walker, R. H., Pirie, P. L., Badger, B. M., Carpenter, J. H., & Geller, B. M. (1994). Mass media and school interventions: Effects two years after completion. *American Journal of Public Health, 84,* 1148–1150.

Gans, J. E. (1990). *Profiles of adolescents health series: Vol. 1. America's adolescents: How healthy are they?* Chicago: American Medical Association.

Glynn, T. J. (1989). Essential elements of school-based smoking prevention programs. *Journal of School Health, 5,* 181–188.

Goodstadt, M. S. (1978). Alcohol and drug education. *Health Education Monographs, 6,* 263–279.

Gortmaker, S. L., Dietz, W. H., & Sobol, A. M. (1987). Increasing pediatric obesity in the United States. *Pediatrics, 141,* 141–535.

Hansen, W. B. (1992). School-based substance abuse prevention: A review of the state of the art in curriculum, 1980–1990. *Health Education Research, 7,* 403–430.

Harvard University Graduate School of Education. (1993). *Coping with violence in the schools: A report of the 1993 summer conference of the Center for School Counseling Practitioners.* Cambridge, MA.

Hill, H. M., Soriana, F. I., Chen, A., & LaFromboise, T. D. (1994). Sociocultural factors in the etiology and prevention of violence among ethnic minority youth. In L. D. Eron, J. H. Gentry, & P. Schlegel (Eds.), *Reason to hope: A psycho-logical perspective on violence and youth* (pp. 59–100). Washington, DC: American Psychological Association.

Holtzman, D., Greene, B. Z., Ingraham, G. C., Daily, L. A., Demchuk, D. G., & Kolbe, L. J. (1992). HIV education and health education in the United States: A national survey of local school district policies and practices. *Journal of School Health, 62*(9), 421–427.

Johnson, C. A., Pentz, M. A., Weber, M. D., Dwyer, J. H., Baer, N., MacKinnon, D. P., Hansen, W. B., & Flay, B. R. (1990). Relative effectiveness of comprehensive community programming for drug-abuse prevention with high-risk and low-risk adolescents. *Journal of Consulting and Clinical Psychology, 58*(4), 447–456.

Jurich, A. P., Polson, C. J., Jurich, J. A., & Bates, R. A. (1985). Family factors in the lives of drug users and abusers. *Adolescence, 20,* 143–159.

Kandel, D. B., & Andrews, K. (1987). Processes of adolescent socialization by parents and peers. *International Journal of the Addictions, 22*(4), 319–342.

Kann, L., Warren, C. W., Harris, W. A., Collins, J. L., Douglas, K. A., Collins, M. E., Williams, B. I., Ross, J. G., Kolbe, L. J. (1995). State and local YRBSS coordinators. Youth risk behavior surveillance—United States, 1993. In CDC Surveillance Summaries, March 24, 1995. *Morbidity and Mortality Weekly Report, 44* (No. SS-1), 1–56.

Kantor, L. M. (1992/1993). Scared chaste? Fear based educational curricula. *Sex Information and Education Council of the US (SIECUS) Report, 21*(2), 1–15.

Kantor, L. M., & Haffner, D. W. (1995). Responding to "the failure of sex education." *Sex Information and Education Council of the US (SIECUS) Report, 23*(3), 17–20.

Kelder, S. H., Parcel, G. S., & Perry, C. L. (1995). Health promotion. In L. Siegel (Ed.), *Advances in pediatric psychology: Behavioral perspectives on adolescent health* (pp. 179–202). New York: Guilford Press.

Kelder, S. H., Perry, C. L., & Klepp, K. I. (1993). Community-wide youth exercise education: Long-term outcomes of the Minnesota Heart Health Program. *Journal of School Health, 64,* 218–223.

Kelder, S. H., Perry, C. L., Klepp, K. I., & Lytle, L. A. (1994). Tracking of adolescent health behaviors. *American Journal of Public Health, 84*(7), 1121–1126.

Kelder, S. H., Perry, C. L., Lytle, L. A., & Klepp, K. I. (1995). Community-wide youth nutrition education: Long-term outcomes of the Minnesota Heart Health Program. *Health Education Research: Theory and Practice, 10*(2), 119–131.

Kirby, D., Barth, R. B., Leland, N., & Fetro, J. V. (1991). Reducing the risk: Impact of a new curriculum on sexual risk taking. *Family Planning Perspectives, 23,* 253–263.

Kirby, D., Short L., Collins, J., Rugg, D., Kolbe, L., Howard, M., Brent, M., Sonenstein, F., & Zabin, L. S. (1994). School-based programs to reduce sexual risk behaviors: A review of effectiveness. *Public Health Reports, 109,* 339–360.

Klein, N. A., Goodson, P., Serrins, D. S., Edmundson, E., & Evans, A. (1994). Evaluation of sex education curricula:

Measuring up to the SIECUS guidelines. *Journal of School Health, 64,* 328–333.

Klepp, K., Halper, A., & Perry, C. L. (1986). The efficacy of peer leaders in drug abuse prevention. *Journal of School Health, 56,* 407–411.

Kolbe, L. J. (1990). An epidemiological surveillance system to monitor the prevalence of youth behaviors that most affect health. *Health Education, 6,* 44–48.

Kolbe, L. J. (1993). An essential strategy to improve the health and education of Americans. *Preventive Medicine, 22,* 544–560.

Larson, J. (1994). Violence prevention in the schools: A review of selected programs and procedures. *School Psychology Review, 23*(2), 151–164.

Luepker, R. V., Perry, C. L., McKinlay, S. M., Nader, P. R., Parcel, G. S., Stone, E. J., Webber, L. S., Elder, J. P., Feldman, H. A., Johnson, C. C., Kelder, S. H., & Wu, M. (1996). Outcomes of a field trial to improve children's dietary patterns and physical activity: The Child and Adolescent Trial for Cardiovascular Health (CATCH). *Journal of the American Medical Association, 275*(10), 768–776.

Lytle, L. A., & Achterberg, C. (1995). Changing the diet of America's children: What works and why? *Journal of Nutrition Education, 27*(5), 250–260.

Lytle, L. A., Kelder, S. H., & Snyder, P. (1993). A review of school food service intervention research. *School Food Research Review, 1,* 7–14.

McGuire, W. J. (1968). The nature of attitudes and attitude change. In G. Lindsey & E. Aronson (Eds.), *Handbook of social psychology* (pp. 236–314). Reading, MA: Addison-Wesley.

McLoyd, V. C. (1990). The impact of economic hardship on black families and children: Psychological distress, parenting, and socioemotional development. *Child Development, 61,* 311–346.

Mercy, J. A., Rosenberg, M. L., Powell, K. E., Broome, C. V., & Roper, W. L. (1993). Public health policy for preventing violence. *Health Affairs, 12*(4), 7–29.

Murray, D. M., McKinlay, S. M., Martin, D., Donner, A. P., Dwyer, J. H., Raudenbush, S. W., & Graubard, B. I. (1994). Design and analysis issues in community trials. *Evaluation Review, 18*(4), 493–514.

Nader, P. R., Sallis, J. F., Patterson, T. L., Abramson, I. S., Rupp, J. W., Senn, K. L., Atkins, C. J., Roppe, B. E., Morris, J. A., Wallace, J. P., & Vega, W. A. (1989). A family approach to cardiovascular risk reduction: Results from the San Diego Family Heart Project. *Health Education Quarterly, 16,* 229–244.

National Center for Injury Prevention and Control. (1993). *The prevention of youth violence: A framework for community action.* Atlanta, GA: Centers for Disease Control and Prevention.

Olson, C. M. (1995). Joint position of the Society for Nutrition Education (SNE), the American Dietetic Association (ADA), and the American School Food Service Association

(ASFSA): School-based nutrition programs and services. *Journal of Nutrition Education, 27,* 58–61.

Pallas, A. M. (1988). School climate in American high schools. *Teachers College Record, 89,* 541–554.

Parcel, G. S., Simons-Morton, B. G., & Kolbe, L. J. (1988). Health promotion: Integrating organizational change and student learning strategies. *Health Education Quarterly, 15,* 435–450.

Parcel, G. S., Simons-Morton, B., O'Hara, N. M., Baranowski, T., & Kolbe, L. J. (1987). School promotion of healthful diet and exercise behavior: An integration of organizational change and social learning theory interventions. *Journal of School Health, 57,* 150–156.

Parcel, G. S., Simons-Morton, B., O'Hara, N. M., Baranowski, T., & Wilson, B. (1989). School promotion of healthful diet and physical activity: Impact on learning outcomes and self-reported behavior. *Health Education Quarterly, 16,* 181–199.

Pentz, M. A. (1994). Directions for future research on drug-abuse prevention. *Preventive Medicine, 23,* 646–651.

Pentz, M. A., Dwyer, J. H., MacKinnon, D. P., Flay, B. R., Hansen, W. B., Wang, E. Y., & Johnson, C. A. (1989). A multicommunity trial for primary prevention of adolescent drug abuse: Effects on drug use prevalence. *Journal of the American Medical Association, 261,* 3259–3266.

Pepler, D. J., & Slaby, R. G. (1994). Theoretical and developmental perspectives on youth and violence. In L. D. Eron, J. H. Gentry, & P. Schlegel (Eds.), *Reason to hope: A psychological perspective on violence and youth* (pp. 27–58). Washington, DC: American Psychological Association.

Perry, C. L., Kelder, S. H., & Klepp, K. I. (1994a). The rationale behind early prevention of cardiovascular disease with young people. *European Journal of Public Health, 4*(3), 156–163.

Perry, C. L., Kelder, S. H., & Klepp, K. I. (1994b). Community-wide cardiovascular disease prevention with young people: Long-term outcomes of The Class of 1989 Study. *European Journal of Public Health, 4*(3), 188–195.

Perry, C. L., Kelder, S. H., & Komro, K. (1992). The social world of adolescents. In S. G. Millstien, A. C. Petersen, & E. O. Nightingale (Eds.), *Promoting the health of adolescents: New directions for the twenty-first century* (pp. 209–241). New York: Oxford University Press.

Perry, C. L., Kelder, S. H., Murray, D. M., & Klepp, K. I. (1992). Community-wide smoking prevention: Long-term outcomes of the Minnesota Heart Health Program. *American Journal of Public Health, 82,* 1210–1216.

Perry, C. L., Stone, E. J., Parcel, G. S., Ellison, R. C., Nader, P. R., Webber, L. S., & Luepker, R. V. (1990). School-based cardiovascular health promotion: The Child and Adolescent Trial for Cardiovascular Health (CATCH). *Journal of School Health, 60,* 406–413.

Perry, C. L., Williams, C. L., Forster, J. L., Wolfson, M., Wagenaar, A. C., Finnegan, J. R., McGovern, P. G., Veblen-Mortenson, S., Komro, K. A., & Anstine, P. S. (1993). Background, conceptualization, and design of a community wide research program on adolescent alcohol use: Project Northland. *Health Education Research Theory and Practice, 8,* 1126-1136.

Perry, C. I., Williams, C. L., Veblen-Mortenson, S., Toomey, T. L., Komro, K. A., Anstine, P. S., McGovern, P. G., Finnegan, J. R., Forster, J. L., Wagenaar, A. C., & Wolfson, M. (1996). Outcomes of a community-wide alcohol use prevention program during early adolescence: Project Northland. *American Journal of Public Health, 86*(7), 956-965.

Petraits, J., Flay, B. R., & Miller, T. Q. (1995). Reviewing theories of adolescent substance use: Organizing pieces in the puzzle. *Psychological Bulletin, 117*(1), 67-86.

Puska, P., Vartiainen, E., Pallonen, U., Salonen, J. T., Poyhis, P., Koskela, K., & McAlister, A. (1982). The North Karelia Youth Project: Evaluation of two years of intervention on health behavior and cardiovascular disease risk factors among 13- to 15-year old children. *Preventive Medicine, 11,* 550-570.

Resnicow, K., Cross, D., & Wynder, E. (1993). The Know Your Body program: A review of evaluation studies. *Bulletin of the New York Academy of Medicine, 70,* 188-208.

Ringwalt, C., Ennett, S. T., & Holt, K. D. (1991). An outcome evaluation of Project DARE (Drug Abuse Resistance Education). *Health Education Research, 6,* 327-337.

Ross, R. R. (1994). The status of fitness programming in our nation's schools. In R. R. Pate & R. C. Hohn (Eds.), *Health and fitness through physical education* (pp. 21-30). Champaign, IL: Human Kinetics Publishers.

Ross, R. R., & Hohn, R. C. (1994). Health-related physical education—A direction for the 21st century. In R. R. Pate & R. C. Hohn (Eds.), *Health and fitness through physical education* (pp. 215-217). Champaign, IL: Human Kinetics Publisher.

Rotheram-Borus, M. J., & Tsemberis, S. J. (1989). Social competency training programs in ethnically diverse communities. In G. W. Albee & J. M. Joffe (Eds.), *Primary prevention of psychopathology* (Vol. XII, pp. 297-318). Newbury Park, CA: Sage.

Rozin, P. (1984). The development of food preferences. In J. D. Matarazzo, S. M. Weiss, J. A. Herd, N. E. Miller, & S M. Weiss (Eds.), *Behavioral health: A handbook of health enhancement and disease prevention* (pp. 590-607). Silver Spring, MD: Wiley.

Sallis, J. F., & McKenzie, T. L. (1992). Physical education's role in public health. *Research Quarterly for Exercise and Sport, 62*(2), 124-137.

Sallis, J. F., & Patrick, K. (1994). Physical activity guidelines for adolescents: Consensus statement. *Pediatric Exercise Science, 6,* 302-314.

Schaalma, H., Kok, G., & Peters, L. (1993). Determinants of consistent condom use by adolescents: The impact of experience of sexual intercourse. *Health Education Research: Theory and Practice, 8*(2), 255-269.

SIECUS. (1991). *Guidelines for comprehensive sexuality education: Kindergarten-12th grade.* New York: National Guidelines Task Force, SIECUS.

SIECUS. (1993). Assessment of state sexuality education programs: Unfinished business. Guidlines for comprehensive sexuality education: Kindergarten-12th grade. *(SIECUS) Report, 21*(4), 21-22.

Silvestri, B., & Flay, B. R. (1989). Smoking education: Comparison of practice and state-of-the-art. *Preventive Medicine, 18,* 257-266.

Simons-Morton, B. G., Parcel, G. S., O'Hara, N. J., Blair, S. N., & Pate, R. R. (1988). Health-related physical fitness in childhood: Status and recommendations. *Annual Review of Public Health, 9,* 403-425.

Slaby, R. G., Barham, J. E., Eron, L. D., & Wilcox, B. L. (1994). Policy recommendations: Prevention and treatment of youth violence. In L. D. Eron, J. H. Gentry, & P. Schlegel (Eds.), *Reason to hope: A psychological perspective on violence and youth* (pp. 447-456). Washington, DC: American Psychological Association.

Spitz, A. M. (1993). Reproductive health information: Pregnancy and birth rates among teenagers, by state United States, 1980-1990: Cumulative cases. *Surveillance Summaries: Morbidity and Mortality Weekly Report, 42*(SS-6), 1-27.

Stone, E. J., Perry, C. L., & Luepker, R. V. (1989). Synthesis of cardiovascular behavioral research for youth health promotion. *Health Education Quarterly, 16,* 155-169.

Strong, W. B., & Kelder, S. H. (1996). Pediatric preventive cardiology. In R. Hennekeus & M. Graziano (Eds.), *Prevention of myocardial infarction* (pp. 433-462). New York: Oxford University Press.

Surveillance United States. (1993). *Morbidity and Mortality Weekly Report 44.*

Sylvester, G. P., Achterberg, C., & Williams, J. (1995). Friend or foe: Television's effect on children's food and nutrition behavior. *Nutrition Today, 30,* 6-15.

Tell, G. S., & Vellar, O. D. (1988). Physical fitness, physical activity, and cardiovascular disease risk factors in adolescents: The Oslo Youth Study. *Preventive Medicine, 17,* 12-24.

Tobler, N. S. (1992). Drug prevention programs can work: Research findings. *Journal of Addictive Diseases, 11*(3), 1-28.

Tolan, P., & Guerra, N. (1994). *What works in reducing adolescent violence: An empirical review of the literature.* Boulder, CO: Center for the Study and Prevention of Violence.

Treboux, D., & Busch-Rossnagel, N. (1990). Social network influences on adolescent sexual attitudes and behaviors. *Journal of Adolescent Research, 5,* 175-189.

U.S. Bureau of the Census. (1992). *Poverty in the United States: 1991.* Current Population Reports. Series P-60, No. 181. Washington, DC: U.S. Government Printing Office.

U.S. Department of Education, Office of Educational Research and Improvement, National Center for Educational Statistics. (1993). *Youth indicators 1993*. NCES 93-242. Washington, DC: U.S. Government Printing Office.

U.S. Department of Justice. (1994). *Partnerships against violence: Promising programs*. Washington, DC: USDJ, OJP, NIJ.

Vartiainen, E., Pallonen, U., McAlister, A., & Puska, P. (1990). Eight-year follow-up results of an adolescent smoking prevention program: The North Karelia Youth Project. *American Journal of Public Health, 80*, 78-79.

Walter, H. J., Vaughan, R. D., Ragin, D. R., Cohall, A. T., & Kasen, S. (1994). Prevalence and correlates of AIDS-related behavioral intentions among urban minority high school students. *AIDS Education and Prevention, 6*(4), 339-350.

Webber, L. S., Osganian, V., Luepker, R. V., Feldman, H. A., Stone, E. J., Elder, J. P., Perry, C. L., Nader, P., Parcel, G. S., Broyles, S. L., & McKinlay, S. M. (1995). Cardiovascular risk factors among third grade children in four regions of the United States. *American Journal of Epidemiology , 141*, 428-439.

Webster, D. W. (1993). The unconvincing case for school-based conflict resolution programs for adolescents. *Health Affairs, 12*(4), 126-141.

Yarber, W. L. (1992). AAHE Scholar's Address: While we stood by … the limiting of sexual information to our youth. *Journal of Health Education, 23*(6), 326-335.

15

Contributions of Health Behavior Research to Community Health Promotion Programs

Caroline Schooler and June A. Flora

Health behaviors and health status are influenced not only by biological and psychological factors, but also by economic, political, and sociocultural factors (Aiken & Mott, 1970; Blum, 1981; Brown, 1984; Flora, Jackson, & Maccoby, 1989; Warren, 1972). For example, leading causes of death in the United States (cardiovascular disease and cancer) have been shown to be related to lifestyle elements such as diet, exercise, and smoking (U.S. Department of Health and Human Services, 1991). Intentional injury is another significant cause of death, especially among youths, that is strongly influenced by environmental and familial characteristics (American Psychological Association, 1993; Elliott, 1994). The important impact that societal factors have on health behavior highlights the significance of health promotion strategies targeting entire communities.

This chapter will examine the contribution of health behavior research to community health promotion by (1) describing essential characteristics of community health promotion programs; (2) reviewing the process of designing, implementing, and institutionalizing behavior change; and (3) highlighting gaps, training needs, and areas for further inquiry to enhance community-based efforts to improve health.

DEFINITION OF COMMUNITY

Defining community has been a major issue of interest to researchers (Chavis & Newbrough, 1986; Chavis, Stucky, & Wandersman, 1983; Newbrough, 1992). Components that have relevance for health behavior include formal organizations such as local government and businesses; educational institutions; voluntary associations such as religious, fraternal, or service groups; informal social networks; families; and individuals (Sanders, 1966; Warren, 1972). Central to the concept of community is that the various components are interrelated and have a potential for being mo-

Caroline Schooler and June A. Flora • Stanford Center for Research in Disease Prevention, Stanford University School of Medicine, Palo Alto, California 94304-1825.

Handbook of Health Behavior Research IV: Relevance for Professionals and Issues for the Future, edited by David S. Gochman. Plenum Press, New York, 1997.

bilized (Rothman & Brown, 1989; Sanders, 1966). Community systems influence health behavior and thereby affect individuals by altering the physical environment (e.g., building more hospitals, reducing the amount of available park space), supporting services or activities (e.g., education, community health programs), and interacting with other systems (e.g., initiating an educational program on reading and comprehending food labels because of a new governmental policy requiring more specific food labeling) (Flora et al., 1989). The complexity of interrelationships among community members, organizations, and institutions means that health promotion strategies need to be comprehensive by focusing on many kinds of change and well integrated so that program components reinforce each other.

COMMUNITY HEALTH PROMOTION PROGRAMS

Community health promotion programs have the potential to influence both the behaviors of individuals and the social systems in which they live. Education campaigns typically use both mass media and direct interpersonal programs to reach the general public and health professionals. In addition, community organization strategies can create institutional and organizational support for behavior change goals. Such health promotion programs can (1) influence the knowledge, attitudes, and behaviors of individuals; (2) modify the environment so that it supports the initiation and maintenance of individuals' healthy actions or, in some cases, prohibits their unhealthy actions; and (3) reduce or eliminate factors in the physical or social environment that are detrimental to health (Farquhar, Flora, & Goode, 1986; Rothman & Brown, 1989).

There are three essential characteristics of community health promotion programs. First, the programs target multiple audiences. Second, the programs use multiple channels of communication. Third, community health promotion programs target multiple health-related outcomes. The timing and placement of individual and envi-

ronmental change efforts must be orchestrated to be mutually reinforcing (Schooler, Flora, & Farquhar, 1993). For example, educational efforts to teach low-income people to prepare nutritious meals using inexpensive ingredients can be hampered by environmental conditions such as high prices for more nutritious foods. Food stamps and the Women, Infants, and Children program are examples of policies designed to reduce economic (environmental) barriers to nutritious diets (Blum, 1982; E. C. Nelson, Keller, & Zubkoff, 1981). This chapter will discuss how health behavior research informs each element of community health promotion.

Multiple Audiences

Community health promotion programs typically target multiple audiences with behavior change strategies. These audiences may include youth, the elderly, women, men, members of various minority groups, and health care providers. Although many interventions focus on individuals, behavior change efforts may also be directed toward families or other groupings of people such as clubs and worksites. Incorporating different audiences enhances the likelihood of influencing community-wide behavior change.

Targeting Subgroups. Health behavior research suggests that segmenting the audience into meaningful subgroups enhances message and program design and contributes to successful behavior change (Lefebvre & Flora, 1988; Slater & Flora, 1991). Traditional segmentation variables include geography (region, county, census tract), demography (age, gender, family size, occupation, ethnic or racial background, socioeconomic status), and social structure (worksites, churches, voluntary agencies, families, legislative bodies) (Kotler, 1975; Murphy, 1984; Novelli, 1984; Weinstein, 1987). For successful program planning, it is important to consider not only the differences between audience groups, but also within-group differences. For example, research demonstrates that efforts to encourage women's use of early detection practices for breast cancer such as breast self-exam and mammography are more successful when different messages and programs are developed for women who are members of ethnic minority groups, who are economically disadvantaged, or who have less educational attainment (Skinner, Strecher, & Hospers, 1994).

Health promotion efforts at all levels, however, whether in individual or group-based programs, schools and other institutional settings, or entire communities, are often more successful with specific audience subgroups (Conrad, 1987; Flay, 1986; Gregg, Foote, Erfurt, & Heinrich, 1990; Luepker et al., 1994; Reynes et al., 1993; Winkleby, Fortmann, & Rockhill, 1992). Health behavior research data suggest that these "more-likely-to-change" persons tend to be better educated, to have higher incomes, to possess greater health knowledge, to be more efficacious about health behavior change, and to have made more changes in the past. Some research suggests that consideration of psychosocial variables such as lifestyle, media use habits, and discussion can improve segmentation and enhance program effectiveness with traditionally underserved and hard-to-reach audiences (Cirksena & Flora, in press; Flora, Slater, & Maibach, 1989; Grunig, 1979; Slater & Flora, 1991). In addition, tailoring programs and messages to audience groups' psychological attributes, such as readiness to change (Campbell et al., 1994; Marcus et al., 1992; Prochaska, Redding, Harlow, Rossi, & Velicer, 1994; Rossi et al., 1994; Skinner et al., 1994) and perceived self-efficacy (Bandura, 1986; Winkleby, Flora, & Kraemer, 1994), enhances program effectiveness and contributes to successful behavior change.

Encouraging Interaction. A defining aspect of communities is that people interact with each other. Community members are connected by family ties, by friendships, as colleagues and coworkers, and as groups involved with certain issues or causes. Social groups are therefore important audiences for behavior change strategies. Health behavior research demonstrates that educational interventions designed to encourage interpersonal discussion among social network members lead to improved preventive health behaviors such as breast cancer screening (Gravell, Zapka, & Mamon, 1985). Moreover, program planners have successfully utilized kin, friendship, and job networks to influence traditionally underserved and hard-to-reach audiences. For example, the Save Our Sisters Project recruited and trained "natural helpers" to influence rural African-American women to seek mammography screening (Eng, 1993). A similar model was used by the Arizona Disease Prevention Center with Yaqui Indian and Mexican-American women (Brownstein, Cheal, Ackerman, Bassford, & Campos-Outcalt, 1992). Training peer leaders was also shown to be effective in promoting HIV preventive behaviors among gay men (Kelly et al., 1991). In addition, a telephone strategy for personal contacts was successful in the American Cancer Society's Tell A Friend program to increase mammography use (Calle, Miracle-McMahill, Moss, & Heath, 1994). The importance of social support and interpersonal influence in shaping individuals' health behaviors suggests that social networks are a key target area for community health promotion programs.

A key characteristic of social systems is that various subgroups interact (Rogers, 1983). Building on natural influence patterns and communication between groups in a community can enhance program effectiveness. Children's health behavior, for example, is strongly shaped by the family environment (Crocket, Mullis, Perry, & Luepker, 1989; Hertzler, 1983; Sallis & Nader, 1988). In addition, teachers and schools have an impact not only on what children learn about health, but also on access to healthful food and recreation options through school lunch programs and fitness activities (Fullen, 1985; Parcel, Simons-Morton, & Kolbe, 1988; Simons-Morton, Parcel, Baranowski, Forthofer, & O'Hara, 1991). Finally, the community and mass media provide health information, as well as disseminate social norms (Parcel et al., 1988).

In the Stanford Five-City Program (FCP), a community-wide cardiovascular disease (CVD) risk reduction program (Farquhar et al., 1985), data demonstrated that family communication, parental behavioral modeling, the FCP education campaign, and personal knowledge and self-efficacy interacted to influence adolescents' diets (Rimal & Flora, 1994). Interactions between families, schools, and children were encouraged in a school-based nutrition and exercise curriculum designed to enhance parental involvement at home in conjunction with classroom activities. Results indicated that parental influences strongly affected children's dietary knowledge and behavior, whereas schools and teachers shaped exercise outcomes (Flora & Schooler, in press). Efforts to encourage parental involvement in youth interventions were also undertaken in the Minnesota Heart Health Program (MHHP), another community-based CVD prevention program (Carlaw, Mittlemark, Bracht, & Luepker, 1984). For example, a correspondence program requiring parents to work with their children led to significantly lowered fat consumption by participating children (Perry, Luepker, Murray et al., 1989). Enhancing interaction between systems to promote diffusion of information among university researchers, school district personnel, and teachers has also been shown to increase the effectiveness of school-based health promotion programs (Dijkstra, de Vries, & Parcel, 1993).

Encouraging social interaction between community components enhances program effectiveness not only by increasing the number of persons reached, but also by building on natural influence and support patterns. For this reason, health promotion efforts may also target whole organizations or institutions. Exploiting the complex interrelationships among various components of a community is the advantage of broad-based programs that incorporate strategies aimed at many different audiences.

Multiple Channels of Communication

Community health promotion programs benefit from using many diverse channels of communication to reach audience members. Channels may include mass media, community organiza-

tions, workplaces, schools, and local businesses such as restaurants and grocery stores. These types of organizations can serve as conduits of information, reinforce the change process, enhance resources applied to communication efforts, and ensure the institutionalization of programs (Flora, Jatulis, Jackson, & Fortmann, 1993). Findings from health behavior research demonstrate that incorporating several communication channels, such as supplementing community-based programs with mass media, enhances the effectiveness of behavior change interventions (Maccoby, Farquhar, Wood, & Alexander, 1977; Worden, Flynn, Merrill, Waller, & Haugh, 1989).

Mass Media. Mass media can serve several different functions in community health promotion programs. First, media messages can be the primary agent for change. Research suggests that media alone can achieve change in some outcomes such as knowledge gain and purchase behaviors, but that other more addictive habits (e.g., smoking) require additional face-to-face interaction (Farquhar et al., 1977; Freimuth, Hammond, & Stein, 1988; Levy & Stokes, 1987; Maccoby et al., 1977). Second, media can supplement other intervention elements. Evidence demonstrates that mass media may be most effective when used in conjunction with complementary messages delivered through other channels, such as school programs, adult education programs, workplace programs, and self-help materials (Brannon et al., 1989; Flay, 1987; Fora & Cassidy, 1990; Maccoby et al., 1977; Puska et al., 1987; Salina et al., 1994; Schooler et al., 1993). Third, media can promote other programs by familiarizing audience members with products and services and encouraging participation (Flora, Fortmann, Taylor, & Maccoby, 1985; Gruder, Warnecke, Jason, Flay, Peterson, 1990; King, Flora, Fortmann, & Taylor, 1987; Klatcher, 1987). Because different types of mass media reach different types of audiences, incorporating many diverse media modalities enhances campaign effectiveness (Flay, Gruder, Warnecke, Jason, & Peterson, 1989; Flora, Roser, Chaffee, & Farquhar, 1988;

McFall et al., 1993; Warnecke, Langenberg, Wong, Flay, & Cook, 1992). Finally, differential reach of media channels suggests that inexpensive vehicles such as inserts in utility bills, grocery bag flyers, and community newsletters can contribute to a campaign's effectiveness in reaching targeted populations.

Worksites. An integral component of community health promotion efforts is the involvement of diverse organizations (Sorensen, Glasgow, & Corbett, 1990). Worksites, places of worship, fraternal and civic organizations, recreation clubs, and other community organizations provide the opportunity to promote knowledge of healthful behaviors, as well as social supports and facilities to encourage behavior change (Lasater, Wells, Carleton, & Elder, 1986; Roberts & Thorsheim, 1987; U.S. Department of Health and Human Services, 1989). Health promotion programs within organizations can motivate participation in the programs. Workplace contests can provide incentives to promote weight loss and smoking cessation, generate good recruitment to programs, and promote interest in health promotion (Brownell et al., 1984; Elder et al., 1987; Felix, Stunkard, Cohen, & Cooley, 1985; Jeffery, Forster, & Schmid, 1989; King et al., 1987; D. J. Nelson, Sennett, Lefebvre, & Loirella, 1987; Pechacek, Freutel, Arkin, & Mittlemark, 1983; Stunkard, Cohen, & Felix, 1989).

Worksites and other organizations can also be the target of change. Institutions can be encouraged to adopt environmental changes such as nonsmoking policies, fitness facilities, or cafeteria modifications that reinforce other health promotion strategies. For example, Wilbur, Zifferblatt, Pinsky, and Zifferblatt (1981) found that making lower-calorie foods available did more to affect food choices than did providing nutrition education materials. Likewise, Jeffery, French, Raether, and Barter (1994) demonstrated that consumption of fruit and salad in a cafeteria increased when the variety of offerings was increased and their prices were reduced. In addition, organizational policy changes such as

smoking bans can contribute to cessation as well as to increased participation in cessation programs (Millar, 1988; Sorensen, Rigotti, Rosen, & Pinney, in press). Organizational changes such as providing fitness facilities, giving employees flexible time to use facilities, and allowing employees to exercise on company time have been shown to promote exercise in both men and women (Blair, Piserchia, Wilbur, & Crowder, 1986; Brill et al., 1991; Iverson, Fielding, Crow, & Christenson, 1985).

Local businesses such as restaurants and supermarkets are important channels for community health promotion programs. Programs aim to inform restauranteurs and supermarket management about the benefits of menu and food item labeling, identify healthful choices, and draw consumers' attention to healthful alternatives with labels, placards, and other promotional devices. Efforts to encourage restaurant menu marking and supermarket shelf labeling have been successful in community CVD risk reduction programs (Albright, Flora, & Fortmann, 1990; Colby et al., 1987; Hunt et al., 1990; Mullis & Pirie, 1988; Mullis et al., 1987; Shannon et al., 1990).

Religious Organizations. Places of worship can also play important roles in community health promotion efforts. The Pawtucket Heart Health Program (PHHP), a CVD risk reduction research and demonstration project (Carleton et al., 1987), showed that a church-based intervention program resulted in significant improvements in diet-related behaviors such as label reading, limiting fats and salt, and modifying recipes (Lasater et al., 1990). Moreover, church programs have been shown to be effective channels for CVD and cancer risk reduction efforts for African-American, inner city, and rural populations (Dressler, 1987; Hatch & Lovelace, 1980; Levin, 1984; Wiist & Flack, 1990). Religious organizations often have characteristics that render them useful channels for health promotion: receptivity to health-related programming, access to large numbers of people, effective communication channels, adequate meeting facilities, and a volunteer orientation (DePue et al., 1990; Lasater, Carleton, & Wells, 1991; Lasater et al., 1990). Research demonstrates, however, that characteristics of churches such as size and educational level of minister influence participation in community health programs (Thomas, Quinn, Billingsley, & Caldwell, 1994).

Schools.   Health promotion programs seeking to influence youth typically involve schools. School-based multiple risk factor programs undertaken in the FCP successfully changed 10th graders' dietary knowledge and behavior, including food availability at home and snack choices at school (Killen et al., 1988; King et al., 1988). The PHHP developed a home economics curriculum involving teachers and students in food selection and recipe modification that was both popular and effective in reducing the risk of high cholesterol (Gans et al., 1990). School-based smoking prevention programs also demonstrated success in the MHHP (Perry, Klepp, & Sillers, 1989; Perry, Kelder, Murray, & Klepp, 1992). Schools do more than provide a channel for curriculum dissemination; their policies also influence the health behavior of students, teachers, and staff. Modifying food availability at school cafeterias, instituting smoking bans, and increasing access to and availability of recreation facilities are examples of environmental changes that can have an important impact on health status (Simons-Morton et al., 1991).

Health Care System.   Health professionals and medical organizations are another important channel of communication in health promotion because many community members turn to their medical leaders when questions arise about new health promotion programs. Health providers can legitimate planned programs and provide technical input, assistance in program leadership and planning, guidance about local health care practices, and encouragement for other community leaders to participate (Luepker & Rastam, 1990; Mittlemark, Hunt, Heath, & Schmid, 1993).

Physicians, nurses, dentists, nutritionists, dieticians, hospitals, clinics, and health agencies are uniquely positioned to provide information to patients about preventive behaviors and maintenance of health (Luepker & Rastam, 1990; Relman, 1982; Wechsler, Levine, Idelson, Rohman, & Taylor, 1982). Such policies of medical institutions as smoking bans send messages to employees, patients, and the general community about the attitude of the institution regarding the importance of not smoking. The involvement and commitment of health professions appears to be essential to obtaining institutional commitment to such health-related policies (Kottke et al., 1985).

There are, however, well-known barriers to professional involvement in health promotion programs, such as lack of remuneration for prevention services, confusion about which preventive measures are appropriate, and inadequate training to deliver effective prevention interventions (Kottke et al., 1992; Mittlemark, Luepker, Grimm, Kottke, & Blackburn, 1988). The PHHP found that a targeted education campaign could involve substantial proportions of practicing community physicians in prevention-oriented continuing medical education (Carleton, Banspach, Block, et al., 1987). Critical components of this program included support and legitimation by local and national professional medical organizations such as medical schools, medical societies, and hospitals. Office-based interventions including training and provision of systems for medical record checklists and reminders have also been shown to increase physicians' delivery of prevention services (Kohatsu, Cramer, & Bohnstedt, 1994; Kottke et al., 1992; McPhee & Detmer, 1993). Finally, mail and telephone follow-up from trained health counselors can increase the effectiveness of health professional behavior change advice (Crouch et al., 1986).

Summary.   Because many components of a community impinge on health behavior, health promotion programs benefit from disseminating programs and messages in many different ways.

Presenting behavior change information through various channels increases the opportunity for achieving effects by capitalizing on interactions among systems. Increasing physicians' delivery of prevention services, for example, can be encouraged by providing training and resources to health care professionals. Changes in the health care delivery system may also result from informing consumers about prevention. In such cases, patient requests promote delivery of prevention services. In addition, worksite insurance policies may also encourage prevention services through cost incentives for healthful behavior change. The interrelationship of community components is therefore an important consideration for health promotion programs.

Multiple Health-Related Outcomes

Communities are complex dynamic entities. The people, institutions, and activities of communities reflect norms, priorities, and attitudes that affect health status. Effective community health promotions programs therefore target multiple health-related outcomes. Individual-level changes such as knowledge and attitudes have often been the focus of health behavior research. Successful community programs, however, also incorporate social-level changes among families, groups, organizations, and institutions. Facilitating environmental changes to enable, reinforce, and encourage healthful behavior change is crucial to improving the health status of communities.

Researchers increasingly acknowledge the need to understand how to bring about healthful changes in social policies and regulations so that people have access to facilities and resources necessary to healthful practices (Altman, Balcazar, Fawcett, Seekins, & Young, 1994; Thompson & Kinne, 1990). Governmental and private institutions influence health behaviors by controlling such matters as funding for health care services, parks and recreational facilities, public transportation, and street lighting; the number and location of liquor stores and the amount of alcohol and tobacco advertising; restrictions on

drinking age and cigarette vending machines; and excise taxes on alcohol and tobacco. In addition, businesses shape health by establishing workplace health and safety policies, providing resources for worksite health promotion programs and facilities, and determining the types of food to be sold in stores and restaurants. Institutional policies also influence health behavior by providing normative sanctions and legitimacy to health innovations. Incorporating diverse change strategies is, therefore, an important characteristic of community health promotion programs.

Qualitative research in the FCP examining smoking policy changes and the potential sources of influence on policy demonstrated that communities have history, norms, political leaders, and resources that place them in different stages regarding readiness to change. Community interventions appear to be able to influence these stages and to advance policy initiatives (Lipari, 1994). Moreover, data from the MHHP indicated that after 5 years of intensive intervention, Bloomington, Minnesota, became the largest municipality in the United States to ban the sale of cigarettes through vending machines (Lando, Bluhm, & Forster, 1991).

One strategy for changing the social and political environment is media advocacy, the "strategic use of mass media to advance social or public policy initiatives" (Pertschuk, 1988). Media advocates seek to influence what is covered by the media to shape public opinion and thus affect policy change (Wallack, Dorfman, Jernigan, & Themba, 1993). In the FCP, analyses demonstrated that frequent, regular, systematic contact with media professionals and provision of materials influenced newspaper coverage of health-related topics (Schooler, Sundar, & Flora, 1996). This study utilized multiple journalistic outcomes to assess the impact of media advocacy efforts; these outcomes included number and prominence of CVD-related articles, presence of prevention-focused themes, and increase in locally written articles (as opposed to wire service or syndicated items). Using these measures to analyze television, newspaper, magazine, or radio content can inform health promotion efforts to shape the media agenda. The success of media advocacy efforts has important implications for community health promotion because of the relationship between media coverage, public opinion, and public policy (Gohzenbach, 1992; Kennamer, 1992; Rogers, Dearing, & Chang, 1991).

Summary. A defining characteristic of communities is that components interact. This interaction means that health promotion programs can influence change at various levels. Individuals may learn health skills through education materials. Worksites can motivate behavior change by providing facilities and incentives. Organizations can encourage healthful practices through social support and policies. Messages and programs directed at many health-related outcomes therefore reinforce each other and promote effective behavior change. Comprehensive, integrated health promotion programs, moreover, can influence lasting changes in communities.

PROCESS OF COMMUNITY HEALTH PROMOTION

Principles and methods for effecting change in communities are central to the practice of health promotion (Minkler, 1990). Rothman (1979) identified three forms of community intervention: (1) social planning, a technical approach using rational empirical processes of data accumulation and persuasion involving experts; (2) social action, an advocacy or conflict strategy entailing mass mobilization of low-power components and use of political pressure; and (3) locality development, a cooperative, broadly based approach involving wide discussion and joint problem solving among many diverse community units.

Empowering Communities

The concept of empowerment is implicit in the process by which community groups are helped to identify common problems or goals, mobilize resources, and develop and implement programs. Empowerment refers to enabling individuals and communities to take control over their lives and their environment (Rappaport, 1984). In other words, community organization can enhance community competence and problem-solving ability and thereby help to effect change in people's lives and environments. Central to this process is building community competence so that various components can collaborate effectively in designing and implementing activities to reach agreed-upon goals (Cottrell, 1983). A key aspect of developing competent communities is the development of leaders who are able to motivate community members and facilitate group communication and activities (Hope & Timmel, 1984). A primary objective of community organization is to foster the capacity and desire of organizations to incorporate health promotion activities into the routines of business, government, and education (Mittlemark et al., 1993). Stimulated by community organization efforts, local health agencies may provide technical expertise, schools may alter curricula, corporate leaders may introduce health promotion at the workplace, and businesses may donate time, contest prizes, space, and other resources.

Health behavior research demonstrates that change agents who begin with a community's felt needs and concerns, rather than an external agenda, will be far more likely to experience success in community organization and in the change process (Nyswander, 1966). This type of community mobilization has been demonstrated to lead to change in health-related behaviors and environmental factors in projects such as the Tenderloin Senior Organizing Project (Minkler, 1985). In this type of locality development process, outside organizers play a facilitative role in helping the community group devise methods and strategies for achieving its objectives. In other situations, health professionals can adapt community organizing methods to heighten community participation and increase the effectiveness of community health programs. In such social planning processes, recognized experts assist community members to identify community needs and implement strategies for change. Moreover, in social action processes, health professionals can participate in community mobilization and activation to accomplish environmental change.

Several major cardiovascular disease interventions have used community mobilization to develop and implement coordinated community-wide health education strategies in order to improve community health-related behavior and reduce CVD-related risk factors and premature disability and death from CVD (Carlaw et al., 1984; Elder, Hovell, Lasater, Wells, & Carleton, 1985; Farquhar et al., 1985; Lefebvre, Lasater, Carleton, & Peterson, 1987; Maccoby & Solomon, 1981; Puska, Salonen, Tuomilehto, Nissinen, & Kottke, 1983; Stunkard, Felix, Yopp, & Cohen, 1985). These comprehensive approaches to community health promotion used strategies of locality development with broad community participation and citizen ownership. For example, the MHHP developed "community partnerships" for health through which community members worked with the research team in decision making and program implementation (Carlaw et al., 1984). In addition, considerable social planning technology was used in community needs assessment and analysis work. Professional planners assisted communities and citizens to determine needs and intervention strategies. Finally, social action strategies were employed in social policy, legislative, and advocacy initiatives (Bracht & Kingsbury, 1990).

Institutionalizing Health Changes. Community participation and involvement in health promotion programs enhance the likelihood that such programs will be sustained after external funding ends. Through the development of an effective network of community groups and support systems, health promotion programs can increase community competence by enhancing the problem-solving capacity of the group (Minkler, 1990). In the MHHP, for example, the members of the research team progressively served as consultants and program resources while the community began assuming planning and even funding roles (Blackburn, 1983). The FCP utilized a capacity-building strategy directed at local health educators to maintain its heart disease education program. Long-term maintenance of CVD prevention activities was achieved by applying a "training the trainers" model and cooperative learning methods to provide professional development, technical assistance, and other resources to a target group of community health educators (Jackson et al., 1994).

Examination of the continuation of programs by community agencies following completion of research projects demonstrates that program incorporation is a dynamic process (Bracht et al., 1994). Community agencies modify programs to meet changing community needs and agency interests. In addition, the limited "shelf life" of programs may necessitate modifying or terminating specific components. To the extent that agencies have the capacity to tailor existing programs and replace outmoded ones, the potential for long-term maintenance of community health promotion programs is enhanced (Jackson et al., 1994).

Summary. Health behavior change research demonstrates that a comprehensive, integrated community health promotion program that includes individual behavior change strategies, community organization and development principles to affect the social and physical environment, and efforts to build public support for policy change such as media advocacy is essential to achieve lasting behavior change. The complexities of planning and implementing health interventions in communities characterized by interactions among policy-making bodies, mass media, organizations, and individuals have prompted behavioral scientists to reconsider models of change that are solely or primarily information-oriented and expert-driven (Fortmann et al., 1995). Community studies have highlighted the importance of the process of intervening—working with communities to plan, develop, and implement appropriate and relevant health promotion programs.

NEW DIRECTIONS FOR COMMUNITY HEALTH PROMOTION PROGRAMS: RESEARCH ISSUES

Health behavior research has clear implications for improving efforts to promote health in community. Health promotion increasingly involves working with communities to ameliorate conditions that contribute to health-related problems such as poor access to services, paucity of low-cost nutritious foods, poor recreational facilities, inadequate housing, overcrowded and underfunded schools, and lack of economic opportunity. These systemic, macro issues directly impinge on health, which means that behavior change strategies need to be linked to community mobilization, policy advocacy, and political action. Three important research issues for enhancing the effectiveness of future health promotion programs are selection of outcomes, understanding interaction, and designing programmatic research.

Selection of Outcomes

A key element in designing a community health promotion program is determining which community components will be targets for change efforts. As discussed, there are many levels of intervention that affect health-related behaviors. Programs focused on individuals are perhaps the most common change strategy . It is important to consider, however, that individuals can also be reached through a variety of groupings, such as families, friendship networks, worksites, places of worship, and community organizations. Likewise, modifying environmental factors is an important program objective because regulations and policies strongly influence people's health behavior.

Selecting relevant and appropriate outcome objectives is informed by several considerations.

First, it is important to review research in a particular behavior change area. In the area of smoking prevention, for example, intervention efforts are increasingly being directed toward policy issues such as limiting youth access to tobacco products via banning free sampling and vending machines, encouraging enforcement of laws limiting sales to minors, raising excise taxes on tobacco products, and regulating advertising and promotion of tobacco products. Policy advocacy is therefore combined with more traditional individual-level programs such as school curricula.

A second important consideration is community interest. Community needs assessments can inform planners about topic areas and approaches that are most likely to garner public support. Integrating community priorities into program planning will enhance participation and contribute to success.

A third area to consider is the relative feasibility of various options. Certain popular programs for example, may be beyond the resources of program planners. Effecting large-scale social change, however, can become a long-term goal of a community health promotion program. Thus, efforts to enhance community capacity to work toward a long-term change goal are very compatible with other program elements.

Understanding Interaction

Community health promotion programs provide an opportunity to develop many types of interventions that can work together to influence health behavior. The number of possible interventions means, however, that programs are often quite complex. There is limited understanding of how program components (e.g., mass media messages, policy advocacy, worksite programs, self-help programs) interact to affect various levels of a community (e.g., individuals, families, organizations). Research demonstrates, for example, that school curricula promote behavior change more effectively when programs incorporate mass media, parental involvement, and school policy changes such as cafeteria selections and recreation programs (Perry & Kelder, 1992). The outcome in many of these studies, however, is individual behavior change. Future research is needed to understand more fully how changes in social norms, organizational policies, or the environment reciprocally affect each other, as well as contribute to individual-level effects.

There are a few constraints that hinder efforts to examine mutilevel health-related outcomes. First, the training of many health educators and researchers focuses on methods for intervening in aspects of individuals such as physiology and psychology. Their understanding of theories and techniques at other levels may therefore be limited. In addition, publishing research that does not include individual behavior change outcomes can be difficult. Many peer-reviewed public health journals favor empirical research that demonstrates validated measures of people's behavior. Another factor that contributes to an emphasis on individual behavior change is the tendency for health behavior research to focus on practical applications; research is often theory-based, but does not explicitly test or develop theory. Thus, there is a lack of models to articulate cross-level influences on community health. The most important constraint, however, is probably resources. Community-wide interventions are very costly. Given limited resources, researchers are encouraged to pursue strategies that are most likely to yield measurable outcomes. This constraint promotes programs focused on individuals. Effecting policy change, for example, is a very complicated, long-term endeavor with uncertain end points.

Despite these barriers, researchers should examine innovative, creative methods to develop a fuller understanding of how various components of a community interact to affect health status. Interdisciplinary projects foster exchange that contributes to theory and research at multiple levels of analysis. The entry of more researchers from fields such as communication and political science into public health provides opportunities to examine processes of exchange between levels. Agenda setting, for example, is a communication theory that explains how mass media messages affect public opinion (McCombs & Shaw, 1972). Research in political science has expanded on these findings to articulate how press coverage influences people's policy and candidate choices (Iyengar, 1991; Iyengar & Kinder, 1987). Now, public health research is beginning to examine how media agenda setting may affect public opinion and policy change in the health arena (Rogers et al., 1991; Schooler, Sundar, & Flora, 1996). This type of interdisciplinary cross-fertilization promises to further understanding of how to improve health in communities more effectively.

Designing Programmatic Research

Developing community health programs that allow for examination of multiple levels of intervention effects is an important next step. Demonstrating clear effects on individual health outcomes has proven challenging in many large-scale community-based interventions (Luepker et al., 1994). In the FCP, MHHP, and the PHHP, however, individual evaluation of numerous intervention components (e.g., smoking cessation methods, self-help kits, restaurant menu labeling programs, school-based dietary interventions) has shown them to be successful risk reduction strategies (Albright et al., 1990; Altman, Flora, Fortmann, & Farquhar, 1987; Crow et al., 1986; Jackson, Winkleby, Flora, & Fortmann, 1991; King et al., 1988; Lando, Loken, Howard-Pitney, & Pechacek, 1990; Murray, Kurth, Mullis, & Jeffery, 1990; Perry et al., 1992). In addition, many of these programs have been adopted and maintained by local groups and have been extended to other prevalent chronic diseases (e.g., cancer, diabetes, osteoporosis) that share common lifestyle correlates (Winkleby et al., 1994).

These results support continued investment in community health promotion programs. Future endeavors should integrate health promotion programs with public policy initiatives. Moreover, incorporating small, more focused studies within large community-wide efforts provides essential information about reaching specific subgroups that are traditionally underserved, such as ethnic minority groups, adults with low literacy, and older women (Winkleby et al., 1994). The three large-scale cardiovascular disease programs discussed in this chapter provide a model for public health research investigating both community-level effects and program-specific outcomes. A framework for evaluation might therefore include ecological analyses of the community environment (e.g., bike racks, exercise facilities, food availability, street lights), policy analysis of relevant institutions (government, education, health care), surveys of opinion leaders and other community members (awareness, skills knowledge, support for policy change, participation in prevention activities including political action), and specific health behavior outcome measures (smoking rates, criminal justice statistics, morbidity and mortality data).

CONCLUSION

It is clear that community health promotion programs can influence healthful changes in individuals, groups, organizations, and social systems. Research demonstrates that innovative programs that build on existing patterns of interaction can shift social norms and promote behavior change (Kelly et al., 1991). The benefits of increased healthful social interaction can be achieved with minimal-contact intervention strategies such as relapse prevention training on the telephone (deBusk et al., 1985; Juneau, Rogers, & DeSantos, 1987). Manipulating people's social environment has also been shown to influence behavior change. For example, Cialdini, Reno, and Kallgren (1990) changed the normative information in natural settings to influence subjects' littering behavior (cf. Reno, Cialdini, & Kallgren, 1993). Coupled with research demonstrating behavioral effects of policy changes, these findings highlight the importance of focusing on the social system to influence health behavior.

Health behavior research demonstrates that incorporating change strategies that target multiple audiences through multiple channels to achieve multiple health-related outcomes enhances the effectiveness of community health promotion programs. It is critical that these efforts be both comprehensive and well-integrated to facilitate synergy among components. Finally, tailoring behavior change strategies to community priorities, preferences, and cultural traditions is key to lasting social change.

REFERENCES

Aiken, M., & Mott, P. E. (Eds.). (1970). *The structure of community power*. New York: Random House.

Albright, C. L., Flora, J. A., & Fortmann, S. P. (1990). Restaurant menu labeling: Impact of nutrition information on entree sales and patron attitudes. *Health Education Quarterly, 17*, 157–167.

Altman, D. A., Flora, J. A., Fortmann, S. P., & Farquhar, J. W. (1987). The cost-effectiveness of three smoking cessation programs. *American Journal of Public Health, 77*, 162–165.

Altman, D. G., Balcazar, F., Fawcett, S., Seekins, T., & Young, J. Q. (1994). *Public health advocacy: Creating community change to improve health*. Palo Alto, CA: Stanford Center for Research in Disease Prevention.

American Psychological Association. (1993). *Violence and youth: Psychology's response, Vol. I: Summary report of the American Psychological Association Commission on Violence and Youth*. Washington, DC: APA.

Bandura, A. (1986). *Social foundations of thought and action: A social cognitive theory*. Englewood Cliffs, NJ: Prentice-Hall.

Blackburn, H. (1983). Research and demonstration projects in community cardiovascular disease prevention. *Journal of Public Health Policy, 4*, 398–421.

Blair, S. N., Piserchia, P. V., Wilbur, C. S., & Crowder, J. H. (1986). A public health intervention model for work-site health promotion. *Journal of the American Medical Association, 225*, 921–926.

Blum, H. L. (1981). Planning as a preferred instrument for achieving social change. In H. L. Blum (Ed.), *Planning for health: Generics for the eighties* (pp. 39–85). New York: Human Sciences.

Blum, H. L. (1982). Social perspective on risk reduction. In M. M. Faber & A. M. Reinhardt (Eds.), *Promoting health through risk reduction* (pp. 19–36). New York: Macmillan.

Bracht, N., Finnegan, J. R. Rissel, C., Weisbrod, R., Gleason, J.,

Corbett, J., & Veblen-Mortenson, S. (1994). Community ownership and program continuation following a health demonstration project. *Health Education Research, 2,* 243.

Bracht, N., & Kingsbury, L. (1990). Community organization principles in health promotion: A five-stage model. In N. Bracht (Ed.), *Health promotion at the community level* (pp. 66–88). Newbury Park, CA: Sage.

Brannon, B. R., Dent, C. W., Flay, B. R., Smith, G., Sussman, S., Pentz, M. A., Johnson, C. A., & Hansen, W. B. (1989). The television, school, and family project: The impact of curriculum delivery format on program acceptance. *Preventive Medicine, 18,* 492–502.

Brill, P. A., Kohl, H. W., Rogers, T., Collingwood, T. R., Sterling, C. L., & Blair, S. N. (1991). Recruitment, retention and success in worksite health promotion: Association with demographic characteristics. *American Journal of Health Promotion, 5,* 215–221.

Brown, E. R. (1984). Community organization influence on local public health care policy: A general research model and comparative case study. *Health Education Quarterly, 10,* 205–233.

Brownell, K. D., Cohen, R. Y., Stunkard, A. J., Felix, M. R., & Cooley, N. B. (1984). Weight loss competitions at the worksite: Impact on weight, morale and cost-effectiveness. *American Journal of Public Health, 74,* 1283–1285.

Brownstein, J. N., Cheal, N., Ackerman, S. P., Bassford, T. L., & Campos-Outcalt, D. (1992). Breast and cervical cancer screening in minority populations: A model for using lay health educators. *Journal of Cancer Education, 7,* 321–326.

Calle, E. E., Miracle-McMahill, H. L., Moss, R. E., & Heath, C. W., Jr. (1994). Personal contact from friends to increase mammography usage. *American Journal of Preventive Medicine, 10,* 361–366.

Campbell, M. K., DeVellis, B. M., Strecher, V. J., Ammerman, A. S., DeVellis, R. F., & Sandler, R. S. (1994). Improving dietary behavior: The effectiveness of tailored messages in primary care settings. *American Journal of Public Health, 84,* 783–787.

Carlaw, R. W., Mittlemark, M., Bracht, N., & Luepker, R. (1984). Organization for a community cardiovascular health program: Experiences from the Minnesota Heart Health Program. *Health Education Quarterly, 11,* 243–252.

Carleton, R., Banspach, S., Block, L., et al. (1987). Physician attitudes and behavior concerning cholesterol: Impact of public education. *CVD Epidemiology Newsletter, 41,* 43.

Carleton, R. A., Lasater, T. M., Assaf, A., Lefebvre, R. C., & McKinlay, S. M. (1987). The Pawtucket Heart Health Program. I. An experiment in population-based disease prevention. *Rhode Island Medical Journal, 70,* 533–538.

Chavis, D. M., & Newbrough, J. R. (1986). The meaning of "community" in community psychology. Psychological sense of community: II. Research and applications (special issue). *Journal of Community Psychology, 14*(4), 335–340.

Chavis, D. M., Stucky, P. E., & Wandersman, A. (1983). Return-ing basic research to the community: A relationship between scientists and citizens. *American Psychologist, 38,* 424–434.

Cialdini, R. B., Reno, R. R., & Kallgren, C. A. (1990). A focus theory of normative conduct: Recycling the concept of norms to reduce littering in public places. *Journal of Personality and Social Psychology, 58,* 1015–1026.

Cirksena, M. K., & Flora, J. A. (1995). Audience segmentation in worksite health promotion: A procedure using social marketing concepts. *Health Education Research, 10*(2), 211–224.

Colby, J. J., Elder, J. P., Peterson, G., Knisley, P. M., & Carleton, R. A. (1987). Promoting the selection of health food through menu item description in a family-style restaurant. *American Journal of Preventive Medicine, 3,* 171–177.

Conrad, P. (1987). Who comes to work-site wellness programs? A preliminary review. *Journal of Occupational Medicine, 29,* 319–320.

Cottrell, L. S., Jr. (1983). The competent community. In R. Warren & L. Lyon (Eds.), *New perspectives on the American community.* Homewood, IL: Dorsey Press.

Crockett, S. J., Mullis, R. M., Perry, C. L., & Luepker, R. V. (1989). Parent education in youth-directed nutrition interventions. *Preventive Medicine, 18,* 475–491.

Crouch, M., Sallis, J. F., Farquhar, J. W., Haskell, W. L., Ellsworth, N. M., King, A. B., & Rogers, T. (1986). Personal and mediated health counseling for sustained dietary reduction of hypercholesterolemia. *Preventive Medicine, 15,* 282–291.

Crow, R. S., Blackburn, H., Jacobs, D. R., et al. (1986). Population strategies to enhance physical activity: The Minnesota Heart Health Program. *Acta Medica Scandinavica, 711 Supplementum,* 93–112.

deBusk, R. F., Haskell, W. L., Miller, N. H., Berra, K., Taylor, C. B., & Berger, W. E. (1985). Medically directed at-home rehabilitation soon after clinically uncomplicated acute myocardial infarction: A new model for patient care. *American Journal of Cardiology, 55,* 251–257.

DePue, J. D., Wells, B. L., Lasater, T. M., et al. (1990). Volunteers as providers of heart health programs in churches: A report on implementation. *American Journal of Health Promotion, 4,* 361–366.

Dijkstra, M., de Vries, H., & Parcel, G. S. (1993). The linkage approach applied to a school-based smoking prevention program in the Netherlands. *Journal of School Health, 63,* 339–342.

Dressler, W. W. (1987). The stress process in a Southern black community: Implications for prevention research. *Human Organization, 46,* 211–220.

Elder, J. P., Hovell, M. F., Lasater, T. M., Wells, B. L., & Carleton, R. A. (1985). Applications of behavior modification to community health education: The case of heart disease prevention. *Health Education Quarterly, 12,* 151–168.

Elder, J., McGraw, S., Rodrigues, A., Lasater, T., Ferreira, A., Kendal, L., Peterson, G., & Carleton, R. (1987). Evaluation of two community-wide smoking contests. *Preventive Medicine, 16,* 221–234.

Elliott, D. (1994). *Youth violence: An overview.* Boulder, CO: Center for the Study and Prevention of Violence, University of Colorado.

Eng, E. (1993). The Save Our Sisters Project: A social network strategy for reaching rural black women. *Cancer, 72,* 1071–1077.

Farquhar, J. W., Flora, J. A., & Goode, L. (1986). *Comprehensive integrated health promotion programs.* Unpublished manuscript.

Farquhar, J. W., Fortmann, S. P., Maccoby, N., Haskell, W. L., Williams, P. T., Flora, J. A., Taylor, C. B., Brown, W. B., Solomon, D. S., & Hulley, S. B. (1985). The Stanford Five-City Project: Design and methods. *American Journal of Epidemiology , 122,* 323–334.

Farquhar, J. W., Maccoby, M., Wood, P. D., Alexander, J. K., Breitrose, H., Brown, B. W., Jr., Haskell, W. L., McAlister, A. L., Meyer, A. J., Nash, J. D., & Stern, M. P. (1977). Community education for cardiovascular health, *Lancet, 1,* 1192–1195.

Felix, M. R., Stunkard, A. J., Cohen, R. Y., & Cooley, N. B. (1985). Health promotion at the worksite. I. A process for establishing programs. *Preventive Medicine, 14,* 99–108.

Flay, B. R. (1986). Mass media linkages with school-based programs for drug-abuse prevention. *Journal of School Health, 56,* 402–406.

Flay, B. R. (1987). Mass media and smoking cessation: A critical review. *American Journal of Public Health, 77,* 153–160.

Flay, B. R., Gruder, C. L., Warnecke, R. B., Jason, L. A., & Peterson, P. (1989). One year follow-up of the Chicago televised smoking cessation program. *American Journal of Public Health, 79,* 1377–1380.

Flora, J. A. & Cassidy, D. (1990). Roles of media in community-based health promotion. In N. Bracht (Ed.), *Health promotion at the community level* (pp. 143–157). Newbury Park, CA: Sage.

Flora, J. A., Fortmann, S. P., Taylor, C. B., & Maccoby, N. (1985). Mediated smoking cessation programs in the Stanford Five-City Project. *Addictive Behaviors, 10,* 441–443.

Flora, J. A., Jackson, C., & Maccoby, N. (1989). Indicators of societal action to promote physical health. In S. B. Kar (Ed.), *Health promotion indicators and actions* (pp. 118–139). New York: Springer.

Flora, J. A., Jatulis, D., Jackson, C., & Fortmann, S. P. (1993). The Stanford Five-City Heart Disease Prevention Project. In T. E. Backer & E. M. Rogers (Eds.), *Organizational aspects of health communication campaigns: What works?* (pp. 101–128). Newbury Park, CA: Sage.

Flora, J. A., Roser, C., Chaffee, S., & Farquhar, J. W. (1988). Information campaign effects of different media: Results from the Stanford Five-City Project. Paper presented at the meeting of the Association for Education in Journalism and Mass Communication, Portland, OR.

Flora, J. A., & Schooler, C. (1995). Influence of health communication environments on children's diet and exercise knowledge, attitudes, and behavior. In G. L. Kreps & D. O'Hair (Eds.), *Communication and health outcomes* (pp. 187–213). Cressfill, NJ: Hampton Press.

Flora, J. A., Slater, M. D., & Maibach, E. W. (1989). Health lifestyles: An analysis of media use and interpersonal communication. Paper presented at the meeting of the International Communication Association, San Francisco, CA.

Fortmann, S. P., Flora, J. A., Winkleby, M. A., Schooler, C., Taylor, C. B., & Farquhar, J. W. (1995). Community intervention trials: Reflections on the Stanford Five-City Project experience. *American Journal of Epidemiology , 142*(6), 576–586.

Freimuth, V. S., Hammond, S. L., & Stein, J. A. (1988). Health advertising: Prevention for profit. *American Journal of Public Health, 78,* 557–561.

Fullen, M. (1985). Change processes and strategies at the local level. *Elementary School Journal, 85,* 391–421.

Gans, K. M., Levin, S., Lasater, T. M., Sennett, L. L., Maroni, A., Ronan, A., & Carleton, R. A. (1990). Heart Healthy Cook-Offs in home economic classes: An evaluation with junior high school students. *Journal of School Health, 60,* 99–102.

Gonzenbach, W. J. (1992). A time-series analysis of the drug issue, 1985–1990: The press, the president and public opinion. *International Journal of Public Opinion Research, 4,* 126–147.

Gravell, J., Zapka, J. G., & Mamon, J. A. (1985). Impact of breast self-examination planned educational messages on social network communications: An exploratory study. *Health Education Quarterly, 12,* 51–64.

Gregg, W., Foote, A., Erfurt, J. C., & Heirich, M. A. (1990). Worksite follow-up and engagement strategies for initiating health risk behavior changes. *Health Education Quarterly, 17,* 455–478.

Gruder, C. L., Warnecke, R. B., Jason, L. A., Flay, B. R., & Peterson, P. (1990). A televised, self-help, cigarette smoking cessation intervention. *Addictive Behaviors, 15,* 505–516.

Grunig, J. E. (1979). Time budgets, level of involvement and use of the mass media. *Journalism Quarterly, 56,* 248–261.

Hatch, H. W., & Lovelace, K. (1980). Involving the Southern rural church and students of the health professions in health education. *Public Health Reports, 95,* 23–25.

Hertzler, A. A. (1983). Children's food patterns—a review: Family and group behavior. *Journal of the American Dietetic Association, 83,* 509–512.

Hope, A., & Timmel, S. (1984). *Training for transformation: A handbook for community workers.* Gweru, Zimbabwe: Mambo Press.

Hunt, M. K., Lefebvre, R. C., Hixson, M. L., Banspach, S. W., Assaf, A. R., & Carleton, R. A. (1990). Pawtucket Heart Health Program point-of-purchase nutrition education program in supermarkets. *American Journal of Public Health, 80,* 730–731.

Iverson, D. C., Fielding, J. E., Crow, R. S., & Christenson, G. M. (1985). The promotion of physical activity in the U.S. population: The status of programs in medical, worksite, community, and school settings. *Public Health Reports, 100*, 21.

Iyengar, S. (1991). *Is anyone responsible? How television frames political issues*. Chicago: University of Chicago Press.

Iyengar, S., & Kinder, D. R. (1987). *News that matters*. Chicago: University of Chicago Press.

Jackson, C., Fortmann, S. P., Flora, J. A., Melton, R. J., Snider, J. P., & Littlefield, D. (1994). The capacity-building approach to intervention maintenance implemented by the Stanford Five-City Project. *Health Education Research, 9*, 385–396.

Jackson, C., Winkleby, M. A., Flora, J. A., & Fortmann, S. P. (1991). Utilization of educational resources for cardiovascular risk reduction in the Stanford Five-City Project. *American Journal of Preventive Medicine, 7*, 82–88.

Jeffery, R. W., Forster, J. L., & Schmid, T. L. (1989). Worksite health promotion: Feasibility testing of repeated weight control and smoking cessation classes. *American Journal of Health Promotion, 3*, 11–16.

Jeffery, R. W., French, S. A., Raether, C., & Baxter, J. E. (1994). An environmental intervention to increase fruit and salad purchases in a cafeteria. *Preventive Medicine, 23*, 788–792.

Juneau, M., Rogers, F., DeSantos, V., & Yee, M. (1987). Effectiveness of self-monitored home-based moderate intensity exercise training in middle-aged men and women. *American Journal of Epidemiology , 60*, 66–70.

Kelly, J. A., St. Lawrence, J. S., Diaz, Y. E., Stevenson, L., et al. (1991). HIV risk behavior reduction following intervention with key opinion leaders of population: An experimental analysis. *American Journal of Public Health, 81*, 168–171.

Kennamer, J. D. (1992). *Public opinion, the press and public policy*. Praeger.

Killen, J. D., Telch, M. J., Robinson, T. N., Maccoby, N., Taylor, C. B., & Farquhar, J. W. (1988). Cardiovascular disease risk reduction for tenth graders: A multiple-factor school-based approach. *Journal of the American Medical Association, 260*, 1728–1733.

King, A. C., Flora, J. A., Fortmann, S. P., & Taylor, C. B. (1987). Smokers' challenge: Immediate and long-term findings of a community smoking cessation contest. *American Journal of Public Health, 77*, 1340–1341.

King, A. C., Saylor, K. E., Forster, S., Killen, J. D., Telch, M. J., Farquhar, J. W., & Flora, J. A. (1988). Promoting dietary change in adolescents: A school-based approach for modifying and maintaining healthy behavior. *American Journal of Preventive Medicine, 4*, 68–74.

Klatcher, M. L. (1987). Prevention of tap water scald burns: Evaluation of a multimedia injury control program. *American Journal of Public Health, 77*, 337–354.

Kohatsu, N. D., Cramer, E., & Bohnstedt, M. (1994). Use of a clinician reminder system for screening mammography in a public health clinic. *American Journal of Preventive Medicine, 10*, 348–352.

Kotler, P. (1975). *Marketing for nonprofit organizations*. Englewood Cliffs, NJ: Prentice-Hall.

Kotler, P., & Zaltman, G. (1971). Social marketing: An approach to planned social change. *Journal of Marketing, 35*, 3–12.

Kottke, T. E., Hill, C., Heitzig, C., Brekke, M., Blake, S., Arneson, S., & Caspersen, C. (1985). Smoke-free hospitals: Attitudes of patients, employees, and faculty. *Minnesota Medicine, 53*, 53–55.

Kottke, T. E., Solberg, L. I., Brekke, M. L., Conn, S. A., Maxwell, P., & Brekke, M. J. (1992). A controlled trial to integrate smoking cessation advice into primary care practice: Doctors Helping Smokers, Round III. *Journal of Family Practice, 34*, 701–708.

Lando, H. A., Bluhm, J., & Forster, J. L. (1991). The ban on cigarette vending machines in Bloomington, Minnesota. *American Journal of Public Health, 81*, 1339–1340.

Lando, H. A., Loken, B., Howard-Pitney, B., & Pechacek, T. (1990). Community impact of a localized smoking cessation contest. *American Journal of Public Health, 80*, 601–603.

Lasater, T. M., Carleton, R. A., & Wells, B. (1991). Religious organizations and large-scale health related lifestyle change programs. *Journal of Health Education, 22*, 233–239.

Lasater, T. M., DePue, J. D., Wells, B. L., et al. (1990). The effectiveness and feasibility of delivering nutrition education programs through religious organizations. *Health Promotion International, 5*, 253–257.

Lasater, T. M., Wells, B. L., Carleton, R. A., & Elder, J. P. (1986). The role of churches in disease prevention research studies. *Public Health Reports, 101*, 125–131.

Lefebvre, R. C., & Flora, J. A. (1988). Social marketing and public health intervention. *Health Education Quarterly, 15*, 299–315.

Lefebvre, R. C., Lasater, T., Carleton, R. A., & Peterson, G. (1987). Theory and delivery of health programming in the community. *Preventive Medicine, 16*, 890–895.

Levin, J. S. (1984). The role of the black church in community medicine. *Journal of the National Medical Association, 76*, 477–483.

Levy, A., & Stokes, R. (1987). Effects of a health promotion advertising campaign on sales of ready-to-eat cereals. *Public Health Reports, 102*, 398–403.

Lipari, L. (1994). Stages of change in public smoking policy: Four California cities. Paper presented at the annual meeting of the International Communication Association, Washington, DC.

Luepker, R. V., Murray, D. M., Jacobs, D. R., et al. (1994). Community education for cardiovascular disease prevention: Risk factor changes in the Minnesota Heart Health Program. *American Journal of Public Health, 84*, 1383–1393.

Luepker, R. V., & Rastam, L. (1990). Involving community

health professionals and systems. In N. Bracht (Ed.), *Health promotion at the community level* (pp. 185-198). Newbury Park, CA: Sage.

Maccoby, N., Farquhar, J. W., Wood, P., & Alexander, J. (1977). Reducing the risk of cardiovascular disease: Effects of a community-based campaign on knowledge and behavior. *Journal of Community Health, 24,* 100-114.

Maccoby, N., & Solomon, D. S. (1981). Heart disease prevention: Community studies. In R. E. Rice & W. Paisley (Eds.), *Pubic communication campaigns* (pp. 105-126). Beverly Hills, CA: Sage.

Marcus, B. H., Banspach, S. W., Lefebvre, R. C., Rossi, J. S., Carleton, R. A., & Abrams, D. B. (1992). Using the stages of change model to increase the adoption of physical activity among community participants. *American Journal of Health Promotion, 6,* 424-429.

McAlister, A., Puska, P., Koskela, K., Salonen, J. T., & Maccoby, N. (1980). Psychology in action: Mass communication and community organization for public health education. *American Psychologist, 35,* 375-379.

McCombs, M., & Shaw, D. (1972). The agenda setting function of mass media. *Public Opinion Quarterly, 36,* 176-187.

McFall, S. L., Michener, A., Rubin, D., Flay, B. R., Mermelstein, R. J., Burton, D., Jelen, P., & Warnecke, R. B. (1993). The effects and use of maintenance newsletters in a smoking cessation intervention. *Addictive Behaviors, 18,* 151-158.

McPhee, S. J., & Detmer, W. M. (1993). Office-based interventions to improve delivery of cancer prevention services by primary care physicians. *Cancer, 72,* 1100-1112.

Millar, W. J. (1988). *Smoke in the workplace: An evaluation of smoking restrictions.* Ottawa, Canada: Minister of Supply and Services.

Minkler, M. (1985). Building supportive ties and sense of community among the inner-city elderly: The Tenderloin Senior Outreach Project. *Health Education Quarterly, 12,* 303-314.

Minkler, M. (1990). Improving health through community organization. In K. Glanz, F. M. Lewis, & B. K. Rimer (Eds.), *Health behavior and health education* (pp. 257-287). San Francisco: Jossey-Bass.

Mittlemark, M. B., Hunt, M. K., Heath, G. W., & Schmid, T. L. (1993). Realistic outcomes: Lessons from community-based research and demonstration programs for the prevention of cardiovascular diseases. *Journal of Health Policy, 14,* 437-462.

Mittlemark, M. B., Luepker, R. V., Grimm, R., Kottke, T. E., & Blackburn, H. (1988). The role of physicians in a community-wide program for prevention of cardiovascular disease: The Minnesota Heart Health Program. *Public Health Reports, 103,* 360-365.

Mullis, R. M., Hunt, M. K., Foster, M., et al. (1987). The Shop Smart for Your Heart grocery program. *Journal of Nutrition Education, 19,* 225-228.

Mullis, R. M., & Pirie, P. (1988). Lean meats make the grade—A collaborative nutrition intervention program. *Journal of the American Dietetic Association, 88,* 191-195.

Murphy, P. E. (1984). Analyzing markets. In L. W. Frederiksen, L. J. Solomon, & K. A. Brehony (Eds.), *Marketing health behavior: Principles, techniques, and applications* (pp. 41-58). New York: Plenum Press.

Murray, D. M., Kurth, C., Mullis, R. M., & Jeffery, R. W. (1990). Cholesterol reduction through low intensity interventions: Results from the Minnesota Heart Health Program. *Preventive Medicine, 19,* 181-189.

Nelson, D. J., Sennett, L., Lefebvre, R. C., & Loisella, L. (1987). A campaign strategy for weight loss at work sites. *Health Education Research, 2,* 21-31.

Nelson, E. C., Keller, A. M., & Zubkoff, M. (1981). Incentives for health promotion: The government's role. In L. K. Y. Ng & D. B. Davis (Eds.), *Strategies for public health: Promoting health and preventing disease* (pp. 218-231). New York: Van Nostrand Reinhold.

Newbrough, J. R. (1992). Community psychology in the postmodern world: Where is community psychology headed? (Special section). *Journal of Community Psychology, 20*(1), 10-25.

Novelli, W. D. (1984). Developing marketing programs. In L. W. Frederiksen, L. J. Solomon, & K. A. Brehony (Eds.), *Marketing health behavior: Principles, techniques, and applications* (pp. 59-89). New York: Plenum Press.

Nyswander, D. (1966). The open society: Its implications for health educators. *Health Education Monographs, 1,* 3-13.

Parcel, G. S., Simons-Morton, B. G., & Kolbe, L. J. (1988). Health promotion: Integrating organizational change and student learning strategies. *Health Education Quarterly, 15,* 435-450.

Pechacek, T., Freutel, J., Arkin, R., & Mittlemark, M. (1983). *The Quit and Win Contest: A community-wide incentive program for smoking cessation.* Paper presented at the World Congress on Behavior Therapy, Washington, DC.

Perry, C. L., & Kelder, S. H. (1992). Models for effective prevention. *Journal of Aging and Health, 13,* 355-363.

Perry, C. L., Kelder, S. H., Murray, D. M., & Klepp, K. I. (1992). Community-wide smoking prevention: Long-term outcomes of the Minnesota Heart Health Program. *American Journal of Public Health, 82,* 1210-1216.

Perry, C. L., Klepp, K. I., & Sillers, C. (1989). Community-wide strategies for cardiovascular health: The Minnesota Heart Health Program youth program. *Health Education Research, 4,* 87-101.

Perry, C. L., Luepker, R. V., Murray, D. M., et al. (1989). Parent involvement with children's health promotion: A one-year follow-up of The Minnesota Home Team. *Health Education Quarterly, 16,* 171-180.

Pertschuk, M. (1988). *Smoking control: Media advocacy guidelines.* Washington, DC: Advocacy Institute for the National Cancer Institute, National Institutes of Health.

Prochaska, J. O., Redding, C. A., Harlow, L. L., Rossi, J. S., & Velicer, W. F. (1994). The transtheoretical model of change and HIV prevention: A review. *Health Education Quarterly, 21,* 471-486.

Puska, P., McAlister, A., Niemensivy, H., Pihu, T., Wijo, J., &

Koskela, K. (1987). A television format for national health promotion: Finland's "Keys to Health." *Public Health Reports, 102,* 263–269.

Puska, P., Salonen, J. T., Tuomilehto, J., Nissinen, A., & Kottke, T. E. (1983). Evaluating community-based preventive cardiovascular programs: Problems and experiences from the North Karelia Project. *Journal of Community Health, 9,* 49–63.

Rappaport, J. (1984). Studies in empowerment: Introduction to the issue. *Prevention in Human Services, 3,* 1–7.

Relman, A. S. (1982). Encouraging the practice of preventive medicine and health promotion. *Public Health Reports, 97,* 216–219.

Reno, R. R., Cialdini, R. B., & Kallgren, C. A. (1993). The transsituational influence of social norms. *Journal of Personality and Social Psychology, 64,* 104–112.

Reynes, J. F., Lasater, T. M., Feldman, H., Assaf, A. R., & Carleton, R. A. (1993). Education and risk factors for coronary heart disease: Results from a New England community. *American Journal of Preventive Medicine, 9*(6), 365–371.

Rimal, R., & Flora, J. A. (1994). *Psychological and familial influences on children's dietary behavior: Perspectives from a health information campaign.* Paper presented at the annual meeting of the International Communication Association, Sydney, Australia.

Roberts, B. B., & Thorsheim, H. I. (1987). A partnership approach to consultation: The process and results of a major primary prevention field experiment. In *The Ecology of Prevention* [Special Issue]. *Prevention in Human Services, 4,* 151–186.

Rogers, E. M. (1983). *Diffusion of innovations* (3rd ed). New York: Free Press.

Rogers, E. M., Dearing, J. W., & Chang, S. (1991). *AIDS in the 1980s: The agenda-setting process for a public issue.* Journalism Monographs No. 126. Columbia, SC: Association for Education in Journalism and Mass Communication.

Rossi, S. R., Rossi, J. S., Rossi-DelPrete, L. M., Prochaska, J. O., Banspach, S. W., & Carleton, R. A. (1994). A processes of change model for weight control for participants in community-based weight loss programs. *International Journal of the Addictions, 29,* 161–177.

Rothman, J. (1979). Three models of community organization practice, their mobilizing and phasing. In F. M. Cox, J. L. Erlich, J. Rothman, & J. E. Tropman (Eds.), *Strategies of community organization* (3rd ed.) (pp. 25–45). Itasca, IL: F. E. Peacock.

Rothman, J., & Brown, E. R. (1989). Indicators of societal action to promote social health. In S. B. Kar (Ed.), *Health promotion indicators and actions* (pp. 202–220). New York: Springer.

Salina, D., Jason, L. A., Hedeker, D., Kaufman, J., Lesondak, L., McMahon, S. D., Taylor, S., & Kimball, P. (1994). A follow-up of a media-based, worksite smoking cessation program. *American Journal of Community Psychology, 22,* 257–271.

Sallis, J. F., & Nader, P. R. (1988). Family determinants of health behaviors. In D. S. Gochman (Ed.), *Health behavior: Emerging research perspectives* (pp. 107–124). New York: Plenum Press.

Sanders, I. T. (1966). *The community: An introduction to a social system* (2nd ed.). New York: Ronald Press.

Schooler, C., Flora, J. A., & Farquhar, J. W. (1993). Moving toward synergy: Media supplementation in the Stanford Five-City Project. The role of communication in health promotion (special issue). *Communication Research, 20*(4), 587–610.

Schooler, C., Sundar, S. S., & Flora, J. A. (1996). Effects of the Stanford Five-City Project media advocacy program. *Health Education Quarterly, 23*(3), 346–364.

Shannon, B., Mullis, R. M., Pirie, P. L., et al. (1990). Promoting better nutrition in the grocery store using a game format: The Shop Smart Game format. *Journal of Nutrition Education, 22,* 183–188.

Simons-Morton, B. G., Parcel, G. S., Baranowski, T., Forthofer, R., & O'Hara, N. M. (1991). Promoting physical activity and a healthful diet among children: Results of a school-based intervention study. *American Journal of Public Health, 81,* 986–991.

Skinner, C. S., Strecher, V. J., & Hospers, H. (1994). Physicians' recommendations for mammography: Do tailored messages make a difference? *American Journal of Public Health, 84,* 43–49.

Slater, M., & Flora, J. A. (1991). Health lifestyles: Audience segmentation for public health interventions. *Health Education Quarterly, 18,* 221–234.

Sorensen, G., Glasgow, R. E., & Corbett, K. (1990). Involving work sites and other organizations. In N. Bracht (Ed.), *Health promotion at the community level* (pp. 158–184). Newbury Park, CA: Sage.

Sorensen, G., Rigotti, N., Rosen, A., & Pinney, J. (in press). The effects of a work-site nonsmoking policy: Evidence for increased cessation. *American Journal of Public Health.*

Stunkard, A. J., Cohen, R. Y., & Felix, M. R. J. (1989). Weight loss competitions at the worksite: How they work and how well. *Preventive Medicine, 18,* 460–474.

Stunkard, A. J., Felix, M. R. J., Yopp, P., & Cohen, R. Y. (1985). Mobilizing a community to promote health: The Pennsylvania County Health Improvement Program (CHIP). In J. C. Rosen & L. J. Solomon (Eds.), *Prevention in health psychology* (pp. 143–190). Hanover, NH: University Press of New England.

Thomas, S. B., Quinn, S. C., Billingsley, A., & Caldwell, C. (1994). The characteristics of northern black churches with community health outreach programs. *American Journal of Public Health, 84,* 575–579.

Thompson, B., & Kinne, S. (1990). Social change theory: Applications to community health. In N. Bracht (Ed.), *Health promotion at the community level* (pp. 45–65). Newbury Park, CA: Sage.

U.S. Department of Health and Human Services. (1989). *Churches as an avenue to high blood pressure control.*

NIH Publication No. 87-2725. Washington, DC: U.S. Government Printing Office.

U.S. Department of Health and Human Services. (1991). *Healthy people 2000. National health promotion and disease prevention objectives*. DHHS Publication No. PHS 91-50212. Washington, DC: U.S. Department of Health and Human Services.

Wallack, L., Dorfman, L., Jernigan, D., & Themba, M. (1993). *Media advocacy and public health: Power for prevention*. Newbury Park, CA: Sage.

Warnecke, R. B., Langenberg, P., Wong, S. C., Flay, B. R., & Cook, T. D. (1992). The second Chicago televised smoking cessation program: A 24-month follow-up. *American Journal of Public Health*, *82*, 835–840.

Warren, R. I. (1972). *The community in America*. Chicago: Rand McNally.

Wechsler, H., Levine, S., Idelson, R. K., Rohman, M., & Taylor, J. O. (1982). The physician's role in health promotion: A survey of primary-care practitioners. *Massachusetts Department of Public Health*, *308*, 97–98.

Weinstein, A. (1987). *Market segmentation*. Chicago: Probus.

Wiist, W. H., & Flack, J. M. (1990). A church-based cholesterol education program. *Public Health Reports*, *105*, 381–386.

Wilbur, C. S., Zifferblatt, S. M., Pinsky, J. L., & Zifferblatt, S. (1981). Healthy vending: A cooperative pilot research program to stimulate good health in the marketplace. *Preventive Medicine*, *10*, 85–93.

Winkleby, M. A., Flora, J. A., & Kraemer, H. C. (1994). Predictors of change during a community-based disease intervention program. *American Journal of Public Health*, *84*, 767–772.

Winkleby, M. A., Fortmann, S. P., & Rockhill, B. (1992). Trends in cardiovascular disease risk factors by educational level: The Stanford Five-City Project. *Preventive Medicine*, *21*(5), 592–601.

Worden, J. K., Flynn, B. S., Merrill, D. G., Waller, J. A., & Haugh, L. D. (1989). Preventing alcohol-impaired driving through community self-regulation training. *American Journal of Public Health*, *79*, 287–290.

16

Health Behavior Interventions with Families

Tom Baranowski and Marsha Davis Hearn

INTRODUCTION

Families are an important social environment within which health-related behaviors occur (Tinsley, 1992). This is particularly true for food-related behaviors. Foods are often purchased, prepared, and consumed in the presence of family members. A fast food restaurant is often selected by family decision, and foods are often selected in the presence of other family members. Some parents use foods as rewards for children's good behaviors. Some couples use a favorite restaurant as a setting for anniversaries and other special occasions. Some characteristics of the family serve to maintain the existing behavior (Neill, Marshall, & Yale, 1978), while other characteristics can be latent forces for change. If health professionals attempt to change an individual's behavior without being informed about the various family influences, the attempt will likely run into many impediments, and thereby fail.

While any of a variety of health behaviors could have been selected, this chapter reviews the literature on interventions with families to promote dietary change and is a companion to Chapter 9 in Volume I of this *Handbook*, which reviewed family correlates of dietary behavior. That chapter demonstrated differences in the purpose and nature of family influences on dietary practices by developmental stage of the children and family and differences by stage in food purchase and availability. This chapter will review the literature of how families have been involved in attempts to change dietary behavior within developmental stages. A major premise of this chapter is that family-based interventions will be more effective if predicated on a better understanding of how families relate to the targeted behavior, which in most cases requires more basic health behavior research.

A stark seriousness descended on the health community (Susser, 1995) with the publication of reports of several large, well-funded, long-term community intervention trials that demonstrated negligible change in the targeted behaviors

Tom Baranowski • Department of Behavioral Science, M. D. Anderson Cancer Center, University of Texas at Houston, Houston, Texas 77030.   **Marsha Davis Hearn** • Department of Nutrition and Dietetics, Georgia State University, Atlanta, Georgia 30303.

Handbook of Health Behavior Research IV: Relevance for Professionals and Issues for the Future, edited by David S. Gochman. Plenum Press, New York, 1997.

(COMMIT Research Group, 1995a,b; Glasgow, Terborg, Hollis, Severson, & Boles, 1995; Lando et al., 1995). Health professionals need, in part, to reconsider what is realistically achievable with current community intervention programs (Fisher, 1995) and, in part, to more carefully scrutinize what the interventions are attempting to do and how to conduct them.

In reviewing the literature on family-based interventions, this chapter reveals that most published articles do not provide sufficient detail on the intervention. While this inadequacy is often due to editorial comments (or to anticipation of such comments) concerning journal space, the level of detail has been insufficient to ascertain how interventions implemented theoretical concepts or involved families. Furthermore, most reports of interventions presented little rationale for the form and nature of the intervention, e.g., why an intervention was designed and implemented in one way rather than in one of many possible alternative ways. Since interventions are not having the desired effects, these details are particularly important to ferret out why some interventions appear to work and others do not and to avoid the mistakes of the past. Also, many interventions have been designed and implemented without being adequately informed of the influences on the targeted behaviors. While the interventions were based on theoretical principles for behavior change, the targeted behavior was often dealt with out of context, i.e., a knowledge of the influences on the targeted behavior. A number of authors have called for more careful targeting of change programs at the factors that maintain the undesired behaviors (Baranowski, Lin, Wetter, Resnicow, & Hearn, 1997; Domel et al., 1993; McLeroy et al., 1993). While families are obvious influences serving to maintain some health behaviors for certain categories of individuals— e.g., children, spousal partners—more needs to be learned about these influences (see Chapter 9 in Volume I).

Families are complex social entities. Professionals are in the earliest stages of understanding how families interact in regard to food or to other health behaviors (Chapter 9 in Volume I). The model of family reciprocal determinism will be used and expanded here to organize and understand the information on family influences on diet (Taylor, Baranowski, & Sallis, 1994; see also Chapter 9 in Volume I). Since little is known about how families influence diet, some researchers have used qualitative techniques in conjunction with theoretical formulations to better understand why family members are not eating the targeted foods, i.e., a theory of the problem (T. Baranowski et al., 1993; Kirby, Baranowski, Reynolds, Taylor, & Binkley, 1995). More qualitative research will further improve this understanding of how families influence diet and thereby provide more insights for promoting change in family interactions in regard to food.

This chapter is limited by the literature available for review. Much of this literature employs a simple experimental–control group design. Such designs are important evaluation tools to assess whether or not a particular program worked. Outcome evaluations of such programs enable professionals to say that this complex intervention with these multiple components developed in this particular way was effective, or was not effective, for this targeted population at this time. While such statements are important, they provide a limited basis for building a body of knowledge about how best to involve families to promote change. Large samples with intensive process evaluations related to compliance with intervention guidelines and outcomes can indicate which components of the programs worked according to design, and which did not, and thereby provide some insight into why the intervention did or did not work. Most intervention studies, however, have not been large, nor have they incorporated substantial process evaluations, thereby limiting the ability to infer why a program worked.

A stronger research design would be to systematically vary one or more components of the intervention, randomly assign participants or social units to condition, and thereby make inferences about the effectiveness of the varied components. Few studies have systematically varied intervention components. An even stronger design would be to identify characteristics of families prior to the intervention and systematically assess which interventions worked with which types of families. Such a design also has not been used. This review of the literature is thus forced to invoke reviewer judgment about why some interventions worked and others did not, and with whom.

WHY INTERVENE WITH FAMILIES WITH CHILDREN?

There has been growing interest in dietary interventions with children to promote cardiovascular health and prevent cancer. The conventional wisdom for such interventions reflects need and opportunity. In regard to need, young children have already been shown to have cardiovascular disease (CVD) (atherosclerotic plaque) (Newman, Freedman, & Berenson, 1986); CVD risk factors (e.g., blood pressure) are elevated among some children, and those with elevated values tend to maintain elevated values across childhood (Nicklas, Webber, Johnson, Srinivasan, & Berenson, 1995) and from childhood into the adult years (called "tracking") (Mahoney, Lauer, Lee, & Clarke, 1991; Nicklas et al., 1995). The adult risk-factor-related behaviors (e.g., fat in the diet) also are elevated and track among children (Shea, Stein, Basch, Contento, & Zybert, 1992) and from childhood into the adult years (Kelder, Perry, Klepp, & Lytle, 1994). All these findings suggest that the risks for adult chronic disease begin among children.

In regard to opportunity, changes in the risk-related behaviors modify the risk factors among children (Gliksman, Lazarus, & Wilson, 1993), and research has indicated that health-enhancing behaviors (e.g., eating more fruits and vegetables) are learned in childhood (Birch, 1993). Child-focused interventions thus have the potential to arrest disease among those children who have it, to disrupt risk-factor and risk-behavior tracking, and to establish lifestyle patterns that

will protect participants into their adult years. All these factors thereby serve to mitigate the ravages of chronic disease in adulthood (Williams, 1983/1985).

Though the rationale for intervening to disrupt smoking initiation among children before the behavior is established is incontrovertible, there has been some controversy about dietary interventions among children. Health behavior researchers have noted that risk-factor tracking over many years beginning in childhood is so low that children with high risk factors do not automatically become middle-aged adults with high risk factors (Van Lenthe, Kemper, & Twisk, 1994). There has also been concern about the extent to which lifestyle changes can be attained among children and maintained into the adult years. Future research must address the extent to which middle-aged adult dietary preferences and practices (e.g., food selections, serving sizes) reflect the preferences and practices of childhood and what the influences are that initiate and maintain these preferences and practices.

DEVELOPMENTAL PHASES

Interventions for dietary change have involved family members across the human developmental span. Because the nature of the targeted behavior and the influences on those targeted behaviors are likely to vary by developmental phase (see Chapter 9 in Volume I), this chapter is organized around phases.

Prenatal

A primary determinant of the health of a newborn is the weight gain of the mother during pregnancy. Inadequate prenatal weight gain can lead to premature birth, low birth weight, and all related complications. It has been proposed that food deprivation at critical stages in pregnancy retards key aspects of fetal development and leads to premature cardiovascular mortality (Barker et al., 1993). Thus, interventions with the pregnant mother have direct implications for the growing fetus, and the mother's family likely influences her behaviors. Since the most appropriate food for infants is breast milk (U.S. Department of Health and Human Services, 1984), getting mothers to initiate breast-feeding soon after delivery requires intervention during the prenatal period. Little literature has appeared on the environmental or personal factors that likely influence mothers' prenatal dietary practices.

Prenatal Weight Gain.   Social marketing techniques were used to enhance prenatal weight gain among lower-income women (Brown et al., 1992). Since parents were anticipated to be important influences on the dietary practices of teenage mothers, a handout was developed to elicit support from parents for teenagers' weight gain. Outcome evaluation revealed that the program may have worked among Euro-American mothers, but not among African-American mothers (Brown, Tharp, & Finnegan, 1996). No process evaluation data were presented on parental social support. To improve the likelihood of success, health behavior research needs to address the sources of influence upon pregnant teenagers' eating practices and perhaps identify different influences in different populations of pregnant teens (e.g., those remaining with families, those getting married, those entering shelters).

Breast-Feeding.   Health behavior research has shown that whether a mother breast-feeds is a function of social support influences (which vary by ethnicity), outcome expectations, and acculturation (Chapter 9 in Volume I). Involving the partners of pregnant Women, Infants and Children participants in an education program using incentives had a substantial impact on the percentage of mothers breast-feeding at hospital discharge and 2 weeks, 6 weeks, and 3 months postpartum (Sciacca, Phipps, Dupe, & Ratliff, 1995). It is not clear from this report whether the effects were due to incentives to attend education classes (thereby increasing mothers' attendance and knowledge), participation of the partner, or

both. Since existing breast-feeding pamphlets do not meet the general guidelines for good promotional literature (Valaitis & Shea, 1993), a self-help manual for encouraging breast feeding among low-income women was developed, but did not affect the dominant influence of the feeding preferences of the mother's significant other (Coombs, Reynolds, Blankson, & Joyner, 1994). A combined television and radio campaign to increase the breast-feeding knowledge of mothers and a professional education campaign to reach health professionals resulted in a substantial increase in the initiation of breast-feeding and in the earlier initiation of breast-feeding, especially among mothers delivering at home (McDivitt, Zimicki, Hornik, & Abulaban, 1994). No process evaluation data were obtained in regard to parents, spouses, or partners for any of these breast-feeding studies.

Implications for Intervention and Priority Research.   Mothers-to-be appear particularly responsive to interventions to promote the health of their child. While support from the spousal partner, or from parents in the case of the single pregnant mother, appears to be important in initiating and maintaining breast-feeding behavior, the crucial elements in obtaining that supportive behavior remain to be clearly delineated. Incentives clearly increase participation rates in educational programs. Whether these incentives undermine participants' intrinsic interest in the issues discussed (Mawhinney, Dickinson, & Taylor, 1989) has not been explored.

Infancy

The infant is dependent on the parents or caretakers for sustenance. Since, as noted, breast-feeding is the most appropriate sole form of infant feeding for at least the first 4–6 months of life (U.S. Department of Health and Human Services, 1984), the mother's behavior directly nourishes the infant. As weaning occurs, there has been some concern about lowering the child's consumption of fat, especially saturated fat.

Breast-Feeding. A summary of intervention programs to encourage breast-feeding in Third World countries (U.S. Agency for International Development, 1991) revealed that early interventions with hospitals (an environmental component) significantly enhanced the ease of and minimized the barriers to in-hospital breast-feeding, resulting in exclusive breast-feeding at discharge increasing from 63% to 91% of mothers. These increases in breast-feeding had substantial other benefits for the health of the children and for cost savings to the hospitals. A Nicaraguan program that involved an early 45-minute contact between the mother and child, or early rooming-in with the child, resulted in greater initiation of breast-feeding; the early rooming-in resulted in marginally higher breast-feeding at 4 months postpartum (Lindenberg, Artola, & Jiminez, 1990). This study did not provide for parents' selection from among rooming-in options, which might have resulted in even greater change.

Social marketing procedures were employed to enhance breast-feeding (Academy for Educational Development, 1991) in Third World countries. The report concluded that general messages reporting the benefits of breast-feeding alone did not work, since they did not help mothers deal with the many barriers that needed to be overcome. The report encouraged the designing of interventions for specific segments of the market of all prenatal and early postnatal women with a concomitant investment in programs with personal contact. At least one project in Africa targeted spousal partners, but results were not available from that campaign. The Healthcom project in Jordan combined in-service training of health professionals with a television and radio campaign targeted at young women and their families (McDivitt et al., 1993). The mass media campaign emphasized the benefits of breast-feeding and advice on managing common problems such as insufficient milk and breast pain, and resulted in earlier initiation of breast-feeding (within hours). Breast-feeding increased among mothers delivering in public hospitals and at home, but not in those delivering at private hospitals (a socioeconomic [SES]-status characteristic). It was not reported whether the higher breast-feeding lasted for any period of time.

Feeding Relationship. An intervention tailored to the individual needs of lower-income mothers of preterm infants involving meetings with the spousal partner, siblings, and parents (the selection being made by the mother) concerning issues of family functioning, social support, and transition to home resulted in fewer depressed mothers, fewer feeding problems, lower grimacing and gagging on the part of the infants, less frequent interruption of feeding, fewer attempts to stimulate the infant's sucking, more vocalization to the infant, more sensitivity to the infant's behavior, more quality of physical contact, and more positive maternal affect (Meyer et al., 1994).

Lower-Fat Diet. Dietary counseling (otherwise unspecified) with families of 7-month-old infants in Finland resulted in no lowering of dietary fat at 13 months in comparison to a control group, but higher polyunsaturated/saturated fat intake ratio and a lower serum total cholesterol value (Lapinleimu et al., 1994).

Implications. Environmental and behavioral interventions can result in increased breast-feeding, improved maternal feeding behaviors, and increased polyunsaturated/saturated fat ratio with concomitant beneficial changes in chronic disease risk factors and other aspects of health. Given the diversity and complexity of the programs reviewed, it is not clear what behaviors, skills, or characteristics of the mother need to be targeted to initiate and maintain such feeding changes; what behavior, skills, or other characteristics of the spousal partner or other family members need to be targeted to help the mother initiate or maintain the changes; or whether these necessary mother's or family behaviors, skills, or characteristics vary by categories of mothers (e.g., SES). Neither is it clear what program components are necessary to achieve all these changes.

Knowing that behavior changes can be achieved should embolden health behavior researchers to conduct more systematic research to elucidate all these factors and thereby enable them to design more efficient and even more effective programs. While consensus meetings of professionals and descriptive research may identify mother and family behaviors, skills, and characteristics necessary for desired feeding behaviors, research systematically varying methods for intervention based on the best available theory and research findings with randomly assigned participants must elucidate how best to promote change.

Toddler and Preschool Years

Nutrition education issues in the toddler and preschool years have emphasized eating a better overall diet, minimizing obesity, and preventing chronic disease risks. The toddler years may be a time when children are more likely to try many kinds of new food (absence of neophobia) and when important food self-control skills are established (Chapter 9 in Volume I).

Improved Diet. A preschool health education project attempted to increase the children's (2-, 3-, and 4-year-olds) consumption of low-sugar snacks (among a variety of health behaviors) through classroom learning activities and 24 different Doing It Together homework activities for the children and parents that corresponded to classroom activities (Bruhn & Parcel, 1982). Unfortunately, among those children who received the curriculum, there was a decline in the percentage of children who selected a fruit snack, but no such decline in the control group (Parcel, Bruhn, & Murray, 1984), even though mothers reported working on this behavior more than any of the others (Bruhn & Parcel, 1982). Perhaps the renowned oppositional behavior of young children may explain this phenomenon. In a series of single-subject experimental designs, children made healthful snack food selections (fruits and vegetables versus cookies and candies) at school, but their doing so did not generalize to home. The children made and maintained desired home snack food selections only when reinforcement training was instituted with parents at home (Stark, Collins, Osnes, & Stokes, 1986).

Obesity. To treat obesity among 2- to 10-year-old children, the major behavioral causes of overeating or inappropriate eating were identified in participating families; corresponding family and home environment modifications were targeted and incentives were identified (Wheeler & Hess, 1976). The treatment for each participating family applied the intervention components most appropriate to that family (often called "tailoring"), resulting in a mean 4.1-lb weight loss, with 71% of treatment children coming closer to their appropriate weight and only 4 moving further away. Unfortunately, no information was provided on the extent to which families complied with the suggested home modifications or what procedures were employed to achieve these home modifications. This paper was an interesting early example of clearly specifying the theory of the problem (i.e., identifying the factors that maintain the undesired behavior) (McLeroy et al., 1993).

A more traditional family-based contingency contracting approach to weight loss for 1- to 5-year-old children involved specifying a diet that was 200 kcal/day lower than usual current consumption, training the parents in using a traffic light diet to assist in making wise food selections, walking a mile each day with their child, using modeling and praise to increase good eating and exercise, using time-out and extinction to decrease negative health habits, and using charts for monitoring behavior to cue parents to provide structured praise and reinforcement for appropriate eating and exercise. The intervention resulted in change averaging from 42.1% overweight at baseline to 26.7% overweight at 2 months and 27.8% overweight at 24 months past initiation of the program (Epstein, Valoski, Wing,

& McCurley, 1986). Again, no process evaluation was reported on the compliance of parents with implementing the specified behavior modification regimen or the incentives or other procedures for attaining these parent behavior changes. Similar contingency training with parents of 1- to 4-year-old food refusers resulted in substantial increases in food acceptance (Werle, Murphy, & Budd, 1993).

Implications. When parents of children in this age range were trained to use behavior modification techniques (both environmental change and contingency approaches), children's dietary behavior changes were obtained. A health education program targeting preschool children's snack behaviors, using homework assignments with parents, did not result in the desired change, and in fact resulted in a decline in consumption of healthy snacks. Children this age thus appear responsive to behavior modification techniques, and young parents may benefit from the provided skills to help control their children's behaviors. The behavior modification approach, however, is labor-intensive. It is not clear whether these behavior modification techniques can be transmitted in a population or public health approach or whether there are sufficient numbers of cases of preschool obesity or failure to thrive to warrant such public health programs. Alternatively, many people believe that food preferences and practices are learned at this early age (Birch, 1990). Behavior modification techniques within a public health program may therefore be appropriate to promote positive dietary changes (e.g., eating more fruits, vegetables, and grains) in all toddlers and preschoolers.

Elementary School Years

Nutrition education among early-school-age children has focused on developing healthful eating patterns for chronic disease and obesity prevention and for treatment of juvenile diabetes mellitus. Different strategies have been used to involve families. Families have expressed a pref-erence for low-intensity materials, versus more intensive methods such as having to attend sessions, as a method for involvement in health behavior change programming (Crockett, Mullis, & Perry, 1988; Dunn, Lackey, Kolasa, & Mustian, 1994).

Chronic Disease Prevention. The school is a common channel for delivery of nutrition interventions because it can reach large segments of elementary-school-age children. Virtually all children this age attend school, thereby providing access to children and their families. The Chicago Heart Health Program (CHHP) was one of the earliest chronic disease prevention programs involving parents. A year-long comprehensive program designed for a multiracial population of 6th-grade students and their families, the CHHP included a parental component that had children bring home materials such as activity logs and newsletter health tips, teacher encouragement to select activities students could do with family members, and student instruction on effective communication styles. Although a 50% participation rate was obtained, no student behavior change was obtained (Petchers, Hirsch, & Block, 1987; Sunseri, Alberti, Kent, Schoenberger, & Dolecek, 1984; Sunseri et al., n.d.).

Providing parent nutrition education in addition to classroom nutrition education for students in kindergarten through 3rd grade increased nutrition knowledge only among younger students, but dietary change was obtained across all grade levels (Kirks, Hendricks, & Wise, 1982). Data at 5-year follow-up revealed that participating families experienced an increase in knowledge, development of positive attitudes toward nutrition, and healthful food purchasing and meal preparation (Kirks & Hughes, 1986). A home-based correspondence course to augment a school-based curriculum achieved high participation in home activities among 3rd-grade children and their families and a significant decrease in consumption of total fat, saturated fat, and monounsaturated fat and an increase in consumption of complex carbohydrates (Perry et al.,

1988). Dietary changes declined, however, after 1 year (Perry et al., 1989).

A nutrition education program for the prevention of hypertension involving a classroom curriculum, a home-based curriculum, or their combination (Luepker, Perry, Murray, & Mullis, 1988) increased knowledge about salt use, with the largest gain in the classroom program, but obtained no behavior change (Luepker et al., 1988). A similar "home team" approach involved parental participation in nutrition and exercise education among 5th- and 6th-graders (Hopper, Gruber, Munoz, & Herb, 1992), wherein each week, for 6 weeks, children took packets home to read with their families. The school-and-home and school-only groups showed significant decrease in skinfold and percentage calories from fat over the control group, but were not significantly different from each other; the school-and-home group had higher nutrition knowledge than both other groups (Hopper et al., 1992). A 50% increase in fruit consumed and qualitative changes in vegetables consumed were obtained among 4th- and 5th-graders using a behavior change curriculum and newsletters to involve parents (Domel et al., 1993). Increased fruit consumption occurred primarily at lunch, however, indicating a need for more intensive efforts to change practices, especially at home.

The school lunch program offers another point for intervention in elementary-school children. One study combined modification of offerings to include a low-fat entree with a parental intervention (Whitaker, Wright, Finch, Deyo, & Psaty, 1994). The offerings included school lunch menus emphasizing the low-fat entrees for students in the treatment group to take home, a one-time mailing to parents containing a newly labeled menu for the coming month, a pamphlet emphasizing the role of parents in modeling dietary habits and providing tips for low-fat eating at home, a letter describing the availability of the daily low-fat entree for their child at school, and encouragement for the family to promote the selection of that entree by their child. While there was an increase in low-fat entree selection compared to the control schools, only 10% of the sample of parents surveyed asked their child to choose a low-fat entree (Whitaker, Wright, Finch, et al., 1994). Children with family members who had an elevated blood cholesterol were more likely to choose the low-fat entree (Whitaker, Wright, Koepsell, Finch, & Psaty, 1994a).

A more intensive 8-week intervention program among Anglo, black, and Mexican-American families with young elementary-school children achieved substantial dietary change (Nader et al., 1983). The San Diego Family Health project targeted Hispanic and Anglo families with 5th- or 6th-grade child with an intensive year-long intervention consisting of 12 weekly sessions and 6 maintenance sessions targeted to culturally specific needs. Hispanic adults and children reported dietary change after participating in the 12-week intervention (Nader et al., 1986). Self-efficacy was the strongest predictor of dietary change (Vega et al., 1988). Direct observation in a standard environment at 1 year indicated generalizability of the intervention effects to an environmental setting: Intervention families consumed fewer calories and less sodium than did control families (Patterson et al., 1988). After 1 year, a modest aggregation of change within families was found, with more aggregation in the behavioral than in the physiological variables; aggregation of change was strongest within generations (e.g., spouse pairs, sibling pairs), suggesting that interventions target families, not individuals (Patterson et al., 1989). Process measures such as attendance, compliance with self-monitoring, achievement of goals, and attitudes toward the sessions only partially mediated intervention effects (Madsen et al., 1993a), with some predictive support for diet self-monitoring among adults (Madsen et al., 1993b). A similar intensive approach among Mexican-American and non-Hispanic white families attending weekly group meetings resulted in changes in eating habits that were maintained 1 year beyond completion of the intervention (Nader et al., 1989).

Modest dietary changes were achieved, however, in a similar intervention involving

African-American families who attended 14 consecutive weeks of educational sessions (T. Baranowski et al., 1990); low participation rates interfered with interpretation of these results.

Mexican-American families offered a year-long intervention consisting of 12 weeks of intensive intervention followed by 6 maintenance sessions distributed over a 9-month period experienced a dramatic drop in attendance over the maintenance period, but maintained dietary change over the year follow-up period (Nader et al., 1992).

A less intensive family intervention in the Child and Adolescent Trial for Cardiovascular Health, based on the work of Perry et al. (1988, 1989) and Nader et al. (1989, 1992), resulted in greater knowledge (Edmundson et al., 1996) but no greater behavioral or risk factor change beyond that achieved by the school-only intervention (Luepker et al., 1996).

Implications. Involving families through homework assignments sent home to parents appears to result in some dietary changes under some circumstances, but the inconsistent findings do not clearly suggest what those circumstances are. It may be that such an intervention by itself will work, but does no better than a classroom program. More intensive programs can achieve substantive dietary changes, but some of these programs experience high dropout rates. The activities or processes that families engage in as a result of these interventions and that result in change need to be clearly specified to facilitate the design of more effective programs.

High-Risk Families. The Heart Clinical Model Program was a school-based program for CVD risk reduction among high-risk children and their families (Johnson et al., 1987). The intervention, including 8 90-minute sessions over 12 weeks, obtained positive changes in eating habits (Johnson et al., 1991). Families at high risk for CVD who received behavioral counseling with an accompanying contract for behavioral change

attained slight changes in total energy, total fat, and saturated fat (Johnson, Nicklas, Arbeit, Webber, & Berenson, 1992). The Dietary Intervention Study in Children (DISC) implemented an intensive dietary intervention for lipid lowering among 8- to 10-year-old children with moderately elevated low-density lipoprotein (LDL) cholesterol. The intensive intervention involved family members, developed personalized eating plans, and used weekly and then monthly group intervention sessions. The group sessions involved several unspecified instructional approaches, cooperative learning experiences, problem-solving activities, behavior modification, and social support (DISC Collaborative Research Group, 1993). DISC attained reduction in dietary fat and cholesterol with a corresponding reduction in LDL cholesterol after 3 years (Writing Group, 1995).

Obesity. A meta-analysis of 41 controlled outcome studies reported that comprehensive behavioral treatments including behavior modification techniques produced better treatment results (Haddock, Shadish, Klesges, & Stein, 1994). Parental participation was not found to be related to treatment outcome. While there is some reason to believe that parental involvement is effective among children up to 10 years of age when the parent attends the sessions with the child, but attends separate sessions after the child is 10 years old, Haddock et al. (1994) concluded that insufficient studies had been conducted to provide an adequate test of this possibility in the meta-analysis. Family therapy for obesity with sessions at 2- to 3-month intervals over a 14- to 18-month period obtained significantly lower mean body mass index at 1-year follow-up among 10- to 11-year old children (Flodmark, Ohlsson, Ryden, Sveger, 1993).

Diabetes Mellitus. Self-management training was used with 9- to 13-year-old children with insulin-dependent diabetes and their parents to alter health care responding and maintain behavior change. Parents and their children met separately for 90-minute sessions once a week for 8 weeks to facilitate discussions of eight differing concerns in the two groups, because of the hesitancy of the children to discuss their concerns in front of their parents. The program resulted in a decline in family arguments and an increase in performance of diabetes self-care behaviors. These changes were maintained at 2- and 6-month follow-ups (Gross, Magalnick, & Richardson, 1985). Over 4 years of treatment, low family cohesiveness and high family conflict were linked to deterioration of glycemic control in boys (Gross et al., 1985). This pattern held for girls initially, but did not persist over the study period. Patients from the least openly expressive families had the highest deterioration of glycemic control. Level of family organization was unrelated to management.

Implications. Intensive interventions with high-risk groups tend to result in dietary change, probably because high-risk populations are motivated to change. The role of the family in such interventions, or how the families facilitated change, has not been delineated. More attention must be given to the role of family functioning characteristics in compliance with guidelines. It may be necessary to tailor different approaches for different gender, ethnic, age, and family functioning groups.

Reciprocal Effects. Children influence many of their parents' activities (M. D. Baranowski, 1978), including the family's food purchasing, preparation, and consumption practices (Chapter 9 in Volume I). As a result, some interventions have trained children to influence the practices of their families.

An intensive classroom health education intervention with low-income elementary-school children resulted in increased health-related knowledge among the parents, including knowledge of dietary sources of tooth decay (Knight & Grantham-McGregor, 1985). Using the elementary-school student as a "health messenger," the families whose student members were trained to assess blood pressure and sent home to take the blood pressures of family members were more likely to have discussions with students on these topics, and such discussion was much more likely to occur among cohesive families (Fors, Owen, Hall, McLaughlin, & Levinson, 1989). Qualitative health behavior research revealed that families more likely to discuss these heart disease–related topics tended to encourage communication with children and to discuss these topics in many locations (not just the dinner table); tended to have a "gentle structure" parenting style wherein rules were enforced in a supportive, encouraging way; and used many forms of positive reinforcement (McLaughlin, Owen, Fors, & Levinson, 1992). The families less likely to discuss these topics reported being very rushed, with little time for interaction. Parents who participated in a school health screening program were more likely to participate in other health behaviors (Resnicow, Cross, Lacosse, & Nichols, 1993). Parents who participated in a 14-session evening education program while their children were participating in a complementary school curriculum were more likely to have positive attitudes toward nutrition than those not attending the sessions (Sunseri et al., 1983).

Implications. Interventions with schoolchildren have implications for the whole family. Elementary-school students can be involved in programs to help change the practices of their family members. Under what circumstances and how this optimally might be done have not been clearly determined. The extent to which school programs targeted at children alone have an impact at home also has not been determined.

Adolescence

With the passage and uncertainties of puberty, the adolescent begins to manifest adult levels of chronic disease risk factors and develop dietary problems unique to this age. The interest in preventing cardiovascular disease remains a key issue, obesity becomes increasingly common, and sufficient cases of juvenile-onset diabetes have accumulated to lead to treatment programs.

Some health behavior research findings suggest that aspects of family functioning and food-related behaviors lead to the development of CVD risk factors and obesity in children (Chapter 9 in Volume I). While family practices may or may not be implicated in the etiology of these disorders, families can be crucial in preventing or treating these problems. In most cases, parents control the family's food expenditures and the entry of many foods into the home. At least one study revealed that parents are strong influences on food selections and practices throughout adolescence (Lau, Quadrell, & Hartman, 1990). Alternatively, a major task of adolescence is achieving independence from the family (Erikson, 1963). Adolescents often take afterschool jobs that provide them with income to purchase foods that meet their taste preferences or frequently get jobs in the fast food industry that enable them to eat, at little or no cost to them, foods that the family may not sanction. Adolescents also often engage in extracurricular activities that allow them opportunities to consume foods that may not be sanctioned by the family. Thus, interventions with families of adolescents are important, but can be expected to have more modest effects than those with younger children.

Chronic Disease Prevention. An early intensive intervention with whole family units using weekly contacts by dieticians to individualize diets for family members resulted in an average 10% reduction in serum total cholesterol in adolescents and their parents and 68% improvements in dietary practices (Witschii, Singer, Wu-Lee, & Stare, 1978). The families were apparently well educated, and this study involved participants with the highest serum cholesterol values in the community, both factors that predisposed to success. An intensive intervention targeted at dietary fat and sodium of 13- to 15-year-old schoolchildren incorporating an unspecified family involvement procedure resulted in substantially lowered dietary fat and sodium consumption, while no such differences were obtained for a less intensive community intervention (Puska et al., 1982). Process evaluations on how families

achieved their changes were not reported for either study.

An intervention to lower the salt in the diets of African-American high school students by lowering salty snacks and increasing fruit and vegetable snacks reached out to the parents through two phone calls and three mailed fliers, attempting to set goals to limit the availability of salty snacks and increase the availability of fruits and vegetables at home (Simons-Morton, Coates, Saylor, Sereghy, & Barofsky, 1984). There was no evidence that this parent intervention had either a separate effect or a synergistic effect combined with the classroom curriculum or media-based components (Coates et al., 1985). Turning the tables, one project used high school students to get more family members to watch a television program on cardiovascular health, but was not able to change parent practices or increase the students' confidence that they could influence their parents (Nader et al., 1982).

Thus, only interventions labeled as intensive resulted in change in dietary practices with families of adolescents. Little attention has been given, however, to clearly specifying why families perform their usual behaviors or how family interventions were designed and implemented.

Obesity. Using three single-subject designs, a family-based intervention resulted in two participants losing 20 lb and 11.5 lb during a 14-week period, with a third control subject gaining 5 lb (Coates & Thoresen, 1981). The intervention employed comprehensive and intensive behavior modification procedures involving both environmental modifications and individual learning procedures. Each experimental child showed different patterns of change, with child 1 demonstrating substantial environmental change in calories available and child 2 demonstrating reductions in foods visually seen in the home. The authors reported that each child's family made the changes most relevant to their family context (Coates & Thoresen, 1981).

In a comparison of an adolescent behavior modification intervention for weight loss with and without parent involvement, parent involvement facilitated earlier (1-year) weight loss, but both groups had comparable outcomes at 2 years (Coates, Killen, & Slinkard, 1982). No differential effects by group were identified for calories or fats consumed. The authors stated that parents reported difficulty in relinquishing control over their adolescents' eating habits, especially in refraining from expressing negative reactions to overeating, and suggested that family therapy become a part of future such interventions. Another study demonstrated that involving the mother in the program separately from the child achieved and maintained weight loss over a year, while involving the mother with the child, and not involving the mother at all, resulted in little or no change (Brownell, Kelman, & Stunkard, 1983). Involving parents separately from the child also resulted in substantial weight loss (Berkowitz & Stallings, 1994).

All the reviewed weight loss studies employed behavior modification techniques (usually highly intensive effort) resulting in weight loss. Involving the mother or parent in the program separately from the child appeared to result in earlier and substantial weight losses.

Diabetes Mellitus. A nutrition education program for adolescent diabetics and their mothers, involving efforts to promote parent–child communication on difficulties in dietary compliance, resulted in greater dietary change and better metabolic control than those in a no-education control group (Elamin, Eltayeb, Hasan, Hofvander, & Tuvemo, 1993). It is possible that the families of these adolescent diabetic patients were more highly motivated than the families in other studies and thereby could benefit from this lower-intensity intervention.

Adulthood

While most of this chapter has considered parental influences on children, spousal pairs constitute a family as well. A substantial amount of work has systematically involved families in interventions for risk factor prevention, risk factor control, and obesity control. Other, more clinical research has examined the role of family factors in surgical efforts to promote weight loss.

Risk Factor Prevention and Control. The Multiple Risk Factor Intervention Trial (MRFIT) involved at-risk men with a spouse or friend in dietary change classes focused on developing a healthy lifestyle, including shopping, cooking, and eating patterns, and on attempting to reach a goal of 8% of calories or less from saturated fat and weight loss for men at or above 115% of desirable weight. The MRFIT experimental group achieved declines in total cholesterol of 12.1 mg/dl, while the control group achieved a decline of only 7.5 mg/dl (MRFIT Research Group, 1982). These modest changes were achieved within 24 months and maintained over 6 years. An intervention wherein one physician and one dietician visit were made with families (mother, father, child) to guide modification of several risk factors resulted in dietary changes among the targeted high-risk men (Knutsen & Knutsen, 1989, 1991). The changes were primarily in lower use of fat spreads and gravies and higher use of skim milk. Another intervention involving periodic nursing visits for family risk factor counseling including diet resulted in somewhat lower blood cholesterols and body mass indices at one year (Family Heart Study Group, 1994). No dietary outcomes were provided for the MRFIT or Family Heart studies. A single visit to the spouse of hypertensive patients at home after a preliminary survey of participants about the kinds of information they would find useful resulted in greater weight control than exit interviews or small group discussions (Morisky, DeMuth, Field-Fass, Green, & Levine, 1985).

From the descriptions provided, it is not clear how intensive these interventions were. The involvement of family in the intervention was unimaginative, essentially including family members in knowledge-based counseling sessions providing suggestions for dietary change. No information was provided on the process of implementing the family intervention or on the processes of patient (non)compliance with the intervention. No results were reported by different sizes, structures, or characteristics of families. Only one study collected any information from families trying to specify factors that influenced diet prior to the intervention, and this one seemed to have the largest impact.

Weight Loss.   Spouses or partners can be particularly useful in weight loss programs when they are involved in food purchasing and preparation and in motivating or otherwise helping the patient to maintain compliance with the program's dietary and physical activity prescriptions when the patient relapses after the initial program. It is not clear that anyone has identified all the skills a partner would need to provide these varied sources of support. A meta-analysis of 14 studies (Black, Gleser, & Kooyers, 1990) revealed that when compared to individual weight loss programs, couples programs resulted in a significantly greater weight loss at posttreatment, but nonsignificant differences afterward. The authors concluded that the kinds of support in which partners were trained varied substantially across studies; many of the studies did not assess partners' compliance with the prescribed supportive mechanisms, and the few that did showed no relationship to outcome. More attention must be paid to studies that assess how best to meet the needs and motivations of participants and how best to involve partners to maintain weight loss.

Surgical Weight Loss.   A related literature has assessed clinical characteristics of the families of patients in surgical weight loss programs. In an early study of patients who underwent intestinal bypass surgery, all patients reported unsatisfactory marriages and, when the male spouse was the patient, dependence on maternal nurturance by the wife. The partners felt threatened by the weight loss, with fears of increased sexual demands and resulting abandonment (Marshall & Neill, 1977). The surgery resulted in substantial sexuality-related marital discord, in-

cluding cessation of sexual relations, impotence, affairs, and bisexuality (Neill et al., 1978). A better-designed study showed that the incidence of divorce was higher (21%) in a sample that was 3 years postsurgery for obesity as compared to a control group (Rand, Kuldau, & Robbins, 1982); the authors reported, however, that the majority reported improved marriages and improved sexual functioning after surgery. A more intensive analysis 5 years postsurgery concluded that marriages that were strong before surgery remained so, but marriages that had serious problems tended to get worse after surgery (Rand, Kowalske, & Kuldau, 1989). Formerly obese patients who had attained normal weight were more likely to relapse in a 5-month period (gain 20% or more of their weight loss) when indicators of marital distress were obtained at baseline (Fischman-Havstad & Marston, 1984).

These clinical studies of interventions to attain weight loss reveal important emotional issues not usually addressed in the dietary change literature. While not all families have these dysfunctional emotional relationships, some do. These studies highlight the complexities of family relationships and how existing behavioral patterns may be maintained by family members in order to maintain other desired characteristics of their lives or to avoid the perceived threats of change. While these findings are highly suggestive, no sophisticated prospective research has addressed these aspects of dietary change.

A MODEL OF FAMILY DIETARY CHANGE

Families are interdependent. Although weight loss is very difficult to achieve, in a group of 92 patients enrolled in a weight loss program, in 47 of the cases in which one member of a family lost weight, a close family relative also lost weight (Franson & Rossner, 1994), with the spouse being the one most likely to do so. Health behavior research needs to elucidate the nature of that interdependence, both to understand the

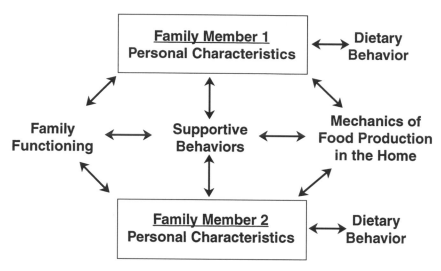

Figure 1. Model of reciprocal determinism relating family and individual characteristics.

mechanisms and to help design more effective interventions. A heuristic model for considering these factors is presented in Figure 1. At a minimum, a family has two members who may be parent–child, sibling–sibling, or a spousal pair. Each family member has important personal characteristics in regard to foods, e.g., preferences, outcome expectations (especially reactions of family members), various aspects of self-efficacy (especially dealing with other family members), skills, attributions of control and success, and emotional strengths and resources. These personal characteristics result in dietary behaviors, which may reciprocally affect these personal characteristics (T. Baranowski, 1990).

Families relate to each other in three general ways that can affect dietary behaviors and dietary change: mechanics of food production in the home, supportive behaviors, and family functioning. The more concrete of this trilogy of family interrelationships is the mechanics of food production. The heart of these mechanics is the following relationship:

food availability → food preparation
→ food accessibility

Food accessibility concerns what foods in what forms and combinations are served at meals or are otherwise immediately accessible for consumption (e.g., fresh vegetable sticks cut up in a plastic bag on the front shelf of the refrigerator). Food accessibility in the home reflects both what foods were initially purchased (availability) or otherwise obtained and brought into the home (e.g., vegetable gardens) and how these foods were prepared. Preparation, of course, can be done on only those foods initially purchased or otherwise made available in the home. An attractive aspect of the family model is that no one person need have all the skills in food purchase and preparation, but that skills in the family can be complementary or compensatory.

The relationship between two people in regard to foods can also be characterized at an interactive behavioral level. Most commonly, the idea of social support captures this item, and support can be positive or negative. Three dimensions of social support with corresponding positive and negative behavioral indicators are listed in Table 1. In part, these socially supportive interactions reflect and shape the characteristics of the individuals and in turn affect the me-

Table 1. Dimensions of Social Support and Their Positive and Negative Behavioral Indicators

Dimensions	Indicators	
	Positive	Negative
Informational/ cognitive	Persuasion Provision of new ideas Reminders	Induction of guilt
Material/ behavioral	Assistance Provision of rewards	Avoidance Noncooperation Hindrance
Emotional/ affective	Praise Listening Comfort	Criticism Denigration Complaints Nagging

chanics of food production in the home. Groups of professionals could be convened to preliminarily identify all the behaviors that a family needs to master to promote the mechanics of production of healthful foods and to identify the supportive behaviors to maintain these food purchase and preparation practices.

At a more profound and pervasive level are characteristics of the relationships in the family. Relationships reflect cognitive, affective, and behavioral adaptations of each person to living with the other, i.e., ways in which each person coexists with the other in general in the attempt to find tolerable to highly attractive life circumstances. Characteristics of family relationships that have received attention in the literature include cohesion, affection, satisfaction, unconditional positive regard, interdependence, and conflict. These patterns of relationship will reflect and shape personal characteristics and provide a broader context within which the supportive behaviors and the mechanics of food production are performed. Since patterns of family functioning reflect stable adaptations on the part of family members to each other, it is likely that older families will have more difficulty changing di-

etary practices than younger families with similar patterns of family functioning.

Figure 1 can be thought of as a clearer specification of the family social cognitive model (Taylor et al., 1994) (see also Chapter 9 in Volume I), with family functioning and supportive behaviors thought of as emergent family characteristics.

At this time, little is known about any of these relationships in regard to food. Given that the patterns of family functioning reflect the full duration of peoples' relationships (often many years) and may even reflect carryover from prior relationships, it is hard to imagine that the common family interventions of low intensity and relatively brief duration (several sessions over weeks or months) can have an impact on dietary behaviors. Health behavior research must determine the nature and extent of relationships among family functioning, supportive behaviors, mechanics of food production, characteristics of the individual, and dietary behaviors. Of particular concern would be how these variables normally interrelate and what the necessary and sufficient conditions at one level for change in others are. Clearly, these relationships will be different for parent–child than for spousal or sibling–sibling pairs.

Given the emerging gender differences in health behaviors and health behavior change (Stone, Baranowski, Sallis, & Cutler, 1995), these relationships may differ in accordance with the gender of the family members. Some people believe that food preferences and practices are established in the earliest years of life (Birch, 1990). A particularly important use of this model will be to identify the components that predict or establish these early preferences and practices and maintain them into the adult years. Adult dietary behaviors may be affected by dysfunctional attachments to the family of origin, or to prior nuclear families, not just their current one.

There has been much recent interest in the transtheoretical model and its concept of stages in an individual's health behavior change (Prochaska, Norcross, & DiClemente, 1994). Within a family context, one family member can initiate dietary changes without the other's support. It is likely, however, that this change will be better maintained if the partner at least supports the family member's change (a stage not in the current model focused on individual change) and even better if both engage in the change. Further research will need to conceptualize and assess stages in a family's health behavior changes, including alternative combinations in each individual's stage of change and joint stages in family change, and what persuasive and other interpersonal influence manipulations are employed by family members to influence each other along the path of change (T. Baranowski, 1992).

There is some reason to believe that some portion of the variance in the ways families interact is genetically determined (Plomin, Reiss, Hetherington, & Howe, 1994). Exactly how and to what extent genes affect family functioning, e.g., a greater need to avoid the arousal associated with conflict, remains to be clearly specified. Genetic variation may affect all components in the model in Figure 1. Since phenotypes reflect gene-by-environment interactions, family-based interventions may have to be tailored to alter environmental factors differently for alternative genotypes.

CONCLUDING COMMENTS

With few exceptions family-based interventions worked primarily among families that had a heightened perceived need or desire to change (e.g., new mothers, families with elevated risk factors or disease) or when the intervenors had an opportunity to collect information on the family and tailor the intervention to documented characteristics of the family (e.g., intensive interventions or social marketing type approaches).

The field would benefit from more theoretically based descriptive health behavior research on how families relate to food (see Chapter 9 in Volume I). The social cognitive model of family dietary behaviors should provide a framework to guide such research, which will identify

processes and mechanisms of family influence, which in turn will identify new points of intervention. Studies of how much the dietary practices are influenced by these processes will help prioritize the points most likely to result in the most change. Of course, knowing these processes does not automatically impart the requisite knowledge of how to change them.

Family interventions will benefit from more sophisticated use of theory in both descriptive and intervention studies. New theoretical formulations (e.g., Rickard et al., 1995; Storer, Frate, Johnson, & Greenberg, 1987) may provide nonlinear, nonobvious approaches to facilitate change in families. There is a need for health behavior research that pits theoretical formulations against each other as competing explanations, thereby eliminating theoretical frameworks that have less explanatory power and helping to refine the successful theories.

Substantial new work has demonstrated that tailoring components of a dietary intervention program to change related characteristics of individuals results in more change than does application of a "one size fits all" intervention (Kramisch Campbell et al., 1994). Tailoring interventions to change related characteristics of families also holds promise for more effective family interventions, but more needs to be learned about what family characteristics are related to change and how to obtain change in these family characteristics.

Research must emphasize designs that systematically decompose previously successful complex interventions to identify the components of the intervention that are critical to success versus those that are not. Sophisticated process evaluations must be mounted to assess whether the programs were implemented as designed (Hearn & Baranowski, 1996), and, if they were not, why not; the extent to which families complied with the directives of the intervention when they received them; whether the level of compliance was related to outcome; and what characteristics of families predicted compliance. Such research will provide clearer guidance for efforts to improve implementation and to better understand when, how, and why families adopt the suggested new behaviors.

Research has shown that consumption of inadequate quantities of selected nutrients (e.g., iron, iodine, calories) impairs children's cognitive functioning (Pollitt, 1987). It will be important to assess how families adapt or respond to such impairments, whether the families' social resources enable the children to compensate for them, and how we might design interventions to help families compensate.

Health-related behaviors in general and dietary practices in particular are related to many outcomes, e.g., cognitive, emotional, fitness-body composition, and social well-being. Some of these outcomes are of more immediate importance to families than long-term cardiovascular disease prevention. It is therefore vitally important to assess the many outcomes of intervention programs, in order to (1) assess the full impact on many aspects of families' lives; (2) assess the possibilities of additive, interactive, or conflicting outcomes; (3) identify more motivators to encourage families' change; and (4) assess the possible interrelationships and regulatory control mechanisms across behaviors and the role the family may play in these interactions.

While families logically need to be involved in attempts to change dietary practices (and other health-related behaviors), more must be learned about how and why families influence these behaviors and about how to promote changes in the factors that affect the behaviors.

REFERENCES

Academy for Educational Development. (1991). *Media promotion of breastfeeding: A decade's experience*. Washington, DC: Academy for Educational Development.

Baranowski, M. D. (1978). Adolescents' attempted influence on parental behaviors. *Adolescence, 52*, 585–604.

Baranowski, T. (1990). Reciprocal determinism at the stages of behavior change: An integration of community, personal and behavioral perspectives. *International Quarterly of Community Health Education, 10*, 297–327.

Baranowski, T. (1992). Interpersonal models for health behavior intervention with minority populations: Theoretical, methodologic and pragmatic issues. In D. Becker, D. R. Hill, J. S. Jackson, D. M. Levine, F. A. Stillman, & S. M. Weiss (Eds.), *Health behavior research in minority populations: Access, design, and implementation* (pp. 112–121). NIH Publication No. 92-2965. Bethesda, MD: NIH.

Baranowski, T., Domel, S., Gould, R., Baranowski, J., Leonard, S., Treiber, F., & Mullis, R. (1993). Increasing fruit and vegetable consumption among 4th and 5th grade students: Results from focus groups using reciprocal determinism. *Journal of Nutrition Education, 25*, 114–120.

Baranowski, T., Henske, J., Simons-Morton, B., Palmer, J., Tiernan, K., Hooks, P. C., & Dunn, J. K. (1990). Dietary change for cardiovascular disease prevention among black-American families. *Health Education Research, 5*, 433–443.

Baranowski, T., Lin, L. S., Wetter, D., Resnicow, K., & Hearn, M. D. (1997). Theory as mediating variables: Why aren't community interventions working as desired? *Annals of Epidemiology* (in press).

Barker, D. J. P., Gluckman, P. D., Godfrey, K. M., Harding, J. E., Owens, J. A., & Robinson, J. S. (1993). Fetal nutrition and cardiovascular disease in adult life. *Lancet, 341*, 938–941.

Berkowitz, R. I., & Stallings, V. A. (1994). Marked obesity in adolescents treated by a behavioral program incorporating a low-calorie diet. *Program of the Annual Meeting of the Society of Behavioral Medicine*, S063.

Birch, L. L. (1993). The control of food intake by young children: The role of learning. In E. Capaldi & T. L. Powley (Eds.), *Taste, experience and feeding* (pp. 116–135). Washington, DC: American Psychological Associate.

Black, D. R., Gleser, L. J., & Kooyers, K. J. (1990). A meta-analytic evaluation of couples' weight-loss programs. *Health Psychology, 9*, 330–347.

Bovbjerg, V. E., McCann, B. S., Brief, D. J., Follette, W. C., Retzlaff, B. M., Dowdy, A. A., Walden, C. E., & Knopp, R. H. (1995). Spouse support and long-term adherence to lipid-lowering diets. *American Journal of Epidemiology, 141*, 451–460.

Brown, J. E., Tharp, T., & Finnegan, J. (1996). Translating social marketing research findings into a prenatal weight gain intervention program: Results of the Healthy Infant Outcome Project. *Journal of Nutrition Education, 28*, 7–14.

Brown, J. E., Tharp, T. M., McKay, C., Richardson, S. L., Hall, N. J., Finnegan, J. R., Jr., & Splett, P. L. (1992). Development of a prenatal weight gain intervention program using social marketing methods. *Journal of Nutrition Education, 24*, 21–28.

Brownell, K. D., Kelman, J. H., & Stunkard, A. J. (1983). Treatment of obese children with and without their mothers: Changes in weight and blood pressure. *Pediatrics, 71*, 515–523.

Bruhn, J. G., & Parcel, G. S. (1982). Preschool health education program (PHEP): An analysis of baseline data. *Health Education Quarterly, 9*, 116–129.

Campbell, M. K., De Vellis, B. M., Strecher, V. J., Ammerman, A. S., De Vellis, R. F., & Sandler, R. S. (1994). Improving dietary behavior: The effectiveness of tailored messages in primary-care settings. *American Journal of Public Health, 84*, 783–787.

Coates, T. J., Barofsky, I., Saylor, K. E., Simons-Morton, B., Huster, W., Sereghy, E., Straugh, S., Jacobs, H., & Kidd, L. (1985). Modifying the snack food consumption patterns of inner city high school students: The Great Sensations Study. *Preventive Medicine, 14*, 234–247.

Coates, T. J., Killen, J. D., & Slinkard, L. A. (1982). Parent participation in a treatment program for overweight adolescents. *International Journal of Eating Disorders, 1*, 37–48.

Coates, T. J., & Thoresen, C. E. (1981). Behavior and weight changes in three obese adolescents. *Behavior Therapy, 12*, 383–399.

COMMIT Research Group. (1995a). Community intervention trial for smoking cessation (COMMIT). I. Cohort results from a four-year community intervention. *American Journal of Public Health, 85*, 183–192.

COMMIT Research Group. (1995b). Community intervention trial for smoking cessation (COMMIT). II. Changes in adult cigarette smoking prevalence. *American Journal of Public Health, 85*, 193–200.

Coombs, D., Reynolds, K., Blankson, M., & Joyner, G. (1994). *Effects of a self-help method on breastfeeding by low income women.* Unpublished manuscript.

Crockett, S. J., Mullis, R. M., & Perry, C. L. (1988). Parent nutrition education: A conceptual model. *Journal of School Health, 58*, 53–57.

DISC Collaborative Research Group. (1993). Dietary Intervention Study in Children (DISC) with elevated low-density-lipoprotein cholesterol: Design and baseline characteristics. *Annals of Epidemiology, 3*, 393–402.

Domel, S. B., Baranowski, T., Davis, H., Thompson, W. O., Leonard, S. B., Riley, P., Baranowski, J., Dudovitz, B., & Smyth, M. (1993). Development and evaluation of a school intervention to increase fruit and vegetable consumption among fourth and fifth grade students. *Journal of Nutrition Education, 25*, 345–349.

Dunn, P. C., Lackey, C. J., Kolasa, K., & Mustian, R. D. (1994). Nutrition education interests of parents of 5- to 8-year old children. *Journal of Nutrition Education, 26*, 284–286.

Edmundson, E., Parcel, G. S., Feldman, H. A., Elder, J., Perry, C. L., Johnson, C. C., et al. (1996). The effects of Child and Adolescent Trial for Cardiovascular Health upon psychosocial determinants of diet and physical activity behavior. *Preventive Medicine, 25*, 442–454.

Elamin, A., Eltayeb, B., Hasan, M., Hofvander, Y., & Tuvemo, T. (1993). Effect of dietary education on metabolic control in children and adolescents with Type I diabetes mellitus. *Diabetes, Nutrition and Metabolism, 6*, 223–229.

Epstein, L. H., Valoski, A., Wing, R. R., & McCurley, J. (1994). Ten year outcomes of behavioral family-based treatment for childhood obesity. *Health Psychology, 13*, 373–383.

Erikson, E. H. (1963). *Childhood and society.* New York: Norton.

Family Heart Study Group. (1994). Randomised controlled trial evaluating cardiovascular screening and intervention in general practice: Principal results of British family heart study. *British Mededical Journal, 308*, 313–320.

Fischman-Havstad, L., & Marston, A. R. (1984). Weight loss maintenance as one aspect of family emotion and process. *British Journal of Clinical Psychology, 23*, 265–271.

Fisher, E. B., Jr. (1995). The results of the COMMIT Trial. *American Journal of Public Health, 85*, 159–161.

Flodmark, C., Ohlsson, T., Ryden, O., & Sveger, T. (1993). Prevention of progression to severe obesity in a group of obese schoolchildren treated with family therapy. *Pediatrics, 91*, 880–884.

Fors, S. W., Owen, S., Hall, W. D., McLaughlin, J., & Levinson, R. (1989). Evaluation of a diffusion strategy for school-based hypertension education. *Health Education Quarterly, 16*, 255–261.

Franson, K., & Rossner, S. (1994). Effects of weight reduction programs on close family members. *International Journal of Obesity, 18*, 648–649.

Glasgow, R. E., Terborg, J. E., Hollis, J. F., Severson, H. H., & Boles, S. M. (1995). Take heart: Results from the initial phase of a work-site wellness program. *American Journal of Public Health, 85*, 209–216.

Gliksman, M. D., Lazarus, R., & Wilson, A. (1993). Differences in serum lipids in Australian children: Is diet responsible? *International Journal of Epidemiology, 22*, 247–254.

Gross, A. M., Magalnick, L. J., & Richardson, P. (1985). Self-management training with families of insulin-dependent diabetic children: A controlled long-term investigation. *Child and Family Behavior Therapy, 7*, 35–39.

Haddock, C. K., Shadish, W. R., Klesges, R. C., & Stein, R. J. (1994). Treatments for childhood and adolescent obesity. *Annals of Behavioral Medicine, 16*, 235–244.

Hearn, M. D., & Baranowski, T. (1996). Doing what comes naturally: Elementary school fidelity to a behavior change nutrition education curriculum. *Journal of Nutrition Education* (submitted).

Hopper, C. A., Gruber, M. B., Munoz, K. D., & Herb, R. A. (1992). Effect of including parents in a school-based exercise and nutrition program for children. *Research Quarterly for Exercise and Sport, 63*, 1–7.

Johnson, C. C., Nicklas, T. A., Arbeit, M. L., Franklin, F. A., Cresanta, J. L., Harsha, D. W., & Berenson, G. S. (1987). Cardiovascular risk in parents of children with elevated blood pressure: Heart Smart Family Health Promotion. *Journal of Clinical Hypertension, 3*, 559–566.

Johnson, C. C., Nicklas, T. A., Arbeit, M. L., Harsh, D. W., Mott, D. S., Hunter, S. M., Wattigney, W., & Berenson, G. S. (1991). Cardiovascular intervention for high-risk families: The

Heart Smart Program. *Cardiovascular Health Promotion,* *84,* 1305–1312.

Johnson, C. C., Nicklas, T. A., Arbeit, M. L., Webber, L. S., & Berenson, G. S. (1992). Behavioral counseling and contracting as methods for promoting cardiovascular health in families. *Journal of the American Dietetic Association,* *92,* 479–481.

Kelder, S. D., Perry, D. L., Klepp, K. I., & Lytle, L. L. (1994). Longitudinal tracking of adolescent smoking, physical activity, and food choice behaviors. *American Journal of Public Health, 84,* 1121–1126.

Kirby, S., Baranowski, T., Reynolds, K., Taylor, G., & Binkley, D. (1995). Children's fruit and vegetable intake: Socioeconomic adult–child, regional, and urban–rural influences. *Journal of Nutrition Education, 27,* 261–271.

Kirks, B. A., Hendricks, D. G., & Wyse, B. W. (1982). Parent involvement in nutrition education for primary grade students. *Journal of Nutrition Education, 14,* 137–140.

Kirks, B. A., & Hughes, C. (1986). Long-term behavioral effects of parent involvement in nutrition education. *Journal of Nutrition Education, 18,* 203–206.

Knight, J., & Grantham-McGregor, S. (1985). Using primary-school children to improve child-rearing practices in rural Jamaica. *Child: Care, Health and Development, 11,* 81–90.

Knutsen, S. F., & Knutsen, R. (1989). The Tromso Heart Study: Family approach to intervention on CHD. *Scandinavian Journal of Social Medicine, 17,* 109–119.

Knutsen, S. F., & Knutsen, R. (1991). The Tromso Survey: The Family Intervention Study—The effect of intervention on some coronary risk factors and dietary habits, a 6-year follow-up. *Preventive Medicine, 20,* 197–212.

Lando, H. A., Pechacek, T. F., Pirie, P. L., Murray, D. M., Mittlemark, M. D., Lichtenstein, E., Nothwehr, F., & Gray, C. (1995). Changes in adult cigarette smoking in the Minnesota Heart Health Program. *American Journal of Public Health, 85,* 201–208.

Lapinleimu, H., Jokinen, E., Myzrinmaa, A., Viikari, J., Ronnemaa, T., Valimaki, I., Linko, L., & Simell, O. (1994). Individualizing dietary counselling of families: Serum cholesterol concentration and growth of children aged 7–13 months. *Acta Paediatrica, 83,* 383–388.

Lau, R. R., Quadrell, M. J., & Hartman, K. A. (1990). Development and change of young adults' preventive health beliefs and behavior: Influence from parents and peers. *Journal of Health and Social Behavior, 31,* 240–259.

Lindenberg, C. S., Artola, R. C., & Jimenez, V. (1990). The effect of early post-partum mother–infant contact and breastfeeding promotion on the incidence and continuation of breast-feeding. *International Journal of Nursing Studies, 27,* 179–186.

Luepker, R. V., Perry, C. L., McKinlay, S. M., Nader, P. R., Parcel, G. S., Stone, E. J., et al. (1996). Outcomes of a field trial to improve children's dietary patterns and physical activity: The Child and Adolescent Trial for Cardiovascular Health (CATCH). *Journal of the American Medical Association, 275,* 768–776.

Luepker, R. V., Perry, C. L., Murray, D. M., & Mullis, R. (1988). Hypertension prevention through nutrition education in youth: A school-based program involving parents. *Health Psychology, 7(Supplement),* 233–245.

Madsen, J., Sallis, J. F., Rupp, J. W., Senn, K. L., Patterson, T. L., Atkins, C. J., & Nader, P. R. (1993a). Process variables as predictors of risk factor changes in a family health behavior change program. *Health Education Research, 8,* 193–204.

Madsen, J., Sallis, J. F., Rupp, J. W., Senn, K. L., Patterson, T. L., Atkins, C. J., & Nader, P. R. (1993b). Relationship between self-monitoring of diet and exercise change and subsequent risk factor change in children and adults. *Patient Education and Counseling, 21,* 61–69.

Mahoney, L. T., Lauer, R. M., Lee, J., & Clarke, W. R. (1991). Factors affecting tracking of coronary heart disease risk factors in children: The Muscatine Study. *Annals of the New York Academy of Sciences, 623,* 120–132.

Marshall, J. R., & Neill, J. (1997). The removal of a psychosomatic symptom: Effects on the marriage. *Family Process, 16,* 273–280.

Mawhinney, T. C., Dickinson, A. M., & Taylor, L. A., III. (1989). The use of concurrent schedules to evaluate the effects of extrinsic rewards on "intrinsic motivation." *Journal of Organizational Behavior Management, 10,* 109–129.

McDivitt, J. A., Zimicki, S., Hornik, R., & Abulaban, A. (1993). The impact of the Healthcom Mass Media Campaign on timely initiation of breastfeeding in Jordan. *Studies in Family Planning, 24,* 295–309.

McLaughlin, J. F., Owen, S. L., Fors, S. W., & Levinson, R. M. (1992). The school child as health educator: Diffusion of hypertension information from sixth-grade children to parents. *Qualitative Studies in Education, 5,* 147–165.

McLeroy, K. R., Steckler, A. B., Simons-Morton, B., Goodman, R. M., Gottlieb, N., & Burdine, J. N. (1993). Social science theory in health education: Time for a new model? *Health Education Research, 8,* 305–312.

Meyer, E. C., Garcia Coll, C. T., Lester, B. M., Bonkydis, C. F. Z., McDonough, S. M., & Oh, W. (1994). Family-based intervention improves maternal psychological well-being and feeding interaction of preterm infants. *Pediatrics, 93,* 241–246.

Morisky, D. E., DeMuth, N. M., Field-Fass, M., Green, L. W., & Levine, D. M. (1985). Evaluation of family health education to build social support for long-term control of high blood pressure. *Health Education Quarterly, 12,* 35–50.

MRFIT Research Group. (1982). Multiple Risk Factor Intervention Trial Risk factor changes and mortality results. *Journal of the American Medical Association, 248,* 1415–1477.

Nader, P. R., Baranowski, T., Vanderpool, N. A., Dunn, K., Dworkin, R., & Ray, L. (1983). The Family Health Project: Cardiovascular risk reduction education for children and parents. *Journal of Developmental and Behavioral Pediatrics, 4,* 3–10.

Nader, P. R., Perry, C., Maccoby, M., Solomon, D., Killen, J., Telch, M., & Alexander, J. K. (1982). Adolescent perceptions of family health behavior: A tenth grade educational activity to increase family awareness of a community cardiovascular risk reduction program. *Journal of School Health, 53,* 372–377.

Nader, P. R., Sallis, J. F., Abramson, I. S., Broyles, S. L., Patterson, T. L., Senn, K., Rupp, J. W., & Nelson, J. A. (1992). Family-based cardiovascular risk reduction education among Mexican- and Anglo-Americans. *Family and Community Health, 15,* 57–74.

Nader, P., Sallis, J., Patterson, T., Abramson, I., Rupp, J., Atkins, C., Roppe, B., Morris, J., Wallace, J., & Vega, W. (1989). A family approach to cardiovascular risk reduction: Results from the San Diego family health project. *Health Education Quarterly, 16,* 229–244.

Nader, P. R., Sallis, J. F., Rupp, J., Atkins, C., Patterson, T., & Abramson, I. (1986). San Diego Family Health Project: Reaching families through the schools. *Journal of School Health, 56,* 227–231.

Neill, J. R., Marshall, J. R., & Yale, C. E. (1978). Marital changes after intestinal bypass surgery. *Journal of the American Medical Association, 240,* 447–450.

Newman, W. P., III, Freedman, D. S., & Berenson, G. (1986). Regulation of serum lipoprotein levels and systolic blood pressure to early atherosclerosis: The Bogalusa Heart Study. *New England Journal of Medicine, 314,* 138–144.

Nicklas, T. A., Webber, L. S., Johnson, C. C., Srinivasan, S. R., & Berenson, G. (1995). Foundations for health promotion with youth: A review of observations from the Bogalusa Heart Study. *Journal of Health Education, 26,* S-18–S-26.

Parcel, G. S., Bruhn, J. G., & Murray, J. L. (1984). Preschool health education program (PHEP): Analysis of educational and behavioral outcome. *Health Education Quarterly, 10,* 149–172.

Patterson, T. L., Sallis, J. F., Nader, P. R., Kaplan, R. M., & Rupp, J. W. (1989). Familial similarities of changes in cognitive, behavioral, and physiological variables in a cardiovascular health promotion program. *Journal of Pediatric Psychology, 14,* 277–292.

Patterson, T. L., Sallis, J. F., Nader, P. R., Rupp, J. W., McKenzie, T. L., Roppe, B., & Bartok, P. W. (1988). Direct observations of physical activity and dietary behaviors in a structured environment: Effects of a family-based health promotion program. *Journal of Behavioral Medicine, 11,* 447–458.

Perry, C. L., Luepker, R. V., Murray, D. M., Hearn, M D., Halper, A., Dudovitz, B., Maile, M. C., & Smyth, M. (1989). Parents' involvement with children's health promotion: A one-year follow-up of the Minnesota home team. *Health Education Quarterly, 16,* 171–180.

Perry, C. L., Luepker, R. V., Murray, D. M., Kurth, C., Mullis, R., Crockett, S., & Jacobs, D. (1988). Parent involvement with children's health promotion: The Minnesota home team. *American Journal of Public Health, 79,* 1156–1160.

Petchers, M. K., Hirsch, E. Z., & Block, B. A. (1987). The impact of parent participation on the effectiveness of a heart health curriculum. *Health Education Quarterly, 14,* 449–460.

Plomin, R., Reiss, D., Hetherington, E. M., & Howe, G. W. (1994). Nature and nurture: Genetic contributions to measures of the family environment. *Developmental Psychology, 30,* 32–43.

Pollitt, E. (1987). A critical view of three decades of research on the effects of chronic energy malnutrition on behavioral development. In B. Schurch and N. S. Scrinshaw (Eds.), *Chronic energy deficiency: Consequences and related issues.* International Dietary Energy Consulting Group.

Prochaska, J. O., Norcross, I. C., & Di Clemente, C. C. (1994). *Changing for good.* New York: William Morrow.

Puska, P., Vartiainen, T., Pallonen, U., Salonen, J. T., Poyhia, P., Koskela, K., & McAlister, A. (1982). The North Karelia Youth Project: Evaluation of two years of intervention on health behavior and CVD risk factors among 13- to 15-year old children. *Preventive Medicine, 11,* 550–570.

Rand, C. S. W., Kowalske, K., & Kuldau, J. M. (1989). Characteristics of marital improvement following obesity surgery. *Psychosomatics, 25,* 221–226.

Rand, C. S. W., Kuldau, J. M., & Robbins, L. (1982). Surgery for obesity and marriage quality. *Journal of the American Medical Association, 247,* 1419–1422.

Resnicow, K., Cross, D., Lacosse, J., & Nichols, P. (1993). Evaluation of a school-site cardiovascular risk factor screening intervention. *Preventive Medicine, 22,* 838–856.

Rickard, K. A., Gallahue, D. L., Gruen, G. E., Tridle, M., Bewley, N., & Steele, K. (1995). The play approach to learning in the context of families and schools: An alternative paradigm for nutrition and fitness education in the 21st century. *Journal of the American Dietetic Association, 95,* 1121–1126.

Sciacca, J. P., Phipps, B. L., Dube, D. A., & Ratliff, M. I. (1995). Influences on breastfeeding by lower-income women: An incentive-based, partner-supported educational program. *Journal of the American Dietetic Association, 95,* 323–328.

Shea, S., Stein, A. D., Basch, C. E., Contento, I., & Zybert, P. (1992). Variability and self-regulation of energy intake in young children in their everyday environment. *Pediatrics, 90,* 542–546.

Simons-Morton, B. G., Coates, T. J., Saylor, K. E., Sereghy, E., & Barofsky, I. (1984). Great Sensations: A program to encourage heart healthy snacking by high school students. *Journal of School Health, 54,* 288–291.

Stark, L. J., Collins, F. L., Osnes, P. G., & Stokes, T. F. (1986). Using reinforcement and cuing to increase healthy snack food choices in preschoolers. *Journal of Applied Behavioral Analysis, 19,* 367–379.

Stone, E. J., Baranowski, T., Sallis, J. F., & Cutler, J. A. (1995). Review of behavioral research for cardiopulmonary health: Emphasis on youth, gender, and ethnicity. *Journal of Health Education, 26,* S9–S17.

Storer, J. H., Frate, D. A., Johnson, S. A., & Greenberg, A. M.

(1987). When the cure seems worse than the disease: Helping families adapt to hypertension treatment. *Family Relations, 36,* 311–315.

Sunseri, A. J., Alberti, J. M., Kent, N. D., Schoenberger, J. A., & Dolecek, T. A. (1984). Ingredients in nutrition education: Family involvement, reading and race. *Journal of School Health, 5,* 193–196.

Sunseri, A. J., Alberti, J. M., Schoenberger, J. A., Kent, N. D., Amuwo, S., Sunseri, J. K., & Vickers, P. (1983). In F. Landry (Ed.), *Health risk estimation, risk reduction, and health promotion* (pp. 617–628). Ottawa, Canada: Canadian Public Health Association.

Sunseri, A. J., Dolecek, T. A., Amuno, S., Kent, N. D., Cullinan, J., & Allendorff, S. (n.d.). Urban families as willing respondents to a school heart-health curriculum. Chicago Heart Association. Unpublished manuscript.

Susser, M. (1995). The tribulations of trials—Interventions in communities. *American Journal of Public Health, 85,* 156–159.

Taylor, W., Baranowski, T., & Sallis, J. (1994). Family determinants of childhood physical activity: A social cognitive model. In R. K. Dishman (Ed.), *Exercise adherence: Its impact on public health* (pp. 319–342). Champaign, IL: Human Kinetics Publishers.

Tinsley, B. J. (1992). Multiple influences on the acquisition and socialization of children's health attitudes and behavior: An integrative review. *Child Development, 63,* 1043–1069.

U.S. Agency for International Development (USAID). (1991). *Breastfeeding: A report on A.I.D. programs.* Washington, DC: USAID.

U.S. Department of Health and Human Services. (1984). *Report of the Surgeon General's workshop on breastfeeding and human lactation.* DHHS Publication No. HRS-D-MC 84-2. Washington, DC: USDHHS.

Valaitis, R. K., & Shea, E. (1993). An evaluation of breastfeeding promotion literature: Does it really promote breastfeeding? *Canadian Journal of Public Health, 84,* 24–27.

Van Lenthe, F. J., Kemper, H. C. G., & Twisk, J. W. R. (1994). Tracking of blood pressure in children and youth. *American Journal of Human Biology, 6,* 389–399.

Vega, W. A., Sallis, J. F., Patterson, T. L., Rupp, J. W., Morris, J. A., & Nader, P. R. (1988). Predictors of dietary change in Mexican American families participating in a health behavior change program. *American Journal of Preventive Medicine, 4,* 194–199.

Werle, M. A., Murphy, T. B., & Budd, K. S. (1993). Treating chronic food refusal in young children: Home-based parent training. *Journal of Applied Behavior Analysis, 26,* 421–433.

Wheeler, M. E., & Hess, K. W. (1976). Treatment of juvenile obesity by successive approximation control of eating. *Journal of Behavior Therapy and Experimental Psychiatry, 7,* 235–241.

Whitaker, R. C., Wright, J. A., Finch, A. J., Deyo, R. A., & Psaty, B. M. (1994). School lunch: A comparison of the fat and cholesterol content with dietary guidelines. *Journal of Pediatrics, 123,* 857–862.

Whitaker, R. C., Wright, J. A., Koepsell, T. D., Finch, A. J., & Psaty, B. M. (1994). Randomized intervention to increase children's selection of low-fat foods in school lunches. *Journal of Pediatrics, 125,* 535–540.

Williams, C. L. (1983/1985). Nutrition intervention and health risk reduction in childhood: Creating healthy adults. *Pediatrician, 12,* 97–101.

Witschi, J. C., Singer, M., Wu-Lee, M., & Stare, F. J. (1978). Family cooperation and effectiveness in a cholesterol-lowering diet. *Journal of the American Dietetic Association, 72,* 384–389.

Writing Group for the DISC Collaborative Research Group. (1995). Efficacy and safety of lowering dietary intake of fat and cholesterol in children with elevated low-density lipoprotein cholesterol: The Dietary Intervention Study in Children (DISC). *Journal of the American Medical Association, 273,* 1429–1435.

17

Stories to Live By

A Narrative Approach to Health Behavior Research and Injury Prevention

Henry P. Cole

INTRODUCTION

An injury prevention research program supported by funding from the U.S. Bureau of Mines (USBM) and the National Institute for Occupational Safety and Health (NIOSH) resulted in the development, evaluation, and dissemination of approximately 70 narrative-based simulation exercises for mining industry workers in the United States (*Catalog of training products*, 1993). More than 400,000 copies of the mining exercises have been used in the United States, and additional copies are used in four other countries (Cole, 1993; Cole et al., 1993). Additional funding from the National Institute for Environmental Health

Sciences (NIEHS), the Office of Surface Mining, the Agency for Toxic Substances Disease Registry, and NIOSH produced interactive–narrative exercises for firefighters, mine reclamation inspectors, hazardous-waste workers, health care providers, and farm family adult and youth workers.

Each exercise is designed to influence workers' knowledge, attitudes, and conduct concerning specific job-related hazards and tasks. The goal is to promote safety attitudes and behavior and to prevent "close calls" and injury events. Based on authentic cases, each exercise presents a problem scenario that requires a series of judgments among alternative actions and provides immediate feedback about the consequences and correctness of the actions selected.

This chapter describes the health behavior theory and research foundation of interactive–narrative exercises designed to educate and empower workers. Examples of the exercises and their structure and content are provided. Their dual role as teaching and assessment devices for critical skills is described. Evaluation of the exercises is summarized, and their impact upon worker safety education is discussed.

Henry P. Cole • Behavioral Research Aspects of Safety and Health (BRASH) Working Group, University of Kentucky, Lexington, Kentucky 40506-0350.

Handbook of Health Behavior Research IV: Relevance for Professionals and Issues for the Future, edited by David S. Gochman. Plenum Press, New York, 1997.

THE EXERCISES
AS INTERACTIVE STORIES

The exercises described in this chapter are interactive stories. Because the exercises faithfully re-create aspects of information gathering and decision making that occur during real-life emergency situations, they are also simulations. Each exercise has its own particular story with which the trainees interact as the plot unfolds. The story includes characters, goals, predicaments, and consequences that result from the interactions of the characters and the simulated workplace environment. The role of the protagonist is usually played by the person(s) working the exercise. The exercise narrative begins before the emergency situation develops, allowing the worker to anticipate, recognize, and eliminate or control potential hazards. From 8 to 15 major decision points are included in each exercise. Each decision point is followed by a series of "correct" actions that experts generally agree will help to prevent or control a pending or ongoing emergency situation. Other plausible but ineffective or counterproductive actions are also listed. These "decision errors" are derived from persons' actions preceding, during, and following actual workplace-injury events as reported in official investigations and as determined by occupational injury epidemiology studies of specific agents, hosts and environments.

Each exercise contains predicaments. For example, a mine section supervisor faced with the first aid care of a critically burned miner may have to deal with a serious underground fire that demands simultaneously organizing a crew, fighting the fire, and escaping from the mine. The supervisor cannot perform all these tasks at once. Other workers present may be well qualified to direct some but not other tasks. As in the real-life cases on which the simulation is based, the supervisor's decisions affect not only the injured miner, but also the well-being of the entire mine-section crew and the safety of other miners elsewhere in the mine (Continuous Miner Fire [*Catalog of training products*, 1993, p. 54]). The exer-

cises encourage discussion of these types of predicaments, help workers to think deeply about such events, and promote proactive strategies to prevent similar life-threatening situations in their own workplaces.

Each simulation is a "problem-posing" exercise (Wallerstein & Bernstein, 1988; Wallerstein & Weinger, 1992). The problems posed are authentic and designed to empower workers to examine and integrate knowledge and attitudes acquired from their personal experience with information learned from working the exercise. As workers complete an exercise, they acquire information from two sources. First, the empirical knowledge that results from analytical investigations of actual workplace disasters and injury events is revealed throughout and following the exercise. Second, the workers' wisdom, attitudes, beliefs, knowledge, and misconceptions are revealed to each other as they interact in small groups of three to five people during the development and resolution of the simulated emergency problem. Empowerment is realized as workers and managers translate this critical analysis of attitudes and knowledge into changed perceptions, behaviors, and work practices that can help prevent injury events within their organizations.

PRIOR RESEARCH
ON SIMULATION EXERCISES

A large body of research exists about simulation training. This research tends to ignore the narrative structure of such simulations, yet much has been learned from this prior work that has relevance for the construction of interactive-narrative simulation exercises. Research from a number of fields suggests that decision-making skills can be assessed and taught by well-designed simulation exercises based on real-world cases (Brener, 1984; Cole, 1994; Giffin & Rockwell, 1984). Decision errors during simulations and real-life problem solving can result from poor engineering and work organization, fatigue, inexperience, lack of knowledge, faulty attitudes (Peters & Wiehagen, 1988), and misconceptions (Passaro, Cole, & Wala, 1994). The simulation exercises discussed in this chapter lend themselves to teaching and assessing knowledge and attitudes, identifying and correcting misconceptions, and promoting strategic thinking to prevent injury events.

A Good Simulation Is an Evocative and True Story. Regardless of its format, a good simulation exercise is like a good story. This principle applies to elaborate flight simulators in which the flight deck crew of a commercial jet plane relive the emergency landing resulting from an actual in-flight engine failure. It also applies to a tabletop paper-and-pencil simulation for firefighters that re-creates a hazardous chemical spill that occurred near a public school just as the children were about to be released for the day. Both simulations require the participants to develop and evaluate strategies and actions for controlling a dangerous situation and preventing a disaster.

Good simulation exercises always have a plot, a theme, characters, goals, and obstacles. As the simulated problem unfolds, predicaments and dilemmas develop. The person working the simulation exercise feels that he or she is experiencing a real problem as it develops, not knowing what might happen next. Unlike a story that is simply to be read, however, the exercise requires the person to gather information, interpret data, remember and use relevant facts and information, make choices and decisions, and experience vicariously the consequences of these decisions. The decisions and their consequences are constrained within the limits of the available resources described in the problem. To be effective, the simulations must deal in a realistic manner with authentic problems and decision alternatives for specific tasks and specific populations of workers (Cole, 1993).

Because the exercises deal with critical thinking and decision making about matters of life and death, they must be more than simply evocative and plausible stories. It is also impor-

tant that they be true stories (Phillips, 1994). The simulation story setting, plot, characters, goals, and predicaments, as well as the correct and incorrect decision alternatives depicted in the story, must be empirically based on investigations and surveillance studies of occupational injury events.

The mining simulation exercises are grounded in a large body of accident investigation reports prepared by the Mine Safety and Health Administration (MSHA). Hundreds of these reports were studied and analyzed, along with statistical summaries of injury and fatality surveillance data (Cole, Mallett, et al., 1988). These health and safety data, and the accident investigations, provide the scenarios for the exercises and insight about the types of errors that are likely to occur before and during actual mine emergencies. When miners work these simulated mine emergency exercises, they vicariously relive an actual injury event or disaster. When miners make plausible but problematic decisions during the simulation, they receive immediate feedback that tells them the consequences of their choices. Likewise, when they make a wise decision, the feedback message reveals the positive outcome(s) for that action and reinforces correct thinking and decisions. Thus, in the safety of a classroom, miners can practice complex problem-solving and decision-making skills and learn from errors that could prove disastrous in real life.

The exercises developed for hazardous-waste workers, firefighters, and farm workers are similarly based on fatality investigations and injury surveillance data. As of the mid-1990s, however, injury surveillance data for these occupations were far less complete than those for mining.

Hindsight versus Forethought. The thinking demanded by simulation exercises is different from the thinking required by case studies and review of accident reports. Case studies analyze disasters with full knowledge of ensuing events through critical hindsight. They usually present a summary of a problem, how the problem arose and was recognized, descriptions of the judgments made and actions taken by the persons who dealt with the problem, and a critique of these actions in terms of their contribution to solving the problem or making it worse. Case studies therefore involve observation and analysis of the decision-making and problem-solving behavior of other persons by observers (the trainees) through hindsight. Making decisions in actual emergency situations requires forethought, which is qualitatively different from hindsight (Halpern, 1984, p. 237). Interactive–simulation exercises are closer to real-life problem solving because they present problem scenarios with incomplete information, unanticipated developments, and contingencies that may complicate solving the problem. Good simulations also provide no knowledge of outcomes until after the trainees have struggled to identify the problem and acted to prevent, correct, or limit its effects. Training with case studies does much to foster critical hindsight, but little to promote the foresight needed to anticipate, prevent, or limit unplanned events that are commonly called "accidents" (Cole et al., 1993; Fischoff, 1975).

Fidelity.   Simulations can be of high or low fidelity or anywhere in between. Simulations can be so realistic that the persons working the exercise can barely distinguish whether they are solving a real problem or working a simulated problem. Examples of such high-fidelity simulations are full-flight-deck simulators that are used to teach pilots decision-making and problem-solving skills. Because of the specialized equipment required, such simulations are costly to develop and use. Lower-fidelity simulations can also be effective training devices. Cognitive processes of problem identification, application of strategic thinking, generation of good decision alternatives, and modification of strategy and tactics in the light of consequences from actions can be effectively taught through simply constructed paper-and-pencil exercises, games, and role play simulations. The cognitive and interpersonal aspects of these lower fidelity simulations can also

be very realistic (Cole, 1993; Jones, 1980). For this reason, a large portion of the simulation training of military personnel in the United States consists of tabletop, paper-and-pencil problem-solving simulations used in combination with high-fidelity simulators and full-scale field simulations (Haliff, Hollan, & Hutchins, 1986). Firefighters and hazardous-material workers also use many lower-fidelity simulation training devices coupled with complex field drills similar to mine rescue contests that are common worldwide (Cole, 1993; Cole, Mallett, et al., 1988).

Formats.   The Behavioral Research Aspects of Safety and Health (BRASH) Working Group exercises for miners and other workers are developed primarily as paper-and-pencil training simulations for classroom instruction. These types of materials are relatively inexpensive to develop, disseminate, and use. The latent-image format is a cost-effective delivery system that requires only a problem booklet, a latent-image answer sheet, and an inexpensive and reusable marking pen for developing the feedback messages for each decision point. In this format, problems are presented in written form with accompanying diagrams and schematics. Drawings depict spatial relationships that are important to comprehend the story narrative accurately (Bower & Morrow, 1990). Moving through the exercise, step by step, the person selects alternative actions at each major decision point and marks choices on an answer sheet with a special pen that develops an invisible ink message (a latent image). The message provides the worker with immediate feedback about the consequences of the action.

Figures 1 through 3 depict three frames from a latent-image exercise that simulates a real-life injury scenario in which a maintenance worker becomes entangled in a large conveyor-belt system at an ore processing plant. The person doing the exercise plays the role of the protagonist—in this case, a coworker who first attempts (unsuccessfully) to prevent a colleague from engaging in a risky shortcut to clean the tail pulley while

Question C

You decide to go to the control panel and lock out and tag the belt drive motor. Half way there you meet Carl. You tell him you are going to lock out the belt so you can clean the tail pulley. Carl says, "Don't bother! I can fix it easy!" Then he walks off toward the tail pulley. What would you do now? (Choose only ONE unless directed to "Try again!")

9. Ask him what he is going to do.

10. Tell him, "OK. Anything to save time!"

11. Sit down and take a break while he takes care of it.

12. Tell Carl he is a fool.

Question C (Latent-Image Answers*)

9.   [Correct! But he says, "Watch me, son, and I'll show you how it's done!"   ]
        [Do the next question.   ]

10.   [Carl may be about to perform an unsafe act. Try again!   ]

11.   [You need to watch out for him. Try again!   ]

12.   [This makes him angry, doesn't help, and may encourage him to do   ]
        [something dangerous. Try again!   ]

*The text between the brackets is the latent image that remains invisible until marked with the special developing pen.

Figure 1. Question and latent-image answers for a decision point in a conveyor-belt injury exercise.

the 4-foot-wide conveyor belt is running. Action alternatives for two of the exercise decision points are shown in the top portions of Figures 1 and 3. The latent-image messages for these actions remain invisible until the person marks the brackets on the answer sheet with the developing pen. These revealed feedback messages are shown in the bracketed text in the lower portions of Figures 1 and 3. The two drawings in Figure 2 depict the events leading up to the injury and the injury event itself. Other decision points in the exercise deal with rescue and first-aid procedures and with prevention strategies, including company policy, work organization, and engineering controls. The exercise concludes with an invitation for workers to critically exam-

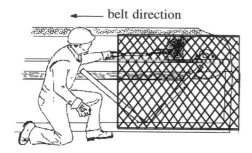

Carl tries to scrape the tail pulley with a shovel

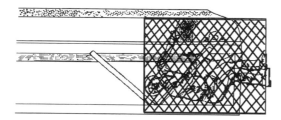

Carl becomes trapped in the pulley and belt guard

Figure 2. Drawings of an in-progress injury event.

ine their own environment and behavior. This last focus helps empower workers and managers to make changes in policy, engineering, work practices, and behavior to reduce risk of a similar injury event at their workplaces.

Figure 4 is a drawing from another latent-image simulation exercise that depicts an actual injury event in which a worker was buried under 80 tons of fine granular material (in this case, coal) in a large bin. This Man in the Bin exercise (*Catalog of training products*, 1993, p. 59) also includes decision points that deal with prevention of such events through implementation of proper engineering, policy, safe work practice, attitudinal, and behavioral controls.

Exercises may be presented in a variety of other formats, including role play, hands-on simulators, interactive video disc, and CD-ROM computer-presented hypermedia with interactive audio, animated color graphics, and text. The two exercises depicted in Figures 1–4, as well as

other exercises, have been produced in interactive hypermedia format (Cole et al., 1992). Similar exercises have been developed in role play format (*Catalog of training products*, 1993, pp. 68–69; Cole, Wasielewski, Haley, & Berger, 1988).

The format of an exercise is not nearly as important as the authenticity of the exercise content and context. The story line, plot, characters, goals, obstacles, predicaments, decision alternatives, and consequences must be part of a well-constructed narrative that is meaningful, believable, and engaging. The exercise must be situated in the cultural context and the everyday lives of the individuals for whom it is designed. It is to provide this authenticity that the exercises are constructed from actual injury events and reports in collaboration with workers engaged in hazardous jobs and occupations. Exercises that meet these design criteria promote "situated cognition in a culture of learning," the efficient and effective acquisition of key knowledge, attitudes, and skills that are readily applied to real-world tasks (Brown, Collins, & Duguid, 1989; Lave & Wenger, 1994). This chapter describes the simulation exercise stories, their use as health behavior interventions, and their grounding in the theory of narrative thinking.

THEORY OF NARRATIVE THINKING

In seminal works that bridge cognitive psychology and the literary arts, Bruner (1986, 1990a) argues that there are two modes of cognitive representation or thinking: the paradigmatic and the narrative. Paradigmatic thinking (also called "propositional thinking") is concerned with the construction of context-free and abstract formal concepts and principles. Paradigmatic thinking is both the goal and method of science, logic, and mathematics. Narrative thinking is basic to both everyday living and scientific inquiry.

Narrative, Life, and Meaning. Throughout the world, stories are universal and powerful

Question E

Before you can do anything, you hear a thump and the shovel comes flying by your head. You see Carl caught between the tail pulley roller and the guard. His face is pushed against the guard. His eyes are open, his mouth is moving, and his face is bloody. (See Figure 2.) What would you do now? (Choose only ONE unless directed to "Try again!")

17. Run and get help.

18. Run back to Carl. Try to reach inside the guard and pull him out.

19. Start removing the guard so you can free Carl.

20. Pull the emergency cord that stops the belt.

Question C (Latent-Image Answers*)

17.　[You need to do something else first. Try again!　　　　　　　　　　　　　]

18.　[You may also become caught in the belt. Try again!　　　　　　　　　　　]

19.　[This would take a long time and expose you to injury. Try again!　　　　　]

20.　[Correct! But the belt doesn't stop! Do the next question.　　　　　　　　]

---

*The text between the brackets is the latent image that remains invisible until marked with the special developing pen.

Figure 3. Question and latent-image answers for another decision point in the conveyor-belt injury exercise.

guides for living and for understanding our own and others' conduct (Holland & Kilpatrick, 1993; Howard, 1991; Robinson & Hawpe, 1986; Rosenthal, 1993; Sarbin, 1986a; Vitz, 1990). Narrative thinking as a process is the translation of one's own and others' experiences into stories that integrate facts, perceptions, emotions, intentions, actions, and consequences into coherent meaning. Storytelling is not the only successful cognitive process for organizing perception, thought, memory, and action, "but within its natural domain of every-day interpersonal experience it is more effective than any other" (Robinson & Hawpe, 1986, p. 123). It is the universal method and root metaphor by which people create, sustain, and transmit meaning about their lives (Sarbin, 1986b). Goals, plans, decisions, and actions are guided by the storied nature of human thinking (Bruner, 1990a). Narrative thinking involves knowing through stories lived, stories heard, and stories told (Howard, 1991).

Unlike paradigmatic thinking, narrative rep-

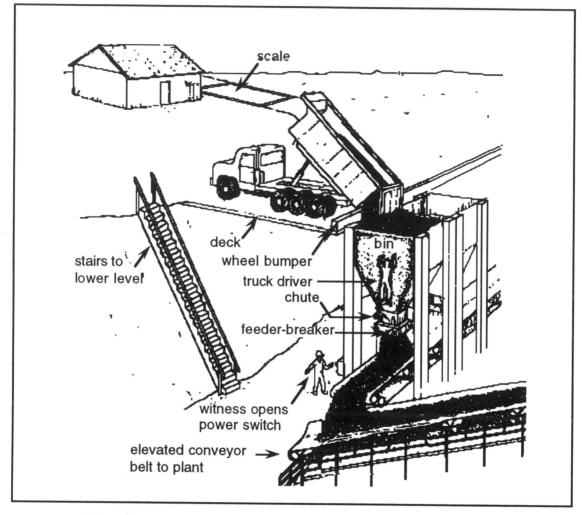

Figure 4. Drawing of the entrapment of a worker and the posing of a rescue problem.

resentation is always contextualized as a story about someone doing something, for some purpose, that results in specific consequences from the actions taken. The narrative mode of thought is well suited to accommodating and making coherent meaning from the incomplete information and inconsistencies that are normal to daily life with all its richness, ambiguities, inconsistencies, and predicaments. The robustness of the life

stories people live, observe, and communicate about cannot be captured in a meaningful way with only the abstract principles of paradigmatic thinking. The complexity of life events and their meanings can be appreciated, comprehended, and used to guide goals and conduct only through narrative thought. As Bruner (1990b, p. 350) says, "Narrative, unlike logic, is not stopped dead by contradiction. Indeed, it thrives on it."

Narrative as Basic to Paradigmatic Thinking. Narrative thinking also provides context, purpose, and perspective for knowing the world through those formal logical concepts that are abstracted from life experience by science, logic, and mathematics. Narrative thought makes it possible to interpret events by constructing coherent causal patterns of meaning that blend what is known about a situation (facts) with relevant conjectures (imagination) (Sarbin, 1986b, p. xxi). This property of narrative thought makes it basic not only to everyday living, but also to causal hypothesis formulation and testing that give purpose and meaning to scientific thinking and paradigmatic inquiry (Mishler, 1986). In this sense, narrative representation as a cognitive process is the foundation for other, more formal modes of thought (Gerrig, 1994). After all, formal paradigms must be abstracted from something, and that something is usually a coherent and contextualized story about some set of personalized life experiences that motivate questing for a higher level of abstract meaning. Thus, narrative thinking is a universal and basic cognitive process of meaning making. It is essential to the many other problem-solving methods used by all people and studied by cognitive psychologists (Bower & Morrow, 1990; Crites, 1986; Sarbin, 1986b).

The theory of narrative thinking is also supported by studies of reading comprehension and artificial intelligence. Researchers who attempted to write computer programs that can read and translate text into meaningful summaries discovered that only about 15% of the information in a typical passage is explicitly stated. The remaining 85% is implicit information and can be understood only when the computer has been programmed to have a huge knowledge base in the form of narrative scripts that define the usual characters, goals, and transactions of persons in particular settings. Earlier researchers independently reached the same conclusion when they studied people's comprehension of prose material. The body of organized narrative knowledge

that both humans and computers need to make meaning from spoken or written language has come to be called, variously, "story grammar" (Schank, 1984), "scripts" (Mayer, 1992), and "event schema" (Bonnet, 1985).

A CONCEPTUAL MODEL FOR HEALTH BELIEFS AND BEHAVIOR

The conceptual model depicted in Figure 5 was derived following a selective review of literature concerned with narrative thinking. Little of the narrative literature deals with health beliefs and safety behavior. Worker health and safety training is dominated by the paradigmatic approach of various health belief models, behavioral analysis, and behavior modification interventions designed to change worker behavior (Cole, Garrity, & Berger, 1998; Irwin, Cataldo, Matheny, & Peterson, 1992; Wallerstein and Bernstein, 1988; Wallerstein & Weinger, 1992). It is also dominated by the didactic instruction of safety rules and facts, especially as these are encoded in federal health and safety laws and regulations and the associated mandatory worker training (Digman & Grasso, 1981; Wallerstein & Weinger, 1992). The narrative conceptual model in Figure 5 is intended to provide a more robust and comprehensive understanding of the cultural, cognitive, and behavioral context of worker

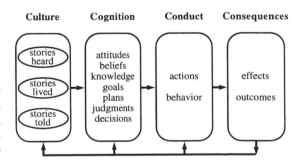

Figure 5. A cultural, cognitive, and behavioral model of health beliefs and safety behavior.

health and safety behavior and education than do the predominant health belief and behavioristic models.

Origin of the Model. The literature on which the model is based is drawn from a variety of disciplines, including life-span human development and personal growth (Hermans, 1992; Vitz, 1990); motivation, goals, and self-efficacy (Bandura, 1989; Baumeister & Newman, 1994; Gerrig, 1994); interpersonal relationships and attributions (Gonzales, Haugen, & Manning, 1994; Murray & Holmes, 1994); mental health and psychotherapy (Crites, 1986; Howard, 1991; Spence, 1986; multiculturalism and professional education (Holland & Kilpatrick, 1993); educational psychology and teacher education (Carter, 1993; Connelly & Clandinin, 1990); and research philosophy and methodology (Josselson & Lieblich, 1993; Mishler, 1986; Phillips, 1994). The model depicted in Figure 5 is particularly indebted to the work of Bruner (1986, 1990a) on literature, narrative, meaning making, and folk psychology; Sarbin's (1986b) conception of the storied nature of human conduct; and Howard's (1991) conception of culture tales as the primary mechanisms that direct human goals, decisions, and actions.

Limitations of Behavioral Approaches. Wallerstein and Weinger (1992) are critical of the pervasive behavioral training interventions administered to workers as part of their mandatory training. In this approach, a job analysis defines specific health risks and problem behaviors. Specific learning objectives are developed to train workers in safe behaviors. Workers then demonstrate and practice the prescribed safety behaviors (e.g., wearing safety goggles, looking before backing vehicles, crossing conveyor belts only at designated places, and keeping walkways clear of liquid spills and clutter). Such behaviors are monitored and reinforced. These types of health and safety interventions can be quite effective in reducing injuries, but often result only in short-term behavior change. Once the careful monitoring and frequent reinforcement of the target be-

haviors ceases, the adherence of workers to the prescribed regimen of safety behaviors tends to return to the baseline levels prior to the intervention (Cole, Garrity, & Berger, 1988; Komaki, Barwick, & Scott, 1978). It is not that behavioral approaches are inappropriate. Rather, they are insufficient by themselves to educate and empower workers to improve workplace health and safety.

Problem of Social versus Personal Relevance. Bruner (1986, 1990a) notes that a universal problem in education is the matter of translating socially relevant information into information that is personally relevant for the individual. Social institutions typically attempt to define and prescribe the most important logical information in a culture as a body of content and skills that individuals need to learn. This body of abstract knowledge is typically codified as didactic information that becomes part of a curriculum presented through compulsory education. Much of the intended value of the knowledge for those persons who are instructed is lost, however, in the teaching of this content (Brown et al., 1989; Resnick, 1987). Many learners who receive didactic instruction in this formally codified and socially relevant knowledge tend to find both the content and the instruction to be burdensome, dull, and boring.

The increasing emphasis on health and safety training of workers as mandated by the Occupational Health and Safety Administration, MSHA, and other federal and state agencies follows this same problematic tradition. Within federal research centers and universities, physical, engineering, medical, social, and behavioral scientists study occupational health and safety. To prevent occupational illness and injury, scholars and legislators translate this knowledge into regulations that deal with engineering, work organization, training, and health and safety standards. Educators and trainers then instruct workers in this content. Like much other formal instruction, safety and health instruction for adults and children tends to be didactic and received with groans and disinterest. This pattern of instruction results in what Whitehead (1929) called "inert knowledge"—facts and figures acquired through formal instruction that are largely put out of mind and seldom used because of their perceived irrelevance to life and living.

Both Bruner (1990a) and Howard (1991) note that interactive narrative, the telling of and participating in powerful and authentic stories, is the age-old and most effective way to translate socially relevant didactic information into compelling and memorable instruction. Under this method of instruction, that which is learned tends to become "active knowledge"—valued, remembered, and used to direct lives and living. For this reason, narrative approaches to instruction (Howard, 1991) and the health and safety narrative–simulation exercises have been called "stores to live by" (Cole, McKnight, Piercy, & McLymore, 1995). The authentic content and context of the exercise narrative invites persons who work the problems to examine, explore, debate, and ponder the risks they face in their own work. The means and resources by which to control these risks, the consequences of injury, and the inconsistencies and misconceptions that may be present in their thinking and behavior are examined critically. Opportunities for generating new ways of thinking, feeling, and acting to promote safety and health are not restricted to individual behavior, but include attention to management practices, engineering, housekeeping, and other controls.

Like the more common behavioral approaches to training, the narrative exercises also translate injury surveillance and epidemiology, federal health and safety laws, and expert knowledge into practical information that can be applied by workers and managers to promote safe work practices and prevent illness and injury. Consistent with Wallerstein and Bernstein's (1988) recommendations, the exercises (1) recognize and draw upon the extensive knowledge and experience of workers; (2) respect adults' preference for real-world, cooperative learning achieved through debate, discourse, and negotiation; (3) present the skills and knowledge to be learned within authentic problem situations; and (4) focus on judgment and decision making.

Integrating Cultural, Cognitive, and Behavioral Contexts. The model in Figure 5 integrates three traditional approaches to studying and explaining human behavior. The two boxes on the right-hand side of the diagram represent the traditional American behaviorism approach. In this tradition, behavior is explained in terms of its consequences, and little attention is given to attitudes, intentions, strategic thinking, or cultural context. It is assumed that in specific contexts, specific behaviors that are reinforced will be exhibited and maintained, that punished behaviors will be inhibited but not extinguished), and that nonreinforced behaviors will be extinguished (Skinner, 1953; Swenson, 1980). In this approach, the material in the two boxes on the left-hand side of the diagram are lumped into "antecedent conditions," which have historically and experimentally been reduced to basic need states and drives (e.g., hunger, thirst, social contact, affection).

This behavioristic conception has been referred to as the "A, B, C model" (Antecedent conditions, Behaviors, and Consequences) of behavior shaping. It has also been called a "deficit motivation model," since the antecedent conditions that motivate behavior are usually seen as resulting from a deficit in some basic physiological, psychological, or social need. This traditional behavioristic model is retained in Figure 5 because reinforcing and punishing contingencies do indeed shape behavior, including the behavior of workers within organizations (Braithwaite, 1985; Cole, 1995). Persons also act out of deficit needs, because they have too little of something they need or want. As many scholars have noted, however, people's behavior and learning are also motivated by many other types of needs, including growth, learning for the sake of learning, self-efficacy, and a sense of mastery, competency, and agency in a complex world (Bandura, 1989; Bruner, 1966; Maslow, 1970; White, 1959).

The second box from the left in Figure 5

recognizes that much human behavior and most decisions are driven by attitudes, intention, goals, and strategies (Halpern, 1984; Lave & Wenger, 1994; Mayer, 1992). Expertise in problem solving and decision making is grounded in a huge store of well-organized knowledge, a great deal of experience, a passion for one's work, and sets of sophisticated strategies. Much strategic thinking includes recognizing in complex real-world situations a coherent pattern (story plot or scenario) as it is developing or may be developed more to one's liking or intentions (Ericsson & Smith, 1994; Halpern, 1984; Mayer, 1992). This perspective is present in the model in Figure 5 because wisdom and expertise in occupational safety and health depend to a high degree on workers' and managers' strategic knowledge that helps them to recognize and prevent problems in proactive rather than reactive ways.

The extreme left-hand box represents the constructs of narrative representation that have been discussed previously. The right-pointing arrows between the boxes depict how culture tales influence the cognitive and behavioral components of human conduct. The upward-pointing arrows below the four boxes in the diagram depict the feedback loops that illustrate the influence of consequences not only on behavior, but also on cognition, and on the narratives that people construct to make meaning from their experiences.

The Model in Action: An Illustration. In keeping with the theme of this chapter, a true story can illustrate the points made thus far to help the reader better comprehend the storied nature of health beliefs and safety behavior as depicted in Figure 5.

On a cold winter day, my daughter-in-law, Tammy, called me. She said Justin, my two-year-old grandson, had burned the palm of his right hand and they had to take him to a hospital emergency department. I asked for more details. She explained that Justin was in the garage with his dad, David. David shut off the kerosene space heater that he had been using to heat the garage.

He and Justin started to leave. Suddenly, Justin ran back to the heater and placed the palm of his right hand directly on the heater's stove top. He screamed and drew back his hand. David immediately dunked Justin's hand into a pail of cold water that was handy. Large blisters soon formed on Justin's palm. Justin's parents gently wrapped his hand in a clean, soft towel, comforted him, and took him to the hospital. There a doctor examined Justin's hand, told his parents it was a second degree burn and that there should be no permanent damage, dressed the burn, and sent them home.

Two days later, Justin and his mom and dad came to my home. Justin ran into the house ahead of his parents, waving his bandaged right hand and saying, "Grandpa! Boo boo! Boo boo!"

I asked, "What happened?"

Justin replied, "Me, Daddy in garage. Daddy stove off! Me touch stove! Boo boo! Boo boo! Go doctor! Better now!"

I asked, "Why did you touch the stove?"

Justin replied, "Other time Daddy stove off, me touch. No hurt!"

I asked, "What happened this time?"

Justin said, "Daddy stove off. Stove hot! Me touch. Make boo boo!"

Justin lived this story, as did his parents. Both parents and Justin told the story to my wife, to me, and to others. I have since heard Justin (who is now four years old) tell others this story, including his younger sister. When he sees the heater, or some similar hot object, he tells his little sister, "Don't touch!," and he often relates the story of his experience. Through this experience, hearing his parents tell the story, and his telling of the story, Justin constructed a meaningful and memorable narrative that he will likely always remember. It is also a coherent narrative by which he abstracted and generalized principles that help him avoid and prevent a similar injury from the heater and other hot objects such as soldering irons, stoves, and toasters.

In the framework of traditional American behaviorism, Justin's injury event contributed to his learning of a specific behavior (don't touch the stove) because of a specific behavioral contingency (a painful burn). His participation in the social activity of constructing and reliving a meaningful story about the event also contributed to a deeper understanding of the physical and social principles involved. Through his narrative meaning making, Justin learned that stoves and other hot objects retain heat after they are "turned off"; that the burn was not intentional on the part of himself, the stove, or his dad, but was an "accident"; that when he is injured his parents become upset, and that he must go to the hospital where other people help him. He learned to respect the stove, but not to fear it. He also learned to feel responsible for protecting himself, his little sister, and others from similar harm. These lessons learned are part of his socialization to be a responsible and safety-conscious member of his family and community. His learning of this complex array of concepts, attitudes, knowledge, beliefs, goals, and intentions can be understood much more adequately by the entire model depicted in Figure 5 than by only the behavioral or the cognitive components. The same argument can be made for the socialization of adult workers to injury prevention attitudes, plans, decision, and actions.

Even adults who are highly skilled in formal methods of analytical thinking tend to speak mainly in terms of narrative when asked to state abstract principles about themselves, their plans, and their accomplishments. Baumeister and Newman (1994) tell an anecdote about a researcher who asked successful businesspeople to explain how they had achieved success. The researcher expected these leaders to respond with generalizations. Instead, he was frustrated when they responded with stories about particular meaningful events in their lives, not with abstractions. The stories these people told were the means by which they ordered, understood, preserved, and communicated information. Studies with thousands of miners and other workers show a similar pattern. When workers are asked about health and safety, they tend to respond, *not* in terms of abstract rules and generalizations that

are common to the Code of Federal Regulations and the language of formal accident investigations, but with specific stories about themselves, their coworkers, and their jobs. Yet, as noted previously, most of their safety and health instruction focuses on the didactic presentation of just such health and safety rules and generalizations.

PROBLEM POSING AND EMPOWERMENT

Freire (1990) developed effective literacy programs that helped Brazilian slum dwellers gain more control over their personal and community lives. His primary method involved first selecting emotionally and socially charged statements, pictures, and issues relevant to the group and presenting these elements as "triggers" for problem-solving tasks. For example, a picture might show children and adults carrying drinking water away from a polluted stream. A caption beneath the picture might say, "Our people are becoming ill from drinking polluted water." He would then listen as people related their stories and experiences with this problem. Then he would encourage dialogue among the community members about the problem, with the "trigger" serving as a focus or lens for peoples' emotions, fears, anger, wishes, and knowledge related to this problem. The empowerment dialogue fosters critical thinking about societal forces, various persons' roles in shaping the quality of individual and community life, and ways to promote change to improve both individual and community life. The empowerment dialogue leads to community members' planning and taking action to improve specific aspects of their lives as they are able to do so within their resources. The initial action is often begun through role play and simulated interactions of community members and other "gatekeepers" inside and outside the community whose perceptions and policies influence the quality of life in the community. This method has become known by a number of names, but especially as "empowerment through problem-posing."

Empowerment in Health and Safety Education. Freire's principles of empowerment through problem-posing triggers and dialogue have been applied to occupational health and safety education, although the method is neither widely appreciated nor embraced by many persons who plan and conduct such training (Wallerstein, 1992; Wallerstein & Bernstein, 1988; Wallerstein & Weinger, 1992). The purpose is to empower workers to better understand the meaning of their own plights and experience and to become more proactive in improving health and safety for themselves and their community of workers.

Wallerstein (1992) reviews a long history of social epidemiology that suggest that when people become more empowered socially and economically, they also become healthier and suffer fewer illnesses and injuries, especially those related to their occupations. She also notes that increased self-efficacy (Bandura, 1989) leads not only to a stronger sense of agency and improvement in the general quality of life, but also to increased proactive identification and elimination of hazards that result in occupational injuries. This result cannot be achieved on an individual basis, but requires social problem solving by communities of workers.

Speaking specifically about the context of health and safety, Wallerstein and Weinger (1992, p. 624) state that:

> ... an educator has many roles: to listen carefully and encourage an environment of trust so that people will share their personal stories and begin to perceive that they are not isolated and alone; to ask questions about how and why these stories fit into the social or organizational context (one of the hardest parts of the dialogue); to synthesize key moments of understanding so that people recognize their learning of new knowledge or their identification of new important themes to pursue; to present information as questions arise that will further the understandings of the health and safety situation, and to urge the group to consider strategies for addressing the problem.

Following the empowerment dialogue in the classroom (p. 621):

> Educators can best support worker actions by working within their organizations to develop institutional structures which can respond to issues identified during the training.

Through this social problem solving, workers and managers are empowered to recognize, eliminate, or control specific occupational hazards that threaten their well-being (Wallerstein, 1992; Wallerstein & Bernstein, 1988; Wallerstein & Weinger, 1992). Wallerstein (1992) also notes that few health and safety instructors know how to teach by this method.

The Exercises, Problem Posing, and Empowerment. The BRASH simulation exercises are problem-posing tasks designed to empower workers and managers. Each exercise begins with a trigger, a situation, a picture, or a predicament that is particularly relevant and emotively arousing to the workers. The simulations are most effective when worked cooperatively by small groups of people. This cooperation provides opportunity for individuals to learn from one another and encourages teamwork in preventing and responding to real-life emergency situations.

The exercises nearly always stimulate a great deal of earnest and passionate dialogue as the individual small groups, and later the whole class and the instructor, discuss and debate the merits of particular actions and the many issues that underlie the development and the prevention of the hazards and injury events depicted. The discussion frequently leads to actions by workers, company instructors, and management involving the recognition and correction of specific conditions or problems.

Empowerment in Action. I was once working with the training staff of a large underground coal mining operation. The company allowed me to field-test, with its entire workforce, a new simulation exercise. During the two days I was present, the simulation exercise was to be administered to 12 different classes of 25 miners each as one part of their annual health and safety refresher training. The company managers and trainers had selected this exercise because it is based on a case that occurred in a setting similar to their mining operation. At 6:30 a.m. on the morning of the second day, the company trainer, who was to conduct the 6 classes with the exercise, was called away by a family medical emergency. Because no one else was available to teach the classes, I was drafted.

The exercise proved to be engaging and productive in terms of the ideas, dialogue, and insights it stimulated among the miners. The simulation problem is about a fire that developed in a large underground coal mine. Two miners became trapped at the mine face (the wall from which the coal is cut as the mine advances). Other people elsewhere in the mine did not know about the fire. One of the trapped miners escaped by donning his emergency breathing apparatus that is usually carried on the belt. His buddy, who had left his breathing device elsewhere, could not travel through the heavy smoke and had to remain in the relatively clear air at the face, but knew this air would soon go bad. On the way out, the first miner found the source of the fire. A maintenance worker had been splicing an electrical cable on a piece of equipment. A rock had fallen from the mine roof, striking the worker in the head and knocking him unconscious. The burning propane torch had started the coal of the mine rib (wall) on fire, and the mine ventilation was fanning the fire. The exercise continues with the miner who escaped making decisions about what to do first (e.g., fight the fire, give first aid to the unconscious miner, try to rescue his friend, or go for help). The predicament is that if he tries to do all these things by himself, he may fail. The fire may burn out of control. His friend and the injured miner may die. Other miners elsewhere in the mine may become trapped. The situation may become much worse.

Every class went well, even though I did not know the miners and they did not know me. The

last class of the day at 10:30 p.m. included a 15-person mine maintenance crew. They liked the exercise and very quickly adopted the appropriate roles and got into the exercise scenario with much enthusiasm and vigorous dialogue. Toward the end of the class, one man (who I later learned was the mine superintendent) stated: "The maintenance worker had no business using an open flame to make repairs near the face!," to which one of the other men said, "Why not! As long as you make a gas check [for methane] and have good ventilation, the law allows the use of an open flame near the face."

The superintendent said, "You had better not be doing this! We don't do this in this outfit! That's why we have cold-splice kits!" (The kits allow electrical cable repairs without flame.)

The second man and several of his colleagues then shouted that they hadn't seen a cold-splice kit in three years, that they had repeatedly asked for the kits and been told there weren't any available. A loud argument followed. The argument was resolved when the superintendent and a maintenance crew worker agreed to go to the supply room and check on the situation. A short time later, both men returned. The superintendent apologized and said that the men were correct. No cold-splice kits had been available for a long time and none had been ordered, but this foul-up was being corrected. A spirited, but productive, discussion followed about how to avoid miscommunication problems like the one just encountered. The author and his colleagues have observed and heard about many similar actions that have been undertaken following the identification and discussion of an issue or problem during a company training class that used one of the simulation exercises.

THE EXERCISES AS DEVICES FOR ASSESSING KNOWLEDGE AND RISK

The narrative exercises described in this chapter are intended primarily as teaching materials. Because they yield performance scores, however, the exercises can measure persons' knowledge, attitudes, and the presence of misconceptions. Portions of the exercises can also elicit information from persons about the frequency with which they have been exposed to hazards similar to those depicted in the exercises. Some exercises also are designed to elicit workers' recollection and reporting of their personal near-injury events (close calls) and actual injuries. These recollections and the discussions of them help workers to apply the information learned from the exercise to their own workplace circumstances to reduce risk of occupational injury and illness. The performance and injury-exposure data gathered by the exercises can be aggregated across samples of workers. Patterns of decision responses, misconceptions, exposures to hazardous agents and conditions, and close calls can be noted. These data can then be used by policy makers and educators to target the identified problem areas for further interventions to reduce injuries. These aspects of the exercises are illustrated with an example from mining and a second example from agriculture.

Misconceptions and Mine Explosions. Coal mines are frequently developed as large sets of independently ventilated entries (tunnels) that are later connected to form what is known as a "retreating longwall." The longwall is a 1200-foot face along which a large machine travels back and forth shearing coal from across its entire width. Moving back and forth, and retreating toward the outside, this longwall mining machine eventually removes all the coal from a horizontal block that is approximately 5000 feet long and 1200 feet wide. The block of coal that is being mined is bounded on both sides by a set of entries (tunnels). One set of entries delivers a constant and large volume of fresh air to the face to dilute and sweep out the explosive mixture of coal dust and methane gas that is often present. After the fresh air sweeps across the face, the other set of entries rapidly carry the contaminated air, with its accumulated methane and dust, out of the mine. The entries also provide access for miners and equipment to travel to and from the longwall and the means to remove the coal from the mine by a large conveyor-belt system.

Before the longwall is established, the entries on each side are independently ventilated. Once the longwall is in operation, the ventilation systems for both sets of entries and the longwall are connected. At this point, the mine ventilation system becomes much more complex, as tens of miles of entries and connections between them are included in one vast ventilation circuit. The size and dynamics of the ventilation system are so complex that it is easy to make conceptual and operational errors that result in poor ventilation of some areas of the mine. Such errors can result in the accumulation of an explosive mixture of methane and air. In the last decade, there have been at least four mine disasters in which these types of errors resulted in massive methane explosions and the loss of many lives (Passaro et al., 1994).

The official disaster investigation reports were obtained for four mine explosions. The mine layout and ventilation systems were modeled by a computer program with a graphic interface. This setup allowed the miners who worked the simulation to see the entries (tunnels) and their connections, measure air flow and methane content, and make adjustments to the ventilation system just as they would do in real life. In short, the computer simulation re-created the circumstances and the decision making that faced the miners who were killed in the actual mine explosions (Wala & Cole, 1987). The computer simulation problem was later converted to a latent-image paper-and-pencil simulation exercise that depicted as an interactive story the developing problems and major decision points of one of the mines.

Both the computer and the latent-image exercise were administered to a few hundred mining engineers, mine foremen, and mine superintendents from five states. These mine personnel are responsible for monitoring and diagnosing ventilation problems and for making changes in the ventilation arrangements to prevent methane explosions. The exercise performance scores from these mine workers revealed that 70% of the sample held a specific set of misconceptions about airflow and airflow measurements when two previously independent circuits are connected to form one much larger ventilation system. In short, the majority of persons who worked the simulation exercise made the same errors at key decision points as did the miners who were involved in the actual explosions (Passaro et al., 1994; Wala & Cole, 1987).

Subsequently, one large company with coal mines throughout the United States and in other countries sent all of its general mine foremen, mine superintendents, and key mining engineers to a workshop in which the Cut-through Mine Ventilation Arrangements latent-image exercise (*Catalog of training products*, 1993, p. 54) was presented by Wala and Cole at a half-day training session. These company leaders then returned home and trained other key persons with the exercise. This pattern was repeated by many other mining companies. The point to be made is that the performance data collected during field tests of the training exercise identified the presence of a dangerous misconception, made this misconception immediately apparent to the persons who worked the exercise, and stimulated their subsequent thinking and action to avoid making these types of potentially disastrous errors in the future in the mines where they worked.

Misconceptions about Avoiding Tractor-Overturn Injuries. Farm work is a major cause of morbidity and mortality among children in the United States. Fatality rates among farm children are 13.7 per 100,000 for 10- to 14-year-olds and 16.8 per 100,000 for 15- to 19-year olds. Injury rates for these same groups are 102 and 154 per 100,000, respectively (Committee on Environmental Health, 1995). Machinery injuries are the leading cause of farm deaths (McKnight & Hetzel, 1985). On the basis of a study of 31 states, Murphy (1992) estimated that approximately 33% of all farm fatalities are related to tractors.

Focus group interviews with 48 farm youths from eight central Kentucky farming counties, and with groups of parents from these countries, revealed that they held a number of misconceptions about tractor overturns and about ways in which an injury could be prevented during such an event. The focus group data also revealed a very high rate of tractor driving at an early age by farm youths (Kidd et al., 1993). Subsequently, an interactive story was developed to promote farm youths' and adults' knowledge, attitudes, and self-protective behavior to reduce risk of injury from tractor-rollover events (Cole et al., 1995). The exercise was field-tested to determine its utility as a knowledge and attitude assessment device and as a training method for farm youths and farm family members. An attached questionnaire was designed to gather demographic, exposure, and safety behavior data with respect to farm tractor operation.

In the tradition of "problem-posing and empowerment" education, the exercise begins with a story called "Tommy's Troubles" and a picture. The story is about a 14-year-old boy and a family decision to let him help his overworked dad by performing a dangerous and difficult task, the "bush hog" mowing of six-foot-tall weeds and brush in a pasture. The task involves using a powerful rotary mower pulled behind the tractor to cut and shred the weeds and brush. Although an experienced tractor driver, the son has never before operated the "bush hog" in such tall weeds, which make it difficult to see hazards such as large rocks, holes, or other objects that can upset the tractor. The tractor is equipped with a roll-over-protection structure (ROPS) (a roll bar) and a seat belt. The first illustration shows Tommy heading into the pasture with the weeds as tall as the tractor. The first question asks persons to identify the hazards faced by Tommy as he works unsupervised at this task. As the problem develops, the mower plugs up. Tommy frequently has to shut down the mower, get off the tractor, and clean out the brush. The tractor seat belt is greasy and dirty. Another decision point is whether Tommy would or would not wear the belt. It is noted that his dad never wears

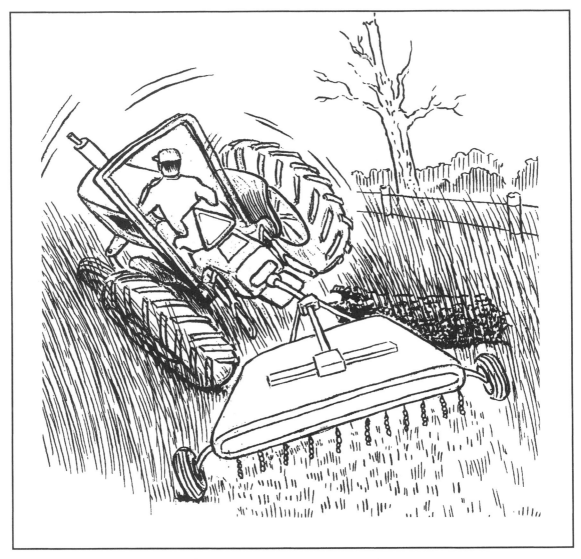

Figure 6. "Trigger" drawing of an overturning farm tractor.

the seat belt, but always admonishes his wife and son to do so.

Figure 6 shows the second graphic "trigger" in the exercise. Under time pressure to complete the task, Tommy increases the speed of the tractor. Suddenly, the right-side wheels of the tractor run up on the stump end of a log that was concealed in the weeds. The picture shows the trac-

tor rolling over to the left. The question posed at this point is, "What can Tommy do to prevent a rollover and keep from being hurt?" The alternatives include: jumping from the tractor before it overturns, pushing in the clutch, shifting his weight to the right, turning the front wheels to the left, and finally the statement, "There is nothing he can do now." Only the last answer is correct. All the other answers are common misconceptions that emerged in discussions and focus group interviews with farm youths and adults. The questions that follow ask what people think would happen to Tommy if he is or is not wearing his seat belt, the nature and severity of any injuries he might sustain, and who else in the family and community will share Tommy's troubles and why. The remainder of the exercise invites farm youths and parents to examine their own risk factors for and exposure to similar injuries and to think about ways to reduce these risks while performing similar chores on their farms.

The exercise was field-tested with 88 youths and 64 adult farm workers. The average age of the youths was 16.1 years (SD = 1.50) and the average age of the adults 37.2 years (SD = 9.93). The youth sample averaged 7.1 years of tractor-driving experience and the adults 22.3 years. In addition to using the exercise as a teaching device, the performance and exposure data were collected and analyzed. Figure 7 plots the frequency of misconceptions related to escaping injury during an ongoing tractor rollover event. The data revealed that the misconceptions were widespread in the adult and youth samples. Significantly more of the youths than of the adults thought they could escape injury by jumping from the over-

turning tractor (a physical impossibility). Otherwise, the pattern of misconceptions was nearly identical. Working the exercise helped farm youths and family members examine these misconceptions and their danger. In the context of the exercise, injury surveillance data about tractor overturns were presented and discussed. In subsequent administrations, field-test data collected from farm community members, like those in Figures 7 and 8, were examined and discussed as part of the exercise.

Figure 8 plots the frequency of near-injury events related to tractors and tractor rollovers as experienced and reported by the sample of 88 youths and 64 adult workers. Data from a short behavioral-practices and risk-exposure questionnaire that accompanies the exercise revealed that only about 9% of the adults and the youths in the field-test sample routinely wore the seat belt when operating a ROPS-equipped tractor, perhaps in part because of their misconceptions about being able to escape injury from an overturning tractor. In the safety of a classroom or community group meeting, farm youths and family members became engaged in the social activity of working through an engaging simulation problem that was situated in their culture, their language, and their everyday experience and

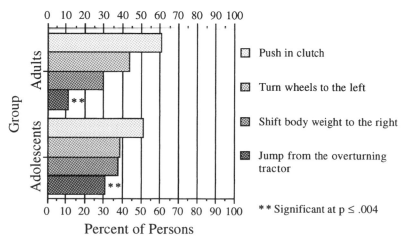

Figure 7. Frequency of misconceptions about preventing injuries during a tractor rollover event.

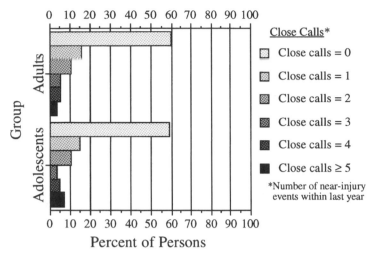

Figure 8. Frequency and distribution of reported tractor-related near-injury events.

concerns. The problem presented empirical information about risk factors, exposure, and effective prevention strategies within the context of a meaningful and memorable "culture tale." The empowerment portions of the exercise invited farm family members to examine their own thinking and behavior toward preventing similar injury events and the many associated troubles that always follow such events.

EVALUATION AND EFFECTIVENESS

In addition to their narrative structure and problem-posing characteristics, the effectiveness of the simulation exercises is based on four additional factors: (1) their practical nature and content, which respects adults' learning styles (Cole et al., 1984); (2) their development, field-testing, and dissemination in collaboration with extensive networks of workers from the target populations and those agencies and persons who provide services and support for these worker groups (Cole, 1993; Cole, Mallett, et al., 1988); (3) equipping leaders, trainers, and instructors in these groups with guides and materials that make it easy for them to use the exercises (Cole, 1993);

and (4) evaluating the exercises by collecting and analyzing data about their effectiveness (Cole, 1993, 1994; Cole et al., 1993).

Evaluation Procedures. Four types of data are routinely collected from the exercises administrations: (1) what workers think about the exercises, (2) what instructors think about the exercises, (3) the performance scores of the workers on the exercises, and (4) demographic characteristics, risk factors, and exposure patterns of the persons who complete the exercises.

The mining exercises were field-tested with a sample of 3658 miners from 14 states. These miners rated the authenticity and worth of each exercise on a number of dimensions. These data were collected and examined for each individual exercise and also pooled across exercises and miners. More than 95% of the miners agreed that the exercises deal with realistic problems that will help them to remember critical information and strategies to prevent or cope with similar mine emergencies and injury events. A sample of 181 instructors who taught these miners were also asked to rate the authenticity and worth of the exercises. More than 99% of the instructors judged the exercises to have appropriate content and objectives for miners' health and safety annual refresher training. Nearly 99% of the instructors wanted additional simulation exercises to use in the future. Approximately 98% of the instructors reported using the exercises in the problem-solving and participatory-learning manner for which they were designed. They also reported that the exercises provided them with new ways of approaching instruction and made their teaching more effective (Cole, 1993; Cole, Mallett, et al., 1988). Similar patterns were found for the exercises developed for surface mine inspectors, hazardous-waste workers, farmers, other groups, and instructors for these groups.

As illustrated previously, performance data are routinely collected for each exercise. These data serve a number of functions, including identifying misconceptions and problematic attitudes that place workers at risk. With these data in hand, additional exercises and other interventions can be developed to address specific problems. The performance data also provide the means by which to calculate the psychometric properties of the exercises as assessment devices. These properties include the reliability of the exercise, item (question) difficulty levels, and the mastery level of critical knowledge and skills attained by the workers in the sample. These data are used to improve exercises and to ensure that they are well designed, reliable, and valid (Cole et al., 1984).

Validity. The validity of the exercises is determined in several ways, including judgments of face validity by experts, the degree to which individual workers' decision alternatives discriminate significantly among persons with high and low total scores on a given exercise, and the ability of the exercise total score to discriminate significantly between groups with high versus low levels of expertise in exercise content. These types of analyses are carried out for each exercise as it is developed, field-tested, and revised. Sometimes exercise performance data are pooled across exercises as a means of assessing their overall effectiveness.

For example, for the mining simulation exercises, it was hypothesized that the more highly trained, experienced, and specially certified mine supervisors and technical personnel would score significantly higher than working miners, who generally have less special training in the non-routine skills that are the focus of the exercises. The performance data were analyzed for 30 exercises with 10 exercises assigned to each of three content areas. Content areas included mine technical training (MTT), first aid training (FAT), and mixture (MIX) problems. The MIX exercises contain both mine technical and first aid training content. Performance data from 2246 miners were converted to standard scores for these exercises. The mean performance scores of supervisors, mine technical personnel, and regular working miners were compared by analysis of variance. Statistically significant differences ($p \le 0.001$) in performance scores were found among these three groups of mine workers in the expected direction for all three categories of exercises. Figure 9 plots these mean standard scores by exercise content type and job category. These and other results reported in the project final report suggested that the simulation exercises

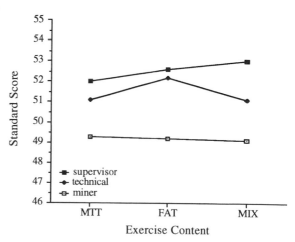

Figure 9. Mean performance scores by job category for 2248 miners on 30 exercises.

are valid (Cole et al., 1993; Cole, Mallett, et al., 1988).

CONCLUSION

The application of the underlying theory, design methods, and effectiveness of narrative-based problem-solving exercises is one method by which to promote increased awareness of hazards and risk factors while also promoting strategic thinking to eliminate injury agents and events. This claim is supported by the field-test results of the mine fire exercise described in this chapter and by similar work completed with many other groups of workers. The problem-solving exercises are also useful measures for assessing existing levels of knowledge, attitudes, and practice in at-risk populations. Data aggregated from exercises administered to large samples of workers can identify attitudes, beliefs, misconceptions, and other variables that place persons at risk. Community interventions can then be designed to inform and influence attitudes and knowledge to reduce exposure to specific injury events from specific agents and environments.

A body of previous research and theoretical literature identifies criteria for the effectiveness of these types of narrative problem-solving exercises. First, they must be accurate with respect to epidemiology and injury surveillance data that define injury events in terms of agents, hosts, environments, the exposure of workers to injury agents, and the frequency and severity of injury events. Second, the exercise narrative must be authentic with respect to the lives, culture, plights, and language of the populations for whom the materials are designed. Third, the exercises should be viewed, designed, and analyzed, not only as educational interventions, but also as reliable and valid tools for assessing attitudes, knowledge, and concepts. Fourth, such materials are most effective when they are used in small groups of persons engaged in collaborative learning and problem solving.

The research and development activity reported in this chapter has had a major impact upon miner health and safety training in the United States and is beginning to have a similar impact upon workers in other occupations. The exercises, and their associated instructor manuals, facilitate teaching and learning through group problem posing and solving. Instructors previously unfamiliar with this approach have learned new ways to teach. Using these narrative simulation exercises, many "train the trainer" workshops have been conducted by BRASH staff, the USBM, the MSHA, and other groups to strengthen the teaching and materials-development skills of hundreds of health and safety instructors from many companies and agencies.

The primary purpose of the simulation exercises is to educate and empower workers and managers to recognize and remove risk factors for occupational illness and injury. The simulation exercises also have potential, however, for program evaluation and policy analysis. During the course of field-testing more than 100 exercises in a wide variety of occupations, much has been learned about the problem-solving skills in which particular groups of workers excel, the skills in which they need more practice, the existence of problematic misconceptions, and the areas in which their ability to perform well is limited by current work practices, equipment design, and availability. The performance data gathered by these and similar exercises can help health and safety professionals to plan and organize future educational intervention activities, as well as to make improvements in work organization, engineering, ergonomics, and enforcement.

ACKNOWLEDGMENTS. Work reported in the chapter was supported by U.S. Bureau of Mines Contract Nos. H0348040, PO 3303440, PO 315477, and PO 325473, NIEHS Contract No. 5 D42 ES 07200-04, and NIOSH Contract Nos. 0009139152, 0009137562, and 0009236852 to the BRASH Working Group, and by NIOSH/CDC Cooperative Agreement No. U07/CCU408035 to the University of Kentucky, Southeast Center for Agricultural Health and Injury Prevention. The author gratefully acknowledges additional grants and contracts from other agencies that also contributed to the work reported, including the National Science Foundation, the American Society of Engineering Education, the Mine Safety and Health Administration, the Kentucky Department of Surface Mining Reclamation and Enforcement, the Office of Surface Mining, the Agency for Toxic Substance Disease Registry, and the Kentucky Department of Health and Human Resources. The assistance of many colleagues within these agencies, the University of Kentucky, other colleges and universities, labor organizations, businesses, and professional organizations is also gratefully acknowledged. Without the help of these many persons, the work reported could not have been conceptualized and completed.

DISCLAIMER. The views and conclusions in this chapter are those of the author and should not be interpreted as necessarily representing the official policies or recommendations of the agencies that supported the work.

REFERENCES

Bandura, A. (1989). Human agency in social cognitive theory. *American Psychologist, 44*, 1175–1184.

Baumeister, R. F., & Newman, L. S. (1994). How stories make sense of personal experiences: Motives that shape autobiographical narratives. *Personality and Social Psychology Bulletin, 20*, 676–690.

Bonnet, A. (1985). *Artificial intelligence: Promise and performance*. Englewood Cliffs, NJ: Prentice-Hall.

Bower, G. H., & Morrow, D. (1990). Mental models in narrative comprehension. *Science, 247*, 44–48.

Braithwaite, J. (1985). *To punish or persuade: Enforcement of coal mine safety*. Albany: State University of New York Press.

Brener, E. S. (1984). Paradigms and problem solving: A literature review. *Journal of Medical Education, 59*, 625–633.

Brown, J. S., Collins, A., & Duguid, P. (1989). Situated cognition and the culture of learning. *Educational Researcher, 18*(1), 32–42.

Bruner, J. S. (1966). *Toward a theory of instruction*. Cambridge, MA: Harvard University Press.

Bruner, J. S. (1986). *Actual minds, possible worlds*. Cambridge, MA: Harvard University Press.

Bruner, J. S. (1990a). *Acts of meaning*. Cambridge, MA: Harvard University Press.

Bruner, J. S. (1990b). Culture and human development: A new look. *Human Development, 33*, 344–355.

Carter, K. (1993). The place of story in the study of teaching and teacher education. *Educational Researcher, 22*(1), 5–12, 18.

Catalog of training products for the mining industry. (1933). Beckley, WV: National Mine Health and Safety Academy.

Cole, H. P. (1993). Developing practical and effective health and safety training for the mining workplace. In P. B. Gilroy (Ed.), *Proceedings of MINESAFE INTERNATIONAL, 1993: An international conference on occupational health and safety in the minerals industry* (pp. 47–64). Perth: Chamber of Mines and Energy of Western Australia.

Cole, H. P. (1994). Embedded performance measures as teaching and assessment devices. *Occupational medicine: State of the art reviews, 9*(2), 261–281. Philadelphia: Hanley & Belfus.

Cole, H. P. (1995, June). *Factors that contribute to some miners committing unsafe acts: A behavioral analysis.* Invited paper presented at the 85th annual convention of the Mine Inspectors' Institute of America, Davis, WV.

Cole, H. P., Garrity, T. F., & Berger, P. K. (1988). Analogs between medical and industrial safety research on compliance behavior. In D. S. Gochman (Ed.), *Health behavior: Emerging research perspectives* (pp. 337–353). New York: Plenum Press.

Cole, H. P., Lineberry, G. T., Wala, A. M., Haley, J. V., Berger, P. K., & Wasielewski, R. D. (1993). Simulation exercises for training and educating miners and mining engineers. *Mining Engineering, 44*, 1397–1401.

Cole, H. P., Mallett, L. G., Haley, J. V., Berger, P. K., Lacefield, W. E., Wasielewski, R. D., Lineberry, G. T., & Wala, A. M. (1988). *Research and evaluation methods for measuring nonroutine mine health and safety skills.* Bureau of Mines Contract No. HO348040 Final Report. Volume 1 (NTIS No. P889-196646/HOM); Volume 2 (NTIS No. P889-196653/HOM). Pittsburgh, PA: U.S. Department of the Interior.

Cole, H. P., McKnight, R. H., Piercy, L. H., & McLymore, R. L. (1995, March). *Interactive narrative and self-protective behavior from tractor roll overs.* Paper presented at the Second National Conference for NIOSH-sponsored Agricultural Health and Safety Centers, Fort Collins, CO.

Cole, H. P., Moss, J., Gohs, F. X., Lacefield, W. E., Barfield, B. J., & Blythe, D. K. (1984). *Measuring learning in continuing education for engineers and scientists*. Phoenix, AZ: Oryx Press.

Cole, H. P., Rubeck, R. F., Lin, B. C., Taylor, R., Lineberry, G. T., Frank, A. L., Wala, A. M., & Haley, J. V. (1992). *Four interactive computer administered problem-solving simulations for teaching critical health and safety skills to mining industry workers.* Bureau of Mines, Mining and Minerals Institute, Title III, Grant No. G-1114121 Final Report. Lexington, KY: Institute for Mining and Minerals Research.

Cole, H. P., Wasielewski, R. D., Haley, J. V., & Berger, P. K. (1988). First aid role play simulations for miners. *Mine*

Safety Education and Training Seminar (Bureau of Mines IC 9185) (pp. 78–124). Library of Congress Catalog No. TN 295.U4. Pittsburgh, PA: U.S. Department of the Interior.

Committee on Environmental Health. (1995). The hazards of child labor. *Pediatrics*, *95*, 311–313.

Committee on Underground Coal Mine Safety. (1982). *Toward safer underground coal mines*. New York: National Academy Press.

Connelly, F. M., & Clandinin, D. J. (1990). Stories of experience and narrative inquiry. *Educational Researcher*, *19* (5), 2–14.

Crites, S. (1986). Storytime: Recollecting the past and projecting the future. In T. R. Sarbin (Ed.), *Narrative psychology: The storied nature of human conduct* (pp. 152–173). New York: Praeger.

Digman, R. M., & Grasso, J. T. (1981). *An observational study of classroom health and safety training in coal mining*. Bureau of Mines Contract No. JO188069 Final Report. Pittsburgh, PA: U.S. Department of the Interior.

Ericsson, K. A., & Smith, J. (1994). *Toward a general theory of expertise: Prospects and limits*. New York: Cambridge University Press.

Fischoff, B. (1975). Hindsight ≠ foresight: The effect of outcome knowledge on judgment under uncertainty. *Journal of Experimental Psychology: Human Perception and Performance*, *1*, 288–299.

Freire, P. (1990). *Pedagogy of the oppressed* (32nd printing). New York: Continuum.

Gerrig, R. J. (1994). Narrative thought? *Personality and Social Psychology Bulletin*, *20*, 712–715.

Gonzales, M. H., Haugen, J. A., & Manning, D. J. (1994). Victims as "narrative critics": Factors influencing rejoinders and evaluative responses to offenders' accounts. *Personality and Social Psychology Bulletin*, *20*, 691–704.

Giffin, W. C., & Rockwell, T. H. (1984). Computer-aided testing of pilot response to critical in-flight events. *Human Factors*, *26*, 573–581.

Haliff, H. M., Hollan, J. D., & Hutchins, E. L. (1986). Cognitive science and military training. *American Psychologist*, *41*, 1131–1139.

Halpern, D. F. (1984). *Thought and knowledge: An introduction to critical thinking*. Hillsdale, NJ: Erlbaum.

Hermans, H. J. M. (1992). Telling and retelling one's self-narrative: A contextual approach to life-span development. *Human Development*, *35*, 361–375.

Holland, T. P., & Kilpatrick, A. C. (1993). Using narrative techniques to enhance multicultural practice. *Journal of Social Work Education*, *29*, 302–308.

Howard, G. S. (1991). Culture tales: A narrative approach to cross-cultural psychology and psychotherapy. *American Psychologist*, *46*, 187–197.

Irwin, C. E., Jr., Cataldo, M. F., Matheny, A. P., & Peterson, L. (1992). Health consequences of behaviors: Injury as a model. *Pediatrics*, *90*, 798–807.

Jones, K. (1980). *Simulations: A handbook for teachers*. London: Kogan Page.

Josselson, R., & Lieblich, A. (Eds.). (1993). *The narrative study of lives*. Newbury Park, CA: Sage.

Kidd, P., Townley, K., Huddleston, S., McKnight, R., Cole, H., & Piercy, L. (1993, October). *Youth perceptions of risk in the farm environment*. Paper presented at the American Public Health Association 121st Annual Meeting, San Francisco.

Komaki, J., Barwick, K. D., & Scott, L. R. (1978). A behavioral approach to occupational safety: Pinpointing and reinforcing safe performance in a food manufacturing plant. *Journal of Applied Psychology*, *63*, 434–445.

Lave, J., & Wenger, E. (1994). *Situated learning: Legitimate peripheral participation*. New York: Cambridge University Press.

Maslow, A. H. (1970). *Motivation and personality* (2nd ed.). New York: Harper & Row.

Mayer, R. E. (1992). *Thinking, problem solving, cognition* (2nd ed.). New York: W. H. Freeman.

McKnight, R. H., & Hetzel, G. H. (1985). Trends in farm machinery fatalities. *Agricultural Engineering*, *55*, 15–17.

Mishler, E. G. (1986). The analysis of interview-narratives. In T. R. Sarbin (Ed.), *Narrative psychology: The storied nature of human conduct* (pp. 233–255). New York: Praeger.

Murphy, D. J. (1992). *Safety and health for production agriculture*. St. Joseph, MI: American Society of Agricultural Engineers.

Murphy, S. L., & Holmes, J. G. (1994). Storytelling in close relationships: The construction of confidence. *Personality and Social Psychology Bulletin*, *20*, 650–663.

Passaro, P. D. (1989). *Miners' misconceptions of flow distribution changes within circuits as a causal factor in underground mining accidents*. Unpublished doctoral dissertation. University of Kentucky, Lexington.

Passaro, P. D., Cole, H. P., & Wala, A. M. (1994). Flow distribution changes in complex circuits: Implications for mine explosions. *Human Factors*, *36*, 745–756.

Peters, R. H., & Wiehagen, W. J. (1988). Human factors contributing to groundfall accidents in underground coal mines. *Mine Safety Education and Training Seminar* (Bureau of Mines IC 9185) (pp. 31–39). Pittsburgh, PA: U.S. Department of the Interior.

Phillips, D. C. (1994). Telling it straight: Issues in assessing narrative research. *Educational Psychologist*, *29*, 13–21.

Resnick, L. B. (1987). Learning in school and out. *Educational Researcher*, *16*, 13–20.

Robinson, J. A., & Hawpe, L. (1986). Narrative thinking as a heuristic process. In T. R. Sarbin (Ed.), *Narrative psychology: The storied nature of human conduct* (pp. 111–125). New York: Praeger.

Rosenthal, G. (1993). Reconstruction of life stories. In R. Josselson & A. Lieblich (Eds.), *The narrative study of lives* (pp. 59–91). Newbury Park, CA: Sage.

Sarbin, T. R. (Ed.). (1986a). *Narrative psychology: The storied nature of human conduct*. New York: Praeger.

Sarbin, T. R. (1986b). The narrative as a root metaphor for psychology. In T. R. Sarbin (Ed.), *Narrative psychology:*

The storied nature of human conduct (pp. 3-21). New York: Praeger.

Schank, R. (1984). Intelligent advisory systems. In P. H. Winston & K. A. Prendergast (Eds.), *The AI business: Commercial uses of artificial intelligence* (pp. 133-148). Cambridge, MA: MIT Press.

Skinner, B. F. (1953). *Science and human behavior*. New York: Macmillan.

Spence, D. P. (1986). Narrative smoothing and clinical wisdom. In T. R. Sarbin (Ed.), *Narrative psychology: The storied nature of human conduct* (pp. 211-232). New York: Praeger.

Swenson, L. C. (1980). *Theories of learning: Traditional perspectives/contemporary developments*. Belmont, CA: Wadsworth.

Vitz, P. C. (1990). The use of stories in moral development. *American Psychologist, 45*, 709-720.

Wala, A. M., & Cole, H. P. (1987). Simulations that teach and test critical skills in mine ventilation. In J. M. Mutmansky (Ed.), *Proceedings of the third mine ventilation symposium at Pennsylvania State University* (pp. 132-141). Littleton, CO: American Society of Mining Engineers.

Wallerstein, N. (1992). Powerlessness, empowerment, and health: Implications for health promotion programs. *American Journal of Health Promotion, 6*, 197-205.

Wallerstein, N., & Bernstein, E. (1988). Empowerment education: Freire's ideas adapted to health education. *Health Education Quarterly, 15*, 379-394.

Wallerstein, N., & Weinger, M. (1992). Health and safety education for worker empowerment. *American Journal of Industrial Medicine, 22*, 619-635.

White, R. W. (1959). Motivation reconsidered: The concept of competence. *Psychological Review, 66*, 297-333.

Whitehead, A. N. (1929). *The aims of education*. Cambridge, England: Cambridge University Press.

18

Health Behavior Research and Communication Campaigns

James W. Swinehart

INTRODUCTION: METHODOLOGICAL ISSUES

Mass media communication campaigns on health topics typically involve the use of television, radio, newspapers, magazines, and other media to convey information or to provide motivation for various actions. Although a large number of such campaigns have been conducted by various governmental, commercial, and voluntary organizations, questions remain about their overall effectiveness and the relative value of their different elements (e g , Atkin & Arkin, 1990; Brown & Walsh-Childers, 1994; Flay, 1987; Rice & Atkin, 1994; Vingilis & Coultes, 1990; Wallack, Dorfman, Jernigan, & Themba, 1993). There are a number of reasons for this uncertainty:

1. In many cases, the possible effects of campaigns have not been adequately assessed, so no conclusions can be drawn concerning their impact.

2. Several well-designed evaluations have shown substantial impact for some campaigns and little or none for others.

3. There are indications that solid progress has been made in several areas, such as the increase in the percentage of patients with adequately controlled hypertension, the reduction in the percentage of adults who smoke, the reduced consumption of foods high in animal fats and cholesterol, and the drop in alcohol-related highway fatalities. Some of these changes are attributed in part to multiyear public education efforts, but there is no way to determine just how much influence these campaigns have had.

4. It is difficult to develop generalizations from experience with campaigns that differ markedly in terms of cost, duration, kinds of results sought, access to media, diversity and accessibility of target audiences, and the themes or appeals used.

5. Some purposive campaigns are aided by the presence of reinforcing messages from other sources; others are undermined by the presence of competing messages from other sources. Examples of such reinforcing or competing messages are paid advertising, other public service advertising, medical news stories, advice col-

James W. Swinehart • Public Communication Resources, 1310 Bolton Road, Pelham Manor, New York 10803-3602.

Handbook of Health Behavior Research IV: Relevance for Professionals and Issues for the Future, edited by David S. Gochman. Plenum Press, New York, 1997.

umns in newspapers or magazines, and portrayals in movies and entertainment programs.

6. Some campaigns are designed to influence certain health behaviors directly, others seek to influence behaviors indirectly through third parties (e.g., parents, teachers, physicians, employers) or by shaping public policy (e.g., more funding for public health clinics, stricter limits on air pollution, mandating child-resistant medicine containers), and still others use a combination of approaches.

7. In some instances, public information or education is used alone; in others, it is one part of a larger effort involving legislation, regulation, or technology (as in the case of, for example, environmental carcinogens, alcohol consumption, immunizations, smoking, highway safety, nutrition labels, and air pollution).

8. Campaign functions differ greatly—e.g., giving people new information, reminding them of something they already know, persuading them to act, providing skills training, increasing public concern about a particular problem, and promoting new laws. When dealing with specific health actions, campaigns may urge people to initiate, cease, alter, or maintain particular behaviors. Some efforts concentrate on reducing the considerable gap between holding "correct" beliefs about healthy lifestyles and engaging in "correct" behaviors.

9. Educational efforts are based on several assumed connections: that campaigns can produce changes in knowledge, attitudes, and skills … which cause changes in behavior … which lead to lower risks and improved physiological states … which produce lower morbidity and mortality. There is some loss of effect in each of these connections, and the losses are much greater for some health problems than for others.

Despite the difficulties inherent in dealing with noncomparable topics and conditions, some generalizations can be drawn. This chapter provides some examples and recommendations regarding the uses of behavioral research in planning, conducting, and evaluating health-related media campaigns.

SETTING OBJECTIVES

How should a target level for desired change be set? There are at least five kinds of standards: *historical* (e.g., this year versus last year versus five years ago), *normative* (e.g., the usual for this agency or this topic area), *theoretical* (what would happen if everything went right, based on previous assessments in controlled situations), *absolute* (the highest possible level, with no consideration of limiting factors), and *negotiated* (usually some combination of the other four kinds of standards). Whatever the basis for the standards used, the choice of objectives obviously has great importance for evaluation, since it can determine whether the actual measures are interpreted as indicating success or failure (Green & Lewis, 1986).

For any given campaign, officials of health agencies should determine whether the effort is to be evaluated in relation to directional objectives (e.g., "an increase in X"), incremental objectives (e.g., "an increase of 10% in X"), what previous efforts of this kind have accomplished, the amount of media coverage obtained, improvements in relationships among organizations in the field, or other factors.

It is worth noting that favorable side effects of a campaign such as greater public awareness of a particular problem, public support for measures to reduce the problem, and improved relations between various organizations may in themselves justify a campaign whether or not it can be proven effective in terms of the outcomes originally intended.

Public information campaigns can be helpful, and sometimes even necessary, in reducing health problems—but no one should expect them to do the job alone. Part of the reason can be seen in a graph (Figure 1) that shows why campaigns never have a one-to-one relationship between efforts and results.

Even when a message is successfully placed (and successful placement should not be taken for granted), it may have little impact (Anderson, 1989). Many people will not even be exposed to

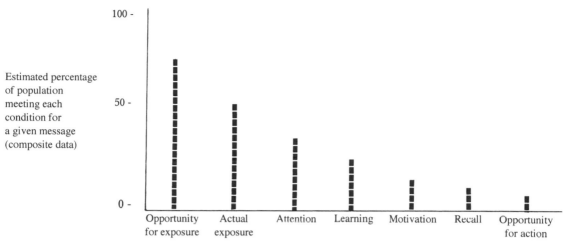

Estimated percentage of population meeting each condition for a given message (composite data)

Figure 1. Declining likelihood of effect.

it; many who are exposed will pay no attention; some of those who pay attention will not understand the message, or not believe it, or not feel that it applies to them; some of those who understand and accept it will not be motivated to act or will soon forget the message; some who intend to act will not have the opportunity to do so. In direct mail campaigns, a 1% response rate is a benchmark of success—but in health campaigns there is an unrealistic desire for a 100% response rate, because every disability day or premature death represents a failure. Aiming for complete success sounds laudable, but from a management standpoint it is unwise, because it almost assures that a campaign will be seen as a failure *in terms of its own objectives.*

The nature of the intended outcome, as well as the size and nature of the intended audience, also need to be taken into account when setting campaign objectives and designing an evaluation plan (see Table 1). Some audiences may be relatively small or unusually resistant to change (e.g., men with detected but untreated hypertension). Some desired outcomes may be time-bound (e.g., occurring before a child enters school, or in the third trimester of a pregnancy, or at a particular time each month). Such circumstances not only

reduce the likelihood that an educational effort will have a demonstrable impact but also have obvious implications for the timing of data collection.

The target audiences listed as examples here were chosen because they have a clear connection with the topics, but greater differentiation would be needed in planning an actual campaign. In the case of smoking, for instance, "current smokers" could be divided into several subgroups on the basis of such factors as their desire to quit, previous efforts to quit, use of low-tar brands, number of cigarettes smoked per day, knowledge of risks related to smoking, and social support for quitting.

The "demand characteristics" of various health behaviors differ greatly; some behaviors are fairly easy to produce and some are quite difficult (see Table 2). For example, getting a parent to have a preschool child immunized against polio should be relatively easy, since the action has a low cost, a high payoff, social support, need be done only once, and so on. On the other hand, getting someone to take medication to control hypertension is hard for a variety of reasons: It must be done daily, the benefits are not apparent, troublesome side effects may oc-

**Table 1. Examples of Messages, Topics, and Target Audiences
for Health Behavior Communication Campaigns**

Some categories of health-related behavioral messages	
1. Learn more about X	7. Don't start doing X (or continue not doing it)
2. Do X once	8. Do less of X
3. Start doing X	9. Stop doing X
4. Continue doing X	10. Encourage someone else to take
5. Do more of X	recommended action (e.g., start, stop,
6. Do X differently	continue)

Examples of topics and target audiences by messages

Topic	Target audiences	Messages
Smoking	Nonsmokers	7, 10
	Former smokers	7, 10
	Current smokers	1, 6, 8, 9
Breast self-examination (BSE)	Those who have not done BSE	1, 3
	Those who have done BSE	4, 10
	Those who do BSE incorrectly	1, 6
Safety belt use	Nonusers	1, 3
	Current occasional users	1, 5
	Current consistent users	4, 10
Nutrition	People with excessive intake of such food components as sugar, sodium, and saturated fat	1, 8, 9
	People with insufficient vitamin A	1, 3, 5
Alcohol/drugs	Nonabusers	7, 10
	Current abusers	1, 6, 9
	Former abusers	7, 10
Immunizations	Parents of preschool children	1, 2, 10
Hypertension	People with undetected hypertension	1, 2
	People with detected hypertension	1, 3, 4
	Families of people with detected hypertension	1, 10
Prenatal care	Pregnant women, concerning:	
	Nutrition	1, 6
	Substance abuse	1, 7, 9
	Prenatal examinations	1, 3, 4
Exercise	People who already exercise	4, 5, 10
	People who don't exercise	1, 3
	People who exercise incorrectly	1, 6
Radon, lead paints, and other environmental hazards	People who have not checked their homes for possible contamination	1, 2, 10

cur immediately, and the financial cost may be significant. Almost every health-related behavior will be high with respect to some facilitating factors and low with respect to others. A problem arises when the inhibiting factors are under-estimated (e.g., in some programs dealing with weight control, smoking cessation, or breast examinations) and as a result too few resources are devoted to the campaign or its goals are set unrealistically high.

Table 2. Factors That Affect the Likelihood of Recommended Health Actions

Factors	Facilitating ←——————————————————→ Inhibiting		
Nature and extent of behavioral change	Maintain	Modify	Initiate or terminate
Purpose of action	Stop symptom	Preclude illness	Increase "wellness"
Beneficiary of action	Family member	Self	Others
Financial cost	Low	Moderate	High
Frequency	Once	Occasionally	Daily
Needed medical facilities available?	Yes	NA	No
Perceived characteristics of health professionals	Positive (e.g., competent, caring)	—	Negative (e.g., careless, cold)
Group norms/values related to action	Support	—	Oppose
Number of competing messages	None	Some	Many
Strength/quality of competing messages	Low	Moderate	High
Number of reinforcing messages	Many	Some	None
Strength/quality of reinforcing messages	High	Moderate	Low
Action consistent with personal values and self-image?	Yes	—	No
Time when health benefits become apparent	Immediately	In weeks or months	In years
Importance of health benefits/magnitude of threat reduced	High	Moderate	Low
Immediacy and importance of nonhealth benefits of action	High	Moderate	Low
Number and importance of negative aspects of action (e.g., painful, boring, inconvenient, frightening, embarrassing, time-consuming)	Low	Moderate	High
Extent to which action is supported by laws, regulations, technology, and in other ways	High	Moderate	Low

CHOOSING AND SEGMENTING TARGET AUDIENCES

Health behavior research can provide answers to a number of questions about the kinds of audiences that need to be reached by a given campaign. The following questions should be resolved at an early stage of planning:

Which groups are most affected by the problem? Are they also the ones in the best position to do something about it, or should the campaign be addressed in part to others? How accessible are they, and how susceptible to influence? What proportion of the people affected have tried previously, and unsuccessfully, to do something about the problem? How much do they know about it? How many people hold incorrect beliefs

about its seriousness, its causes, or intervention methods? How many are afraid of it, or apathetic about it, or merely resigned? How many regard the problem as more important than other problems? What people will have the ability and opportunity to influence others? For each kind of audience, what information sources are most trusted and accepted? What channels or media do they use most often, and for what purposes? Why aren't they already doing what they are supposed to do—what are the personal or situational or financial constraints on their actions?

For each target audience selected, the answers to these questions can be summarized on a page indicating the importance of the audience, objectives, barriers to recommended actions, communication strategies/themes/appeals, spokespersons, media/channels/vehicles, and method of measuring results. This task is difficult but worthwhile because it imposes order and data-based rationality on the process of campaign design.

Level of receptivity to health information is a crucial factor in segmenting audiences for health campaigns and in choosing the kinds of content and media to be used (Swinehart, 1991; Zillman & Bryant, 1985). Just as relatively few people can be expected to maintain a general preventive orientation, relatively few will make special efforts to find and use health information on a regular basis. Four categories of receptivity and estimates of their size appear in Table 3.

These categories are somewhat arbitrary, and there are many exceptions to the general pattern, but they are a reminder that exposure to health information is more often inadvertent than deliberate. Such segmentation can also be useful in setting expectations for program impact.

Table 3. Categories of Receptivity to Health Information

Categories	Estimated percentage of the population
Seekers: People who actively look, even while asymptomatic, for health information presented in the mass media and by consulting health professionals	5%
Acceptors: People who will pay attention to health information when they encounter it and who tend to accept statements by medical authorities, but do not actively seek such information	30%
Tolerators: People who pay little attention to health information, do not seek it, and tend to be skeptical of any such information they happen to counter	50%
Avoiders: People who actively avoid health information, whether presented in the mass media or directly by health professionals	15%

SELECTING MEDIA AND VEHICLES

In addition to choosing which media (e.g., television, radio, newspapers) to use for a given campaign, planners must decide which "vehicles" (particular kinds of materials) to use within each medium. The vehicles most often used in public service campaigns are television and radio spots, posters, feature articles, video news releases, transit cards, billboards, and various kinds of pamphlets or handouts. Which of these, or others, should be used in a particular case depends on such factors as ease or difficulty of access, production cost, distribution cost, staff time required, production capabilities required, amount of control over the final product, tie-in possibilities, timing flexibility, and the context in which the audience will be exposed to the message. For example, a planner using magazines may choose to prepare feature articles rather than display advertisements on the grounds that the former are more likely to receive donated space, more likely to attract readers' attention, and more able to convey detailed information.

Of course, the most important considerations are the potential audience size, or "reach," and the frequency of exposure (Jones, 1992). Estimates can be based on data provided by media outlets (typically without charge to potential advertisers) regarding the size and characteristics of their audiences, or on data obtained directly from target audiences regarding their media usage habits.

FORMATIVE OR BACKGROUND RESEARCH IN DEVELOPING CAMPAIGNS AND MATERIALS

The years since 1980 have seen increasing use of a "social marketing" approach by various agencies (Atkin & Arkin, 1990; Bauman et al., 1988; Fox & Kotler, 1980; Karsten, Bowler, Kasab, & Arkin, 1992; Lefebvre & Flora, 1988; Maibach & Parrott, 1995; Meade, McKinney, & Barnas, 1994; Public Health Service, 1990; Worden et al., 1988).

Following are some examples of research on target audiences that was used in shaping campaign decisions:

1. In planning to increase immunization of inner-city children in Philadelphia, it was assumed that a high proportion of these children were entirely unvaccinated and that the reasons they were not were that parents did not know or did not believe that immunizations were needed and that parents could not afford the cost of vaccines. Health behavior research conducted by the Annenberg School for Communication and Albert Einstein Medical Center showed, however, that all three assumptions were wrong. About three-fourths of the inner-city children studied had incomplete but substantial levels of protection. Parents and others caretakers were generally knowledgeable about the need for vaccinations, but typically were not aware of the timetable for shots and whether their child was up to date; as a result, they missed many opportunities to get shots for their children during clinic visits. It was also found that the cost of shots was not a major problem, since everyone in the study was either insured or had access to free vaccinations. As a result of this health behavior research, the plan to conduct a public information campaign was replaced by efforts to change the operation of the clinics in several ways: Reduce long waiting times, make appointments and follow them up more aggressively, promote vaccination of children who come into clinics when sick or without appointments, and maintain registries that would tell providers when particular children need immunizations (Annenberg School for Communication, 1994).

2. Health behavior research at the University of Maryland assessed the strategies used by African-Americans to obtain health information. Family members, friends, and coworkers were the major sources of health information; African-American sources and health pamphlets were trusted more than general circulation newspapers and other sources. The least-educated African-Americans were the most pessimistic about surviving cancer, indicating that the message about the value of early diagnosis and treatment had not reached this segment of the population. The study findings provided the basis for designing new messages and selecting appropriate channels for disseminating them (Freimuth, 1990).

3. The Partnership for a Drug-Free America has made considerable use of health behavior research in developing messages for various target audiences (G. Marston, 1995, personal communication). Some examples:

- After a survey showed that only 51% of teenagers believed that they could become addicted to cocaine, a television spot showing an addicted white rat was used to make the point that cocaine is the most highly reinforcing substance known.
- The finding that most young teenagers vastly overestimate the number of their peers who use drugs led to a television spot emphasizing that nonusers are a majority among preteens and young teens, thus undermining the belief that "everybody does it."
- When a majority of parents were found to believe that their children were not vulnerable to drug experimentation (partly because drug use was viewed as occurring in cities but not in suburbs), a message aimed at parents was produced to make the point that drug abuse is a problem in every kind of community.
- To counteract the belief of many young teens that marijuana carries few risks, a young user talking about the changes in his life conveyed the message that use of this drug is associated with having trouble in school and in family relationships.

4. Research for a television program on breast cancer found that many women were reluctant to do self-examinations or to have a mammogram because they were afraid of detecting cancer and of the possible consequences—dying, or losing a breast, and becoming "less feminine" or sexually unattractive. As a result, a documentary style was used with a breast cancer patient and her family to demonstrate that a

woman who has had a mastectomy can continue to have an active and fulfilling life in all respects (Mielke & Swinehart, 1976).

5. Research for a program on mental health indicated that blue-collar workers were unlikely to seek help for a problem because they were worried about the cost of treatment for mental illness, the effectiveness of treatment, and the reactions of their friends. In the program, an actual case history was used to demonstrate that company benefits will often cover the cost of treatment, that appropriate therapy can restore a troubled person to a normal and happy life, and that most people now accept the idea of seeking treatment for depression or similar illnesses (Mielke & Swinehart, 1976).

6. The Minnesota Department of Health has used market research at several stages in planning and implementing antismoking campaigns aimed at adolescents and young women. Messages and media choices have been based on health behavior research using telephone surveys, classroom surveys, and focus groups, as well as reviews of published research. Focus groups were used before ads were created to help develop message concepts and to segment the target groups, to pretest rough versions of ads, to find out during the campaigns how the ads were being received, and to refine questions used in periodic surveys to assess the results. (The preparatory research indicated that rather than focus on health, the messages should stress the short-term social and personal consequences of smoking. Youngsters who experimented with smoking at age 13 or younger typically smoked with a same-age friend; they said they smoked to be accepted, to look and feel older, and to take risks. Both boys and girls greatly overestimated the percentage of others their age who smoke, and both genders indicated that their smoking behavior would be strongly influenced by a boyfriend or girlfriend who disapproved of smoking. These findings led to ads for this age group that emphasized acceptance by the opposite sex, peer pressure to smoke, the fact that most of their peers do not

smoke, and bad breath.) Research also shaped the decision to reach this age group via broadcast television, cable television, radio, bus stop ads, and posters. Placement schedules were based on data showing the highest listening/viewing periods for teens and the kinds of formats—Contemporary Hit Radio, Album-Oriented Rock, VH-1, MTV—that draw large teen audiences. Parallel findings about women aged 18–24 were used to develop messages designed specifically for them and to make similarly tailored media choices (Minnesota Department of Public Health, 1991).

7. On the basis of data on smoking prevalence, California developed a control program for several segments of the population: children aged 10 and under, preteens and teenagers 11–18, adult smokers, pregnant women, smokeless-tobacco users, and four ethnic minorities (African-Americans, Latinos, Native Americans, and Asian-Pacific Americans). Beginning in 1990, the effort included a media campaign along with other major components designed to influence the public climate and policies regarding smoking. Extensive formative research (109 focus groups in the first year) was used to pretest all advertising messages, to shape the campaign strategies (deglamorizing tobacco use, emphasizing negative health effects during pregnancy, promoting cessation behavior, and providing information-oriented messages), and to determine the choice of media (television, radio, newspapers, magazines, posters, bus shelter cards, and extensive community outreach efforts). By using a large amount of paid advertising (about $20 million in the first year) as well as negotiating an additional $6.6 million worth of free television and radio time, the campaign reached 97% of all teens an average of 75 times during the first 8 months. Multiwave evaluation surveys indicated that the campaign reduced the number of students who smoked or intended to smoke (California Department of Health Services and Department of Education, 1990).

8. In planning a public education campaign

on drinking and driving, a group in Vermont conducted extensive research to identify high-risk audiences and the most effective ways to influence them. Repeated roadside surveys covered demographic information, drinking patterns, sources of messages received about alcohol and highway safety, knowledge concerning problem drinking and the effects of alcohol, opinions about drinking and driving, and a measure of blood alcohol level. These health behavior assessments were used to shape decisions regarding media and message themes as well as to track the effects of the campaign. The primary target audience (young men) proved to be interested primarily in messages that gave them positive information in a simple, straightforward manner; for example, they preferred a message about how to avoid arrest and its consequences to negative themes such as the chances of getting killed on the highway (Worden, Waller, & Riley, 1975).

9. An initial assumption in planning a campaign on hypertension was that people needed to be informed that they could have high blood pressure without knowing it—that the condition was often asymptomatic. Health behavior research showed that previous educational efforts had convinced a large majority of people that this was true—so the point no longer needed to be made—and in fact that emphasizing it could be counterproductive. The message was changed to stress the value of family enjoyment and role responsibilities as reasons for taking medication for high blood pressure: People who control their hypertension stay alive to enjoy and support their families (National Heart, Lung, and Blood Institute, 1986).

10. The Stanford Heart Disease Prevention Program was a pioneering effort to use a combination of media campaigns and face-to-face counseling to produce changes in high-risk levels of blood pressure, weight, and plasma cholesterol. Extensive audience research was used to develop the form and content of both kinds of interventions (Maccoby & Alexander, 1980).

In addition to obtaining information about target audiences, data on "gatekeepers" (e.g., media personnel, school and clinic officials) can also prove valuable. For example:

1. Interviews with public service directors and program directors at a number of radio stations found a strong preference for "live announcer copy" over prerecorded public service announcements. This was a doubly useful finding, since live-copy versions of the messages were both more likely to be aired and much cheaper to produce (UniWorld Group, 1982).

2. The Healthy Mothers/Healthy Babies Coalition pretested a series of posters for pregnant women using fantasy photographs, which were strongly admired by the target audience. They were not pretested, however, with physicians and nurses on the staff at low-income clinics. When the posters were distributed, these providers were found to dislike the posters as "too pretty"—but consented to use them when shown the pretest results (E. B. Arkin, 1995, personal communication).

3. A study of ways to reach high-risk adolescents found that radio would be the most efficient medium; that if television were used, messages should be placed in or around music videos, on MTV, and in televised movies; that such magazines as *Seventeen* and *Teen* would reach white females; that African-American girls and boys could be reached through *Ebony* magazine; and that *Sports Illustrated* would reach high-risk African-American and white adolescent boys, and also many girls (Klein et al., 1993).

CAMPAIGN EVALUATION

Evaluation of communication programs normally involves (1) *formative* or developmental evaluation (such as pretesting of informational materials) and (2) *summative* evaluation (assessing outcomes or impact). Some assessments also include a look at *process*. The various kinds of measures used are sometimes classified in terms of their thoroughness and cost, ranging from Level I (lowest) to Level III (highest). For example, a Level I intermediate outcome evaluation of the placement of informational materials could involve a count of the ads or articles placed; Level II could entail monitoring of placements through tracking services; Level III could involve both of these kinds of activities plus sample surveys covering awareness and recall of the materials.

Pretesting

In recent years, it has become fairly common to use focus groups, mall intercepts, theater tests, or other research formats to pretest prototype versions of campaign materials (Atkin & Freimuth, 1989). Using various levels of "finish," from concept through rough sketches to polished work, reactions are obtained from a small number of people who are representative of the intended audiences for the materials.

In most cases, pretesting should include measurements of comprehension, incorrect inferences, recall of message, recall of referral information (if any), overall appeal, appeal of specific elements, perception of message as accurate or misleading, perception of self-relevance of message, perceived value of message, attitude change, behavioral intentions, actual behavior (as feasible), and recall of message source (as desired).

Typically, prototype materials are pretested only once because time and money are limited. If the initial results indicate that major changes are needed, however, a second or even a third pretest is in order to check the success of revisions. Pretesting does not guarantee success, but the process makes it possible to identify problems at a stage at which they can still be corrected at relatively little cost. Some examples:

1. A television spot that was intended to dramatize the risks of using cocaine showed a young man taking a white gun from a desk and placing the barrel against his temple. This spot was never used because pretest research showed that about one-third of teens misunderstood it to suggest that suicide is an option for a depressed addict (G. Marston, 1995, personal communication).

2. A pretest of alternative warning symbols for contact lens cleaning solution found that one design was interpreted as meaning the product was to be used in the eye, rather than the opposite. The results as a whole provided a basis for dropping the misunderstood design and combining desirable elements from several others (Public Communication Resources, 1989).

3. A pretest of a booklet about condoms led to replacing the words "safer sex" with the words "less risky sex." Although the denotative meaning is identical, the connotation turned out to be quite different: The first phrase was perceived as conveying the idea of safety and reassurance, while the second conveyed the notion of risk and the need for caution (Public Communication Resources, 1988). This pretest, like many others, also led to improvements in text wording, illustrations, sequence of topics, title, and cover design.

4. The National Institute on Drug Abuse (NIDA) planned a media campaign to counter growing use of cocaine by young adults in the early 1980s. Pretests indicated that the planned theme line, "Cocaine's Insane," was well received by the target audience. Subsequently, however, focus groups with adolescents, who were not the primary audience but would be exposed to the public service ads, showed that teenagers interpreted "insane" as meaning "really cool." NIDA then changed the campaign theme to "Cocaine: The Big Lie" (E. B. Arkin, 1995, personal communication).

5. The Federal Division of Maternal and Child Health pretested its "Health Diary," designed as a tool to help low-income pregnant women negotiate prenatal care and health care systems more effectively. An unexpected result was the women's strong preference for a book that was spiral-bound for ease of entering notes. On the basis of the results, the division printed a book that was more expensive but far more appealing to the intended users (E. B. Arkin, 1995, personal communication).

6. Extensive audience research shaped a number of decisions concerning a large-scale effort to reduce cigarette smoking among adolescents. Examples of these decisions include the selection and refinement of various television spots, the use of an approach that emphasized modeling of desired behaviors rather than simply providing information about risks, the avoidance of exhortation, and omitting the use of identifying tags on television spots so they would not appear to be from a single campaign (Flynn, Worden, Secker-Walker, Badger, Geller, & Costanza, 1992).

Assessing Process and Outcomes

Some questions that should be covered by a communication program evaluation that deals with both process and outcomes are listed below. Possible methods of answering each question are indicated following the question; other methods, such as reviewing available records or interviewing expert informants, should also be used when appropriate. Although these questions apply to a purposive program (such as a public information campaign to encourage treatment seeking), they can be adapted for use with any kind of information dissemination effort.

1. Were the program materials scientifically accurate? This can be determined through a review by scientists, both inside and outside the originating agency.

2. Were the materials regarded as appealing and understandable by the target audiences? These questions can be answered through small-group studies with representatives of the designated target audiences.

3. Were the materials regarded as appealing and appropriate by media gatekeepers? Answers to these questions can be obtained through interviews or questionnaires, or both, with public service directors of television networks and stations, cable systems, radio networks and stations, magazine and newspaper editors, and others as appropriate.

4. Were the materials regarded as appeal-ing and appropriate by officials and volunteers in cooperating organizations? Interviews or questionnaires or both should be used with officials and volunteers in cooperating organizations.

5. Did the materials achieve a level of distribution and placement that gave the target audiences adequate opportunities for exposure to them? Data concerning this question should be obtainable through reports from persons in agencies distributing these items, plus monitoring of on-air placements by a commercial service. These sources can be supplemented by interviews/reports from persons in agencies distributing spots, ads, articles, and other items, as well as interviews/reports from other intermediaries as appropriate.

6. How satisfactory were the procedures that were used in making program decisions (e.g., setting objectives, choosing target audiences and communication strategies, developing materials)? What changes, if any, should be made in planning future efforts of a similar nature? A set of specific questions should be used to conduct interviews with participants in the process, and their comments can also be solicited informally. In either case, they should be given assurances of anonymity.

7. How satisfactory were the arrangements used to obtain cooperation from private sector organizations and to coordinate activities with them? This question can be answered through the same steps stated in answer to question 6, but with agency staff, state coordinators (if any), and local and national representatives of nongovernmental organizations involved in the campaign.

8. To what extent did the target audiences notice the materials and pay attention to them? These assessments will depend largely on agency capabilities and budgets. If funds are available, for example, a series of three surveys could be conducted a 2-month intervals among samples representative of designated target audiences, assessing both unaided and aided recall of campaign materials. The sources of inquiries prompted by the campaign could be determined through the use of keyed box numbers or other identification on campaign materials. A continuing survey of persons submitting inquiries or requests could be conducted by enclosing a reply card or brief questionnaire when fulfilling information requests, perhaps in 1/10 or fewer of the packages sent out, depending on the total number of requests received.

9. To what extent did the campaign alter the beliefs, attitudes, and behavioral intentions of the target audiences in the direction intended? Did any changes occur that were opposite to the ones intended? One possibility here would be to conduct a series of three surveys: 1 month before the campaign begins, at its midpoint, and 1 month after it ends.

10. To what extent did the campaign alter the actions of the target audiences in the direction intended? Did any changes occur that were opposite to the ones intended? These questions call for multiple assessments. One might be a series of surveys with samples representative of the designated target audiences, scheduled as follows: 1 month before the campaign, at its midpoint, 1 month after it ends, 1 year later, and 3 years later. Another might involve an analysis and summary of volunteered comments from persons noticing or using campaign materials.

11. To what extent did the campaign stimulate inquiries or requests for more information? This can be tracked through a month-by-month tally of inquiries, classified by topic, source, and other relevant characteristics — such tracking to begin at least a month prior to the start of the campaign and continuing for a year after it ends.

12. To what extent did the campaign stimulate related activities on the part of schools, voluntary organizations, business firms, and units of local or state government? To what extent did the campaign prompt greater cooperation among such entities? Did the campaign have any negative impact on state and local activities or coordination? These questions can be answered through a combination of methods:

an analysis and summary of monthly reports from state and local officials, plus interviews with these officials at the end of the campaign; interviews with representatives of governmental and nongovernmental organizations, and a continuing survey of persons submitting inquiries or requests for information.

Campaign Objectives and Evaluation Objectives

It is useful to distinguish these two kinds of objectives from one another, although they will match in many cases. A campaign that has as its ultimate objective a behavioral change will have a number of intermediate objectives, such as producing specified changes in attitudes or beliefs. Evaluation objectives can include not only the extent to which the intermediate and ultimate campaign objectives are achieved, but also assessment of the relative effectiveness of various media components (e.g., television spots, radio spots, news releases), message sources, and other campaign elements. In the case of a single message in one medium, such as a particular television spot, the process objectives can be listed in a temporal sequence as follows:

1. Acceptance or clearance of spot by networks or stations
2. Actual broadcast of spot (time, day, frequency, program context)
3. Size and characteristics of potential audience
4. Size and characteristics of actual audience (those exposed to the spot)
5. Awareness of and attention to the spot
6. Understanding and acceptance of the message
7. Changes in attitudes, beliefs, and/or motivation to take recommended action(s)
8. Commitment to act, initiation of action, maintenance of action
9. Change in health status, risk status, life expectancy, and other characteristics

The first three items in this list constitute the major differences between assessment of mass communications and assessment of other interventions such as the use of presentations to various organizations. At a meeting, the audience is known and in some cases self-selected because they are interested in the topic; in the case of a mass communication campaign, the potential audience always includes a large number of persons who are never actually exposed to the message or who pay little attention to it.

Choosing Evaluation Methods

Various evaluation methods that could be used to assess any campaign should be compared with regard to the extent to which they meet the following kinds of needs:

1. Determining the extent to which subobjectives (i.e., intermediate or instrumental goals) are achieved.
2. Demonstrating a clear connection between campaign effort and any measured effects.
3. Providing data that can serve as a basis for estimating the cost-effectiveness of each campaign element or segment.
4. Detecting unexpected campaign effects, including possible negative consequences as well as those regarded as desirable.
5. Producing conclusions concerning process as well as outcomes.
6. Measuring delayed or cumulative effects as well as short-term effects, and effects that are small but significant.

Research Designs

When pretesting or pilot-testing educational materials, it is possible to employ true experimental designs (and thus assess the influence of such potential contaminants as the sensitizing effect of a premeasure or any maturation that occurs among respondents between baseline and postmeasure). In most actual campaigns, however, such designs can only be approximated; health agencies can arrange the timing and audiences for measurements, but normally

cannot randomize or control exposure to a campaign. It is necessary, however, to use at least a quasi-experimental design such as the "equivalent time samples" design or the "equivalent materials samples" design if one is to attribute any observed changes in a target audience to a particular campaign rather than to concurrent influences from other sources (e.g., parallel campaigns from other agencies, changes in laws or regulations, school programs, or media coverage of related issues).

Once placement information is available, estimates of the probable audience reached through each medium can be obtained from the media outlets using the materials, firms such as Nielsen Media Research or Simmons Market Research Bureau, school officials, and officials of voluntary groups cooperating with the campaign.

To obtain better information about *actual* exposure, and at the same time obtain measures of attention, learning, attitude change, and the like, specialized surveys are needed. Such surveys permit identification of the characteristics of persons who do or do not notice the materials, pay attention to them, learn from them, and so on. Interviews that tap both unaided and aided recall can be used to clearly differentiate people who remember the messages from those who can only recognize them and those who can do neither. These specialized surveys need to be carried out by professional survey organizations, but agencies may be able to keep costs down by providing questions for surveys conducted by others, e.g., the National Health Interview Survey. It may also be possible to identify a commercial client for surveys that would permit a health agency to add several questions to some of its surveys at little or no cost.

"Social Indicator" Measures

While most informational materials in a campaign are designed to influence individuals directly, there are other influence mechanisms that can also be promoted indirectly. For example, in a campaign by a government agency to reduce drinking by young people, some additional "intermediate" objectives might be to reduce the number of places where alcoholic beverages can be purchased by young people; to increase taxes on beer, wine, and liquor, to increase federal, state, and local appropriations for alcohol education; to institute more restrictive regulations governing alcohol advertising; to increase the number of pediatricians advising their preteen patients about the risks of using alcohol and other drugs; to increase the number of health departments and voluntary organizations sponsoring educational programs; and to increase funds for research related to drinking by preteens and adolescents. Each of these outcomes has the advantage of being measurable with relatively "hard" data, and indicators of change in one or a combination of them might prove to be better predictors of reduced or delayed drinking by preteens and adolescents than measures of beliefs or attitudes in these population groups.

RESEARCH PROBLEMS

The three major types of studies on health communications have complementary strengths and weaknesses. *Laboratory experiments* help to identify important variables and show how they interact, but the settings and controls used necessarily limit the generalizability of findings. Large-scale *surveys* can show how various characteristics are distributed in target populations, but it is not feasible to include all relevant factors in such surveys. *Field experiments* can measure the results obtained with programs based on information gained in laboratory studies and surveys, but they are relatively costly and their manipulations are subject to real-world variability. Taken together, however, findings produced by these kinds of studies provide the basis for the recommendations presented elsewhere in this chapter.

Many excellent studies have been conducted, but others have limitations that are noted here in the hope that future work in this area will produce more definitive results.

1. Many studies have failed to treat adequately the complexity of information seeking and information handling. These behaviors are often seen as momentary events, rather than as parts of a process, and little attention is given to the time dimension—the duration or imminence of a health threat conveyed by a message, the temporal context in which it occurs, or the effects of a decision or action upon subsequent responses. The role of motivation in influencing reactions to information is given slight emphasis; as a result, little is known about the particular functions served by the seeking or avoidance of information under varying circumstances. When an uncertain outcome involves an element of danger, as is true of any threat to health, the seeking of relevant information obviously entails a risk and hence some degree of conflict for the persons affected. Their motivational states, interacting with such personality characteristics as risk-taking propensity and tolerance of ambiguity, shape the quality and form of any related attention, perception, selective learning and forgetting, decision making, and problem solving.

2. Experimental situations are often highly artificial; e.g., they use communication content on topics of slight interest, provide little or no opportunity for the audience to avoid or ignore communications, and study people who are unrepresentative of high-risk populations.

3. Many analyses using demographic variables do not combine them with psychological variables (and vice versa) in predicting selective exposure to health information. As a result, little is known about either the reasons for apparent differences among population segments or the distribution of relevant variables in large populations.

4. Little emphasis is placed on the interaction of the message and the recipient; most studies focus more narrowly on message content (e.g., fear arousal value), source (e.g., correlates of credibility), or recipient (e.g., personality

traits). Since within-study variations in message topic are also rare, very little is known about the effects on various behaviors of many possible combinations of source, appeal, topic, medium, and recipient. For example, a given fear appeal may produce a momentary but not habitual change in behavior, it may have lasting effects on behavior related to cancer but not to heart disease, or it may be effective in one medium but not in another.

5. An undifferentiated concept of "health threat" is often used, with little specification of its major dimensions (e.g., duration, intensity, visibility, and preventability).

6. The possibility of curvilinear effects is often ignored; level of fear or anxiety, for example, is frequently dichotomized rather than scaled. This approach precludes testing the idea that a moderate level of fear leads to more adaptive behavior than do either high or low levels of fear, as some evidence indicates.

7. The range of responses studied is often narrow, and frequently these responses are assessed by only one method (such as self-report) with no independent validation of the measures used.

TOPICS THAT NEED FURTHER RESEARCH

Following are some examples of questions relevant to health behavior that are viewed as deserving attention from research professionals, ideally in collaboration with health education practitioners.

Exposure Thresholds and Dose-Response Relationships. The "right" medicine in too small a dose has no effect, but too large a dose can cause other problems. Is a certain amount of exposure to a health message required before it "registers" and has some potential impact? Should the criteria used in commercial advertising (for which some studies indicate that at least three

exposures in a short period of time are necessary for minimum awareness) be applied to health messages if exposure to them cannot be controlled by the agencies that produce them? How can minimum, optimum, and excessive (wasteful or counterproductive) levels of exposure be established for health messages in the mass media?

Sequence of Presentation. In a communication that uses both threat and reassurance, for example, which should come first: the threat (because it arouses concern, and thus interest in the rest of the message) or the reassurance (because it may make the person less likely to "tune out" the message as unpleasant)?

Positive/Negative Balance. Where should greater emphasis by placed—on the benefits of taking a recommended action or on the consequences of failing to do so? The latter are usually easier to describe because they are specific, whereas "not getting sick" is a vague nonevent. Although these are really two versions of the same thing, it would be useful to know how many people respond more adaptively to positive phrasing than to negative phrasing.

Information Persistence after Learning. How long after a message is received should its effects be measured? As the interval increases, ability to recall learned information declines, but there is also greater opportunity for people to take a recommended action. There is a need to know more about the frequency and timing of reinforcing messages in order to produce both sustained knowledge gain and maximum adaptive actions.

Behavior Thresholds. Research to identify the thresholds at which information or motivational appeals produce actual behavior deserves a relatively high priority. Some people are prompted to act by low levels of information or motivation, while others resist even high levels. Greater knowledge of the nature and correlates of these individual differences should make it possible to design mass media programs that would be more effective as well as more efficient.

Density of Information.   The number of information points per unit of time or space can have important effects on attention, learning, recall, and action. High density of a television spot or a print ad tends to decrease attention, but produces greater learning in individuals who do attend. Experiments that manipulate information density as an independent variable, if they are to produce findings that apply to the usual mass media situation, must provide an opportunity for subjects to avoid (i.e., not attend to) the material presented. This option is not made available in most experiments in which groups of subjects are recruited to represent target audiences.

Program Design Features.   Which elements or formats produce the most learning and which produce the most behavior? The features that promote one sometimes undermine the other, as when vivid graphics or striking uses of humor are memorable but overwhelm the point of the message. Stressing risks may be necessary to get the attention of an audience, while stressing ways to reduce risks may be needed to motivate action. The features that promote both learning and motivation need to be identified. (The self-test, in which viewers can score their own knowledge while reading a pamphlet or watching a television program related to the test, is one format that appears to both attract attention and convey information effectively.)

Relative versus Absolute Levels of Perceived Susceptibility and Perceived Seriousness.   Is there some level of perceived susceptibility or perceived seriousness (e.g., 90% certainty of experiencing "extremely serious" effects) that almost invariably produces behavior change, or does this threshold vary with circumstances? What are the effects of various combinations and levels of perceived susceptibility, severity, benefits of action, and barriers to action?

Variable Interactions and Distributions.   In what ways do psychological variables such as risk-taking propensity and tolerance of ambiguity interact with experiential variables such as media usage and health behaviors? How much influence do psychological variables have on such decisions as postponing the diagnosis of a symptom? How are the relevant psychological variables distributed in high-need target populations and across standard demographic groups?

Message–Recipient Interactions.   More studies are needed that use as an independent variable the state produced in a person by a message, rather than the characteristics of the message itself or of the recipient. Particularly in experiments on very serious diseases, the appropriate analytical variable is not the amount of threat applied but the amount of fear produced.

Familial Determinants of Health Decisions.   Too little is known about the circumstances that enable one family member (spouse, child, other relative) to influence the health behavior of another. The same is true of "third parties" such as neighbors, friends, or employers.

Use of Indirect Appeals.   The qualifying "indirect" denotes appeals to values not related to health (such as saving money, gaining social approval, or fulfilling parental role expectations) that can be invoked as inducements to take preventive health actions. Most people want to avoid being seen as hypochondriacal or too self-protective, and providing alternative reasons to follow medical recommendations may be more effective than the commonly used health appeals. The effectiveness of indirect appeals has been demonstrated in antismoking programs for children and youths, who have trouble imagining long-term health consequences (while bad breath and social disapproval are immediate social consequences), but their effectiveness for adults is less clear.

Conflict Resolution. The decision about whether or not to have a symptom diagnosed typically involves an approach–avoidance conflict, because the diagnosis may resolve the ambiguity either favorably or unfavorably. The conflict is greatest, of course, when the potential health problem may be life-threatening. It would be helpful to know how communications about such problems could be designed to reduce this conflict and thus increase subsequent willingness to take diagnostic tests. Providing reassurance (such as by emphasizing the efficacy of treatment and the value of early intervention) is the most commonly used approach, but its effectiveness may be limited by the presence of other factors not yet identified.

Seriousness and Utility. To what extent is receptivity to information about a health problem influenced by the perceived seriousness of the disease and the perceived usefulness of the information provided? Some research indicates that there are striking individual differences in the relationship between these factors and that for some people the availability of useful information on ways to handle a threat may actually increase rather than decrease the impact of that threat. Denial and feelings of helplessness are of no help in resolving a health problem, of course, but they clearly provide some psychological relief; if "nothing can be done," the person is freed of a sense of responsibility for the outcome.

Comparison of Appeals. What is the relative effectiveness of various appeals in altering the anxiety value of disease topics? In the case of cancer, for example, is it easier to reduce anxiety by emphasizing the value of early detection, the efficacy of treatment, or other appeals?

Consequences of "Informedness." Is there something intrinsic to the possession of health knowledge that predisposes people to seek more knowledge? If so, is the converse true of a lack of knowledge? If felt ignorance maintains itself by prompting avoidance of information, this is an

additional barrier to raising the currently low level of knowledge among some population groups. On the other hand, an awareness of ignorance about health matters (relative to what others are believed to know or to what one should know) probably motivates some people to seek information. Thus, the question for health behavior research as well as for public health practice is this: As a means of inducing people to seek health information, is it more effective to make them feel relatively ignorant or relatively informed?

RECOMMENDATIONS FOR FUTURE HEALTH CAMPAIGNS

Research findings are always subject to modification by the results of later studies, and changes in health problems and the media environment will dictate adaptations in any "prescription" for campaign success. The following recommendations are offered with the understanding that they will need to be updated as conditions warrant. Most are based on personal experience and conversations with practitioners as well as published findings, and they have some elements in common with recommendations produced by others (e.g., Backer & Rogers, 1993; Backer, Rogers, & Sapory, 1992; DeJong & Atkin, 1995; Edwards, Tindale, Heath, & Posavac, 1990; Freudenberg, 1989; Glanz, Lewis, & Rimer, 1990; Graeff, Elder, & Booth, 1993; Maibach & Parrott, 1995; Rice & Atkin, 1994; Sutton, 1982; Wallack et al., 1993).

1. Campaigns should probably be planned to operate on a continuing basis, i.e., from year to year, rather than for only a few weeks or months. This may be difficult to achieve in view of the limited resources available and the fact that most agencies must deal with a variety of health topics. It is unrealistic, however, to expect very brief or limited campaigns to markedly increase public awareness of a particular problem or to exert a sustained influence on the actions of high-risk target groups. In this regard, it is interesting to

consider the antismoking campaigns that have been conducted by one agency or another in this country since the Surgeon General's Report in 1964. Year-to-year changes were too small to measure, so the efforts were viewed as failures, yet the cumulative effect over three decades—during which the proportion of adults who smoke has fallen from 50% to less than 30%—is one of the great success stories in the history of public health. Information campaigns, along with school programs and many other efforts, have contributed to this result.

2. Whether a campaign is produced by in-house staff, by an outside firm under contract, or by a combination of the two, lines of authority and responsibility should be clearly established before campaign planning is begun. If an outside contractor is used to produce mass media materials, considerable time should be allowed for staff of the sponsoring agency to monitor decisions and products at all stages of development.

3. Although most health agencies prefer to produce their own mass media materials, in some cases it is possible to reduce campaign costs by reproducing (with permission) materials developed previously for other organizations. A review of such materials is recommended as a useful step in preparing to conduct a campaign, whether or not the review leads to adoption of any of the items.

4. The desirability and feasibility of involving top management in campaign decisions depend upon such factors as the degree of autonomy of the health education staff, the personal interest of agency executives in the planning and execution of campaigns, and the importance of educational activities to the overall work of the agency. Involving management in campaign decisions typically requires additional time for meetings and clearances, but the investment can be worthwhile if it helps to maintain support at an appropriate level.

5. At least 3 months should be allowed for planning most campaigns. Whenever possible, the schedule of other campaign activities (e.g., materials design, pretesting, production, distri-bution, evaluation) should include safety margins to cover unanticipated delays.

6. Responsibility for public education regarding health is often shared by several agencies. In addition, some commercial organizations (such as insurance firms) and many voluntary organizations have a continuing interest in health promotion. Greater coordination among public agencies, and between such agencies and various groups in the private sector, is recommended as a means of (a) increasing the total amount of health communication to the public, (b) ensuring that messages on any given topic are consistent with one another and thus mutually reinforcing, and (c) increasing the amount of media coverage or placement by scheduling the release of materials in a noncompetitive way. Greater coordination would entail a perceived loss of autonomy for some organizations, but should make it possible to achieve greater impact at lower cost.

7. Although the choice of a theme or motivational appeal is one of the most critical decisions faced by planners of health campaigns, little is known about the relative effectiveness of various appeals (e.g., personal risk, avoidance of pain, social approval) in stimulating appropriate actions on the part of various target groups. Thus, a recommendation for future research is that controlled field experiments be conducted to provide a reliable basis for selecting campaign themes or appeals. In the meantime, the developmental phase of new campaigns should include at least small-scale research on the potential effectiveness of alternative appeals.

8. In planning campaigns, target audiences should be characterized in considerable detail so that appropriate materials can be developed for them and distributed through the channels most likely to reach them. There is a particular need to identify "barriers"—psychological and situational factors that inhibit the taking of recommended actions, such as cost, fear, lack of social support, inability to visualize benefits, negative side effects, and lack of facilities—so that such factors can be addressed directly in campaign materials.

9. The selection of target audiences for any particular campaign should take into account their contribution to the problem, their accessibility, their estimated susceptibility to influence, their opportunity to influence others, and their beliefs or actions regarding the problem being treated. It is clearly an unwise use of resources to design materials for groups that either already take the recommended actions or are extremely unlikely to do so. Health statistics, surveys, expert informants, focus groups, and reviews of previous studies can all help to identify the population segments that should be reached by a given campaign.

10. Whenever possible, specialized materials should be prepared for various target audiences (e.g., teenagers, employers, physicians, pregnant women), rather than a single message intended to reach such diverse groups. The information content, style, and motivational appeal should be tailored to the interests and tastes of each audience, and the choice of distribution channels should be based on each audience's media usage habits and use of time. These factors should be considered in relation to age, gender, and ethnicity in every case.

11. Although many campaigns are addressed directly to various target audiences in the hope of changing their health-related behaviors, some campaigns also seek to influence such behaviors indirectly by addressing potential "influence agents"—friends, employers, physicians, family members, and others who may persuade someone to take appropriate self-protective actions. Since personal influence is believed to have greater impact than mass media materials, which are necessarily impersonal, expanded use of the "influence agent" approach is recommended.

12. To increase the likelihood that materials will be appealing and understandable, preliminary versions of such items as television and radio spots, print ads, pamphlets, and posters should be pretested with representatives of the audiences these materials are designed to reach. If the exposure of materials depends upon approval by "gatekeepers" (e.g., public service directors of radio and television stations or officials of clinics or schools), having several such people review preliminary versions of materials permits revisions to be made prior to final production and helps to assure that the materials will be acceptable for use.

13. Some agencies, particularly at the state level, have been able to buy media time and space for health messages. (Some have also negotiated rates so that paid spots are supplemented by free placements.) When budgets are adequate, this tactic allows planners to control the placement of their materials and to obtain enough exposure to produce greater impact. Most agencies have little control over placement, however, because they still use only contributed time or space in the media; some agencies cannot afford to purchase time or space, and others have a policy that prohibits the use of paid advertising, but both free-media and paid-media campaigns can be cost-effective (Murry, Stam, & Lastovicka, 1996). In some cases, it is possible to obtain funds for the production or distribution of materials from commercial organizations without compromising the purpose or content of a campaign, and consideration of this step is recommended. Alternatively, some firms produce their own materials and seek an endorsement from health agencies; since both sides can benefit, this step is also recommended. (Insurance companies and drug firms, for example, have conducted health campaigns both independently and in collaboration with public agencies.)

14. No specific recommendation can be offered with regard to the quantity of materials that should be distributed or the amount of media time or space needed in order to achieve campaign objectives. These decisions will depend on such factors as the kind of topic addressed, the number and diversity of target audiences, the nature of campaign objectives, the duration of the campaign, and the possible reinforcing effect of similar public education efforts by other organizations. Most agencies try for maximum exposure, but find it hard to get enough media access to be noticed at all; as a practical matter, they

never have to ask "How much is enough?" A definitive answer to this question would require a number of field experiments in which campaign scale or intensity is varied while all other factors are controlled.

15. Personal contact with media personnel is generally regarded as the best way to obtain placement or use of campaign materials (National Cancer Institute, 1989). Some planners feel that personal contact should be made by local volunteers, others believe that it should be made by staff members of public agencies, and some feel it should be made by advertising agency personnel who also buy time or space for commercial campaigns. There appears to be little empirical evidence regarding the relative effectiveness of these differing approaches. There is general agreement, however, that materials are used more if they are delivered in person and described as having substantial *local* importance; thus, both steps are recommended. (Importance can be shown by citing surveys, other statistics, comments by lay people and public officials, and endorsements by concerned organizations or companies.) Health agencies should supply a brochure or fact sheet about themselves and offer to handle any requests for information that are received directly by the media as a result of using their materials. A script should be provided with each radio spot and a storyboard or photoboard with each television spot, plus a prepaid response card. Each spot should be clearly labeled with length, title, source, and intended audiences. Several lengths should be provided to match station availabilities, and each spot should have a local tag.

These suggestions apply particularly to placement of public service announcements, but they should also help to obtain media access in general and to increase the number and accuracy of stories on health topics. The use of a personal approach and local emphasis generally applies to newspapers as well as to broadcast outlets, although newspapers are much more likely to carry news releases and less likely to provide space for advertising.

16. Most health organizations find it difficult to obtain accurate measures of the extent to which their materials are used by broadcast and print media. Current methods tend either to provide incomplete data (as in the case of reply cards sent along with tapes to radio and television stations, which seldom achieve response rates exceeding 25–30%) or to be fairly costly (as in the case of commercial monitoring services). Developments in technology, however, have lowered the cost and improved the accuracy of tracking ad placements in the electronic media, and such improvements are likely to continue. Agencies can also reduce the cost of monitoring by sharing services and, at the local level, by using volunteers to clip articles and advertisements in newspapers.

17. In view of the difficulty of obtaining adequate amounts of public service advertising time or space, health campaigns should also utilize other means of reaching target audiences (e.g., exhibits, feature articles in newspapers and magazines, presentations to groups, direct mail to opinion leaders, video news releases, and online computer services). Cooperation from business and voluntary organizations should also be sought for such forms of assistance as distributing materials to employees or members, endorsing campaign objectives, and providing time for presentations at meetings.

18. Whenever possible, evaluations of health campaigns should cover not only *ultimate objectives* (e.g., changes in observed behavior, reductions in morbidity), but also *intermediate objectives* (e.g., distribution of materials, exposure of target audiences to materials, attention, learning), *quality* of materials (appeal and intelligibility to intended audiences, technical accuracy), and *process* (e.g., cooperation across organizational units, clearance procedures, selection and monitoring of contractors, and scheduling). If designed and conducted appropriately, such evaluations can provide useful diagnostic information as well as a measure of campaign impact. The evaluation process should also be broad enough to include indirect effects, such as changes

in laws or regulations that may result from heightened public awareness of a problem.

19. Especially if comprehensive evaluations of this kind are conducted, persons responsible for health campaigns should characterize in detail the methods and approaches used in these campaigns. Doing so would make it possible to relate various campaign elements to measured results. At present, such documentation is rarely feasible because detailed information is not available on most campaigns, and the evaluation designs used vary so widely that direct comparisons of results have little meaning.

RECOMMENDATIONS FOR PREPARING MEDIA MATERIALS ON HEALTH

1. In terms of frequency of use, 30 seconds appears to be the optimum length for radio and television public service announcements (California Department of Health Services and Department of Education, 1990; Swinehart, 1981; Worden et al., 1988). Longer materials such as 60-second spots, and video news releases that may run 3–5 minutes, are harder to place but obviously provide greater opportunity to explain health issues and to develop involvement on the part of the audience. Since no single length offers an ideal combination of characteristics, agencies should produce materials in a variety of lengths tailored to station preferences and availabilities.

2. The following recommendations pertain specifically to television spots and are based on commercial research as well as studies of public service announcements:

- Use direct delivery of dialogue among the characters shown.
- Integrate audio and visual elements so that they reinforce one another.
- Mention the problem or main issue several times.
- Identify the problem or issue within the first 10 seconds.

- Emphasize a solution as well as a problem.
- Make the message understandable from the visual elements alone.
- If possible, demonstrate as well as describe. (Illustrate cause and effect in sequence. Show the benefits of taking a recommended action.)
- Use authentic settings.
- Keep the message simple and eliminate extraneous elements.
- Summarize the main message or theme at the end.

3. Any information presented should be current and technically accurate.

4. Language and style should be appropriate to the intended audience.

5. Technical terms should be avoided whenever possible. When such terms must be used, they should be explained clearly and without condescension.

6. In general, the tone of health messages should be serious rather than flip or frivolous. A humorous approach can attract attention and be entertaining, but special care should be taken to ensure that the overall tone is consistent with the topic, the information presented, and the public image of the agency presenting the material.

7. Whenever possible, the intended audience should be identified in the material. This will increase its perceived relevance to the people it is designed to reach and will avoid alienating those for whom it is inappropriate.

8. Each message should be simple—several points in a pamphlet, but no more than one or two in a poster, television spot, or radio spot.

9. Avoid exaggeration and moralizing, since either can cause the audience to reject the entire message. The sample caveat applies to assumptions or guesses presented as facts.

10. Avoid the use of well-known facts or examples.

11. Messages should offer a direct benefit— a reason for taking the recommended action— stated strongly, specifically, and in a way that makes it easy for the audience to visualize the

benefit. Whenever feasible, new aspects of the action or benefit should be emphasized.

12. The content of messages should be personal and specific to the concerns of the intended audience (rather than, for example, simple factual information about a particular health topic).

13. Special care should be taken to choose a spokesperson who is appropriate to both the message and its source and who will be believed by the target audience—someone who will be seen as knowledgeable, unbiased, likeable, noncontroversial, similar to the audience in some respects, and having the best interest of the audience at heart. For one message, a parent with a small child might be the best spokesperson; for another, an African-American physician; for another, a well-known person who has a particular health problem; and so on.

14. The results of using threat or fear appeals depend upon the situation, the audience's initial level of anxiety about the topic, the number of threats posed, the perceived effectiveness of actions that can be taken, and many other factors. Some amount of fear arousal increases the likelihood that people will act, but specifying (and inducing) the optimum level is extremely difficult. When dealing with high-fear topics such as cancer or AIDS, it may be better to offer reassurance than to emphasize risk, to *allay* fear rather than *arouse* it. Strong fear appeals seem to work better when they pose a threat to the audience's loved ones (rather than a direct personal threat), are presented by a highly credible source, deal with topics that are somewhat unfamiliar to the audience, and are directed to people with relatively low income and education, high self-esteem, and low perceived vulnerability to danger. If fear appeals are used at all, the audience should be in a position to take immediate action on the recommendations and should be given explicit instructions to help them do so.

15. If a message includes referral information (mail address, e-mail address, and/or phone number for inquiries), this information should be repeated, or left in sight for 5 seconds or longer, so the audience will have the opportunity to write it down. In the case of messages that last 30 to 60 seconds, it is often worthwhile to alert the audience at the outset that a number or address will be provided. Brief messages obviously cannot convey detailed information about a health problem or recommended behavior, but by providing toll-free phone numbers and Internet addresses they enable the most interested members of the audience to obtain such information directly.

REFERENCES

Anderson, R. (1989). Reassessing the odds against finding meaningful behavioral change in mass media health promotion campaigns. In C. Botan & V. Hazelton (Eds.), *Public relations theory*. Hillsdale, NJ: Erlbaum.

Annenberg School for Communication (1994). Immunizing inner-city minority children. *Newslink*. Philadelphia, PA: Annenberg School for Communication.

Atkin, C. K., & Arkin, E. B. (1990). Issues and initiatives in communicating health information. In C. Atkin & L. Wallack (Eds.), *Mass communication and public health: Complexities and conflicts* (pp. 13–40). Newbury Park, CA: Sage.

Atkin, C. K., & Freimuth, V. (1989). Formative evaluation research in campaign design. In R. E. Rice & C. K. Atkin (Eds.), *Public communication campaigns* (2nd ed.). Thousand Oaks, CA: Sage.

Backer, T. E., & Rogers, E. M. (Eds.). (1993). *Organizational aspects of health communication campaigns: What works?* Thousand Oaks, CA: Sage.

Backer, T. E., Rogers, E. M., & Sopory, P. (1992). *Designing health communication campaigns: What works?* Thousand Oaks, CA: Sage.

Bauman, K. E., Brown, J. D., Bryan, E. S., Fisher, L. A., Padgett, C. A., & Sweeney, J. M. (1988). Three mass media campaigns to prevent adolescent cigarette smoking. *Preventive Medicine, 17*, 510–530.

Brown, J. D., & Walsh-Childers, K. (1994). Effects of media on personal and public health. In J. Bryant, & D. Zillman (Eds.), *Media effects: Advances in theory and research* (pp. 389–415). Hillsdale, NJ: Erlbaum.

California Department of Health Services and Department of Education (1990). *Toward a tobacco-free California*. Sacramento: California Department of Health Services and Department of Education.

DeJong, W., & Atkin, C. K. (1995). A review of national television PSA campaigns for preventing alcohol-impaired driving, 1987–1992. *Journal of Public Health Policy* (Spring), 59–80.

Edwards, J., Tindale, R. S., Heath, L. & Posavac, E. J. (Eds.) (1990). *Social influence processes and prevention*. Ann Arbor, MI: Society for the Psychological Study of Social Issues.

Flay, B. R. (1987). Evaluation of the development, dissemination and effectiveness of mass media health programming. *Health Education Research, 2*, 123–130.

Flynn, B. S., Worden, J. K., Secker-Walker, R. H., Badger, G. J., Geller, B. M., & Constanza, M. C. (1992). Prevention of cigarette smoking through mass media intervention and school programs. *American Journal of Public Health, 82*, 827–834.

Fox, K. F. A., & Kotler, P. (1980). The marketing of social causes: The first ten years. *Journal of Marketing, 44* (Fall), 24–33.

Freimuth, V. S. (1990). Narrowing the cancer knowledge gap among blacks. Report prepared for the National Cancer Institute.

Freudenberg, N. (1989). *Preventing AIDS: A guide to effective education for the prevention of HIV infection.* Washington, DC: American Public Health Association.

Glanz, K., Lewis, F. M., & Rimer, B. K. (Eds.) (1990). *Health behavior and health education.* San Francisco: Jossey-Bass.

Graeff, J., Elder, J. P., & Booth, E. M. (1993). *Communication for health and behavioral change.* San Francisco: Jossey-Bass.

Green, L. W., & Lewis, F. M. (1986). *Measurement and evaluation in health education and health promotion.* Palo Alto, CA: Mayfield.

Jones, J. P. (1992). *How much is enough? Getting the most from your advertising dollar.* New York: Lexington Books.

Karsten, S., Bowler, A., Kasab, D., & Arkin, E. (1992). *Prospective evaluation of unified approaches to health communication.* Silver Spring, MD: Birch & Davis.

Klein, J. D., Brown, J. D., Childers, K. W., Oliveri, J., Porter, C., & Dykers, C. (1993). Adolescents' risky behavior and mass media use. *Pediatrics* (July), 24–31.

Lefebvre, C., & Flora, J. (1988). Social marketing and public health intervention. *Health Education Quarterly, 3*, 299–315.

Maccoby, N., & Alexander, J. (1980). Use of media in lifestyle programs. In P. Davidson & S. Davidson (Eds.), *Behavioral medicine: Changing health lifestyles* (pp. 351–370). New York: Brunner/Mazel.

Maibach, E., & Parrott, R. L. (Eds.) (1995). *Designing health messages: Approaches from communication theory and public health practice.* Thousand Oaks, CA: Sage.

Meade, C. D., McKinney, W. P. & Barnas, G. P. (1994). Educating patients with limited literacy skills: The effectiveness of printed and videotaped materials about colon cancer. *American Journal of Public Health* (January), 119–121.

Mielke, K. W., & Swinehart, J. W. (1976). *Evaluation of the "Feeling Good" television series.* New York: Children's Television Workshop.

Minnesota Department of Public Health (1991). *Minnesota tobacco-use prevention initiative 1989–1990.* Minneapolis: Minnesota Department of Public Health.

Murry, J. P. Jr., Stam, A., & Lastovicka, J. L. (1996). Paid- versus donated-media strategies for public service announcement campaigns. *Public Opinion Quarterly, 60*, 1–29.

National Cancer Institute. (1989). *Making health communication programs work.* NIH Publication No. 89-1493. Bethesda, MD: National Cancer Institute.

National Heart, Lung & Blood Institute. (1986). *National high blood pressure education program annual report.* Bethesda, MD: National Institutes of Health.

Public Communication Resources. (1988). Reactions of intended users and STD clinic counsellors to the FDA booklet *About Condoms.* Pelham Manor, NY: Public Communication Resources.

Public Communication Resources. (1989). Reactions of soft contact lens users to prototype package labels for homemade saline solution. Pelham Manor, NY: Public Communication Resources.

Public Health Service. (1990). *Promoting healthy diets and active lifestyles to lower-SES adults: Market research for public education.* Washington, DC: U.S. Department of Health and Human Services.

Rice, R. E., & Atkin, C. (1994). Principles of successful public information campaigns. In J. Bryant & D. Zillman (Eds.), *Media effects: Advances in theory and research* (pp. 365–387). Hillsdale, NJ: Erlbaum.

Sutton, S. (1982). Fear-arousing communications: A critical examination of theory and research. In J. R. Eisner (Ed.), *Social psychology and behavioral medicine* (pp. 303–337). New York: Wiley.

Swinehart, J. W. (1981). *A descriptive review of selected mass media campaigns on highway safety.* Washington, DC: National Highway Traffic Safety Administration.

Swinehart, J. W. (1991). Tailoring the message to the audience. In A. Fisher, M. Pavlova, & V. Covello (Eds.), *Evaluation and effective risk communications* (pp. 73–81). Washington DC: Environmental Protection Agency.

UniWorld Group. (1982). Study of radio station preferences regarding programming and public service announcements. Bethesda, MD: UniWorld Group.

Vingilis, E., & Coultes, B. (1990). Mass communications and drinking-driving: Theories, practices and results. *Alcohol, Drugs and Driving* (April–June), 61–81.

Wallack, L., Dorfman, L., Jernigan, D., & Themba, M. (1993). *Media advocacy and public health.* Thousand Oaks, CA: Sage.

Worden, J. K., Flynn, B. S., Geller, B. M., Chen, M., Shelton, L. G., Secker-Walker, R. H., Solomon, D. S., Solomon, L. J., Couchey, S., & Constanza, M. C. (1988). Development of a smoking prevention mass media program using diagnostic and formative research. *Preventive Medicine, 17*, 531–558.

Worden, J. K., Waller, J. A., & Riley, T. J. (1975). The Vermont public education campaign in alcohol and highway safety: A final review and evaluation. Montpelier: Vermont Department of Mental Health.

Zillman, D., & Bryant, J. (1985). *Selective exposure to communication.* Hillsdale, NJ: Erlbaum.

IV

TOWARD THE FUTURE

An Integration

Part IV begins with a chapter that integrates the content of this volume on the relevance of health behavior research for professional training and applications. A second level of integration is presented in a chapter that examines four social (or behavioral) science disciplines that have major involvements in health behavior research. In addition to identifying the ways in which health psychology, medical anthropology, medical geography, and medical sociology have contributed to understanding health behavior, the chapter provides an integrating discussion of the issues they face as they pursue their investigations into the

21st century, particularly around the common factor of their relationship with medicine. The chapter then analyzes issues of the identity of health behavior and offers recommendations that will heighten and secure this identity. The chapter culminates with a proposed "work-in-progress" matrix for organizing health behavior knowledge.

The Glossary of health behavior concepts and definitions integrates material from all four volumes of this *Handbook*. Finally, this volume provides an Index to Volumes I–IV.

19

Relevance of Health Behavior Research

An Integration of Applications

David S. Gochman

This chapter integrates major points and findings presented in Volume IV. Although its contents reflect primarily the contributions to this volume rather than the larger body of scholarship about the relevance of health behavior research, the contents are nonetheless congruent with such knowledge. The nature of this volume precludes using the same matrix organizing structure underlying the integrations in Volumes I through III. It proved unwieldy to coordinate categories of health behaviors with personal, social, and institutional systems as levels of analysis for these applications.

The chapter discusses the relevance of health behavior research for professional practice, its place in professional socialization, and its relevance for planned interventions. It continues with discussion of some common themes and issues and concludes by identifying some directions for future research.

PROFESSIONAL PRACTICE

Relevant Knowledge and Theory

The importance for health professionals of empirical findings and conceptual models from health behavior research is discussed throughout the other volumes of this *Handbook*, but it is treated more systematically and documented more explicitly in this one. Knowledge of every type of health behavior, and of all the personal, social, and health institutional influences upon them, is meaningful and relevant to a broad spectrum of professional applications.

For example, Bruhn (Chapter 1) calls attention to the professional's need to understand health cognitions, including the diverse meanings of health for different people, the role of such meanings within an individual's total cognitive framework, and the relationship between

David S. Gochman • Kent School of Social Work, University of Louisville, Louisville, Kentucky 40292.

Handbook of Health Behavior Research IV: Relevance for Professionals and Issues for the Future, edited by David S. Gochman. Plenum Press, New York, 1997.

personal values and engaging in health-promoting behavior. He further emphasizes the importance for health professionals of understanding the concept of risk perception; the linkage between high uncertainty and erroneous attributions of illness with delay in care seeking; and the factors that underlie people's reluctance to give up gratifying behavior.

Bruhn stresses the importance for professionals of understanding that health behaviors have multiple determinants and are particularly influenced by developmental levels, the family, social networks, community institutions, and cultural values; that prevention occurs at multiple levels; and that behaviors can be risk factors as well as vehicles for restoring and maintaining health. The importance for health professionals of understanding the family's role in protecting an individual against the emergence of a risk behavior is particularly noted, as is the linkage between adherence to regimens and the patterns of interaction between professionals and patients, particularly data showing the inappropriateness of the traditional model of an active professional and a submissive patient.

Although health professionals themselves are often role models for health behaviors, they remain only one part of healing and health maintenance (Bruhn). Furthermore, health professionals often do not feel competent in fostering preventive behaviors and believe that health promotion is too time-consuming (Bruhn). Health care institutions themselves fail to reward the preventive and health-promoting activities of health professionals and instead reward curing disease (Bruhn).

Medicine. Health behavior research, stressing as it does the human agency and its social context, is a marked contrast to the mechanistic disease model that has traditionally served as a model for medicine and medical education (Reed, Moore-West, Jernstedt, & O'Donnell, Chapter 2; Wiese & Gallagher, Chapter 4). According to this model, sometimes referred to as "Pasteur's doctrine of specific etiology," there is no need to

know about any individual patient (Wiese & Gallagher). There is, however, continuing accrual of evidence that the medical model is insufficient to account for differential responses to conditions or for the very broad range of patient and family behaviors that come into play in illness. Heightened awareness that this model cannot deal with the inadequacies of medical care (e.g., Reed et al.), the burden of chronic conditions, changes in mortality patterns (Flipse, Chapter 3), increased and deep patient dissatisfaction, and changing social attitudes about health care (e.g., Wiese & Gallagher) mandate a shift away from it.

Good communication between patient and physician is a critical factor in the interrelated issues of adherence, remaining in care, and patient satisfaction (DiMatteo, this *Handbook*, Volume II, Chapter 1). Health behavior research is important not only for developing improved communication between physicians and patients in clinical encounters, but also for strengthening community service programs (Reed et al.). Wiese and Gallagher observe that patients' perceptions of their relationships with physicians are more important to them than their physicians' technical skills. Yet, they point out, while improved communication is so vital, especially in interviewing, and inadequate communication can lead to dissatisfaction and malpractice litigation, physicians ignore opportunities for improving communication, such as the times when they obtain informed consent, explain pathology and pharmacology, or prescribe medicines.

Flipse emphasizes the role of health behavior research in establishing the importance of the meanings that patients and their families attach to an illness or condition, how the patient has been "educated about illness," the patient's explanatory models, and the difference between local, regional, and national perceptions of different health issues. Such meanings and perceptions underlie the decision processes that lead to the negotiation of a successful treatment plan. They are also related to the physician's ability to assess how a patient will respond to a regimen. She further notes the importance of recognizing cultural differences in languages of distress and use of folk terminology.

Health behavior research findings suggest the need for physicians to recognize the relativity of their own perceptions about illness, to appreciate that chronic pain and intensive-care-unit psychosis are issues in perception rather than physiology, and to be able to gauge the patient's own ability to understand (Wiese & Gallagher). Wiese and Gallagher also stress the importance of physicians understanding culture-specific frameworks for medical practice and the culture-specific nature of stigma for conditions such as obesity, and of recognizing a floating set point for patients' interpretations of symptoms for conditions such as goiter and obesity. Health behavior data on perceptions of waiting time, encroachments on personal modesty and privacy, the importance of child care arrangements, and the activities of patient advocates provide compelling rationales for more user-friendly institutions, in order to generate higher levels of patient satisfaction with care (Wiese & Gallagher). Moreover, health behavior research shows that stigma, along with the patient's occupying a less powerful role, can subvert therapies (Wiese & Gallagher).

Flipse points to the role of the health belief model and other perceptual variables in attempts at changing individual behavior and to the barriers to such change presented by unrealistic optimism. Such health behavior research is an important component of the model curriculum at the University of Miami School of Medicine, which Flipse describes. Health behavior research also increases the ability of physicians to understand the determinants of care-seeking behavior and the role played in this behavior by interpersonal crises and individual and cultural variation in symptom perception, and to reach underserved populations, particularly in terms of the role of demographic factors in use of free screenings (Flipse). Health behavior research also sheds light on health institution factors, such as health promotion campaigns that lead to an "epidemic of apprehension" and inappropriately assign re-

sponsibility for health status to the individual (Flipse).

Wiese and Gallagher also emphasize the importance of beliefs, perceptions, and other cognitions, calling attention to the relativity of such cognitions as well as their cultural contexts. They note in addition the importance of health behavior research in broadening physicians' perspective on definitions of health, illness, and stigma.

Nursing. More so than practitioners of the other clinical health professions, nurses have embraced health behavior research, have found it relevant to a wide range of their activities, and have contributed substantially to its knowledge base. Knowledge about perceptions of health and illness, belief structures, attitudes toward health practices and treatment regimens, social support, and barriers to behavior have been used to develop individualized nursing interventions directed at improving patient self care and health status, as well as health promotion interventions to maintain and improve the health of well persons (Blue & Brooks, Chapter 5). Conceptual models from health behavior research, particularly the health belief model, social cognitive theory, the theory of reasoned action, and locus of control models, have proven especially suitable for nursing health promotion activities at the community health level, more so than for "supportive" nursing care (Blue & Brooks). Health behavior research has been used to guide the development of "relationship models," health promotion models, interaction models, theory of care-seeking models, self-care system models, and resource models of preventive behavior (Blue & Brooks).

Nursing has taken methodological initiatives resulting in the development of diverse instruments, such as measures of cognitions related to breast self-examination; perceptions of benefits of and barriers to exercise; self management; social support; self-efficacy measures related to diabetes, cardiac rehabilitation, and epilepsy; health-promoting lifestyles; and health self-determination. It has also operationalized knowledge from health behavior research in the development of specific nursing diagnoses, which constitute a classification system for structuring nursing knowledge, guiding nursing research, and directing nursing care (Blue & Brooks). Among the diagnostic categories that are directly linked to health behavior research are health maintenance, health-seeking behavior, risk for injury, management of regimen, and noncompliance. These categories all include the issue of client–professional interaction, itself an important area of health behavior research.

Social Work. Health behavior research can provide social workers with knowledge about developmental, family, social, and community factors that underlie adherence to regimens (Levy, Chapter 6). It thus informs their efforts to provide physicians with knowledge about patients and families relevant to ability to adhere, particularly family characteristics that may be barriers to adherence. Levy further notes findings showing that adherence is increased to the degree that professionals convey a sense of caring and to the degree that patients become involved in their own treatment.

Knowledge about organizational, institutional, and community determinants of health behavior is also relevant to the role of the social worker as an advocate for social change. Social work recognizes the importance of perceptions, particularly of opportunities to improve health, of the health problem itself, and of the meanings attached to the problem. Furthermore, social work draws on health behavior research in increasing its understanding of the impact of illness on individuals and families, of risk behaviors, and of the cultural determinants of perceptions of suffering.

Social workers are involved in interventions in a number of areas such as risk behaviors, especially substance abuse, prevention of pregnancy, and reducing high-risk sex behaviors in gay men; use of emergency rooms; coping with diseases such as AIDS and cancer; patient education; and

community-based health promotion, all of which draw heavily upon knowledge generated by health behavior research. Particularly relevant to social work are social learning and sick role concepts (Levy).

Health behavior knowledge about the impact of cultural norms and family beliefs on the choice of caregiver enables social workers to increase their clients' perceptions of alternative care-seeking patterns and treatments. Moreover, health behavior research has the potential of improving the attempts of social workers to tailor interventions specifically to individuals (Levy).

Health behavior research knowledge has sensitized social workers to multiple drug use in the elderly and has led them into working cooperatively with pharmacists to initiate and use "medication" profiles. Knowledge generated by health behavior research has also drawn social workers into collaborative arrangements with dentists around prevention and into women's health issues such as irritable bowel syndrome and inappropriate urological procedures (Levy).

Dentistry. Dentistry has been involved in health behavior research since the 1950s, and the relevance of such research has been especially recognized in the areas of compliance and prevention, since most oral diseases are preventable (Gift & White, Chapter 7). Furthermore, oral health professionals have long been concerned with patients' disproportionate fear of dental visits, especially as this fear is related to developmental characteristics of younger patients. Health behavior research has helped dentists understand some of the factors that underlie the anxieties of dental visits, particularly the factors related to gender. It has also shown dentists the importance of recognizing pain as a perceptual issue rather than as an issue of tissue damage (Gift & White).

Though dentists are concerned with problems in adherence and have been actively involved in compliance research, there have been few studies dealing with the role of the dentist as a factor in increasing compliance (Gift & White).

Dentists deny that communication is as important as technical skill; they focus on compliance rather than on collaboration. The structure of dental care itself reinforces a traditional model of the practitioner–patient role that negates the value of the communication necessary for successful adherence. Dentists are not confident of their own abilities to deal with patients' anxiety and fears. Although good communication can reduce dentists' problems with young patients, dentists tend, instead, to label such youngsters as "problem children." Health behavior research has shown that adherence to orthodontia is related to the patient's motivation, to the perceptions of the value of the treatment, to cognitive competence, and to a patient's having some knowledge of oral health (Gift & White).

Health behavior research has shown that despite an abundance of information, people in general are still unable to identify symptoms of dental disease (Gift & White). It has also shown that a dentist's own preventive orientation, provision of preventive services, and oral hygiene instruction by a professional, as well as a facilitative environment, are important factors in increasing levels of preventive behavior and oral health. Too often, however, dentists do not recognize that instruction alone is not sufficient. Health behavior research has also shown dentists that preventive behaviors cluster. Brushing, flossing, use of fluoride, trauma protection, avoidance of alcohol and tobacco, and asymptomatic dental visits all seem to be correlated with one another. They are all also related to developmental levels, but are not as much related to a person's beliefs as they are to social supports and social norms (Gift & White).

In addition to their concern about dental hygiene behaviors, oral health professionals are increasingly concerned about risk behaviors such as use of alcohol and tobacco (Gift & White). Few oral health professionals, however, have appropriate levels of training in smoking cessation. They believe they should be good role models, but are less certain of strategies for risk reduction (Gift & White).

The health services utilization model has been useful to dentists in understanding preventive behavior (Gift & White). A decrease in the population's fatalistic beliefs about dental diseases and increased access to dental care has not translated to an increase in asymptomatic dental visits. Preventive dental visits have been found to be linked to perceived need and knowledge of the system; regularity of care-seeking has been found to be related to beliefs about self-efficacy. Availability of transportation and location of facilities are linked to the likelihood of using services. A dentist's negative attitudes, or lack of experience and knowledge of populations with disabilities or of populations with stigmatized conditions such as AIDS/HIV, are often barriers to care seeking in such populations (Gift & White).

Gift and White further indicate that although oral health issues have been an important focus of health behavior research, and dentists have long been involved in developing and conducting such research, findings have not been incorporated appreciably into dental practice. For example, dental practitioners have been slow to grasp the replicated evidence that single instructional sessions are insufficient to support behavioral changes necessary for maintaining and improving oral health. While dentists have increased their provision of preventive services, their use of hygienists, and their provision of information about diet, nutrition, and plaque control, the profession itself does not foster a level of collaborative work with other professionals that would increase levels of preventive behavior. Moreover, what happens during a dental visit—the nature of the encounter between dentist and patient—has not been extensively studied (Gift & White).

Public Health. Knowledge generated by health behavior research is germane to a number of areas within public health (Buchanan, Chapter 9). Knowledge about personal risk factors is especially appropriate for school- and community-based programs, occupational health and safety, and environmental health. Public health draws upon behavioral theories such as the health belief model, social learning theory, social marketing, and community organization.

Buchanan notes the importance for public health professionals of health behavior knowledge of family and social factors that can increase a person's resistance to the emergence of a risk behavior as well as to some types of peer pressure that encourage such behavior. At the same time, Buchanan notes that the level of evidence for such resilience and protective factors is minimal compared to the evidence on the impact of biological risks. Knowledge related to resistance to change is especially related to issues of maternal and child health, particularly in developing countries (Buchanan).

The public health analogy of the medical model is Koch's Postulates, which stipulate a single agent, with uniform impact, for every disease (Buchanan). As in medicine, this model, though it served very well for acute, infectious diseases, has been insufficient to account equally for the realities of chronic conditions, for which probabilistic models, acknowledging the role of the host and of behavioral risk factors, are more valid.

Buchanan observes, moreover, that British data strongly indicate that socioeconomic conditions contribute more substantially to risk than do lifestyles and that material factors, rather than the behavior of the human host, should be a focus for public health professionals. Buchanan also notes the United States Surgeon General's reports in which national health status objectives are linked to a large array of modifiable behaviors. The assumption that information (or knowledge) leads to actions, which underlies the recommendations stemming from these reports, is rendered untenable by health behavior research. For example, as Buchanan notes, health behavior research has shown that personal beliefs, particularly about control over risk, affect an individual's interpretation of knowledge and information and thus a person's perception of risk. Health behavior knowledge indicates that public health behavioral interventions at the population

level are of greater consequence than those targeted only at individuals (Buchanan).

Health behavior research has also increased understanding of the population's overreaction to exposure to certain types of toxic substances that carry very low levels of risks in relation to the lack of any reaction at all to other types of exposures that often pose much greater risks (Buchanan). These overreactions are related to whether such exposure is perceived to be under the individual's control; those exposures over which persons have no control tend to generate the overreaction. The media also promote much confusion about food and nutritional patterns in their reporting of contradictory findings. Such coverage generates public skepticism about scientific knowledge and subsequently vitiates behavioral change (Buchanan).

Health Promotion and Health Education. Health behavior research is at the core of health promotion and health education (HP/HE) efforts (Glanz & Oldenburg, Chapter 8). Such efforts have drawn on the health belief model, social learning theories, the theory of reasoned action, and stages of change models. At the same time, Glanz and Oldenburg acknowledge that there is no full empirical assessment of the degree to which health behavior knowledge affects professional practice in these areas. The literature, they report, reflects innovations rather than "normative" practice.

More important are Glanz and Oldenburg's observations that behavioral change in communities often occurs independently of planned interventions, challenging the magnitude of the impact of these interventions, raising questions about their underlying assumptions and conceptual frameworks, and cautioning against widespread adoption of intervention models in the absence of health behavior data on their impacts. Glanz and Oldenburg suggest that health promotion and health education interventions and programs be multilevel; that they have clinical, family, community, and worksite components; and that they not be driven by any single health behavior theory or model, but draw broadly on a number of such theories and models.

Barriers to incorporating health behavior research knowledge in HP/HE include the quality of instruction in teaching these concepts, basic gaps in health behavior knowledge, the lack of linkages between the concepts and the real world, inadequacies in the planning of interventions and in theoretical research, and on underestimation of barriers to diffusion and implementation (Glanz & Oldenburg). Especially critical gaps in health behavior knowledge exist in relation to underserved populations; little is known about the health behavior of Asian-Americans and other ethnic populations. Questions arise about whether frameworks such as the health belief model and others that were normed largely on nonethnic, middle-class Americans will have as much value for other groups (Glanz & Oldenburg).

Health Management and Health Policy. Although health behavior research has great potential for health administration, management, and policy, health care managers have had little in the way of health behavior data to guide their decisions and actions and have drawn to a greater degree from the larger body of general consumer behavior research (Daugherty, Chapter 10). Although a body of research exists on physician–patient interactions and their outcomes and on how organizational policies affect care seeking, there has been minimal parallel investigation of how various aspects of management behavior are linked to organizational outcomes. Health behavior research has likewise not addressed the implications of the movement of care—especially managed care—away from hospitals into community settings or the influences of an interorganizational service delivery system on care seeking, adherence, or satisfaction with care.

To the great detriment of the effectiveness of health policies, relevant findings from health behavior research have been largely ignored by policy makers. Robertson (Chapter 12) and Cummings (Chapter 13) both point out that accumulated health behavior research data showing the relatively minimal benefits of programs and interventions to change individual risk behaviors compared to the benefits of making changes in the "system" have had little or no impact on policies relating to injury reduction or smoking. Yet data show the more appreciable impact of institutional changes, e.g., those relating to use of seat belts and production of safer windows. Media campaigns directed at helmet use and jaywalking often ignore accumulated and available health behavior data. Moreover, Robertson questions the validity of the assumption underlying many programs that knowledge about behavioral risks produces changes in behavior.

Drawing upon health behavior knowledge, Robertson calls attention to the importance of differentiating between risk taking and risk denial. Persons often engage in "risk behavior," not as a result of a conscious decision to take a risk, but in the absence of an awareness that the act is dangerous. Evidence that it is easier to initiate or change a one-time behavior than to change an ongoing one affirms the far greater importance for injury control of a decision to purchase a safer vehicle than of use of seat belts (Robertson). Health behavior research also reveals that persuasion campaigns aimed at increasing safety and reducing injuries can have unintended opposite results. Encouraging participation in a driver education program had no impact on reducing injuries; instead, although the percentage of fatal crashes remained the same, the driver safety program increased the number of inexperienced drivers on the road and thus increased the overall number of fatalities. Finally, Robertson notes the degree to which institutional factors, such as media and corporations, mislead the public about safety and injury control issues.

Smoking policies are too often based on the assumption that smoking is an informed choice, and although there is limited empirical support for some cognitive models of smoking, health behavior data show that it is an addiction and that the assumption is untenable (Cummings). Noncognitive theories underscore the smoker as a victim in need of help. The policy implications of this view remain largely ignored. Governmental smoking policies remain geared to providing the individual with information necessary for an informed decision, in the hope that this information will lead to behavioral change, even though health behavior data show the weakness of negative future events as determinants of behavior compared to the strength of present satisfaction. Instead, governmental policies should be based on the knowledge that smoking is an addictive behavior, appropriately subject to governmental regulation and control. Rather than simply provide information, policies should provide for tort damage against cigarette manufacturers, as well as for free or low-cost smoking cessation clinics, protection of nonsmokers, and limitations on smoking behavior. Health behavior knowledge relevant to tobacco policies also includes evidence that increasing numbers of young women are initiating smoking, as well as evidence for the inverse relationship between smoking and tobacco use and social class and for the increased use of smokeless tobacco (Cummings).

Available data also would have indicated to policy makers that the overly lengthy and small warnings on cigarette packages would have no impact on reducing smoking, while increasing cigarette taxes would have an impact, but such data are ignored in policy formulation and change. Other data have begun to suggest that institutional changes such as smoke-free environments, lowering insurance premiums for nonsmokers, and restrictions on sales to minors do have an impact on smoking reduction, as have the increased number of product liability suits. In addition, such policy changes are seen as symbolizing and reinforcing social antismoking norms (Cummings).

Nilstun (Chapter 11) cautions about the ethical issues—derived more from social theory and philosophy than from health behavior research—involved in implementing social policy such as restrictions on smoking behavior. Nilstun calls

attention to the paternalism and infringement on personal autonomy often inherent in such policies and raises questions about whether health behavior data justify such paternalism.

Summary: A Potential Ignored

The chapters in this volume together with much material in Volume II of this *Handbook* indicate that while health behavior research knowledge has great potential for enriching professional activities, it has yet to be appreciably incorporated into a large number of these activities, particularly in medicine, dentistry, and health management and policy. Confirming this lack is Flipse's observation (Chapter 3) that literature searches do not support the obviousness of the relevance of health behavior research. The entire domain of communication, and the importance of appreciating a range of personal and social systems, are two salient points for health professionals.

Communication. Of great relevance to medicine, dentistry, nursing, and social work are health behavior research findings on the encounter between professionals and patients, particularly knowledge about communication and the factors that communication can improve. Yet communication skills remain ignored by and large in medicine and dentistry. "Cognitive" services, including those involving good communication, receive lower reimbursements than technological ones (Wiese & Gallagher, Chapter 4). Nursing, more than the other professions, incorporates health behavior knowledge about communication in clinical as well as community health promotion interventions (Blue & Brooks, Chapter 5). Social work emphasizes communication and interpersonal skills, but has not systematically drawn upon health behavior research as a foundation for increasing and improving communication in health settings (Levy, Chapter 6).

Personal and Social Systems. Of great relevance to public health, HP/HE, and health man-

agement and policy interventions are health behavior research findings showing the interaction
between different personal and social systems—
or social entities—and populations and sub-
populations. Yet with few exceptions, knowledge about how such systems affect behavior
remains ignored in the development of interventions, programs, and policies.

Prevalence in Professional Socialization

Medicine. Despite the relevance of health
behavior research to producing a new breed of
physician better equipped to foster the promotion of healthy lifestyles and to empower people
as competent consumers of health services (Bruhn,
Chapter 11), health behavior research is neglected or overlooked in medical training and
socialization and occupies a minimal and marginalized place in the medical curriculum. At the
same time, there is strong consensus about the
inappropriateness of the traditional mechanistic,
pathogenic, medical model for understanding
and dealing with the health issues of the 1990s
and early 21st century; thus, there is a great need
for change and restructuring within medical education, particularly to counterbalance the narrow emphasis on technology (Bruhn, Reed et al.,
Chapter 2; Flipse, Chapter 3; Wiese & Gallagher,
Chapter 4). Yet despite waves of self-examination,
no real change has occurred (Bruhn). There is
little time available in the curriculum to offer
basic health behavior content such as material on
community health promotion or patient education, and students report inadequate coverage of
behavioral science content (Reed et al.).

Major barriers to real change include not
only the prevailing, yet discredited, mechanistic
medical model, but also the manner in which a
good share of medical education is financed,
whereby payments are given to teaching hospitals for clinical services and research activities
rather than for less tangible components of care
(Reed et al.). Moreover, the decentralized decision making of medical school faculties makes

overall curricular change difficult (Reed et al.).
Furthermore, an admissions process that typically overvalues competence in basic hard sciences at the expense of communication and interpersonal skills (Reed et al., Wiese & Gallagher,
Chapter 4) does little to encourage entry of persons with appropriate interpersonal skills.

Reed et al. also observe that there are a
diminishing number of departments of behavioral sciences in United States medical schools
and that behavioral sciences are often contained
within departments of psychiatry and family
medicine rather than diffused throughout the
institution. If health behavior research is to
be incorporated into the curriculum, it must be
valued and used by the physicians and medical
educators who serve as role models for medical
students (Flipse). Yet physicians who have themselves survived the gauntlet of medical training
have little interest in changing it or in increasing
student exposure to community clinical experiences, prevention, or epidemiology (Wiese &
Gallagher). Wiese and Gallagher further note that
medical schools and hospitals are self-sustaining
microcosms, and thus insensitive to pressures to
change, and that administrators of large teaching
hospitals have capital investments in maintaining
the institutional status quo.

The Flexner Report, which rationalized
medical practice and established standards for
medical training in the United States, also led to
the removal of students from regular contact
with the community—where they would have
had an opportunity to observe the social context
of their patients' lives and behavior—and to their
insulation and isolation within hospitals (Wiese
& Gallagher). Teaching hospitals, in which so
much medical education is conducted, expose
students to the sickest of the sick and not to the
95% of the population that they will eventually
serve (Flipse).

Nursing. Nursing education is moving away
from a narrow clinical definition of the role of
nursing and toward a role that increases nursing's
involvement in health promotion and disease

prevention (Blue & Brooks, Chapter 5). Nearly all baccalaureate programs in nursing include health behavior concepts, although there is no unanimity about how critical these concepts are to nursing education (Blue & Brooks). While graduate-level training provides nurses with knowledge of health behavior conceptual and theoretical models, Blue and Brooks suggest that such models need to be incorporated within the baccalaureate generalist programs to supplement the health behavior concepts already taught. Moreover, they suggest that nursing curricula should reflect a broad spectrum of health behavior knowledge at all levels. Undergraduate programs are oriented to concepts of illness behavior and sick role behaviors, but not to behaviors related to maximizing health. Graduate programs should require content that will generate at least some understanding of health promotion concepts and should integrate the theoretical models that underlie health promotion and health-protecting behavior throughout the curriculum, not just include them in discrete health promotion courses. Although Blue and Brooks note a lag in textbook treatment of health behavior knowledge, they observe that texts are increasingly incorporating health behavior material, particularly in relation to community-level interventions.

Social Work. Although health behavior content *may* be found throughout the curriculum in terms of issues related to diversity and to personal, family, social, and cultural factors as determinants of behavior, there is generally little formal attention to health behavior research content as such (Levy, Chapter 6). Social work as a profession has historically been skeptical of empiricism and has been reluctant to become involved with, or endorse, research.

Dentistry. Dental education is conducted almost exclusively within dental schools, as opposed to community settings, and has a highly technological focus. Curriculum guidelines contain expectations about behavioral science, but this coverage is not mandated (Gift & White,

Chapter 7). Gift and White estimate that the total behavioral science context (not broken down into health behavior versus other behavioral material) in dental curricula is about 3% and that there is little evaluation of students' behavioral science competency. Findings from health behavior research have thus not moved appreciably into dental education and training.

Dental students themselves are conventional, conforming, and technology-oriented, and they seek a professional career that will grant them relative independence (Gift & White). To the degree that dental education disproportionately fosters their interest in technology, it does not enhance their communication or interpersonal skills. Nor do faculty seem to be mentoring such skills.

Public Health. Schools of public health are required to demonstrate that their curricula develop professional competence in "identifying the role of cultural, social and behavioral factors in determining disease, disease prevention, health promoting behavior, and medical service organization and delivery" (Sorenson & Bialek, Faculty/Agency Forum, cited in Buchanan, Chapter 9). All public health professionals are thus expected to have a working knowledge of health behavior research.

Health Promotion and Health Education. Although competency guidelines exist for professional training at the undergraduate level in HP/HE, these guidelines do not explicitly refer to health behavior content; such material may be either pervasive or minimal (Glanz & Oldenburg, Chapter 8). Glanz and Oldenburg estimate that the reality is somewhere between these extremes, with concrete knowledge about health disease and related behavioral factors being a more likely focus than theory, research, and data.

At the graduate level, although there is no analogous competency framework, the Council on Education for Public Health requires courses in health behavior theory and relevant research methods. Yet Glanz and Oldenburg report that only about a third of the HP/HE programs in schools of public health and far fewer outside formal schools of public health require a program-planning course in which this content would reasonably be expected. Such findings may underestimate this content, since many schools have full courses in health behavior, and several departments of health promotion and health education have added "health behavior" to their names. Regardless of these findings, coverage of health behavior content has increased since the early 1980s, not only in North America but also in Australia and in a number of European countries, particularly the Netherlands (Glanz & Oldenburg).

Health Management and Health Policy. There are no formal health behavior research components in the training of health management or health policy makers. As a matter of fact, there are generally no requirements for any level of knowledge or skill of any sort for such positions or activities (e.g., Daugherty, Chapter 10).

Programmatic Interventions: Health Promotion and Health Education

Health behavior research has great relevance for health promotion programs, yet interventions directed at schools, communities, families, and worksites often draw on health behavior knowledge in a random, unsystematic way.

School-Based Programs. Recognizing the risks that adolescents face for social morbidities, such as unintended pregnancies, sexually transmitted diseases, homicides, suicides, injuries related to violence, and substance abuse, and for behavioral morbidities, such as poor nutrition, inadequate exercise, and tobacco use, Kelder, Edmundson, and Lytle (Chapter 14) show the way in which health behavior research can successfully drive school-based programs. The traditional assumption that if students understand the negative consequences of behaviors they will decide not to engage in them is contradicted by

health behavior research showing the failure of intervention models based on this assumption. The credibility of interventions has been undermined by programs conveying myths and inaccuracies, such as those that make use of the movie "Reefer Madness."

Successful school-based programs aimed at smoking, alcohol and drug use, nutrition, exercise, and sex education tend to be those that draw upon multiple sources of health behavior knowledge—knowledge about human development, about families, about peer influences, and about social, institutional, and community factors—and incorporate all or nearly all of these factors in an intervention or series of interventions. Health behavior research has shown the value of direct modeling by adults based on social learning theory, social cognitive theory, and inoculation techniques, and of continuous rather than one-shot interventions. For example, health behavior research has shown that fostering parent education and in-home learning, with the parents involved in activities with the child, increases program effectiveness. Parental attitudes are themselves observed to be linked to risk behaviors, and parents have some control over peer group influences. Health behavior research showing that a family's food context is shaped more by parents' preferences and habits than by their nutritional knowledge is also relevant to school-based interventions.

Health behavior research showing how social pressures affect the initiation of risk behaviors, particularly substance abuse, are also relevant to school-based programs, as is research showing that minority/majority differences in violent behaviors disappear when socioeconomic status is controlled (Kelder et al.). Health behavior research has shown the importance of considering multiple levels of community institutions, the role of endorsement by health care institutions in legitimating programs and interventions, and the inclusion of practitioners' office-based components in increasing their success (Schooler & Flora, Chapter 15).

While health behavior research has also

proven useful in shaping the curricular parts of school programs, it has also shown the failure of programs that are based purely on imparting knowledge and information (Kelder et al.). School programs increase in effectiveness to the degree that they go beyond imparting information and incorporate mass media, parental involvement, and school policy changes in areas such as cafeteria food selections and nutritional standards, recreational programs, school-wide smoking bans, parental fines, and loss of athletic eligibility for fighting (Kelder et al.; Schooler & Flora). In particular, programs with community components and reinforcement are better able to catch students who leave school, who are usually those at greatest risk. Health behavior research has also shown the strength of cultural values as barriers to implementation of sex education programs and of data collection in relation to sex. These barriers have led to inadequate curricular material on gender and sexual orientation biases.

In addition, health behavior research has been helpful in identifying behaviors that are resistant to interventions, such as the onset of use of alcohol, and in pointing out the relative lack of success of programs based solely on providing information or knowledge, or on self-esteem, or values clarification, and of slogan-driven, marketing-focused programs such as the large-scale and highly touted DARE (Kelder et al.).

Community-Based Programs.   Schooler and Flora (Chapter 15) note the value of health behavior research in identifying multiple audiences for specifically tailored interventions in community-based health promotion programs and the characteristics of persons most likely to change their behaviors. Health behavior research data on social characteristics enable community intervention programs to encourage interactions among social networks and community subgroups to foster behavior change. Health behavior research data on ethnicity and other subcultural differences, and on educational levels, facilitate tailoring different messages to different community segments.

Health behavior research data on the distinc-

tive characteristics of different channels of communication, on the differential impact of different media, and on how media interact with other community institutions also increase the success of community-based programs (Schooler & Flora; Swinehart, Chapter 18). Health behavior research data further emphasize the importance of beginning with the community's own definition of its needs; of empowering and mobilizing the community as a social entity; of focusing on changes in institutions such as schools, worksites, restaurants, markets and shops, religious facilities and houses of worship; and of changes in laws and policies (Schooler & Flora). Furthermore, health behavior research has demonstrated the importance of incorporating components of the community's health care system, including office-based programs, into interventions to provide them with legitimation (Schooler & Flora).

Family-Based Programs.   Family-based interventions are often based on an assumed rather than a demonstrated understanding of family health behavior (Baranowski & Hearn, Chapter 16). Very few of the large number of family-based interventions undertaken by health professionals have been proven to be effective; the larger number generate equivocal data of success, particularly for behavioral modification programs. Yet health behavior research knowledge has the potential to increase the effectiveness of such interventions.

Available data do suggest, however, that the degree of family member involvement and of social network support has an impact on changing both feeding and breast-feeding behaviors (Baranowski & Hearn). Moreover, institutional encouragement of breast-feeding within the hospital leads to increased rates in developing countries. Baranowski and Hearn also note that knowledge of the "oppositional stage" in child development could have been relevant to increasing the success of some family-based programs.

Worksite-Based Programs.   Health behavior research data on workers' reactions to actual workplace disasters, derived from a large body of mine safety reports, form the basis for narrative interventions designed to improve occupational safety (Cole, Chapter 17). Narratives, or stories, are powerful ways of translating what is socially relevant into what is personally relevant; they integrate cultural tales with cognitive and behavior components. Data emerging from health behavior research suggested that purely behavioral interventions were insufficient to improve workplace safety behavior and that stories that had authenticity in terms of the lives, culture, plight, and language of workers might be more effective in generating behavioral change. Their effectiveness, moreover, would be increased to the degree that the interventions were also informed by health behavior knowledge of variability in individual decision-making processes and skills, fatigue, inexperience, lack of knowledge, "faulty" attitudes, and misconceptions, and by knowledge of workers' anticipation and recognition of potential hazards. Cole also draws attention to the organizational and engineering antecedents of decision-making errors.

Media and Communication Campaigns. Data from health behavior research have relevance for media campaigns targeted at behavioral change. Such data show that audiences may not actually receive the message, may ignore it, may misinterpret it, or may not believe it (Swinehart, Chapter 18). Health behavior research data about the ease or difficulty of changing behaviors and about the segmentation of an audience are also relevant to increasing the success of a media campaign. Furthermore, health behavior research data can often point out erroneous assumptions held by professionals about audience beliefs; e.g., parental beliefs and understanding of immunizations, and thus change the shape of a campaign (Swinehart).

Swinehart presents some cogent examples of how health behavior research improved media campaigns. Data on African-Americans' perceptions and beliefs about cancer, on women's specific fears about breast cancer, on workers' beliefs about mental health treatment, and on teenagers' beliefs about addiction changed the

nature and thus enhanced the effectiveness of media campaigns directed at these respective target audiences.

COMMON THEMES

Themes that emerge from a number of chapters include those related to conceptual and methodological issues, changing professional perspectives and roles, and range of focus.

Conceptual Issues

Major conceptual issues include the complexity of interventions, the role of information, and paradigms.

Complexity. A major conceptual issue relates to the complexity of determinants of health behavior and the consequent complexity of interventions. There is broad consensus that health behaviors are determined by personal, family, social, cultural, community, institutional, and provider factors. Thus, the success of attempts to change health behaviors hinges on including these multiple factors. Buchanan's ecological model (Chapter 9) is one framework that captures this complexity. (The description of this model affirms the underlying organization of Volumes I and II of this *Handbook*, as well as the 1988 work from which this *Handbook* evolved.) Parallel with this complexity is the emerging consensus that diseases and health conditions are themselves complexly determined, that the single agent or germ theory, the Pasteur or Koch or medical model, is insufficient to understand the emergence of disease, and that characteristics of the host must be considered as well (Bruhn, Chapter 1; Wiese & Gallagher, Chapter 4; Buchanan).

In addition, health behavior research indicates that there is no single conceptual model applicable to all health behaviors. The diversity of models available in the mid-1990s—in comparison to the few available in the mid-1970s—provides a theoretical potential of sufficient richness for future investigations. Furthermore, questions arise about whether knowledge derived from most available frameworks, such as the health belief model or social cognitive theory, can be appropriately generalized to diverse and underserved populations (Glanz & Oldenburg, Chapter 8).

Information. A major theme common to a number of chapters is the insufficiency of providing information or knowledge in changing health behaviors. There is consensus that information by itself is insufficient (e.g., Bruhn, Chapter 1; Gift & White, Chapter 7). "Knowledge does not cause action" (Buchanan, Chapter 9); simply demonstrating the effectiveness of a behavior or a program does not readily translate into its adoption (Robertson, Chapter 12); smoking is not merely "an informed choice" (Cummings, Chapter 13); giving students information is ineffective in reducing their risk behaviors (Kelder et al., Chapter 14); the assumptions that information is veridically received and interpreted are inappropriate (Swinehart, Chapter 18). Successful attempts at changing behaviors involve an understanding of the personal, family, social, cultural, and institutional contexts in which the information is provided, received, and processed.

Paradigms. A need for a shift in the way interventions are conceptualized becomes clear as Cole (Chapter 17) urges a switch from "paradigmatic" to "narrative" thinking, basing his argument on a rich array of literature in cognitive psychology. Paradigmatic thinking involves context-free and abstract formal concepts and is the normative model for science, logic, and mathematics (Cole). Narrative thinking, in contrast, "is always contextualized as a story about someone doing something, for some purpose, that results in specific consequences" (Cole) and contains the inconsistent, incomplete, ambiguous information that makes up life's stories. Yet, as Cole demonstrates, narrative thinking is more understandable than paradigmatic thinking to laypersons dealing with their own health and safety issues. Thus, it is narrative thinking that

generates the most successful intervention programs.

Methodological Issues

Two levels of methodological issues are relevant to the application of health behavior research. One is the manner in which health behavior research itself is conducted; the second is the manner in which the interventions or programs are developed and implemented.

Health Behavior Research Methods. Health behavior research too often reflects characteristics of the majority community and does not reflect the increasing diversity of community populations (e.g., Reed et al., Chapter 2; Wiese & Gallagher, Chapter 4). The database for substance abuse programs, for example, is largely white and middle-class (Kelder et al., Chapter 14). Health behavior knowledge is often insufficient as a base for programs aimed at minority, underserved, and stigmatized populations. Moreover, reports of research findings are often not linked directly to the needs of practitioners; made explicitly relevant to them, particularly in relation to health education and health promotion; or disseminated in ways that have special implications for diverse populations (Glanz & Oldenburg, Chapter 8).

Questions are also raised about whether knowledge about health behavior is best derived and increased from continued collection of data or whether already existing data should be analyzed more fully and formally. Reed et al. indicate that meta-analyses of studies already conducted might be equally valid and appropriate, and they urge that journals change their requirements for reporting data so that meta-analyses can be more readily conducted in the future.

Intervention Methods. Too many interventions are conducted in a health behavior knowledge vacuum. Health educators and health promotion professions often have difficulty keeping abreast of research reports and thus fail to use health behavior theory and data in their programs, drawing instead on their own sense of what seems to work (Glanz & Oldenburg, Chapter 8). The failure of many interventions to consider the culture, developmental stages, lifestyles, and community decision-making contexts of targeted individuals (Bruhn, Chapter 1) is a major methodological issue. Many programs that target families, for example, reflect no conception of family process and are often based on theoretical models that are irrelevant to the family as a social entity or that fail to address issues of family functioning and relationships (Baranowski & Hearn, Chapter 16).

Furthermore, there often is no use of any design to evaluate the impact of programs. Standard experimental–control group designs are rarely used to evaluate the impact of injury control policies (Robertson, Chapter 12). Similarly, it is nearly impossible to evaluate the differential impact of policies on behaviors such as use of tobacco (Cummings, Chapter 13). Reports of a number of interventions are often too ambiguous about the details, or contain too few details, to permit either appropriate replication or appropriate generalizations of findings (Baranowski & Hearn). At the same time, a slavish overdependence on simple experimental–control group designs may be a limiting factor in a number of interventions (e.g., Baranowski & Hearn).

Contrasted with these points is Buchanan's concern (Chapter 9) about conducting research or conducting untried interventions on populations that are typically underserved. Buchanan raises questions about the ethics of doing do.

Changing Professional Perspectives and Roles

There is a strong consensus that the traditional models of understanding diseases, responses to illness, and health maintenance behaviors are too narrow and that physicians' perspectives on these health concerns must be broadened (e.g., Wiese & Gallagher, Chapter 4), as must be conceptions of the roles of health professionals. For example, the traditional clinical role of the physician or nurse is increasingly expanding to embrace the role of health educator (Bruhn, Chapter 1; Wiese & Gallagher; Blue & Brooks, Chapter 5).

Complementing this shift is the changing role of the patient, who is becoming more of an informed consumer and less of a passive, uninformed layperson (e.g., Wiese & Gallagher), with implications for changes in the dynamics of the patient–physician relationship. At the same time, interventions that increase the empowerment of laypersons, particularly in the area of workplace safety, often meet with resistance by management professionals (Cole, Chapter 17).

Moreover, as medicine becomes enmeshed in managed care, physicians will find additional infringements on their professional autonomy with concomitant changes in their interactions with patients. Such changes in medicine will mandate a different role for physicians in relation to pharmacists, administrators and management personnel, organizational and governmental policies, and insurance companies (Daugherty, Chapter 10).

Occurring along with modifications of professional roles is a movement toward phenomenological perspectives and issues of meaning. Flipse (Chapter 3) notes the inadequacy of statistical data as a basis for understanding care seeking and urges that physicians attempt to understand the meanings that patients attach to their illnesses. Gift and White (Chapter 7) make particular note of the relevance for professionals of the meanings that people attach to oral health.

Range of Focus

There is broad consensus that health behavior research and health professionals can no longer conceptualize problems or the locus for behavior change solely within individuals, but must locate problems and targets for change within a broader context, including multiple social and cultural factors and the health providers—professions and institutions—themselves. It follows that for maximum success, interventions directed at health behavior change must involve and affect multiple social and institutional environments.

Levy (Chapter 6) points to social work's goals of changing social policy and social institutions, not only to generate behavioral change, but also to offset negative perceptions of health professionals held by clients and patients. Robertson (Chapter 12) and Cummings (Chapter 13) both note the relative inadequacy of focusing on individual behavior change compared with changing social and institutional policies and practices in relation to injury control and tobacco use. Robertson particularly notes the need to eradicate the "pluralistic ignorance" that too often characterizes corporate behavior. Schooler and Flora (Chapter 15) point to the need to change institutional, governmental, and social policies as more appropriate steps in changing individual risk behaviors. They underscore the need to understand community processes such as agenda setting by the mass media, and the role that the media play in shaping public opinion. At the same time, they recognize that professional training disproportionately focuses on the individual, and that the acceptability of reports for publication often depends on demonstrating individual behavior changes.

Related to shifting away from a focus on individual behaviors is the shift in locale of health interventions. Medicine, for example, has moved away from small-scale solo practice to become part of team practice within larger and more complex health care organizations (Wiese & Gallagher, Chapter 4) and has moved, as well, from being based in hospitals and clinics to being part of community-based "interorganizational service delivery systems" (Daugherty, Chapter 10).

Finally, diversity itself must be a focus. Wiese and Gallagher stress the importance of diversity as a concept, and several authors emphasize the increasing diversity of the population as well as of medical students (Reed et al., Chapter 2), together with geographic mobility and multiculturalism. Such diversity mandates curricular materials that increase reaching out to minorities, and underserved, disabled, and stigmatized elements of the population (Wiese & Gallagher).

FUTURE RESEARCH DIRECTIONS

Future directions for increasing the relevance of health behavior research include those that relate to provider issues and to methodology.

Provider Issues

One major focus for future health behavior research is the changes in the health care system and in provider roles. Important topics would include the impact of the following changes on care seeking, adherence and other responses to illness, self-management, and satisfaction with care:

1. New competencies and skills demonstrated by health care professionals (e.g., Bruhn, Chapter 1; Reed et al., Chapter 2; Flipse, Chapter 3; Wiese & Gallagher, Chapter 4; Blue & Brooks, Chapter 5).
2. Increased understanding by health professionals of the family, social, lifestyle, and cultural influences on such behaviors (e.g., Bruhn; Reed et al.; Flipse; Wiese & Gallagher; Blue & Brooks; Levy, Chapter 6; Gift & White, Chapter 7).
3. Increased long-term interactions between medical students and patients (Reed et al.; Flipse; Wiese & Gallagher).
4. Increased managed care as opposed to fee-for-service practice and changes in the interorganizational service delivery system (e.g., Daugherty, Chapter 10).
5. Provider behaviors taking place outside the illness experience and behaviors that reflect interprovider and interphysician interactions and influence (Daugherty).
6. Physicians undertaking their own health behavior research with their own patients (Flipse).
7. Greater understanding of community needs (Flipse).

Another focus is the patient–professional encounter. This would include research on:

1. What actually happens during the encounter (Gift & White).
2. The degree to which provider attitudes serve as barriers to successful interactions (Gift & White).

Other topics include the impact of the following changes on prevention, risk reduction, and lifestyle change:

1. Increased involvement of different segments of the community (Kelder et al., Chapter 14; Schooler & Flora, Chapter 15).
2. Increased specificity of the tailoring of messages, programs, and interventions (Swinehart, Chapter 18; Glanz & Oldenburg, Chapter 8; Kelder et al.; Schooler & Flora; Baranowski & Hearn, Chapter 16).
3. Increased understanding of the multiple social risks presented by the environment (e.g., Buchanan, Chapter 9; Kelder et al.).
4. Increased understanding of the complexity of information-seeking and processing (Swinehart).

Methodological Directions: The "Boilerplate"

A discussion of future directions for health behavior research would be incomplete if it did not include a restatement of "boilerplate" themes, although many of these themes are the mirror images of the earlier discussion of methodological issues. To increase its applicability and relevance, future health behavior research must be multitargeted and multilevel, and it must include, to a far greater degree, underserved and hard-to-reach populations. In addition, future research might devote greater attention to meta-analysis as a method and to the specification of outcomes.

Meta-Analysis. Future research should also include more meta-analyses of existing studies (Reed et al., Chapter 2). Meta-analyses would help both researchers and practitioners appreciate more fully the impact of a cumulative body of knowledge—an impact that is not immediately apparent from the results of single studies.

Outcomes. A major methodological issue for future research involves the specification of outcomes. Too many health behavior research applications inadequately identify or narrowly specify behavioral outcomes. Schooler and Flora (Chapter 15) urge that outcomes be specified not only at the level of individual behavior, but also in terms of social, institutional, and community changes. Future research should thus examine how planned health behavior applications affect larger system variables such as social norms, organizational policies, governmental regulations, and the physical environment of institutions and communities (Schooler & Flora).

SUMMARY

This chapter has demonstrated the relevance and potential relevance of health behavior research findings for health professionals. It has also demonstrated the degree to which such relevance remains ignored or unincorporated into professional practice and training, especially in medicine and dentistry. The chapter has pointed to the value of multilevel interventions involving health behavior research knowledge not only about individuals and families, but also about social networks, institutions such as schools and worksites, communities, and health care professionals.

The chapter identifies some common themes that are emerging from applications of health behavior research, including the recognition that information by itself is insufficient in changing behaviors, and some directions for future research, including the impact on health behavior of changes in the roles of health professionals and in the delivery of health care.

20

Health Behavior Research, Cognate Disciplines, Future Identity, and an Organizing Matrix

An Integration of Perspectives

David S. Gochman

HEALTH BEHAVIOR RESEARCH: A MULTIDISCIPLINARY UNDERTAKING

Health behavior research is multidisciplinary. It is not exclusively the turf or domain of any single discipline or profession and is conducted by persons trained in a number of these disciplines. This chapter describes and discusses four major cognate disciplines that inspire and generate health behavior research: health psychology, medical anthropology, medical geography, and medical sociology. There is danger, of course, in designating these as "four major cognate disciplines"; it may well be argued that there are other "major" ones. Literature reviews, suggest, however, that the phrase, and its implied limitations, are appropriate.

David S. Gochman • Kent School of Social Work, University of Louisville, Louisville, Kentucky 40292.

Handbook of Health Behavior Research IV: Relevance for Professionals and Issues for the Future, edited by David S. Gochman. Plenum Press, New York, 1997.

The term "cognate" connotes an underlying relationship or commonality. Each of the four disciplines is a social (or behavioral) science, and each deals with a broad range of phenomena related to health, illness, and health behavior. The domain of each discipline includes (1) persons who either are defined as being ill or are concerned about health or illness, (2) persons who are defined as having the capacity to heal the illness or address the health-related concern, and (3) interactions between these two groups of persons. The overlap can be seen in major texts in health psychology (e.g., DiMatteo, 1991; Stone, Cohen, & Adler, 1979), medical anthropology (e.g., Helman, 1990), medical geography (e.g., Shannon & Dever, 1974), and medical sociology (e.g., Cockerham, 1995; Wolinsky, 1988), all of which cover the issues of patient–professional interactions, care-seeking behavior, and illness behavior.

Historically, the major characteristics that have differentiated the four disciplines have been their independent variables and, to some degree, their methods. For health psychology, the independent variables are largely at the individual level: personality and belief factors, individual histories, and lifestyle; for medical geography, the independent variables are: location, distance, space, and place; for medical anthropology: cultural meanings of illness and healing; for medical sociology: social organization, structure, roles, and power relationships. Increasingly, these disciplines demonstrate overlap in independent variables—and in some instances in method. There is often little difference, for example, in the methods with which medical anthropologists and medical sociologists study health professionals (McElroy & Townsend, 1989, p. 66).

A brief definition of each discipline is followed by a section identifying the health behaviors it has emphasized, a discussion of some of the dominant issues it faces in relation to health behavior, and suggestions for areas for future research. The chapter then analyzes some issues common to the disciplines related to the identity of health behavior research, and concludes with a "work-in-progress" proposal for a matrix-type framework for organizing the growing body of health behavior knowledge.

The chapter is not intended to be a minitext. It does not cover knowledge, concepts, and issues in these fields comprehensively; instead, it is highly selective, dealing primarily with matters deemed most salient to health behavior research. Furthermore, it must be understood that despite his training in "personality and social psychology"; past involvement in the American Psychological Association's Division of Psychologists in Public Service and its Section on Health Research; active role in initiating—and charter membership in—the Division of Health Psychology, which evolved from that section; the author does not identify strongly with health psychology (or, for that matter, with any of the other disciplines).

A great deal of health behavior research is also conducted by dentists, epidemiologists, nurses, physicians, public health educators, social workers, and other health professionals. This chapter is not intended to devalue their investiga-

tions as much as it is to elaborate on the disciplinary basis for much of it. The conceptual framework and methods that drive the health behavior research undertaken by these professionals come largely from one or another of the cognate disciplines. For example, much of the excellent work done by nurses on patient education and prevention is derived from frameworks such as the health belief and locus of control models (health psychology) or sick role theory (medical sociology).

Health Psychology

Health psychology is the youngest of the cognate disciplines. Until the late 1960s, psychology as an institution and discipline showed little interest in somatic, nonmental health. Schofield's work (American Psychological Association, Task Force on Health Research, 1976; Schofield, 1969) provided the impetus for a Section on Health Research to be established within the Division of Psychologists in Public Service, out of which emerged, in 1979, a full-fledged Division of Health Psychology.

Definition

The appearance in 1979 of *Health Psychology—A Handbook* (Stone, Cohen, & Adler, 1979) is thought to mark the first time that a book had borne that title (Stone, 1979). Yet beyond a statement that health psychology reflected the activities of psychologists within the health system, that volume did not provide an explicit definition of health psychology. A year later, health psychology was explicitly defined as "the aggregate of the specific educational, scientific, and professional contributions of the discipline of psychology to the promotion and maintenance of health, the prevention and treatment of illness, the identification of etiologic and diagnostic correlates of health, illness and related dysfunction" (Matarazzo, 1980, p. 815). The definition was later reframed as "any aspect of psychology that bears upon the experience of health and illness, and the behavior that affects health status" (Rodin &

Stone, 1987, pp. 15–16). The discipline embraces basic study of psychophysiological mechanisms that link environmental events with health and of the structure and content of communications designed to alter health behaviors (Rodin & Stone, 1987, p. 16), together with "the analysis and improvement of the health care system and health policy formation" (Stone, 1987, p. 27). This conception of health psychology has remained fairly stable (e.g., Taylor, 1990).

Behavioral Medicine: A Related Field

Closely related to health psychology is *behavioral medicine*. This has been defined as the "field concerned with the development of behavioral science knowledge and techniques relevant to the understanding of physical health and illness and the application of this knowledge and these techniques to prevention, treatment and rehabilitation" (Schwartz & Weiss, 1978).

Health Behavior Emphases

Psychology has been an important source of theoretical and conceptual frameworks for health behaviors and of investigations of the role of stress in illness and illness behavior, the cognitive representations or images people have about health and illness, and the ways in which people cope with illness and the determinants of their adjustment to it. As a matter of history, the health belief and health locus of control models preceded the formal institutionalization of health psychology, but health behavior research has made ample use of these and other more recent frameworks, such as behavioral intention theories (the theory of reasoned action and theory of planned behavior), protection motivation theory, and transtheoretical/stage models of adoption. Health psychology has contributed extensively to health behavior research, primarily in the areas of reducing risk behaviors such as consumption of fat, sodium, and excessive calories; smoking; unprotected sexual activity; adherence to and acceptance of regimens related to lifestyle, such as exercise, and to management of diseases

such as hypertension, diabetes, and renal dialysis. These are all instances of the involvement of health psychology in health promotion through its facilitation of behavioral change (e.g., Taylor, 1990). Two other research areas, equally critical but—from reviewing the literature—less dominant in health psychology, are cognitive representations of illness and the role of social support in adherence.

Issues

Three issues appear to dominate debate in health psychology in relation to health behavior research: whether health psychology is a profession or a discipline, whether it deals with health or illness, and the consequences of its focus on the individual.

Profession or Discipline. There is continuing debate over whether health psychology is a health care profession, a scientific discipline, or both (e.g., Enright, Resnick, DeLeon, Sciara, & Tanney, 1990). Landmark reports (e.g., Taylor, 1987, 1990) of the accomplishments of health psychology document its extensive involvement in clinical activities. The literature reveals a number of reports of well-conducted, rigorous behavioral intervention trials designed to increase acceptance of conditions; to increase adherence to regimens; to reduce stress in illness, and thus make adherence more likely; and to increase health-promoting lifestyles.

Taylor (1987) wonders whether health psychology has been perhaps too zealous in its clinical and professional involvements to the detriment of its evolving as a discipline. Others (e.g., Ford, 1990) question whether health psychology is a field with its own body of knowledge or whether it is just an application of psychology to the area of health.

Health or Illness. It could be argued that "health psychology" is a misnomer; "illness psychology" is a more apt title for the activities of most health psychologists. One could legitimately question whether health psychology has become overidentified with behavioral medicine; whether it has, in fact, become identical to behavioral medicine; and whether, as a consequence, it has uncritically accepted the medical model. The bundling of health psychology with behavioral medicine is apparent in the marketing of its major journal (*Health Psychology*). Health psychology appears to be disproportionately more concerned with illness and pathology than with health (e.g., Evans, 1989; Taylor, 1987, 1990). Using the technology of health psychology to increase people's acceptance of their conditions (e.g., Taylor, 1990) is, in other terms, a way of using that technology to increase the power and authority of the medical profession's diagnoses and labeling.

Individual Focus. Health psychology focuses on the individual and tends to ignore the social and cultural context in which individual behavior occurs. This focus holds not only for its clinical interventions, but also for basic research. Landrine and Klonoff (1992) point out the failure of researchers in health psychology, uninformed by knowledge generated by sociology and anthropology, to grasp important cultural differences in cognitive representations or schemata of illness.

Future Research

Four areas suggest themselves for the future: risk behaviors, responses to illness and treatment, cognitive representations and models, and conceptual development.

Risk Behaviors. Health psychology will enter the 21st century repeating in large measure what it has been doing: behavioral interventions designed to reduce risk behaviors and improve adherence to regimens. Of particular importance, however, will be its use of behavioral technologies in the area of sexual risk behaviors to reduce the spread of AIDS/HIV infection (Chesney, 1993), to improve lifestyle behaviors to reduce risks (American Psychological Association, Sci-

ence Directorate, 1995), and, in the area of conflict and impulse control, to reduce levels of violent behavior and its correlative risks (American Psychological Association, Science Directorate, 1992).

Responses to Illness. Chesney (1993) identifies several other items for this future agenda, including rethinking nonadherence itself as an issue. Health psychologists need to examine trade-offs between quality of life and the costs, including debilitating side effects, of adherence to experimental and other medications. In addition, Chesney suggests that health psychology will need to explore the behavioral issues emerging from technological advances in early detection and to study the nonacceptance of fear-arousing messages. Responses to early detection are closely related to adherence.

Additional future research agendas would include increased understanding of the major context in which health psychology operates: physician–patient relationships, usually in hospitals and other institutional settings (e.g., Enright, Welch, Newman, & Perry, 1990; Matheson, 1983). The impact of these contextual factors on health behavior has often been neglected by health psychology.

Cognitive Representations and Models. Health psychology should also increase its attention to "everyday" or "mundane" issues, including cognitive schemata for health and illness, and the cognitive mapping of a range of health-related phenomena (Taylor, 1990). Future health behavior research by health psychologists should involve systematic use of data from sociology and anthropology to increase understanding of how societal and cultural factors affect these health cognitions (Landrine & Klonoff, 1992). Health psychology would thus increasingly participate in interdisiplinary health behavior investigations.

Conceptual Development. Finally, future health behavior research development by health psychologists should include enlarging its conceptual framework or, as Ford (1990) terms it, its "propositional glue" (p. 980). Ford proposes that while health psychology recognizes the limitations of mind–body dualism, it has not yet developed and made explicit its own axiomatic base. Among the assumptions that could be incorporated into this base are that humans are self-organizing and self-constructing systems and that interventions—whether through diet, drugs, surgery, exercise, or education—can only facilitate a person's self-organizing and self-constructing tendencies. Additionally, Ford suggests that "feed-forward" processes, a proactive complement to reactive "feedback" processes, need to be incorporated in any model designed to understand human purposive, goal-directed behavior. This suggestion recollects Allport's (1960) conception of adult, nonpathological persons as being proactive rather than reactive in nature.

Medical Anthropology

Definition

Medical anthropology, although a relatively new branch of anthropology with origins in the early 1960s (e.g., Foster & Anderson, 1978; Helman, 1990), is nonetheless older than health psychology. It has also garnered a wider range of definitions. For example, one definition is "a study of medical thought and problem solving, the acculturation process of the healer and physician in diverse cultural settings, and the social and cultural context of medicine" (Romanucci-Ross, Moerman, & Tancredi, 1991, p. ix).

Alternatively, medical anthropology has been defined "as a biocultural discipline concerned with both the biological and sociocultural aspects of human behavior, and particularly with the ways in which the two interact...to influence health and disease" (Foster & Anderson, 1978, pp. 2–3). Foster and Anderson further elaborate on their definition of medical anthropology as "the term used by anthropologists to describe (1) their research whose goal is the comprehen-

sive description and interpretation of the bio-cultural interrelationships between human behavior, past and present, and health and disease levels, without primary regard to practical utilization of this knowledge; and (2) their professional participation in programs whose goal is the improvement of health through greater understanding of the relationships between bio-sociocultural phenomena and health, and through the changing of health behavior in directions believed to promote better health" (p. 10).

Medical anthropology has also been defined as the study of "how people in different cultures and social groups explain the causes of ill-health, the types of treatment they believe in, and to whom they turn if they do become ill ... and how these beliefs and practices relate to biological and psychological changes in the human organism in both health and disease" (Helman, 1990, p. 1). By another definition, it has as a primary concern "the way health and disease are related to the adaptation of human groups over a wide geographic range and across a broad span of time, from prehistory to the future" (McElroy & Townsend, 1989, p. 2).

Ethnomedicine: A Related Field

Closely entwined with medical anthropology is *ethnomedicine*. This term refers to "those beliefs and practices relating to disease which are the products of indigenous cultural development and are not explicitly derived from the conceptual framework of modern medicine" (Hughes, 1968, p. 88). The term is also sometimes used to denote the methods that generate knowledge about these beliefs and practices.

Health Behavior Emphases

Beliefs and practices relating to ill health are a central feature of any culture, and healer groups are found in every society (Helman, 1990, p. x). "Culture," "illness," and "healing" and the relationships between them have been critical focal points for medical anthropological research in health behavior. Medical anthropology has provided numerous investigations of the relationships between religion and health beliefs, of the coexistence of "scientific" or Eurocentric biomedical models and "folk" or indigenous models within a culture, and of the persistence of indigenous beliefs in the face of the infiltration of Eurocentric biomedicine into non-Eurocentric societies (Hill, 1985). Medical anthropologists have explored the linkages between cultural beliefs and diet, drugs, and medication, as well as the role of cultural ritual in dealing with illness, and have been especially interested in the selection, training, concepts, values, and internal organization of a society's healers (e.g., Helman, 1990, 1991). Medical anthropologists have studied the relationship between culture and the recognition and labeling of symptoms and seeking of care (e.g., Angel & Thoits, 1987), and culture-bound syndromes such as "falling out" or "high blood" among African-Americans (e.g., Weidman, 1988) or *espanto* (fright, soul loss) among the *Ladinos* of Chiapas (Fabrega & Hunter, 1978).

Issues

Three major interrelated issues confront health behavior research within medical anthropology. Two of these issues—the medical model and "critical" theory—have remained prominent for some time, continue to generate considerable debate, and in no way seem to be moving toward resolution. The third, alternative systems, generates fewer polemics.

The Medical Model. The Western, or Eurocentric, biomedical model for understanding and treating disease is major point of difference among medical anthropologists. McLean (1990), arguing that medical knowledge is produced by living actors who are shaped by their social and historical contexts, and is not a reflection solely of either the natural world or of larger social and economic factors, urges a critical look at what passes for "scientific" medical knowledge. In particular, she points out that the assumptions of the medical establishment are themselves reflections

of the cultural system of which physicians are part and argues for rigorous questioning of the validity of the assumptions themselves.

Similar critical stances are urged by M. Singer (1990), who notes medical imperialism in the differential status given Western biomedical and non-Western systems. The former is considered as science, with its successful treatments accorded organic explanations; the latter are considered as components of culture, and their treatments marginalized by being given "psychological" or nonorganic explanations. Scientific medicine is seen to belittle alternative approaches, even though these alternatives may have the same level of rationality, efficaciousness, and empiricism and the same sanctions of age and coherence within a lay theory of disease (Atkinson, 1979).

Nichter (1992), however, cautions against an "imperialist nostalgia" (p. xiv) that may draw attention to healing rituals and away from power relationships. Such nostalgia may lead to the communication skills and competence of traditional healers being perceived in a disproportionately more favorable light and as far more congruent with their patients than data would support, at the same time that biomedical practitioners are criticized for their lack of such skills and their lack of similarity to, and familiarity with, their patients.

The paradox of the attractiveness of the medical disease model in the face of its inadequacy is discussed by Stein (1990) in an analysis of alcohol and chemical addictions. A good part of the appeal of the medical model lies in its congruence with social myths about these conditions and its support for marginalizing pariah groups—especially in a time of "social regression" in the United States, with its resurgence of social Darwinism and withdrawal of compassion—and its emphasis on technological rather than other types of solutions. Scheper-Hughes (1990) criticizes the overidentification of much of medical anthropology with the interests of conventional biomedicine; McLean (1990) criticizes the perceived neutrality of the biomedical model that reduces patients to physical bodies and ignores the pain and suffering they experience in their illnesses.

The values of physicians are a related issue. These values are often quite different from those of patients and are shaped by physicians' cultural and social background and their socialization into the profession (MacCormack, 1994).

Critical Theory. Very much related to concerns about the medical model are debates about critical theory or, more explicitly, about critical anthropology, critical medical anthropology, and clinical anthropology, the definitions of which, as Baer (1990) notes, are themselves subject to debate. The essence of "critical anthropology" appears to be willingness to recognize and commitment to recognizing social and cultural institutions as being reflections and reinforcers of particular social, economic, and political systems. "Critical medical anthropology" is thus a perspective that recognizes medicine, physicians, and other components of health institutions as representatives of, and reinforcers of, larger social, economic, and political systems, the primary concerns of which are advancing the interests of these systems (e.g., Baer, 1990; Scheper-Hughes, 1990; M. Singer, Baer, & Lazarus, 1990). Critical medical anthropology thus focuses on aspects of the macrosystem, on forces such as world capitalism, as the dominant factors in understanding clinical interactions.

Critical medical anthropology thus sees clinical events such as physician–patient interactions largely in terms of power relationships in which physician power, sanctioned by medical institutions, attempts to assure that patient behavior is compatible with the interests of the ruling class (e.g., Baer, 1990; M. Singer et al., 1990). Within the critical perspective, the locus of the sickness or condition lies not in the individual patient, but rather in the power relations between social groups or classes (McElroy & Townsend, 1989, p. 68). Baldwin (1990) recognizes the economic factors that underlie the diagnostic process in his analysis of how sources of institutional funding generate pressures to create sicker patients: patients with more severe diagnoses.

Wright and Morgan (1990) note that the critical perspective is at least one view of understanding the creation of problem patients, i.e., those patients who end up labeled as deviant. Alternatively, they suggest that patient beliefs and perceptions are themselves important determinants of the nature of the clinical encounter—that patient beliefs and the meanings that patients attach to their conditions and their treatments are major factors in the encounter and in negotiating the power relationship.

M. Singer (1990) observes that capitalism has transformed a particular model of ethnomedicine into a worldwide system in which illness-related behaviors are seen as compensatory responses to onerous conditions. The consequent "medicalization" of "medical anthropology," in which medical interests determine domains of study, impedes the proper study of the nonmedical political behavior of the medical profession that relates to its seeking and securing power. In contrast, Scheper-Hughes (1990) observes that much of "critical medical anthropology" is a Marxist analysis that fails to account for or deal with the highly subjective content of illness and healing as events lived, having particular meanings for, and felt by people. Scheper-Hughes, however, also notes the importance of challenging the materialist premises of biomedicine.

Press (1990) cautions medical anthropology against an extreme critical position that would overinterpret the impact of any single element in clinical interactions. Press stresses the complexity of such interactions, noting that physicians and patients often share some cultural medical and economic values and that overemphasis on the macrosystem impedes understanding of the role of the patient's support network and of individual factors such as the patient's unique experiential response to disease. Pappas (1990) makes important distinctions between power as a general phenomenon present in a large number of social interactions, and power as domination and exploitation, and discusses the complementarity and commonalities of critical and other perspectives. Pappas notes that the critical perspective often ignores the functionality or content of the physician–patient encounter, while noncritical or action perspectives tend to ignore the exploitive role of power both within the encounter and in the larger social system.

Possible linkages between anthropology and epidemiology are viewed through the filter of critical theory. The interests of epidemiology in identifying behavioral risks have been misperceived as efforts of vested interests to develop data that could be used in victim blaming, and these misperceptions have been barriers to collaborative relationships between the two disciplines (Inhorn, 1995).

Alternative Systems. The treatment of alternative healing systems is a third issue facing medical anthropology. Stoner (1986) reaffirms the existence of multiple medical or healing systems in many different cultures, with indigenous "traditional" systems coexisting with more Eurocentric and "cosmopolitan" biomedical systems, and points to the importance of recognizing and analyzing the use of such traditional systems along with the use of the biomedical ones to provide a more comprehensive picture of use of a range of healing options. Scheper-Hughes (1990) makes a parallel point in her criticism of the double standard whereby institutional skepticism is raised about alternative healers, while orthodox biomedicine is viewed uncritically. (This point is, of course, the other side of Nichter's caution, cited earlier in this chapter, that it is the alternative healers who are likely to be viewed uncritically.)

Future Research

Four areas suggest themselves for future research by medical anthropologists: the phenomenal world, healing cultures, community issues, and feminism.

The Phenomenal World. Medical anthropology should increase its understanding of the phenomenal world. In particular, future research

would include studies of beliefs related to traditional healing methods (Anderson, 1992; Hill, 1985; Stoner, 1986); laypersons' explanatory models of disease (e.g., Helman, 1991), which are linked to the cognitive representations undertaken by health psychology (Lau, this *Handbook*, Volume I, Chapter 3); and lay definitions of community health needs (Hill, 1985). Related to this research would be research on the cultural construction of "diseases" such as hyperactivity (e.g., Romanucci-Ross et al., 1991, p. x), and the meanings attached to nonbiological models of healing (Scheper-Hughes, 1990).

Charmaz (1990) emphasizes the importance of using grounded theory in such phenomenological studies. At the same time, Dressler and Oths (this *Handbook*, Volume I, Chapter 17) note the tension in anthropology between attempts to systematize and quantify the study of culture and attempts to limit anthropology to describing or documenting cultural differences. Health behavior research, they suggest, will be advanced more by the former than by the latter.

Other phenomenal dimensions worthy of future research are the cultural stereotypes of physicians and other health professionals and the relationship between staff perspectives and physician perspectives (Press, 1990). Kroeger (1983) encourages the anthropological study of beliefs that determine self-care.

Closely related to phenomenology are the different languages used to communicate about health and illness. Helman (1991), among others, suggests the need for future investigations of different languages of distress, the terminology as well as nonverbal cues that patients use to present their conditions to health professionals.

Healing Cultures. The total healing culture, including both biomedical and alternative approaches, should be a focus of future research. Of particular value would be studies examining the culture of medicine (e.g., Foster & Anderson, 1974), particularly the professional behaviors that are relevant to system maintenance and the status quo (e.g., M. Singer, 1990); the proliferation of rituals within biomedicine and, related to this proliferation, how much of medical activity is directed to answering patients' needs and how much to relieving stress among physicians and other professionals (MacCormack, 1994); and the effects of these behaviors, rituals, and activities on patient care seeking, choice, adherence, and satisfaction. Stoner (1986) urges that the often unacknowledged range of alternative choices that underlie use of services be studied. Finally, the hospital should be examined as a socially constructed space (Scheper-Hughes, 1990).

Community Issues. Future health behavior research should include the application of anthropological methods to determine what communities perceive their own health and medical needs to be, in contrast to the needs identified by health professionals (Helman, 1991; Hill, 1985; Whiteford 1985). Moreover, there is also a need for research on the impact of different community histories, such as escape or encampment experiences among refugees, and their responses to screening, parasitic infestations, and new diets (Whiteford, 1985). Coreil and Mull (1988) advise further medical anthropological research in developing countries on community definitions and terminology for diarrhea and other conditions in order to devise appropriate, culturally valid educational materials.

Feminism. There is also a need for future research in a feminist anthropology that moves the healing role of women beyond midwivery and childbirth. McClain's (1989) suggestion of a greater focus on women's role as healers in medical and religious systems has implications for understanding the impact of women as healers on a range of health behaviors.

Medical Geography

Definition

Medical geography is the oldest of these four disciplines, with a history going back to the work of Finke's *An Attempt at a General Medical-Practical Geography* (Finke, 1792–1795, referred to in Barrett, 1993). As initially envisioned, Finke's work sought to provide a medically relevant description of the inhabited countries of the late 18th-century world (Barrett, 1993). These descriptions would include information about soil, air and atmosphere, water, food, morals and habits that affect health or disease, discourse on diseases, and customary remedies as these characteristics vary from country to country (Barrett, 1993; Shannon & Dever, 1974, p. 2).

Two centuries later, abstracting from several definitions and in language more congenial to the Zeitgeist, medical geography can be broadly defined as the study of the relationships between spatial and locational characteristics and the distribution of disease, health resources, health behaviors, and the interactions and decision making of patients and professionals (e.g., Duncan, Jones, & Moon, 1993; Earickson, 1990; Pol & Thomas, 1992; Shannon & Dever, 1974). Kearns and Joseph (1993) make an important distinction in medical geography between the geography of disease and the geography of health care—characterizing the former as being more concerned with ecology and environmental determinants of particular pathologies; the latter, with the spatial correlates of delivery systems and with their accessibility, utilization, and planning. The relevance of medical geography to health behavior lies more in the geography of health care—or the geography of health—than in the geography of disease.

Health Behavior Emphases

In relation to health behavior, the geography of health care has provided important insights into the impact of distance. Shannon and Dever (1974, pp. 89–90) report on studies that show that as distance from health facilities increases, perception and recognition of symptoms also increase. Persons removed from ready access to health care, e.g., in wilderness areas, are apparently more sensitive to cues that have the potential to indicate illness. Although increased physical distance is simultaneously related to decreased use of services, the relationship is complex and varies with the severity of the condition; utilization does not decline uniformly with increased distance. Although a distance gradient (e.g., Shannon & Dever, 1974, pp. 92–93) is an important concept in medical geography, distance and spatial locations by themselves, without consideration of social factors, have not proven to be sufficient predictors of utilization (e.g., Béland, Philibert, Thouez, & Maheux, 1990; Eyles, 1990; Friss, Friedman, & Demakis, 1989; Scarpaci & Kearns, this *Handbook*, Volume II, Chapter 5; Shannon & Dever, 1974, p. 93).

Medical geography has also provided knowledge about spatial locational characteristics related to perceived health needs and health status in communities (e.g., Kearns & Joseph, 1993). According to Kearns and Joseph, the sociogeographic structure of cities and of the prevailing system of service delivery profoundly shapes the patterns of treatment opportunities. In a study of a New Zealand community, for example, Kearns and Joseph (1993) demonstrated the implications of such characteristics for appropriate planning and provision of community health services.

Duncan et al. (1993) explored the spatial and locational correlates of a range of risk behaviors in the United Kingdom and found that while communities and regions themselves differed in the prevalence of smoking and drinking, such differences were not readily attributable to geography as such. The geographic effects by themselves apparently interacted with social and personal variables such as social class, gender, and age.

Armstrong's (1985) analysis of space and time in British general practice moves issues of space and distance from the macro level to the level of the physician's surgery. Armstrong notes the relocation and reconfiguring of the surgery from being a part of the physician's own living quarters—perhaps separated by a curtain—to being a special office attached to these quarters, to being located in a special annex separated from the home, to being part of a community-based health center. Parallel with these changes, Armstrong notes, came the decreasing frequency with which the physician encountered the patient in the patient's own living space. Armstrong links these spatial and locational changes with changes in the perception of illness, the separation of illness from the patient's personal and social life, and the treatment of specific illness rather than of the patient as a human entity.

Issues

Two dominant issues in mid-1990s medical geography are the construction of space and the concept of landscape. Each has implications for health behavior.

Construction of Space. A major issue in mid-1990s medical geography is the construction of space and the interplay of personal and social factors. Kearns and Joseph (1993) identify different conceptions of space as focal points of medical geography. Geometric space represents the purely physical concerns for distance and location that underlie spatial analysis. Space can also be viewed as a medium in which human and social transactions take place. Finally, it can be viewed as a product of such transactions; as such, it acquires personal and social meaning. Scarpaci (1993), Scarpaci and Kearns (this *Handbook*, Volume II, Chapter 5) and Kearns and Joseph (1993) urge that the human and social meanings of space, or space as it is experienced, or the "sense of place" as they refer to it, is a more critical variable in understanding health behavior, particularly use of services, than is space in the geometric or physical sense. "Place" as a set of meanings attached to a setting and viewed as emerging from an interplay of personal and social forces, as opposed to space in its purely physical and spatial dimensions, is considered to have implications for attracting or repelling services and facilities.

Landscape Concepts. Gesler (1992) uses a set of landscape concepts, borrowed from cultural geography, to account for different types of healing environments. In a traditional sense, the concept of landscape denotes the physical environment, both natural and humanly imposed, in which behavior is enacted. In relation to health and illness, Gesler identifies "landscapes of despair"—sick places, settings in which disease is pervasive and feared—and "therapeutic landscapes"—places in which treatment or healing takes place.

Rustic settings, spas, and special curative springs have typically been identified as therapeutic landscapes. These landscapes are also generally associated with rural areas, which are believed to be essentially healthy. This conception reflects the traditional attribution of healing powers to certain parts of the physical environment, such as medicinal plants, fresh air and pure water, mineral springs, and beautiful scenery. Herbs, barks, water, mineral springs, and rivers, usually found in the countryside, have historically been viewed as having healing powers. This view contrasts markedly with that of urban areas, which are believed to be relatively unhealthful. The facts contradict these views; residents of rural areas in many countries, including the United States, have poorer health status than their urban counterparts. Gesler (1992) argues that in addition to some of these "natural" symbols of healing, an important component of therapeutic landscapes is made up of the humanistic and cultural meanings attached to the setting. According to Gesler, humanistic landscapes are settings that encourage or support subjectivity, individuality, meaning, and value. Humanistic therapeutic landscapes would be landscapes in which patients can relate their experiences and feelings and in which providers are sympathetic to the patient's narrative.

The structural component of landscapes refers to those characteristics of settings that reflect issues of physician hegemony versus patient resistance; legitimation versus marginalization of the patient's ideology, territoriality, and private interests; and social inequalities. Structural dimensions of therapeutic landscapes are those

that reflect how physicians manifest their power and authority, either as a profession or as individual professionals. As a major agent of social control, replacing religion and law, medicine demonstrates the hegemony of the political and economic interests it often serves through increasing the medicalization of everyday life, increasing the consumption of medical goods, and using increasingly privatized health care services (Gesler, 1992).

The structural landscapes of health-related settings thus reflect a medical model and are often at variance with the therapeutic landscapes of these settings (Gesler, 1992). Both the humanistic and the structural dimensions of therapeutic settings must be considered in understanding how individuals use and respond to them.

The "sense of place" is a critical concept within such landscapes. It "connotes the meaning, intention, felt value, and significance that individuals and groups give to places" (Gesler, 1992, p. 738). Medical geographers are urged to consider the ease with which a hospital or clinic or community lends itself to meaning, the ease with which patients attribute meaning to it and are able to express themselves within it and relate to it. Individual differences in levels of impairment, independence, financial resources, and social supports affect the degree to which a landscape will be therapeutic and the degree to which the environment will provide hope and be sustaining. At the same time, landscapes differ in the degree to which they convey symbols of caring, cleanliness, power to heal, and concern for the individual.

Future Research

Future research by medical geographers might involve a reconceptualization of space and an examination of the nature of therapeutic landscapes. Each of these areas has implications for health behavior.

Reconceptualization of Space. Medical geographers can be expected to increase their understanding of the ways in which the interrelationships among people, places, and socioeconomic factors affect use of services (Kearns & Joseph, 1993). Future health behavior research undertaken by medical geography will deal, in all likelihood, with reconceptualized space, moving away from the purely physical (Kearns & Joseph, 1993; Scarpaci & Kearns, this *Handbook*, Volume II, Chapter 5). It will include investigations of the personal, social, and cultural factors that determine the "sense of place," or place as it is experienced by individuals and by communities (Kearns & Joseph, 1993). It should examine the linkages between "place" as a social construction and risk behaviors, prevention, and lifestyle behaviors (e.g., Duncan et al., 1993).

Therapeutic Landscapes. Future health behavior research in medical geography should examine the elements that create a therapeutic landscape. It should show the degree to which components of the health care delivery system such as hospitals and clinics are experienced as places and the meanings they convey as therapeutic landscapes (e.g., Gesler, 1992). It should explore the ways in which such landscapes affect patient–professional interactions in terms of negotiation and influence, as well as patient care seeking, adherence, satisfaction with care, and perceptions of health professionals (e.g., Gesler, 1992). Of particular value would be studies that show the degree to which treatment centers represent places of failure, threats, and being unwanted (Gesler, 1992).

Medical Sociology

Definition

Older than either health psychology or medical anthropology, medical sociology has roots going back to the late 1950s (Bloom, 1990). It has been defined as "the subfield of sociology which applies the perspectives, conceptualizations, theories, and methodologies to phenomena having to do with human health and disease ... it encompasses a body of knowledge which places health and disease in a social, cultural and behavioral context" (Committee on Certification in Medical Sociology, 1986, cited in Wolinsky, 1988, p. 28). Its subject matter includes descriptions, explanations, and theories dealing with the distribution of diseases among various population groups; the social contexts of health behaviors and health-related attitudes and beliefs; analyses of medical occupations and the delivery of medical care; medicine as a social institution; cultural values and societal responses related to health, illness, and disability; and the way in which social factors affect the etiology of diseases, especially those that are seen as stress-related (Wolinsky, 1988, p. 28).

Mumford (1983, p. 1) provides a complementary definition of medical anthropology: It "studies how people define themselves as sick as well as the ways they use to avoid feeling that something is wrong with them. It also studies the means a society has developed to reassure people that they will get better, as well as the ways to obtain cure or relief from pain or disability. Medical sociology deals with social responses and the management of emotional defenses in the presence of diseases; it deals with the social arrangements, institutions, and occupations societies develop to deal with disease and the threat of it. Medical sociology also investigates the distribution of disease as well as the distribution of occupations and facilities for the treatment and prevention of disease."

Health Demography: A Related Field

A closely related field is *health demography*, which melds medical sociology, epidemiology, and demography. Health demography involves "the application of the content and methods of demography to the study of health status and health behavior" (Pol & Thomas, 1992, p. 1). In its predictions and analyses, it makes use of a range of socially relevant characteristics including, but not limited to, age, marital status, gender, race, ethnicity, educational levels, and income.

Health Behavior Emphases

In relation to health behavior, a major contribution made by medical sociology lies in numerous studies of the patient–professional relationship and of the sick role concept (Parsons, 1951). The sick role concept embraces the role and power issues in this relationship and the linkage between this relationship and the larger social system, particularly its values. Medical sociology has examined the professional training and socialization not only of physicians, but also of a range of health professionals, including nurses, dentists, midwives, and physician assistants, and has examined how their training relates to their behavior with patients. It has examined the social organization of health care institutions, hospitals, clinics, and emergency rooms, as well as the organization of medical care in a society, and the implications of these organizational characteristics for client, layperson, and patient behavior. It has examined care-seeking behavior and the utilization of health services. It has examined the patient as consumer, as well as "alternative" healing forms that coexist with established biomedical treatments, and why these alternatives are sought.

Issues

Four dominant issues in medical sociology are structure versus meaning, the medical model, social construction, and feminism. Each of these issues has implications for health behavior.

Structure Seeking versus Meaning Seeking. Pearlin (1992) suggests that divisions within medical sociology are based on illusions that there are clearly defined centers of difference. Pearlin uses the broad categories of "structure-seekers" and "meaning-seekers" to discuss some differences in perspectives. Structure seekers are concerned with the arrangement of parts of a social system, with factors such as social stratification and institutional organization. Meaning seekers are concerned with the phenomenal and cognitive worlds of persons interacting within a social system. These two different perspectives generate two different approaches to data collection and analysis — one more statistical and based on sociologists' preconceived categories, the other more "qualitative" and presumably closer to human reality. The structuralist perspective is productive, for example, in determining regularities in the way risk behaviors and interactions with professionals are associated with different social positions; the meaning perspective, in determining the personalized experiences of illness, loss, and suffering, and the perceptions of medical encounters.

The Medical Model. Just as the Western, biomedical model of disease is a major point of divergence among medical anthropologists, it has been a major issue for medical sociologists for some time. Gold (1977) noted some time ago that medical sociology in the United States, Great Britain, and Germany had been criticized as being subservient to the interests of the medical establishment. Gold demonstrated that the research literature itself showed substantial bias in favor of medical rather than sociological perspectives in terms, for example, of defining illness as deviance and the medical system as an agent of social control; of medicalizing complex social phenomena such as alcohol consumption and extramarital pregnancy by viewing them as pathologies; and of assuming the appropriateness of adherence and utilization behaviors.

The medicocentrism of the sick role concept itself generated considerable debate (e.g., Gallagher, 1976; Parsons, 1975). Did this enormously heuristic concept imply uncritical acceptance of the assumptions of the medical model? Levine (1987) pointed out that medical sociology had made attempts to get medicine to examine its own perspectives more critically, but implied that medicine has not readily embraced these attempts. Gerhardt (1989) noted, however, that in attacking "medical imperialism," medical sociology is itself indulging in a form of imperialism, since in doing so it is serving its own interests.

Social Construction. The phrase "social construction," one that has many applications, appears as an issue in medical sociology that is parallel to that of critical theory in medical anthropology. Brown (1995) insightfully discusses plural definitions of "social construction" and notes, on one level, the degree to which social construction is involved in the diagnostic process and in the interplay of social interaction and the personal experiences of symptoms or disorders, particularly in relation to psychiatric diagnoses. An extreme version of social constructionism would rule out any objective biomedical events, arguing that all diagnoses are totally the result of social interactions. Yet, at another level, Brown notes that medical knowledge itself is socially constructed, that professional beliefs and the diagnostic process reflect how health providers are socialized and how professional and institutional practices reflect larger social factors, such as patriarchalism, criteria for professional advancement, and labor market needs, that are often imperialist or capitalist.

Waitzkin (1989) argues that the medical encounter reflects the ideology of the larger system, that physicians are part of an ideological state apparatus, which he likens to other forms of repressive state mechanisms such as the police. By focusing on a very narrow range of the patient's experience during the clinical interview—the somatic complaints that are congruent with biomedical interests—the physician deemphasizes the patient's concerns with personal, social, and economic issues and the linkage between these concerns and the presenting symptoms. In this instance, the diagnostic process can be intepreted as an impediment to dealing with these larger social problems.

Feminism. Feminist issues reflect a special aspect of social construction, and the degree to which males have disproportionately influenced both medicine and the scientific process is a fourth dominant issue in medical sociology. Medicine is often viewed as a patriarchal institution (VanScoy, this *Handbook*, Volume III, Chapter 7)

that has medicalized a number of women's issues that are more appropriately reflections not of physiological factors but of women's political, social, and economic marginalization. In the context of linking feminist scholarship with the emergence of women's health issues into a more prominent place in national policy debates, Auerbach and Figert (1995) particularly note the social construction of illness around conditions such as PMS (premenstrual syndrome), which the medical establishment had attempted—in the absence of evidence—to designate as a psychiatric condition. Auerbach and Figert also observe that the seeming "naturalness" of the scientific biomedical model masks the social and cultural components of what seems to be neutral, scientific knowledge.

Future Research

Four highly related areas suggest themselves for future research: medicine as a profession, medicalization, feminism, and nonclinical arenas. Each of these areas has implications for health behavior.

Medicine as a Profession. Elinson's (1985) response to announcements of the "end of medicine"—and, with it, of medical sociology—identifies some critical future directions for health behavior research. Research on use and nonuse of service, for example, can reveal the "unmet needs for health care." In addition, Elinson points to the continuing change both in society and in the health professions as points for study. Health behavior research would investigate the impact of these changes on decisions to seek care, particularly if health care becomes more competitive.

Elinson also indicates the importance of considering "quality of life" in relation to medical care, as do a number of others (e.g., Levine, 1987). Although Elinson's major research concern is the impact of medical interventions on quality of life, quality of life needs to be studied as a major factor underlying decisions to accept care or to adhere to regimens. Other future research would explore the degree to which medical diagnostic and treatment decisions in fact result from social decision making by people engaged in social roles, guided by social values, and acting in particular social settings, as Levine suggests, and determine the differential responses of patients to, and their differential levels of adherence to and satisfaction with, these decisions.

Although medicine as a profession is slow to change, particularly in its training of future physicians and its use of health behavior and other nontechnological knowledge, it faces mandates for change from alterations in its economic context. Movements toward managed care, societal resistance to the increasing costs of care, and demands by both patients and payors for greater accountability are altering the way in which medicine is practiced. The emergence of an administrative elite that shares power with the existing knowledge elite (Hafferty & Light, 1995) raises important research questions about the future nature of professional roles and professional–patient interactions, with ultimate implications for patient adherence, continuance in care, and perceptions of satisfaction.

In conjunction with the changing nature of medicine, and following Light (1988), among others, health behavior research might move away from purely social psychological assessments of medical students' and physicians' professional beliefs and social attitudes and toward analyzing the organizational factors—characteristics of medical schools, teaching hospitals, and professional associations—that impinge on, and often impede, satisfactory interactions between physicians and patients. These changes in direction invite medical sociologists to reconceptualize the institutions that deliver care and to develop new models that account for innovation within medical institutions (Flood & Fennell, 1995).

Medicalization. If medical sociology is in fact held captive by larger social forces that have as their goal the imposition of a different set of values on the people studied (e.g., Gold, 1977),

future research might well focus on the degree to which medicine does in fact impose its values on the population. One way of doing this might be to make a more systematic assessment of Waitzkin's (1989) position that the physician–patient encounter reflects and reinforces physician bias against examination of social and economic issues as factors in illness—a bias manifested in the physician's avoidance of discussion of work and family matters by keeping the discourse focused strictly on medical issues. Pescosolido and Kronenfeld (1995) further argue that medical sociology puts its own research agenda at risk if it continues to service medical interests uncritically.

Feminism. The linkage between medicalization and women's health issues (Auerbach & Figert, 1995) suggests another important set of questions for future research. To what degree will women's health behavior, particularly care seeking and conceptions about health and illness, change as medicine as a profession and the scientific process that underlies it become less patriarchal? To what degree will the increase in the numbers and proportions of women physicians change care seeking, adherence, and satisfaction with care on the part, not only of women, but also of men.

Nonclinical Focus. The movement of medical sociology away from hospitals and clinical sites and toward nonclinical community settings such as workplaces (e.g., Pescosolido & Kronenfeld, 1995) provides opportunities for generating new research insights into use of services, participation in screenings, and adherence and other responses to illness. It also creates opportunities to study patterns of broad connections between social institutions, including insurance structures, and the implications of these patterns for health behavior.

Pescosolido and Kronenfeld (1995) encourage medical sociology to keep abreast of research models and technologies from other disciplines. In relation to health behavior, doing so would particularly involve sharpening its conceptions and assessments of cultural and health belief variables, which are considered to lag appreciably behind their development in other social sciences.

PRESENT INTO FUTURE: ISSUES OF IDENTITY

Major issues and challenges that face health behavior research and the disciplines that conduct it involve its identity and the organization of the corpus of knowledge it generates.

Health behavior research has its own definition and purpose independent of its practical applications, and must move toward establishing an identity not yet solidly secured. There are few institutional arrangements, i.e., departments or programs, that attract numbers of health behavior researchers. Most health behavior researchers work in relative isolation from one another and do not have the opportunity for the face-to-face interaction that generates conceptual breadth and enhances methodological strengths. Health behavior often "falls between the cracks," institutionally and organizationally. Identity issues must thus be satisfactorily resolved for health behavior research to move productively into the future. Of particular relevance to the identity of health behavior research are its relationship to medicine, as well as the issues of interdisciplinary collaboration, ideology, and co-optation.

Health Behavior and Medicine

Critical Theory: Whether of or in Medicine

All four disciplines face at least one common identity issue: their relationship to the field of medicine. Medical anthropologists and medical sociologists have been quite explicit about this issue, raising questions about whether they are involved in the anthropology or sociology *of* medicine or in anthropology or sociology *in*

medicine (e.g., Cockerham, 1995, pp. 11–12; Mumford, 1983, p. 93; Wolinsky, 1988, pp. 32–38). The differences in preposition reflect concerns about whether these scholars are independent observers of physicians, the medical profession, the medical model, and medical and health care institutions or whether they are part of the profession itself. To the degree that they have become part of the profession, i.e., to the degree that they are *in* rather than *of* medicine, they are at risk not only for diminished objectivity but also for having their research agendas compromised or co-opted by the interests of medicine and the social, political, and economic institutions it serves. Within both disciplines, there are appreciable proponents of "critical theory" voicing grave concerns about the conflicts of interest inherent in overidentification with medicine.

Although literature reviews do not show that the issue has emerged as extensively in medical geography, it appears in concerns about the inappropriate, or at least poorly thought-through, use of spatial analyses for political purposes to serve economic and other vested interests. In an examination of how formal analyses use space as a consumer focus, as a basis for interprofessional activity, and as a resource, Moon (1990) raises the question of whether such formal analyses are strictly neutral or whether they in fact lend themselves to use by governmental and other agencies with interests in retaining or increasing administrative control over certain locations and areas. Moon employs the phrase "critical medical geography" and encourages theoretical debate in what has traditionally been viewed as an empirical field.

Health psychology, in contrast to the other three disciplines, is apparently "in denial" about this issue. Although there have been occasional criticisms of the role of health psychology in relation to medicine and health promotion (e.g., Evans, 1988), there is little extensive discussion in *Health Psychology*, the major journal for United States health psychology, of a "critical health psychology" or a "critical behavioral medicine" or of the relationship of psychology to medicine. Although each of the cognate disciplines has a clinical aspect, clinical applications are appreciably more extensive for health psychologists, who serve as direct service providers to a greater degree than do members of the other three disciplines. Possibly this greater clinical involvement has resulted in their being socialized more thoroughly by, and more adherent to, the norms of medicine. Psychology in general, as a discipline, is urged to become more interested in building health than it has typically been (Cowen, 1991), and health psychology in particular should consider doing so.

Health or Illness: Directional Definitions

In addition to the concern about being *in* or *of* medicine, each of the disciplines faces the question of whether its focus is health, medicine, or illness. Historically, the term *medical* or *medicine* has been an essential part of the name of three of the disciplines: medical anthropology or anthropology of medicine, medical geography or geography of medicine, and medical sociology or sociology of medicine. Yet within each discipline, there is both questioning of whether the focus should remain on medicine and the medical and recognition of the value of focusing on health. Only health psychology has the word "health" in its title, an irony in light of its disproportionate concern for illness.

McElroy and Townsend (1989), for example, recognize that medical anthropology has roots that extend beyond medicine and include nursing and public health as well (p. 68). They raise the questions of whether medical anthropology should not focus more broadly on health rather than on illness and whether it might be time to consider an "anthropology of health" as an alternative to, or in addition to, the established terms "medical anthropology" and "anthropology of [illness] medicine."

Levine (1987), describing changes within medical sociology, ponders whether it might more appropriately be labeled the "sociology of health." Alternatively, as part of his development

and reconceptualization of the sick role concept, Segall (this *Handbook*, Volume I, Chapter 14) proposes the label "health sociology."

Kearns and Joseph's (1993) distinction between two branches of medical geography—a geography of disease and the geography of health care—provides support for a "geography of health" or "health geography" that would focus attention on the locational, physical, and spatial dimensions of health or well-being. In a far earlier analysis, Terris (1975) argued in parallel fashion for an "epidemiology of health" as a complement to the more typical and traditional epidemiology of disease and risk factors. Such an epidemiology would examine behaviors as varied as the intake of supplemental protein in developing countries and the academic and physical performances of schoolchildren in developed ones.

Although it is possible that changing a word in the title of a discipline or subdiscipline from *medicine* or *medical* to *health* will have no implications for health behavior research, more likely it will. Definitions differ not only in substance, but also in vector. Definitions have labeling qualities that guide or impel movement along selected paths (e.g., Gochman, 1982). Health behavior researchers who identify with behavioral medicine are thus more likely to accept and build upon the medical model, to conduct research addressing medical problems, and to subordinate *basic research interests* to interests with immediately discernible *medical applications*. Health psychology remains a cogent example of the exception that proves the rule. Its birth was preceded by the emergence of "behavioral medicine"—an attractive and potent "label" with the capacity to "direct" research activities selectively, a label that continues to adhere to and guide a number of health psychologists—and an organization of persons who selected "behavioral medicine" as a label, many of whom then moved into leadership positions in the newly formed Division of Health Psychology of the American Psychological Association. Unquestionably, behavioral medicine research has considerable practical and human value, but it does not routinely advance *basic* health behavior research—knowledge about the behavior itself. Basic research in health behavior will be productively developed and conducted to the degree that it can resist being labeled as "behavioral medicine."

Medical School Settings

Programs that generate health behavior research, regardless of how they are labeled, are often located within medical schools, usually in departments of community or behavioral medicine or of behavioral science. Such programs have often produced research of high quality and great practical value. Research of similar quality and value is often conducted in professional schools of dentistry, nursing, and public health. Understandably, the primary objectives—clinical instruction and research needs—of schools of medicine (and dentistry, nursing, and public health) are often incongruent with, or in conflict with, the objectives and needs of nonclinical, academic departments and programs. To the degree that such incongruence or institutionally generated conflict exists, the objectives and needs of nonclinical academic departments, especially those perceived as "soft science," are likely to be subordinated to those of the clinical departments, particularly those involved in high-technology medicine. This subordination will be true regardless of the ultimate practical value for training and practice of the knowledge generated by such basic research. Instances of some of the effects of these conflicts and of subordinate status can be found in the chapters in this volume by Reed, Moore-West, Jernstedt, and O'Donnell (Chapter 2), Flipse (Chapter 3), and Wiese and Gallagher (Chapter 4).

Questions thus arise about the sustained effects of locating health behavior research within medical (and other professional) schools. For example, what are the effects of the subordinate status of health behavior research, in relation to the status of clinical programs, on allocation of funds, personnel, and space? What are the effects of this subordinate status on the vitality of basic health behavior research? Despite their having compiled some impressive research track records, how productive might such programs have been if they had been located elsewhere? Such questions are more salient for health behavior than for programs such as, say, biochemistry and microbiology, because the latter branches of science have no similar need to establish their identities.

It might be argued that locating health behavior research in medical school settings would foster the integration of health behavior knowledge into medical curricula. However, the continued low priority of such content, and its lack of meaningful incorporation into the training of physicians, as related in this volume by Bruhn (Chapter 1), Reed et al. (Chapter 2), Flipse (Chapter 3), and Wiese and Gallagher (Chapter 4), make this argument unconvincing.

While there are sometimes expedient reasons (i.e., political, economic, funding) for some health behavior research activities to be embraced by a "behavioral medicine" label and to be conducted in medical school settings, the continuation of health behavior research in these settings provides an arena for institutionally generated conflict between the legitimate requirements of medicine and the needs of health behavior research to establish basic knowledge and understanding for its own sake.

Health Behavior Research: An Interdisciplinary Undertaking

In addition to its *multidisciplinary* character, health behavior research is and must be *interdisciplinary*. It must be conducted *collaboratively* by scientists in anthropology, dentistry, epidemiology, geography, health promotion and health education, medicine, nursing, nutrition, physical education, psychiatry, psychology, public health, social work, and sociology. Each of these fields offers unique perspectives, skills, and interests. Productive, rigorous, basic health behavior research requires borrowing among, and sharing the broad spectrum of, theories, concepts, and methods. Such interdisciplinary collaboration enhances the likelihood of increasing basic health behavior knowledge.

Integration of Approaches and Methods

Collaborative efforts and the sharing of concepts and methods inhere in the interdisciplinary character of health behavior research and are thus part of its identity. Yet few studies reflect such collaboration. Mechanic (1979) attributed the failure of such research to yield appreciable findings to the lack of such collaborative efforts. His point remains equally valid in the mid-1990s. Mechanic identified two rather distinct "literatures": (1) theoretical studies of sociocultural, organizational, and psychosocial factors that used small, intensively interviewed samples and paid attention to subjective experiences and (2) multivariate, cross-sectional studies that used less detailed measures, but more powerful statistical techniques and large samples. Mechanic urged that future research combine these two broad approaches to maximize the likelihood of nontrivial findings.

Similarly, Eckert and Goldstein (1983) and Landrine and Klonoff (1992) urged an integration that would combine, say, the broad concepts derived from anthropology with the methodological precision of the techniques of psychology. Greater linkages between anthropology and epidemiology, for example, might not only improve the identification of risk behaviors in a population, but also help in reframing the discourse on risk away from pathology and toward prevention and health (Inhorn, 1995). Increased conceptual and methodological integration in the future, and the synergism that is likely to result when researchers from several disciplines bring their varied perspectives together, are necessary to improve the study of specific health behaviors.

In the context of dental research, J. E. Singer (1981, p. 351), suggested that "dentistry should be part of a larger field of health behavior" and encouraged persons trained in a relevant health behavior discipline, who are adept and thoroughly immersed in the methods and concepts of that discipline, to conduct research with an oral health focus. In addition, Singer urged that such research be truly interdisciplinary and reflect a breadth of health behavior perspectives rather than a single theoretical point of view.

Additional areas for future interdisciplinary research might involve collaborative efforts by psychologists and medical (or health) geographers to determine the impact of landscape characteristics and of dimensions of socially and culturally constructed space on the acceptance of regimens and satisfactions with care. Other productive collaborative efforts might emerge from medical geographers working with medical sociologists to examine the impact of such characteristics as well as other locational characteristics on power relationships between professionals and patients, and the subsequent implications of such impact for regimens and satisfaction.

It is worth noting that when such interdisciplinary partnerships are on occasion identified in "health psychology," they include "epidemiologists, physiologists, pharmacologists, physicians, and the like" (Baum, 1989, p. 2). They do not include nurses or dentists, or disciplines or professions that focus on larger social, community, or environmental systems, such as anthropology, geography, public health, social work, or sociology. This enumeration of the disciplines and professions that remain closest to biological and physiological dimensions can be interpreted as another reflection of the essentially medical perspective of health psychology.

The Methodological "Boilerplate"

Interdisciplinary efforts are appropriate to provide the "boilerplate" of methodological issues—more and better research—that exists in any area at any time, reflecting the tentativeness of all scientific "knowledge." It is thus redundant to say that more and better research is needed in health behavior. Yet failure to acknowledge this need could be construed as either oversight, negligence, or gross lack of understanding. There is a standard litany that appears in critical evaluative reviews, declaring the need for: larger, more representative samples; greater precision in measurement; more controlled research designs; increasingly complex multivariate design; more frequent replications; and so forth. Having dutifully stated these needs on behalf of health behavior research, this chapter can resume discussion of identity issues in this research.

Academic Programs in Health Behavior

Basic health behavior research requires organizational and institutional structures that encourage interdisciplinary efforts, facilitate the interaction of researchers representing relevant disciplines and professions, and establish and reinforce health behavior's identity. *Ideally*, such institutional structures would be departments or programs of "health behavior" made up of persons from several of these disciplines and professions who are engaged in and committed to basic health behavior research. *Ideally*, their interdisciplinary research activities would be recognized as essentially scholarly in nature, rather than as adjuncts to community service or to solving personal or community health and medical problems. *Ideally*, such structures would be located within the basic arts and sciences units of universities, with strong linkages to scholarly, substantive doctoral programs in relevant areas, as well as to professional training programs in dentistry, medicine, nursing, and social work.

In settings such as these, basic research would go hand in hand with graduate-level instruction both in doctoral programs in health behavior and in the disciplines that participate in it. Establishment of such programs would reduce the isolation that health behaviorists experience. Relatively few such programs exist. Many more are needed.

Location of health behavior research elsewhere than in medical schools, especially if it were integrated with rigorous doctoral programs, would in all likelihood increase the status

accorded to it and thus increase the integration of health behavior knowledge with the training programs of medical and other health professionals. Furthermore, the "administrative identity" that would result from acknowledging such a department or program would foster its recognition and increase its visibility as a basic interdisciplinary and multidisciplinary activity. Moreover, its intellectual respectability would increase to the degree that it was seen as overlapping with and representing basic, traditional academic disciplines, rather than as an adjunct of medicine or as an essentially applied science. Such recognition, visibility, and academic respectability would appreciably strengthen its identity.

An intriguing and constructive federal mandate for academic centers for prevention research might provide a mechanism for linking health behavior research findings with applications in medicine and public health (e.g., Conner & Livengood, 1991). Such centers, however, are located in schools of either medicine or public health, and their agenda is determined by applied interests in prevention rather than by basic research.

Health Behavior and Ideology

While partisans of one model or another (e.g., health belief model, locus of control, cosmopolitanism–parochialism, explanatory models, critical theory) have emerged from time to time in the history of health behavior research, such partisanship has never assumed the fanaticism of the debates within related disciplines (e.g., behaviorism versus psychoanalysis versus gestalt theory within psychology; Marxism versus structural functionalism within sociology). Basic research is rarely served by such polemics. The viability and productivity of health behavior research will be enhanced to the degree that such ideological overkill can continue to be avoided in the future.

Moreover, the ideological neutrality mentioned in Chapter 1 of Volume I in relation to individual responsibility for health must similarly be demonstrated in relation to social, societal, and cultural factors and to policy factors that determine health behaviors. The research process must not be prevented—on the political grounds that such knowledge might be used to excuse the failure of governmental structures or private agencies to adopt or change social policies related to health care and health services or to exert undue influence on individuals—from developing new knowledge about the personal factors that determine health actions.

Much health behavior research, however, even those studies conducted with large systems, *has* focused on inducing changes in individuals or on generating knowledge that ultimately increases the likelihood of such individual change. Borrowing and generalizing from Bynder and New's (1976) analysis of the imbalance between micro- and macrosociological concepts in disability research, one can argue that health behavior research must not accept the "therapeutic" role of improving its technologies simply to change the individual, rather than pursue its role of developing knowledge to change the professions and policies *themselves* that have traditionally sought to change the individual. Nor must research be prevented from developing new knowledge of the role of social, policy, and structural variables, on the moral or religious grounds that such knowledge might be used to excuse the reluctance or failure of individuals to assume responsibility for their own actions.

On the other hand, knowledge of individual determinants of health actions—particularly in relation to behavioral consistency and stability—can be taken into account in the formulation of policy in order to improve estimates of the eventual impact of policy changes and thus improve the effectiveness of the policies themselves. Similarly, knowledge about the social and institutional context of individual behavior can improve the effectiveness of programs based on the premise that individuals *can* assume responsibility for their behavior and thus increase the effectiveness of programs designed to generate behavioral changes.

Co-optation: Politics and Profits

Kinston's (1983) analysis of health services research in Great Britain described how ideology and political interests have had a chilling and nullifying effect on basic research processes. Health behavior researchers should be increasingly sensitized to such pressures and not be co-opted by political factors to advance any single presumed correct perspective or approach. To the degree that such political co-optation occurs, it will place scientific research values in a subordinate position and will ultimately devalue and destroy the credibility of the research process.

Political co-optation can take another form: subordination to funding sources. Much funding for health behavior research in the United States has come from federal and state governments that continually reassess (a polite way of saying "change") their own priorities in the light of changing political climates, regardless of whether these priorities are in the public interest or not.

Such linkage of health behavior investigations with fluctuating governmental priorities raises questions about the degree to which the scientific process is subordinated to political or economic interests. Questions must be also be raised about the impact of continually changing governmental policies and priorities on basic *longitudinal* research. Moreover, hurrying research proposals toward premature completion to meet new and trendy priorities raises additional questions about their thoroughness, thoughtfulness, clarity of concepts, and other characteristics, all of which relate to their essence as *basic* investigations.

In the mid-1990s, however, looking toward the 21st century, the very existence of such government funding, regardless of priorities, becomes doubtful. Corporate for-profit agencies such as hospitals and insurance companies may become the major funding sources for much health behavior research, and their economic and political interests may well determine what and how research is undertaken.

A MATRIX FOR ORGANIZING HEALTH BEHAVIOR KNOWLEDGE

A Taxonomy for Health Behavior Research

A half century of health behavior research has generated a number of productive theoretical models, vast amounts of data unevenly and inequitably distributed across and among numerous populations, at least hundreds of supported and unsupported predictions, and a host of interventions and programs (too often unimpressive, unsuccessful, or both) directed at changing behavior. However, the findings of the past 50 years are inchoate and thus minimally useful to health professionals. The broad theoretical and conceptual models described in Volumes I and II have been excellent in focusing research efforts, but such focus does not by itself allow for organizing a broad body of knowledge. Similarly, the health behavior findings for diverse populations and at different developmental stages described in Volume III fail to comprise an organized body of knowledge. Critical to any organizing framework is an encompassing taxonomic model.

Building upon Kasl and Cobb and Other Pioneers

A "work-in-progress" draft of such a taxonomy emerges from a convergence of two paths. The first is the route established in Kasl and Cobb's (1966a,b) seminal taxonomy of health behavior, illness behavior, and sick role behavior. This benchmark conceptualization, which has remained a critical taxonomic model for four decades, embraces a large number of behaviors identified throughout this *Handbook*. Other scholarly works that have enriched the taxonomy of health behaviors are those of Harris and Guten (1979), who use the term "health protective behaviors" to refer to actions that people engage in to protect their health whether medically approved or not (Harris & Guten, 1979), and Langlie's (1977, 1979) distinction between "direct risk" and "indirect risk" preventive behaviors.

Gochman (this *Handbook*, Volume I, Chapter 1), provides a more detailed treatment of the meaning of these categories.

A second route to the proposed working draft was the assimilation of the large numbers of findings presented throughout this *Handbook* with the goal of developing common integrational frameworks for Volumes I through III. (Presentation of health behavior findings was not an objective of this volume, and incorporating the taxonomy systematically would far exceed the scope of an integrating chapter.) Working on such an integration for Volume I showed that nearly all the findings presented by the contributors could be encompassed by a taxonomy of six broadly defined categories: health-related cognitions; care seeking; preventive, protective, and safety behaviors; risk behaviors; responses to illness, including sick role and adherence; and lifestyle. Four of these categories encompassed nearly all the findings presented by the contributors to Volume II. Risk behaviors and health-related cognitions were rarely discussed in their own right in Volume II, but emerged in the contexts of other categories. For example, satisfaction with care—an important health cognition—emerges in the contexts of adherence to regimens, a reframing of the category of responses to illness, and of care seeking. The six categories again worked well for the contents of Volume III.

Kasl and Cobb's "health behaviors" and Harris and Guten's "protective behaviors" would fall under the "preventive, protective, and safety" category of this taxonomy. The actions embraced by Langlie's "direct risk" and "indirect risk preventive behavior" categories would be subsumed under either the "preventive, protective, and safety" category or the "lifestyle" category.

The matrix proposed here as a framework for organizing health behavior knowledge thus draws upon two of the major organizational principles of this *Handbook*: the preliminary attempt at grouping health behaviors into categories, and the use of a range of personal, social, and institutional systems as levels of analysis. The categories are identified and exemplified in Table 1. They clarify and codify the definition and descriptions given to contributors about the range of actions and cognitions that are embraced by health behavior. They also include, albeit within a different organization, the numerous behaviors identified in Chapter 1 of Volume I, "Health Behavior: Definitions and Diversity."

An Editorial Caveat

The intellectual tasks of developing the conceptual model for, and completing both the editing and the writing required by, this four-volume *Handbook* have led to clarification and refinement of my own thinking. The six categories of health behaviors that served as part of the organizational framework for the integrating chapters in Volumes I through III were used in an unelaborated way, and without clear definitions. Much as I might have preferred to be totally consistent and to continue to use them in the same way, the development of a conceptual matrix to organize health behavior knowledge challenged this usage and demanded rethinking, in the course of which a seventh category was added to the original six. Though this revised seven-category framework was used as the outline for the clarifying definitional discussion of the behavioral categories in this chapter, applying it retroactively would have necessitated some minor organizational changes in the final chapters of Volumes I through III. Since the initial framework worked well for the purposes of those chapters and there was little if any gain to be realized by applying the revised framework, the editorial objective of consistency was eclipsed by the objective of timely completion.

Categories of Health Behavior

At first glance, the categories are not as mutually exclusive as good nominal scaling requires. For example, a number of lifestyle behaviors such as getting proper nutrition and exercise can as reasonably be considered to be preventive behaviors. The absence or a low amount of a risk behavior might be considered as an instance of a healthy lifestyle or preventive behavior. In a number of instances, the lifestyle behavior is the reverse of the risk behavior.

This working model thus requires a greater degree of precision if it is to qualify as a nominal scale. Although "health cognitions" as a category is fairly straightforward and doesn't overlap with others, clarifications of the other six are necessary.

"Care seeking" denotes behavior that involves the services of some other person, either a layperson, health professional, or healer; it may itself be preventive as well as a response to illness symptoms but involves a direct encounter with a person rather than mere participation in a screening or prevention program. "Risk behavior" denotes and is restricted to *the initiation and/or maintenance* of some action, or *nonengagement* in some action, such as not using a seat belt, that increases the likelihood of a negative health status outcome. It does not include efforts to diminish that action that would fall into the "preventive, protective, and safety behaviors" category. Moreover, in this working model it makes sense to divide "risk behavior" into "nonaddictive" and "addictive" categories.

"Lifestyle" denotes behaviors that avoid risk *in general* and are directed toward what might be called "fitness" or "wellness" or "health seeking" rather than toward avoidance of specific diseases, illnesses, or injuries. "Responses to illness/adherence" denotes behaviors related to adherence, self-management, and reduction of risks attributed to a specific behavior, e.g., reducing fat, sodium, or caloric intake, that result from a disease diagnosis. A number of what are ordinarily thought of as lifestyle behaviors are thus included under responses to illness if they result from such a diagnosis. "Preventive, protective, and safety behavior" denotes a specific illness, disease, condition, or health or safety hazard together with a specific action that reduces its likelihood (primary prevention, e.g., immunizations, use of seat belts) or its impact (secondary prevention, e.g., screenings for early detection).

The point of this elaboration and these caveats is not so much to develop and proclaim watertight categories as it is to try to organize

Table 1. Categories, Definitions, and Selected Examples of Health Behaviors: A Work-in-Progress Model

Categories of health behaviors	Health cognitions	Care seeking	Risk behaviors		Lifestyle	Responses to illness/adherence	Preventive, protective safety
			Nonaddictive	Addictive			
Definition	Thought processes that serve as frames of reference for organizing and evaluating health, illness, disease, and sickness	Actions to involve some other person in health-related issue; can be for preventive reasons or response to illness	Initiation/maintenance of actions amenable to conscious control that increase likelihood of negative health outcome; nonengagement in actions that reduce such likelihoods	Actions that are beyond conscious control that increase likelihood of negative health outcomes	Actions to avoid general risk, or directed toward health/fitness; not undertaken in response to illness in relation to specific diseases	Actions undertaken to restore or maintain health in the face of a diagnosis	Specific actions undertaken to avoid identifiable negative health outcomes; early detection of disease

Examples							
Definitions: health, illness, am I sick? Perceptions of symptoms Representations: images, schemata, interpretations of illness Perceptions, expectations, beliefs: e.g., perceived health status, perceived vulnerability, perceived threat; beliefs about control; intentions Appraisal processes Attitudes, evaluations, satisfaction with care Values, motives, preferences: health as a motive, motives or values related to health Decision processes: when and where to seek care, and from whom; decisions to accept care (see also Care seeking)	When care is sought From whom care is sought: biomedical physician, alternative healer, other health professionals; clergy, counselors; laypersons: family members, social support network Consumerist behavior: physician shopping	Consumption of excess salt, fats, calories Unsafe sex behaviors: failure to use contraception; failure to use condoms Nonuse of seat belts or safety helmets Nonuse of worksite safety equipment Nonuse of smoke detectors Use of car telephone while driving Initiation of smoking: use of tobacco, alcohol, drugs Suicide; suicide attempts	Smoking; use of tobacco, alcohol, drugs	Nonsmoking/ smoking cessation; reducing alcohol/drug consumption Consumption of dietary fiber; eating breakfast Safe sex behaviors: contraception; careful use of condoms Acceptance of lifestyle/fitness program Sufficient sleep Skills for coping, problem solving, stress reduction	Acceptance of diagnosis, medication, total regimen Self-management; self-care, self-regulation of treatment Returning for treatment/care, appointment keeping Seeking or use of social support (caregivers)	Immunizations Use of seat belts; motorcycle helmets Use of safety helmets, safety equipment in workplace Use and maintenance of smoke detectors Injury preventive behavior: wearing football helmets, appropriate athletic safety equipment Purchasing, using safe vehicles Flossing; dental prophylaxis Use of sunscreen "Non-medically endorsed" actions: praying, saying mantras; taking laxatives, emetics; eating garlic and onions; drinking herbal teas; taking Turkish baths Screenings for early detection: TB, BSE, mammography; Pap tests; testicular self-examination

knowledge, and this matrix must be considered a very tentative, very preliminary model for doing so. Finally, the categories are at best a nominal scale rather than an ordinal one. In their current format, they resist any ordering. No one category has "more" or "less" of some characteristics or quality than any other.

Personal and Social Systems as Levels of Analysis

For all their inadequacies, these categories do form one axis of the matrix. The second axis is formed by an elaboration of the range of personal and social systems. Table 2 presents their intersection: the proposed matrix for any one population. A separate matrix could be used for each population group for which health behavior data exist. It may make sense, at the same time, to incorporate all findings into a single matrix. Virtually all the health behavior research findings reported in these volumes and elsewhere can be categorized into at least one cell of the matrix. Moreover, investigations in the four cognate disciplines—either individually or collaboratively—embrace this range of systems.

This matrix would be helpful not only in organizing such knowledge, but also in making it easier for researchers and health behavior theorists and scholars to see the differential importance of the various personal and social systems in determining health behaviors. This matrix could serve as an analogue to the use of a scatterplot to see whether certain types of determinants have greater impacts than others on a selected category. Such insights should ultimately be of relevance to health professionals, whether in clinical or in programmatic interventions.

Multidisciplinary and Interdisciplinary Publication: A Journal of Health Behavior Research

Health behavior as a multidisciplinary, interdisciplinary research activity needs its own scholarly journal. Several journals of superb quality publish reports of health behavior investigations, but these journals—*Social Science and Medicine*, *Journal of Health and Social Behavior*, *American Journal of Public Health*, and *Health Psychology*—do not have domains that are coterminous with that of health behavior as a basic, research discipline. They each contain much that is *not* relevant to health behavior, and each has a special focus that precludes publishing much basic interdisciplinary research. There is no journal that focuses on and is dedicated to health behavior research. An international scholarly journal dedicated to basic multidisciplinary and interdisciplinary research in health behavior would not only provide a suitable vehicle for publishing, but also further establish the identity of health behavior research. Such a journal would thus encourage contributions on the characteristics of the personal, family, social, institutional, community, and health care provider systems that affect health cognitions; care seeking; addictive and nonaddictive risk behaviors; lifestyle; responses to illness and adherence; and preventive, protective, and safety behaviors. Furthermore, such a journal could periodically present the organizing matrix, locating all the primary data and other findings reported or referred to in its articles in the appropriate cells. Having health behavior research findings made available in such an organizational matrix would make them more relevant to health professionals in clinical settings and in planned interventions.

SUMMARY

The four cognate disciplines of health psychology, medical anthropology, medical geography, and medical sociology have contributed substantially to the growth of health behavior research. Each discipline has to deal with its own issues of focus and subordination to medical and other interests. If health behavior research is to develop and mature as a focus of multidisciplinary and interdisciplinary inquiry, it must resolve issues related to its identity, particularly in relation to medicine, and to being located within medical schools.

Ideally, health behavior research programs should be located in arts and sciences units of

Table 2. A Matrix for Organizing Health Behavior Knowledge

Interdisciplinary and multidisciplinary health behavior research undertaken by health psychology, medical anthropology, medical geography, medical sociology, and other health behavior disciplines provides knowledge related to:	Categories of health behaviors						
Personal/social systems—levels of analysis	Health cognitions	Care seeking	Risk behavior		Lifestyle	Responses to illness/ adherence	Preventive, protective safety
			Nonaddictive	Addictive			
Personal Demographic	Data/findings						
Personal Personality							
Personal Cognitive							
Family							
Social Group characteristics							
Social Social role							
Social Gender role							
Institutional/organizational							
Community							
Cultural							
Health providers/ Interactional Perceptions							
Health providers/ Interactional Roles and power							
Health providers/ Structural Organizational							
Health providers/ Structural Environmental/ locational							

universities and should be linked with basic scientific disciplines as well as with the helping
professions. This chapter has presented a work-
in-progress proposal for a matrix for organizing
health behavior research knowledge generated
by the cognate disciplines, and by other disciplines and professions, that integrates seven categories of health behaviors with a range of personal, social, and institutional levels of analysis.
The matrix has implications for the future development of health behavior knowledge as well as
for increasing the value of such knowledge for
health professionals. It could become a major
organizational principle of a new international
multidisciplinary and interdisciplinary journal
that would publish basic health behavior research findings.

REFERENCES

Allport, G. W. (1960). The open system in personality theory.
    In G. W. Allport (Ed.), *Personality and social encounter*
    (pp. 39–54). Boston: Beacon Press.
American Psychological Association, Science Directorate.
    (1992). *The human capital initiative: Report of the Na-
    tional Research Agenda Steering Committee, Behavioral
    Science Summit*. Washington: American Psychological As-
    sociation.
American Psychological Association, Science Directorate.
    (1995). *Doing the right thing: A research plan for healthy
    living—A Human Capital Initiative strategy report*.
    Washington: American Psychological Association Human
    Capital Initiative Coordinating Committee.
American Psychological Association, Task Force on Health
    Research. (1976). Contributions of psychology to health
    research. *American Psychologist, 31*, 263–274.
Anderson, R. (1992). The efficacy of ethnomedicine: Re-
    search methods in trouble. In M. Nichter (Ed.), *Anthro-
    pological approaches to the study of ethnomedicine* (pp.
    1–17). Amsterdam: Gordon & Breach.
Angel, R., & Thoits, P. (1987). The impact of culture on the
    cognitive structure of illness. *Culture, Medicine and Psy-
    chiatry, 11*, 465–494.
Armstrong, D. (1985). Space and time in British general prac-
    tice. *Social Science and Medicine, 20*, 659–666.
Atkinson, P. (1979). From honey to vinegar: Lévi-Strauss in
    Vermont. In P. Morley & R. Wallis (Eds.), *Culture and
    curing* (pp. 168–188). Pittsburgh, PA: University of Pitts-
    burgh Press.

Auerbach, J. D., & Figert, A. E. (1995). Women's health re-
    search: Public policy and sociology. *Journal of Health and
    Social Behavior, 36*, (Special Issue), 115–131.
Baer, H. (1990). The possibilities and dilemmas of building
    bridges between critical medical anthropology and clinical
    anthropology: A discussion. *Social Science and Medicine,
    30*, 1011–1013.
Baldwin, D. M. (1990). Meeting production: The economics
    of contracting mental illness. *Social Science and Medicine,
    30*, 961–968.
Barrett, F. A. (1993). A medical geographical anniversary.
    Social Science and Medicine, 37, 701–710.
Baum, A. (1989). Preface. In A. Baum (Ed.), Proceedings of the
    National Working Conference on Research in Health and
    Behavior. *Health Psychology, 8*, (Special Issue), 629–630.
Béland, F., Philibert, L., Thouez, J.-P., & Maheux, B. (1990).
    Socio-spatial perspectives on the utilization of emergency
    hospital services in two urban territories in Quebec.
    Southern Medical Journal, 30, 53–66.
Bloom, S. W. (1990). Episodes in the institutionalization of
    medical sociology: A personal view. *Journal of Health and
    Social Behavior, 31*, 1–10.
Brown, P. (1995). Naming and framing: The social construc-
    tion of diagnosis and illness. *Journal of Health and Social
    Behavior, 36*, (Special Issue), 34–52.
Bynder, H., & New, P. K.-M. (1976). Time for a change: From
    micro- to macro-sociological concepts in disability re-
    search. *Journal of Health and Social Behavior, 17*, 45–52.
Charmaz, K. (1990). "Discovering" chronic illness: Using
    grounded theory. *Social Science and Medicine, 30*, 1161–
    1172.
Chesney, M. (1993). Health psychology in the 21st century:
    Acquired immunodeficiency syndrome as a harbinger of
    things to come. *Health Psychology, 12*, 259–268.
Cockerham, W. C. (1995). *Medical sociology* (6th ed.). Engle-
    wood Cliffs, NJ: Simon & Schuster.
Committee on Certification in Medical Sociology. (1986).
    *Guidelines for the certification process in medical soci-
    ology*. Washington, DC: American Sociological Association.
Connor, S. P., & Livengood, J. R. (1991). Academic centers for
    prevention research: Making prevention a practical reality.
    American Psychologist, 46, 525–527.
Coreil, J., & Mull, J. D. (1988). Introduction: Anthropological
    studies of diarrheal illness. *Social Science and Medicine,
    27*, 1–3.
Cowen, E. J. (1991). In pursuit of wellness. *American Psy-
    chologist, 46*, 404–408.
DiMatteo, M. R. (1991). *The psychology of health, illness, and
    medical care: An individual perspective*. Belmont, CA:
    Brooks/Cole.
Duncan, C., Jones, K., & Moon, G. (1993). Do places matter? A
    multi-level analysis of regional variations in health-related
    behaviour in Britain. *Social Science and Medicine, 37*,
    725–733.

Earickson, R. (1990). Introduction. *Social Science and Medicine*, *30*(1), vii–ix.

Eckert, J. K., & Goldstein, M. C. (1983). An anthropological approach to the study of illness behavior in an urban community. *Urban Anthropology*, *12*, 125–139.

Elinson, J. (1985). The end of medicine and the end of medical sociology. *Journal of Health and Social Behavior*, *26*, 268–275.

Enright, M. F., Resnick, R., DeLeon, P. H., Sciara, A. D., & Tanney, F. (1990). The practice of psychology in hospital settings. *American Psychologist*, *45*, 1059–1065.

Enright, M. F., Welch, B. L., Newman, R., & Perry, B. M. (1990). The hospital: Psychology's challenge in the 1990s. *American Psychologist*, *45*, 1057–1058.

Evans, R. I. (1988). Health promotion—science or ideology. *Health Psychology*, *7*, 203–219.

Evans, R. I. (1989). The evolution of challenges to researchers in health psychology. *Health Psychology*, *8*, 631–639.

Eyles, J. (1990). How significant are the spatial configurations of health care systems? *Social Science and Medicine*, *30*, 157–164.

Fabrega, H., & Hunter, J. E. (1978). Judgements about disease: A case study involving *Ladinos* of Chiapas. *Social Science and Medicine*, *12*, 1–10.

Flood, A. B., & Fennell, M. L. (1995). Through the lenses of organizational sociology: The role of organizational theory and research in conceptualizing and examining our health care system. *Journal of Health and Social Behavior*, *36* (Special Issue), 154–169.

Ford, D. H. (1990). Positive health and living systems frameworks. *American Psychologist*, *45*, 980–981.

Foster, G. M., & Anderson, B. G. (1978). *Medical anthropology*. New York: Wiley.

Friss, L., Friedman, B., & Demakis, J. (1989). Geographic differences in the use of Veteran's Administration hospitals. *Social Science and Medicine*, *28*, 347–354.

Gallagher, E. B. (1976). Lines of reconstruction and extension in the Parsonian sociology of illness. *Social Science and Medicine*, *10*, 207–218.

Gerhardt, U. (1989). The sociological image of medicine and the patient. *Social Science and Medicine*, *29*, 721–728.

Gesler, W. M. (1992). Therapeutic landscapes: Medical issues in light of the new cultural geography. *Social Science and Medicine*, *34*, 735–746.

Gochman, D. S. (1982). Labels, systems and motives: Some perspectives for future research. In D. S. Gochman & G. S. Parcel (Eds.), *Children's health beliefs and health behaviors*. *Health Education Quarterly*, *9*, 167–174.

Gold, M. (1977). A crisis of identity: The case of medical sociology. *Journal of Health and Social Behavior*, *18*, 160–168.

Hafferty, F. W., & Light, D. W. (1995). Professional dynamics and the changing nature of medical work. *Journal of Health and Social Behavior*, *36* (Special Issue), 132–153.

Harris, D. M., & Guten, S. (1979). Health protective behavior: An exploratory study. *Journal of Health and Social Behavior*, *20*, 17–29.

Helman, C. G. (1990). *Culture, health and illness* (2nd ed.). London: Wright/Butterworth.

Helman, C. G. (1991). Limits of biomedical explanation. *Lancet*, *337*, 1080–1083.

Hill, C. E. (Ed.). (1985). *Training manual in medical anthropology*. Washington: American Anthropological Association.

Hughes, C. C. (1968). Medical care: Ethnomedicine. In D. L. Sills (Ed.), *International encyclopedia of the social sciences* (pp. 88–92). New York: Macmillan & The Free Press.

Inhorn, M. C. (1995). Medical anthropology and epidemiology: Divergences or convergences? *Social Science and Medicine*, *40*, 285–290.

Kasl, S. V., & Cobb, S. (1966a). Health behavior, illness behavior, and sick-role behavior: I. Health and illness behavior. *Archives of Environmental Health*, *12*, 246–266.

Kasl, S. V., & Cobb, S. (1966b). Health behavior, illness behavior, and sick-role behavior: II. Sick-role behavior. *Archives of Environmental Health*, *12*, 531–541.

Kearns, R. A., & Joseph, A. E. (1993). Space in its place: Developing the link in medical geography. *Social Science and Medicine*, *37*, 711–717.

Kinston, W. (1983). Pluralism in the organisation of health services research. *Social Science and Medicine*, *17*, 299–313.

Kroeger, A. (1983). Anthropological and socio-medical health care research in developing countries. *Social Science and Medicine*, *17*, 147–161.

Landrine, H., & Klonoff, E. A. (1992). Culture and health-related schemas: A review and proposal for interdisciplinary integration. *Health Psychology*, *11*, 267–276.

Langlie, J. K. (1977). Social networks, health beliefs, and preventive health behavior. *Journal of Health and Social Behavior*, *18*, 244–260.

Langlie, J. K. (1979). Interrelationships among preventive health behaviors: A test of competing hypotheses. *Public Health Reports*, *94*, 216–225.

Levine, S. (1987). The changing terrains in medical sociology: Emergent concern with quality of life. *Journal of Health and Social Behavior*, *28*, 1–6.

Light, D. W. (1988). Toward a new sociology of medical education. *Journal of Health and Social Behavior*, *29*, 307–322.

MacCormack, C. (1994). Ethnological studies of medical sciences. *Social Science and Medicine*, *39*, 1229–1235.

Matarazzo, J. D. (1980). Behavioral health and behavioral medicine: Frontiers for a new health psychology. *American Psychologist*, *35*, 807–817.

Matheson, G. (1983). Health psychology: An opportunity, a responsibility. *Ontario Psychologist*, *15*(2), 4–10.

McClain, C. S. (1989). Reinterpreting women in healing roles.

In C. S. McClain (Ed.), *Women as healers: Cross-cultural perspectives* (pp. 1–19). New Brunswick, NJ: Rutgers University Press.

McElroy, A., & Townsend, P. K. (1989). *Medical anthropology in ecological perspective* (2nd ed.). Boulder, Co: Westview.

McLean, A. (1990). Contradictions in the social production of clinical knowledge: The case of schizophrenia. *Social Science and Medicine, 30,* 969–985.

Mechanic, D. (1979). Correlates of physician utilization: Why do major multivariate studies of physician utilization find trivial psychosocial and organizational effects? *Journal of Health and Social Behavior, 20,* 387–396.

Moon, G. (1990). Conceptions of space and community in British health policy. *Social Science and Medicine, 30,* 165–171.

Mumford, E. (1983). *Medical sociology* (1st ed.). New York: Random House.

Nichter, M. (Ed.). (1992). *Anthropological approaches to the study of ethnomedicine.* Amsterdam, The Netherlands: Gordon & Breach Science Publishers.

Pappas, G. (1990). Some implications for the study of the doctor–patient interaction: Power, structure, and agency in the works of Howard Waitzkin and Arthur Kleinman. *Social Science and Medicine, 30,* 199–204.

Parsons, T. (1951). *The social system.* Glencoe, IL: Free Press.

Parsons, T. (1975). The sick role and the role of the physician reconsidered. *Milbank Memorial Fund Quarterly: Health and Society, 53*(Summer), 257–278.

Pearlin, L. I. (1992). Structure and meaning in medical sociology. *Journal of Health and Social Behavior, 33,* 1–9.

Pescosolido, B. A., & Kronenfeld, J. J. (1995). Health, illness, and healing in an uncertain era: Challenges from and for medical sociology. *Journal of Health and Social Behavior, 36*(Special Issue), 5–33.

Pol, L. G., & Thomas, R. K. (1992). *The demography of health and health care.* New York: Plenum Press.

Press, I. (1990). Levels of explanation and cautions for a critical clinical anthropology. *Social Science and Medicine, 30,* 1001–1009.

Rodin, J. & Stone, G. C. (1987). Historical highlights in the emergence of the field. In G. C. Stone, S. M. Weiss, J. D. Matarazzo, N. E. Miller, J. Rodin, C. D. Belar, M. J. Follick, & J. E. Singer (Eds.), *Health psychology: A discipline and a profession* (pp. 15–26). Chicago: University of Chicago Press.

Romanucci-Ross, L., Moerman, D. E., & Tancredi, L. R. (Eds.). (1991). *The anthropology of medicine: From culture to method* (2nd ed.). New York: Bergin & Garvey.

Scarpaci, J. L. (1993). On the validity of language: Speaking, knowing and understanding in medical geography. *Social Science and Medicine, 37,* 719–724.

Scheper-Hughes, N. (1990). Three propositions for a critically applied medical anthropology. *Social Science and Medicine, 30,* 189–197.

Schofield, W. (1969). The role of psychology in the delivery of health services. *American Psychologist, 24,* 565–584.

Schwartz, G. E., & Weiss, S. M. (1978). (Eds.), Proceedings of the Yale conference on behavioral medicine. Department of Health, Education and Welfare Publication No. (NIH) 78-1424. Washington, DC: U.S. Government Printing Office.

Shannon, G. W., & Dever, G. E. A. (1974). *Health care delivery: Spatial perspectives.* New York: McGraw-Hill.

Singer, J. E. (1981) Some themes, perspectives, and opinions on a national research conference on oral health behavior. *Journal of Behavioral Medicine, 4,* 349–357.

Singer, M. (1990). Reinventing medical anthropology: Toward a critical realignment. *Social Science and Medicine, 30,* 179–187.

Singer, M., Baer, H. A., & Lazarus, E. (1990). Introduction: Critical medical anthropology in question. *Social Science and Medicine, 30*(2), v–viii.

Stein, H. F. (1990). In what systems do alcohol/chemical addictions make sense? Clinical ideologies and practices as cultural metaphors. *Social Science and Medicine, 30,* 987–1000.

Stone, G. C. (1979). Health and the health system: A historical overview and conceptual framework. In G. C. Stone, F. Cohen & N. E. Adler (Eds.), *Health psychology* (pp. 1–17). San Francisco: Jossey-Bass.

Stone, G. C. (1987). The scope of health psychology. In G. C. Stone, S. M. Weiss, J. D. Matarazzo, N. E. Miller, J. Rodin, C. D. Belar, M. J. Follick, & J. E. Singer (Eds.). (1987). *Health psychology: A discipline and a profession* (pp. 27–40). Chicago: University of Chicago Press.

Stone, G. C., Cohen, F., & Adler, N. E. (Eds.). (1979). *Health psychology—A handbook: Theories, applications, and challenges of a psychological approach to the health care system.* San Francisco: Jossey-Bass.

Stoner, B. P. (1986). Understanding medical systems: Traditional, modern, and syncretic health care alternatives in medically pluralistic societies. *Medical Anthropology Quarterly, 17*(2), 44–48.

Taylor, S. E. (1987). The progress and prospects of health psychology: Tasks of a maturing discipline. *Health Psychology, 6,* 73–87.

Taylor, S. E. (1990). Health psychology: The science and the field. *American Psychologist, 45,* 40–50.

Terris, M. (1975). Approaches to an epidemiology of health. *American Journal of Public Health, 65,* 1037–1045.

Thouez, J.-P., Foggin, P., & Rannou, A. (1990). Correlates of health-care use: Inuit and Cree of Northern Quebec. *Social Science and Medicine, 30,* 25–34.

Waitzkin, H. (1989). A critical theory of medical discourse: Ideology, social control, and the processing of social context in medical encounters. *Journal of Health and Social Behavior, 30,* 220–239,

Weidman, H. H. (1988). A transcultural perspective on health behavior. In D. S. Gochman (Ed.), *Health behavior: Emerging research perspectives*. New York: Plenum Press.

Whiteford, L. M. (1985). Community health assessment and evaluation. In C. E. Hill (Ed.), *Training manual in medical anthropology* (pp. 21–39). Washington, DC: American Anthropological Society.

Wolinsky, F. D. (1988). *The sociology of health: Principles, practitioners, and issues* (2nd ed.). Belmont, CA: Wadsworth.

Wright, A. L., & Morgan, W. J. (1990). On the creation of "problem" patients. *Social Science and Medicine, 30,* 951–959.

Concepts and Definitions

A Glossary for Health Behavior Research

With few exceptions, the definitions in this Glossary are either taken verbatim, paraphrased, or abstracted from this *Handbook*. Specific chapters and, where appropriate, sources cited herein are identified. Italicized terms within a definition denote additional Glossary entries.

Consistent with the focus of this *Handbook* on health *behavior*, the Glossary does not routinely define diseases or medical treatments. Space limitations preclude defining every "named" intervention or program, or every social or behavioral science model that is not especially focused on health behavior. A number of these programs and models, however, are listed in the Index.

acceptance See *adherence; compliance.*

access framework A conceptual refinement of the *health services utilization model* that predicts the use of and satisfaction with health care; basic components are health policy, the organizational and accessibility characteristics of the delivery system, and *predisposing, enabling,* and *need factors* (Aday & Andersen, 1974, in Aday & Awe, I, 8). See *utilization framework.*

action stage In the *transtheoretical model*, the phase in which persons have modified their behavior and are participating in the appropriate health practice (Prohaska & Clark, III, 2).

active coping In health contexts, a tendency or motivation to exercise personal control, reflecting preference for decision making in health care, preference for behavioral involvement, and low expectations that health care professionals can control one's health (Christensen, Benotsch, & Smith, II, 12).

active patient orientation See *mutual participation model.*

active prevention See *prevention, active.*

activities of daily living (ADL) Instrumental and basic behaviors necessary for everyday life (Prohaska & Clark, III, 2).

adherence Practice of following health care provider recommendations (Clark, II, 8; Chrisler, II, 17); "an interdependent network of regimen behaviors rather than a single behavior" (Wysocki & Greco, II, 9); following recommended screening procedures (Rimer, Demark-Wahnefried, & Egert, II, 15); congruence between patient behaviors and advice or instructions provided by health care providers; medical adherence: how closely a patient's medication-taking behaviors match instructions prescribed by a physician (Creer & Levstek, II, 7). The concept embraces total adherence and acceptance, as well as degrees thereof; in relation to smoking, it includes not only total cessation, but also participation in cessation activities, as well as the actions of change agents (Glasgow & Orleans, II, 19). It connotes active, voluntary behavior designed to produce a therapeutic effect (Chrisler, II, 17). See *compliance.*

ADL See *activities of daily living.*

affective behavior, physician's Comprises acts aimed at establishing a relationship with patients in which the physician accepts the patient as a human being whose anxiety-arousing problems cannot be alleviated by technical procedures; it involves the physician attributing therapeutic importance to, and engaging in warm, open relations with the patient; being attentive to problems that may not be related to disease, gathering information about personal and family problems and social relations; and explaining the rationale of the diagnosis and treatment (Ben-Sira, II, 2).

AIDS Acquired immunodeficiency syndrome: a condition in which exposure to the *HIV* (human immunodeficiency virus) leads to the destruction of the body's natural defenses against infection (Thomason & Campos, III, 8).

analytical framework for the study of child survival A conceptual model designed to understand morbidity and mortality in children in developing countries; basic components are maternal factors, environmental contamination, nutrient deficiency, and injury and personal illness control (Mosley & Chen, 1984, in Coreil, III, 9).

anthropology of medicine See *medical anthropology*.

appropriate interventions/care Lists of indications for use of procedures consensually generated by nationally recognized experts (Rand Corporation/McGlynn, Kosecoff, & Brook, 1990, in DiMatteo, II, 1). Compare *inappropriate/unnecessary care*.

attributable risk Amount of disease (disability or mortality) in a population group that could be eliminated if a risk factor were eliminated (Prohaska & Clark, III, 2).

authority, physician The physician's power over others (Haug, II, 3).

autonomy, physician The physician's power or ability to resist or withstand being compelled by others (Haug, II, 3).

autonomy, principle of A moral standard stressing the obligation to respect rights to self-determination (Nilstun, IV, 11).

autonomy, self-care See *self-care autonomy*.

availability bias A concept that explains safety and risk avoidance behaviors, denoting the inclination to be inordinately influenced by dramatic events that have low probabilities of happening but are vivid in memory; ease of recall being a function of saliency, recency, and emotional impact (Slovic, 1978, in Cohen & Colligan, II, 20).

behavioral epidemiology The study of the relationships between lifestyles and mortality and morbidity patterns in a population (Rakowski, III, 5).

behavioral model See *health services utilization model*.

beneficence, principle of A moral standard stressing the obligation to benefit others, especially not to harm them (Nilstun, IV, 11).

bruxism Spasmodic grinding of the teeth in other than chewing movements (Gift & White, IV, 7).

caregiver, informal Layperson who provides personal care to an older, ill family member or close friend (Wright, III, 13).

care-seeking behavior, theory of A conceptual framework in nursing, incorporating components of the *health belief model*, *theory of reasoned action*, and Triandis's theory of interpersonal behavior; designed to predict preventive rather than illness-related behaviors; basic components are affective arousal, perceived utility, *social norms*, and habits (Lauver, 1992a, in Blue & Brooks, IV, 5).

central place theory A conceptual framework based on land economics that is used to relate a hierarchy of levels of health care services to concentrations of population and distances (Scarpaci & Kearns, II, 5).

children's health belief model A conceptual framework for understanding children's health behaviors, incorporating components of the *health belief model*, environmental variables, and readiness factors (O'Brien & Bush, III, 3).

chronic Referring to an illness or condition that is incurable and lasts through a person's lifetime (Gallagher & Stratton, III, 11).

cognitive appraisal The process of intellectually evaluating and deciding on available options to engage in a particular behavior (Cowell & Marks, III, 4).

cognitive developmental theory A conceptual framework for understanding the development of children's thinking; assumes that children take an active rather than a passive role in constructing their own knowledge and understanding of health and illness and that they move through universally recognized sequences in doing so (O'Brien & Bush, III, 3).

cognitive representations Personal images or schemata of illness, disease, and being healthy, and the meanings attached to these images; persons develop their own individualized images or schemata in relation to symptoms and illness that are often different from the representations of physicians and the medical community (Lau, I, 3).

coming out Disclosure of nonheterosexual identity by a lesbian or a gay man (VanScoy, III, 7); can also mean self-recognition of such identity.

commonsense representation of illness The images or schemata of illness, disease, or symptoms held by a layperson; the images include an identity, a set of consequences, a time-line, a cause, and a cure or control (Lau, I, 3).

communication Exchange of meaning, either verbally or nonverbally, between people to establish a commonality of thought, attitude, feeling, and ideas (DiMatteo, II, 1).

communication campaign Use of mass media on a health topic, typically involving television, radio, newspaper, magazines, and other channels to convey health information or to provide motivation for health actions (Swinehart, IV, 18).

community A social entity or system made up of individuals together with formal organizations, such as local government, businesses, and educational institutions, and voluntary organizations, such as religious, fraternal, or service groups; informal social networks; and families. Critical to the concept is the premise that various components are related to each other and have the potential for being mobilized in relation to health promotion programs (Schooler & Flora, IV, 15).

community health promotion Interventions for effecting change in communities that involve social planning, social action, and locality development (Rothman, 1979, in Schooler & Flora, IV, 15).

community organization An intervention strategy designed to empower a community and to enhance its competence and problem-solving ability; of particular importance for increasing the success of a *health promotion* program (Schooler & Flora, IV, 15).

compadrazgo A system of selecting *comadres* (female friends) and *copadres* (male friends) for one's children; levels of perceived support from these friends are related to health status and health behavior (Dressler & Oths, I, 17).

competence gap The difference in health-related knowledge and skill between physicians and other health professionals and their patients or clients (Haug, II, 3).

compliance Degree of correspondence between the physician's prescription and the patient's behavior (Sackett & Haynes, 1976, in DiIorio, II, 11; Morisky & Cabrera, II, 14); congruence between medical recommendations and the degree to which a patient takes medicine, follows a diet, or changes lifestyle behaviors (Trostle, II, 6); an ideology that transforms a physician's theories about patients' behavior into research strategies and potentially coercive interventions that strengthen physicians' authority (Trostle, II, 6). See also *adherence*.

conscientiousness factor A theoretical personality dimension reflecting "will to achieve," "dependability," and "self-control" thought to be related to medication adherence in renal dialysis patients (Christensen et al., II, 12).

consciousness raising A component of the *transtheoretical model*, denoting a process by which people move from not being ready to initiate a behavior to being ready to initiate it (Rakowski, III, 5).

consumerism A framework for viewing physician–patient interactions that argues for patient autonomy and sole decision making as essential in combating physician paternalism (DiMatteo, II, 1), or in which an "activist" patient approaches health care as a problem-solving endeavor that requires active coping (Pratt, 1978, in Wiese & Gallagher, IV, 4).

contemplation In the *transtheoretical model*, the stage in which people are aware that a problem exists and are seriously thinking about overcoming it (Prohaska & Clark, III, 2)

contracting Use of a written document, resulting from the negotiation of a treatment plan between a patient and medical personnel, that identifies the reinforcements the patient will receive contingent on performing the behaviors stipulated in the treatment plan (Creer & Levstek, II, 7).

control beliefs See *locus of control*.

control demand model A conceptual framework developed to understand how workplace characteristics are related to health behaviors such as smoking, alcohol use, exercise, and self-protective behavior; basic components are levels of control over work, psychological demands, and social support (Eakin, I, 16).

control, perceived behavioral See *perceived behavioral control*.

convergence hypothesis A proposition that suggests that as gender roles become more similar, gender differences in health behavior decrease or disappear (Waldron, I, 15).

conversation model A conceptual framework for viewing physician–patient interactions in which the patient continually provides the physician information about values, preferences, and constraints and the physician engages in "thinking out loud" about possible courses of action, recommended interventions, and their implications, using language that is understood by the patient (DiMatteo, II, 1).

coping appraisal   Evaluation of adaptive responses to threat; a component of the *protection motivation theory* (Rogers & Prentice-Dunn, I, 6).

coping mode   Way of responding to threat messages (Rogers & Prentice-Dunn, I, 6). See *protection motivation theory*.

cue to action   A stimulus, either internal or external, that can trigger health-related cognitive processes or health actions (Strecher, Champion, & Rosenstock, I, 4).

cultural consensus model   A conceptual framework to assess the degree to which a body of information is shared within a social group; provides an estimate of shared beliefs related to health and illness (Dressler & Oths, I, 17).

culture   A set of interlocking cognitive schemata that literally construct much of what people do on a daily basis; the manner in which a social group stores and transmits information; a system of symbols or abstract elements that are learned and patterned socially (Dressler & Oths, I, 17).

damaging cycle   A chain of events in which a somatic disturbance leads to a detrimental appraisal of health, which then precipitates stress, which then increases the risk of further somatic disturbance (Ben-Sira, II, 2).

decisional balance theory   A conceptual framework for understanding how persons make specific choices, based on comparisons of perceived positive and negative aspects of a behavior, and including gains and losses to self and others and approval or disapproval of self and others (Janis & Mann, 1977, in Marcus, Bock, & Pinto, II, 18).

demography, health   See *health demography*.

deskilling   Transference of work functions once controlled exclusively by physicians or nurses to positions lower down on the occupational hierarchy (Salloway, Hafferty, & Vissing, II, 4).

developing country   A designation based on economic, demographic, and social/health indicators, given to a nation that is relatively poor, with a relatively young and fertile population and relatively scarce health and social resources (Coreil, III, 9).

developmental model of diabetes self-management   A conceptual framework for understanding

the responsibilities that patients and families can assume in monitoring, evaluating, and adjusting treatment for insulin-dependent diabetes mellitus; basic components include demographic factors, family functioning, psychological stress, and interactions with providers to acquire necessary skills (Wysocki & Greco, II, 9). See *self-management, childhood diabetes*; *self-regulation/self-regulatory skills*.

diagnosis   Naming of a condition by medical professionals; represents the interplay of social, institutional, and cultural factors together with personal symptoms through which time and location at which medical professionals and other parties determine the existence and legitimacy of a condition (Brown, 1995, in Gochman, IV, 20).

diagnosis related group/diagnostic related group (DRG)   One of 438 groupings of patient conditions that have been the basis for federal reimbursements to hospitals for Medicare patients since 1983 (Daugherty, IV, 10); hospitals are paid a fixed amount for a given DRG regardless of length of stay and services provided.

disease   A biological/organic abnormality; not identical to illness (Lau, I, 3); the measurable deviation of an organic system from some independently defined optimum (Dressler & Oths, I, 17).

doctrine of specific etiology   See *specific etiology, doctrine of*.

DRG   See *diagnosis related group*.

drinking culture   Group norms, particularly within work settings, that encourage and support consumption of alcohol; closely related to *occupational culture* (Eakin, I, 16).

ecological model   A conceptual framework that integrates five levels of personal and social systems: intrapersonal, interpersonal, organizational, community, and public policy in public health efforts (Buchanan, IV, 9).

edentulous   Without teeth; toothless (Gift & White, IV, 7).

effectiveness   Benefits of medical care measured by improvements in health (Aday & Awe, I, 8).

efficiency   A relationship between improvements in health and the resources required to produce them (Aday & Awe, I, 8).

elaboration likelihood model   A conceptual framework to predict attitude change; persuasion is proposed to be a function of the audience's active involvement in processing a message and the importance of the message's topic to the audience (Petty &

Cacioppo, 1986, in Rogers & Prentice-Dunn, I, 6; Wiese & Gallagher, IV, 4).

emic Denotes a way of knowing reflecting an internal or cultural "insider" perspective (Weidman, 1988, in Gochman, I, Part V); emic behavior is behavior that a person believes to be related to health, regardless of whether it is externally validated (Eakin, I, 16). Compare *etic*.

empowerment Enabling individuals, families, and communities to take control over their lives and their environment (e.g., Rappaport, 1984, in Schooler & Flora, IV, 15).

enabling factor A resource characteristic, such as family income or community availability, that predicts use of health services; a component of the *health services utilization model* (Aday & Awe, I, 8).

energized family A conceptual framework for understanding the family as a social system; basic components are regularity of interaction among members, contacts with the larger community, working together to advance members' interests, and coping with and mastering their lives. Energized families tend to encourage autonomy, rather than use "autocratic" parenting, and to socialization methods, resulting in children with better levels of health behaviors (Pratt, 1976, in Gochman, I, 10; Tinsley, I, 11).

epidemiology "Study of the distribution and determinants of diseases and injuries in human populations" (Inhorn, 1995, in Gochman, IV, 20).

epidemiology, behavioral See *behavioral epidemiology*.

epidemiology, psychosocial See *psychosocial epidemiology*.

equity The degree to which the benefits and burdens of medical care are fairly distributed in a population (Aday & Awe, I, 8); the degree to which participants (either patients or professionals) believe that the ratio of benefits received to their efforts and resources expended is equal or skewed in their favor (Daugherty, IV, 10).

etic Denotes a way of knowing reflecting an external or cultural "outsider" perspective (Weidman, 1988, in Gochman, I, Part V). Etic behavior is behavior that external observers believe to be related to health, independent of the behaving individual's beliefs (Eakin, I, 16). Compare *emic*.

eudaimonistic health A state of exuberant well-being (Lau, I, 3).

exercise Physical activity of moderate intensity (Marcus et al., II, 18).

explanatory model A cognitive framework of health processes based on both cultural knowledge and idiosyncratic experience that is used to understand health status, illness, and sickness; basic components include etiology, timing of onset of symptoms, pathophysiology, course of sickness, and treatment. Explanatory models exist at both lay and professional levels (Kleinman, 1980, & Kleinman, Eisenberg, & Good, 1978, in Dressler & Oths, I, 17).

facilitative environment An environment in which "nonsmoking cues and cessation information are persistent and inescapable" (Glynn, Boyd, & Gruman, 1990, in Glasgow & Orleans, II, 19).

familism Importance of family and relatives in a person's live, particularly in relation to care-seeking behavior (Geertsen, I, 13).

family aggregation A concept denoting intrafamilial similarities in health variables compared to nonfamilial similarities (Sallis & Nader, 1988, in Gochman, I, 10).

family code A system of norms for a family's behavior, including core assumptions, beliefs, family stories, myths, and rituals (Tinsley, I, 11).

family concordance Degree to which members of a family exhibit similarity in a specified health behavior (Baranowski, I, 9).

family, energized See *energized family*.

family health culture The unique combination of family experiences, beliefs, perceptions of symptoms, and reactions to the perceptions that influences the way in which families seek care or treatment (Black, 1986, in Gochman, I, 10).

fighting the illness A posture of gritty defiance as a way of dealing with a chronic illness (Gallagher & Stratton, III, 11)

fixed role hypothesis A proposition suggesting that men's more structured role obligations, compared with women's, may make it more difficult for men to engage in care-seeking behavior and thus accounts for women's greater use of health services (Marcus & Siegel, 1982, in Gochman, I, Part IV).

Flexner Report An analysis and recommendations relevant to United States medical education, prepared by Abraham Flexner in 1910, that became the basis for the reform of and standardization of medical training; remains a critical foundation for late 20th-century medical education (Weise & Gallagher, IV, 4).

folk illness A shared interpretation of a cluster of symptoms within a social group that is at variance with a biomedical framework (Dressler & Oths, I, 17).

framework of relationships model   A conceptual scheme for understanding compliance behavior, especially for epilepsy; basic components are the *health services utilization model*, the *health belief model*, and health education, with an emphasis on adequate financial and community resources (Di Iorio, II, 11).

gay   Without a gender qualifier, refers to a homosexual, a person who engages or desires to engage in sexual behavior with a person of the same gender (Kauth & Prejean, III, 6).

gay man   A male who engages or desires to engage in sexual behavior with another male; a homosexual (Kauth & Prejean, III, 6).

gender role   The social roles, behaviors, attitudes, and psychological characteristics that are more common, more expected, and more accepted for one sex or the other; includes a group of interrelated behaviors, attitudes, and psychological characteristics that influence a variety of risk and risk-taking behaviors as well as care-seeking behaviors (Waldron, I, 15).

GOBI   Acronym for *G*rowth monitoring, *O*ral rehydration, *B*reast-feeding and *I*mmunization, the four cornerstone child survival interventions in developing countries (Coreil, III, 9).

grazing   Snacking throughout the day (O'Brien & Bush, III, 3).

group ties   See *social ties*.

habit   A behavior that does not require conscious effort but is set in motion by situational cues (Schneider & Shiffrin, 1977, in Maddux & DuCharme, I, 7) and is less under the control of conscious cognitive processes and deliberate decisions.

healing   The social processes and actions brought to bear to deal with a condition of disease or illess (Fabrega, I, 2).

healing culture   The totality of institutions involved in treatment of disease, including biomedical and alternative approaches and the range of choices available, and the culture of medicine and its rituals and stresses (e.g., Foster & Anderson, 1978, in Gochman, IV, 20).

healmeme   A unit of symbolic cultural information that gives meaning to the domain of health, well-being, sickness, and healing; underlies and constitutes a society's health-related beliefs and behaviors (Fabrega, I, 2).

health   A state of being, almost impossible to define satisfactorily; includes components of physiological, psychological, and social functioning (Gochman I, 1; Lau, I, 3). What is considered to be health is appreciably determined by societal and cultural factors (Fabrega, I, 2). A continuous variable reflecting a capacity or ability to perform, as well as the use of that capacity to achieve expectations and to negotiate the demands of the social and physical environment (Tarlov, 1992, in Reed, Moore-West, Jernstedt, & O'Donell, IV, 2); "an individual or group capacity relative to potential to function fully in the social and physical environment" (Tarlov, 1992, in Flipse, IV, 3).

health behavior, formal   Actions taken for the prevention or treatment of a condition or for the maintenance or enhancement of health that involve the use of institutionalized services such as physicians and hospitals (Pol & Thomas, III, 1).

health behavior, informal   Actions taken for the prevention or treatment of a condition or for the maintenance or enhancement of health that do not involve the use of institutionalized services such as physicians and hospitals; these actions include self-care, tooth brushing, and use of over-the-counter medications (Pol & Thomas, III, 1).

health belief model   A conceptual framework designed to predict preventive actions and eventually used to predict illness and sick role behaviors; basic components of the model are perceived susceptibility to some illness, perceived severity or seriousness of that condition, perceived benefits of taking a specified action, and perceived barriers to taking such action (Strecher, Champion, & Rosenstock, I, 4).

health care management   See *management, health care*.

health care manager   See *manager, health care*.

health culture   A society's repertoire of patterns for cognition, affect, and behavior in relation to health, sickness, and well-being (Weidman, 1988, in Gochman, I, Part V).

health demography   Application of the content and methods of demography to the study of health-related phenomena; analyzes the influence of demographic factors such as age, marital status, and income on the health status and health behavior of poplations and the differential impact of health-related phenomena on demographic groupings; focuses on the implications of population change for health care (Pol & Thomas, III, 1). See *behavioral epidemiology*; *psychosocial epidemiology*.

health education Efforts to change behavior in order to improve health (Glanz & Oldenburg, IV, 8); "any combination of learning experiences designed to facilitate voluntary adaptations of behavior conducive to health" (Green, Kreuter, Deeds, & Partridge, 1980, p. 7, in Glanz & Oldenburg, IV, 8).

health input–output model See *input-output model, health*.

health maintenance organization (HMO) A prepaid group practice for delivering comprehensive health care from a specific set of providers. See *managed care*.

health policy Aggregate of federal, state, and local laws, rules, and regulations that govern the financing, regulation, and organization of health care (Aday & Awe, I, 8).

health-promoting self-care system model A conceptual framework for nursing, integrating self-care deficit nursing theory, the *interaction model of client health behavior*, and the *health promotion model of nursing*, designed to predict individual autonomy and responsibility for health-promoting behaviors (Simmons, 1990a, in Blue & Brooks, IV, 5).

health promotion "any combination of health education and related organizational, economic, and environmental supports for behavior of individuals, groups, or communities conducive to health" (Green & Kreuter, 1991, in Glanz & Oldenburg, IV, 8); "the science and art of helping people change their lifestyle to move toward a state of optimal health ... by a combination of efforts to enhance awareness, change behavior, and create environments that support good health practices" (O'Donnell, 1989, in Glanz & Oldenburg, IV, 8); "the process of enabling people to increase control over, and to improve, their health ... a commitment to dealing with the challenges of reducing inequities, extending the scope of prevention, and helping people to cope with their circumstances ... creating environments conducive to health, in which people are better able to take care of themselves" (Epp, 1986, in Glanz & Oldenburg, IV, 8). The term was seldom used prior to 1980.

health promotion model, nursing A conceptual framework for nursing, similar to the *health belief model*, used to predict engaging in behaviors that maintain or improve well-being, rather than prevent disease; basic components are importance of health, perceived control of health, perceived *self-efficacy*, definition of health, perceived health status, *perceived benefits* of health-promoting behaviors, and *perceived barriers* to health-promoting behaviors (Pender, 1982, in Blue & Brooks, IV, 5).

health psychology "The aggregate of the specific educational, scientific, and professional contributions of the discipline of psychology to the promotion and maintenance of health, the prevention and treatment of illness, the identification of etiologic and diagnostic correlates of health, illness and related dysfunction" (Matarazzo, 1980, p. 815, in Gochman, IV, 20); "any aspect of psychology that bears upon the experience of health and illness, and the behavior that affects health status" (Rodin & Stone, 1987, pp. 15-16, in Gochman, IV, 20).

health-seeking process model A conceptual framework for understanding people's experiences with sickness holistically as natural histories of illness; basic components are symptom definition, illness-related shifts in role behavior, lay referral, treatment actions, and adherence (Chrisman, 1977, in Dressler & Oths, I, 17).

health service system Arrangements for the potential rendering of care to consumers, including the volume and distribution of services and their accessibility and organization (Aday & Awe, I, 8). See *health services utilization model*.

health services utilization model A conceptual framework designed to predict use of health care, such as visits to physicians and dentists and use of medications and clinical facilities; basic components are *predisposing*, *enabling*, and *need factors* (Aday & Awe, I, 8); sometimes referred to as the *behavioral model*.

heterosexism An assumption, especially among health providers and institutions, that heterosexuality, or male-female sexual expression, is normative and superior to others (VanScoy, III, 7).

HIV See *AIDS*.

HMO Acronym for *health maintenance organization* (Daugherty, IV, 10). See *managed care*.

homeless assistance act, Stewart B. McKinney A 1987 federal law that extended the National Health Care for the Homeless Initiative to a total of 109 cities (Wright & Joyner, III, 10).

homeless, literally Persons who spend their nights either in outdoor locations, in temporary overnight shelters, or in other places not intended for human habitation (Wright & Joyner, III, 10).

homelessness No agreed-upon definition (Wright & Joyner, III, 10). See *homeless, literally*; *housed, marginally*.

homophobia An irrational fear of homosexuality (Eliason, Donelan, & Rundall, 1992, in Vanscoy, III, 7).

housed, marginally Persons with a claim to some minimal housing, but who are at high risk of being *homeless* (Wright & Joyner, III, 10).

illness The subjective experience of some biological/organic/social/emotional abnormality; not identical to disease (e.g., Lau, I, 3); the social and psychological concomitants of putative physiological problems (Conrad, 1990, in Gochman, I, 1); incapacity for role performance (Gerhardt, 1989a, in Gochman, I, 1); motivated deviance (Segall, I, 14); the individual experience of suffering or distress, or disvalued states of being and functioning (Dressler & Oths, I, 17).

illusion of safety Workers' practicing of safe behavior under supervision but of unsafe behavior, such as taking shortcuts and engaging in risky actions, in the absence of supervision; convinces management that it has done its job and that safety regimens are being followed when in reality they are not (Cohen & Colligan, II, 20).

image theory A conceptual framework for decision making based on the fit between alternative choices and an individual's images, plans, or principles (Mitchell & Beach, 1990, in Rogers & Prentice-Dunn, I, 6).

inappropriate/unnecessary care A medical intervention with risks that exceed the potential benefit to the patient (DiMatteo, II, 1). Compare *appropriate intervention/care*.

informal caregiver See *caregiver, informal*.

information seeking A generic process that underlies behavior change and comprises a cluster of behaviors including but not limited to reading articles about health, attending to media programs on health, and reading food package labels (Rakowski, III, 5; Swinehart, IV, 18).

information vigilance factor A tendency or motivation to attend actively to threat-relevant information and sensory experiences related to health and treatment, reflecting *information seeking*, internal health *locus of control*, and monitoring of sensory information (Christensen et al., II, 12).

inoculation theory A conceptual framework suggesting that providing persons in advance with information and counterarguments enables them to resist persuasive and pressuring appeals to engage in risk behaviors; sometimes termed "social inocula-

tion theory" (McGuire, 1968, in Kelder et al., IV, 14; Bruhn, IV, 1).

input–output model, health A framework combining external factors such as the physical and community environments and the macrosocial structure with internal biological–genetic–psychic factors as predictors of role fulfillment and well-being (Tarlov, 1992, in Flipse, IV, 3).

inreach Directing health promotion and prevention strategies at persons already in the health care system (Rimer et al., II, 15).

intention, behavioral A person's subjective probability or prediction of performing a specified behavior; a basic component of the *theory of reasoned action*/theory of planned behavior. It has been inaccurately defined as what a person intends or plans to do and the degree to which a person has developed conscious plans to enact some behavior in the future (Maddux & DuCharme, I, 7). See *self-prediction*.

interaction model of client health behavior A conceptual framework in nursing to explain and predict a range of health behaviors; basic components are elements of client singularity, such as background, motivation, cognitive appraisal, and affective responses, and elements of client–professional interactions, such as affective support, health information, decisional control, and professional competence (Cox, 1982, in Blue & Brooks, IV, 5).

interfamilial consensus A concept denoting the degree of similarity in illness-related conceptions in randomly selected pairs of persons (Susman et al., 1982, in Gochman, I, 10).

intrafamilial transmission A concept denoting the degree of similarity in illness-related conceptions found in parent–child pairs (Susman et al., 1982, in Gochman, I, 10).

justice as fairness A conceptual framework applied to health issues that stipulates that each person has an equal right to liberty, that persons with similar abilities and skills should have equal access to services, and that social and economic institutions should be arranged to benefit maximally the least well off (Nilstun, IV, 11).

justice, principle of A moral standard stressing the obligation to act fairly in the distribution of burdens and benefits, especially not to discriminate against anyone (Nilstun, IV, 11).

KAP (acronym for *K*nowledge, *A*ttitudes, and *P*ractices) A standardized measure to assess knowledge of disease risk factors, use of a health service, and perceptions of therapeutic efficacy; used extensively in *developing countries* (Coreil, III, 9).

landscape, therapeutic A combination of physical and humanly imposed environmental characteristics of treatment settings that facilitate the healing process (Gesler, 1992, in Gochman, IV, 20).

language of distress Terminology as well as nonverbal cues that patients use to present their conditions to health professionals (Helman, 1991, in Gochman, IV, 20).

lay-intelligible cues An action on the part of the physician that serves as a basis for the patient's understanding of a condition and its treatment and for the patient's evaluation of the physician's treatment and competence (Ben-Sira, II, 2).

lay referral system The informal network of family members, friends, and community contacts who provide information and advice about the care-seeking process prior to use of a professional (Geertsen, I, 13).

learned resourcefulness Tendency to apply self-control skills in solving behavioral problems, e.g., use of strategies to delay gratification or tolerate frustration (Rosenbaum, 1980, in Christensen et al., II, 12).

lesbian A woman who engages or desires to engage in sexual behavior with another female; the preferred term is "lesbian identity," denoting a woman whose identity is defined by other women (VanScoy, III, 7).

lesbian epistemology A way of knowing the world that reflects a lesbian's own identity and constructions of reality, including of health and illness, in contrast to patriarchal, heterosexist constructions (VanScoy, III, 7).

lesbian invisibility The degree to which lesbian health issues or lesbian identity are hidden or ignored in health services and in the lesbian's interactions with the health care system (VanScoy, III, 7).

libertarianism A conceptual framework applied to health issues that emphasizes the liberty of all individuals to do what they please with themselves and their property, provided they do not interfere with the like liberty of others (Nilstun, IV, 11).

lifespan A framework for individual development that includes chronological age as well as biological and social role transitions (Prohaska & Clark, III, 2).

lifestyle Utilitarian social practices and ways of living adopted by an individual that reflect personal,

group, and socioeconomic identities. A health lifestyle involves decisions to live or not to live healthfully; decisions about food, exercise, coping with stress, smoking, alcohol and drug use, risk of accidents, and physical appearance; and reflects social norms and values (Cockerham, I, 12).

lifestyle changes Modifications of behavior resulting from negotiated agreements rather than physician's orders (Chrisler, II, 17).

locality development A cooperative, broadly based approach to community health promotion interventions involving wide discussion and joint problem solving among many diverse groups (Rothman, 1979, in Schooler & Flora, IV, 15).

locational attributes Proximity, centrality, and convenience of health care facilities (Scarpaci & Kearns, II, 5).

locus of control, internal Beliefs that things that happen are a result of one's own ability to influence events as opposed to being the result of chance or fate or of powerful other forces; has been used to predict varied health behaviors (Reich, Zautra, & Erdal, I, 5).

managed care A form of delivering health services in which an organization assumes total responsibility and financial risk for its participants' health, providing all needed services and treatments on a prepaid, capitation basis; an outgrowth of *health maintenance organizations (HMOs)* (Daughtery, IV, 10).

management, health care Tasks of planning, organizing, directing, communicating, coordinating, and monitoring organizational functions in health settings by persons specifically designated and empowered to do so; execution of these tasks through an orderly institutional process carried out by persons designated as managers, regardless of their specific titles (Daugherty, IV, 10).

manager, health care An administrator, executive, director, or chief; anyone who has, or shares in, the legal authority and responsibility for the functions, direction, and achievements of a health organization (Daugherty, IV, 10).

media advocacy Use of mass media to advance a social or public policy objective (Pertschuk, 1988, in Schooler & Flora, IV, 15).

medical anthropology The study of cultural factors related to disease and its explanations, and to healing, treatment, responses to illness and interactions between healers and persons who are sick (Gochman, IV, 20).

medical geography The study of physical, climatic, and locational factors related to disease and its explanations and to healing, treatment, responses to illness, and interactions between healers and persons who are sick (Barrett, 1993, in Gochman, IV, 20).

medical model A framework for looking at illness that is based largely on the 19th-century linkages of germ theory and acute diseases and that accords physicians and medical institutions primacy in diagnosis and treatment; an overdependence on medical metaphors in dealing with behavioral variability and problems in living.

medical pluralism Existence of a multiplicity of medical systems, usually biomedical plus varied indigenous ones, within a society; alternatively, a multiplicity of healing techniques, rather than of medical systems (Durkin-Longley, 1984, in Gochman, I, Part V; Stoner, 1986, in Gochman, IV, 20).

medical sociology The study of social and societal factors related to disease and its explanations and to healing, treatment, responses to illness, and interactions between healers and persons who are sick (Gochman, IV, 20).

medicalization Expansion of the jurisdiction of the profession of medicine to include many problems not previously defined as medical entities (Gabe & Calnan, 1989, in Gochman, I, Part IV).

medication event monitor system A device attached to a medication bottle that records the date and time of every opening, for use in studying adherence (Di Iorio, II, 11).

medicocentrism Practice of viewing health- and illness-related phenomena solely from the point of view of the physician, particularly in reference to *sick role* (Segall, I, 14).

meme A unit of symbolic cultural information (Fabrega, I, 2). See *healmeme*.

mental illness, severe (SMI) A diagnosis in the family of schizophrenic or any other psychotic disorders, or any bipolar disorder, as well as any other medical disorder that is of at least 2 years' duration and disables the patient in at least two major areas of life (Hawley, III, 12).

mutual participation model A framework for physician–patient interaction in which the patient takes an active role in care and both parties share the goal of the patient's well-being (Szasz & Hollender, 1956, in DiMatteo, II, 1).

narrative representation Presentation of materials in the context of a story about someone doing something, for some purpose, that results in specific consequences; used in interventions to increase safety and reduce injury (Cole, IV, 17).

narrative thinking Translation of personal experiences into stories that integrate facts, perceptions, emotions, intentions, actions, and consequences into coherent meaning; involves knowing through stories lived and stories heard and told; contrasted with *paradigmatic thinking* (Howard, 1991, in Cole, IV, 17).

National Health Care for the Homeless An initiative take in 1984 by the Robert Wood Johnson Foundation and the Pew Charitable Trusts to establish health care clinics for the homeless in 19 United States cities (Wright & Joyner, III, 10).

need factor A characteristic such as health status or illness that predicts use of health services; a component of the *health services utilization model* (Aday & Awe, I, 8).

negotiating An intervention to increase adherence that involves medical personnel and the patient jointly discussing and agreeing upon the treatment plan (Creer & Levstek, II, 7).

negotiating model of decision making A framework for physician–patient interaction in which physician and patient belief systems and expectations are given equal value (Reed et al., IV, 2).

occupational culture Group norms and practices within work settings that often shape the discourse on health, including how workers define situations of threat and danger, and influence risk behaviors such as smoking and alcohol use (Eakin, I, 16).

operational research model A way of conducting investigations that begins with a practical, problem-focused question rather than with a conceptual framework; characteristic of research in international health (Coreil, III, 9).

oral rehydration therapy (ORT) An intervention to treat diarrheal conditions in *developing countries* (Coreil, III, 9).

organizational barrier A structural problem within the health care system that hampers a patient's perceptions of availability and accessibility of care; organizational barriers may include compromised quality of care, patient's perceptions of inhospitable facilities, distance and transportation problems, waiting time, inflexible hours, dearth or lack of bilingual or bicultural staff, and exclusionary policies (Morisky & Cabrera, II, 14).

organizational culture   See *occupational culture*.

outcome expectancy   A person's beliefs about the consequences of some behavior (e.g., Maddux & DuCharme, I, 7; Baranowski, I, 9); perceived value of the consequence of a given behavior (Di Iorio, II, 11).

pain   A multifaceted noxious experience involving sensory, cognitive, and emotional dimensions (Gift & White, IV, 7).

paradigmatic thinking   Cognitive processes concerned with the construction of context-free and abstract formal concepts and principles; both the goal and method of science, logic, and mathematics, in contrast to *narrative thinking* (Cole, IV, 17).

parochialism/cosmopolitanism   A conceptual framework for understanding social ties within families and families' relationships to the larger community. Parochial families are presumed to demonstrate strong commitment to family (usually paternal) tradition and authority and to have enduring friendships primarily with persons whose backgrounds are similar to their own; cosmopolitan families demonstrate less commitment to family authority and expand their friendships over time, including persons with diverse backgrounds. This typology has guided some research into use of health services and attitudes toward health professionals, but its value has been limited (Suchman, 1965, in Geertsen, I, 13).

passive prevention   See *prevention, passive*.

paternalism   Characterizing an act by a person or a group, *P*, intended to avert some harm or promote some good for a person or a group, *Q*, where *P* has no reason to believe that the act agrees with the current preferences, desires, or dispositions of *Q*, and *P*'s act is a limitation of *Q*'s right to self-determination (Nilstun, IV, 11).

patient role   The component of the sick role that involves interaction with health professionals and/or the formal health care system, in contrast to *self-care* and informal care behaviors (Segall, I, 14).

perceived barriers   A person's belief that a specified health action has negative value, particularly in terms of impediments or costs; a component of the *health belief model* (Strecher et al., I, 4).

perceived behavioral control   A person's belief in the relative ease or difficulty of performing a specified health action; importance increases as volitional control decreases (Maddux & DuCharme, I, 7); similar to *self-efficacy*.

perceived benefits   A person's belief that a specified health action has positive value, particularly in reducing the threat of an illness or health condition; a component of the *health belief model* (Strecher et al., I, 4).

perceived health competence   Belief in one's ability to influence one's personal health outcomes effectively (Christensen et al., II, 12).

perceived severity/seriousness   A person's belief that an illness or health condition would have negative consequences; a component of the *health belief model* (Strecher et al., I, 4).

perceived social norm   A person's belief about how other people view and evaluate a behavior (e.g., Maddux & DuCharme, I, 7).

perceived susceptibility   A person's belief about risk for an illness or health condition; a component of the *health belief model* (Strecher et al., I, 4).

perceived threat   A function of perceived susceptibility and perceived seriousness providing an impetus for taking some action; a component of the *health belief model* (Strecher et al., I, 4); also a component of *protection motivation theory*.

physician authority   See *authority, physician*.

physician autonomy   See *autonomy, physician*.

poverty   An exceptionally low standard of living officially defined by the U.S. Bureau of the Census, based ultimately on cost of food and adjusted annually for inflation (Wright & Joyner, III, 10).

power, patient   The degree to which patients exert control over encounters with physicians and other health care professionals; basic factors are the patient's age, gender, race, education and knowledge, and health status (Haug, II, 3).

power, physician   Dominance of and control by the physician over patients and other health professionals; basic factors are the physician's age, gender, race, practice style, and social status (Haug, II, 3).

precaution adoption process model   A conceptual framework to predict protective or risk-reducing behavior; identifies five basic stages—unaware, aware but not personally engaged, engaged but deciding on a course of action, planning to act but not yet doing so, and acting—plus a maintenance stage (Weinstein & Sandman, 1992, in Gochman, I, Part II). See *transtheoretical model*.

PRECEDE   Acronym for part of a conceptual framework for developing and evaluating health education programs, denoting the basic terms: *Predisposing, Reinforcing,* and *Enabling Causes in Educational Di-*

agnosis and *Evaluation* (Green, Kreuter, Deeds, & Partridge, 1980, in Glanz & Oldenberg, IV, 8). See *PROCEED*.

precontemplation   In the *transtheoretical model*, the stage at which there is no apparent intention to change behavior (Prohaska & Clark, III, 2).

predisposing factor   A characteristic such as a health belief, family composition, or social position of family that predicts use of health services; a component of the *health services utilization model* (Aday & Awe, I, 8).

preparation   In the *transtheoretical model*, the stage at which a person has taken small steps to engage in some behavior but has not yet taken effective action (Prohaska & Clark, III, 2).

PREPARED™   Acronymic name of a system of improving provider–patient communication and patient self-efficacy and satisfaction; denotes the basic components: recommended *Procedure*, *Reason for it*, patient's *Expectations*, *Probability* of achieving them, *Alternative* treatments, *Risks*, *Expenses*, prior to making a *Decision* (DiMatteo, II, 1).

prevention, active   Individual actions to eliminate or reduce the likelihood of a negative health outcome, in contrast to *passive prevention* (Gauff & Miller, 1986, in Gochman, I, 1).

prevention, passive   Societal, institutional, or governmental activities to eliminate or reduce the likelihood of a negative health outcome, in contrast to *active prevention* (Gauff & Miller, 1986, in Gochman, I, 1).

prevention/preventive behavior   Any activity (medically recommended or not) undertaken to eliminate or reduce the likelihood of contracting a disease or incurring a negative health outcome, or of detecting a disease at an early, asymptomatic stage (Gochman, I, 1).

prevention, primary   Reduction or elimination of risk factors (Last, 1987, in Buchanan, IV, 9).

prevention, secondary   Asymptomatic detection of a disease in its early stages (Gochman, I, 1).

principle of justice   See *justice, principle of*.

problem-based learning   An approach to professional education in which curricular materials resemble problems that students will face as practitioners (Bruhn, IV, 1).

PROCEED   Acronym for part of a conceptual framework for developing and evaluating health education programs, denoting the basic terms: *Policy*, *Regulatory*, and *Organizational Constructs for Educational and Environmental Development* (Green et al., 1980, in Glanz & Oldenburg, IV, 8). See *PRECEDE*.

professional role   See *role, physician/provider*.

protection motivation theory   A conceptual framework to determine the effects of threatening health information on attitude and behavior change; basic components are internal and external sources of information, cognitive mediating processes of *threat appraisal* and *coping appraisal*, and adaptive or maladaptive coping modes (Rogers & Prentice-Dunn, I, 6).

psychosocial epidemiology   Application of epidemiological methods to determine health-related personal and social characteristics in a population, e.g., people's perceptions of social support, religiosity, and health (Rakowski, III, 5).

public health   Collective actions of society to assure the conditions for people to be healthy (Institute of Medicine, 1988, in Buchanan, IV, 9).

reactance   Workers' tendency to be defiant about safety and risk behaviors as a way of maintaining their control when they believe their behavior is being manipulated (Cohen & Colligan, II, 20). See *illusion of safety*.

reciprocal determinism   A concept expressing the constant interaction between a person, the person's behavior, and the person's family and social environment in the development and maintenance of health behaviors (Baranowski, I, 9; Baranowski & Hearn, IV, 16).

relapse   In the *transtheoretical model*, the movement from one stage to a previous stage (Prohaska & Clark, III, 2); in the context of regimens of dental flossing and brushing for plaque removal, defined as *adherence* at less than 43% (McCaul, II, 16).

relapse prevention model   A conceptual framework, derived from *social learning theory*, for understanding how and why people backslide from a path of behavior change (Marlatt & Gordon, 1985, in Marcus et al., II, 18).

relative risk   Ratio of adverse health consequences of a specified behavior accruing to groups who do and do not perform that behavior (Prohaska & Clark, III, 2).

resource model of preventive health behavior   A conceptual framework in nursing to predict health actions; basic components are health resources, including perceived health status, energy level, concern about health, feelings about taking care of one's health; and social resources, such as educational level and income (Kulbok, 1985, in Blue & Brooks, IV, 5).

response efficacy Belief that adopting a behavior will reduce some threat (Strecher et al., I, 4).

risk behavior, sexual Any behavior that increases the likelihood of a sexually transmitted disease (STD), including *AIDS*; such behaviors include sexual intercourse without latex protection, actions that expose open sores or cuts to infected bodily fluids, and sharing intravenous drug use apparatus (Thomason & Campos, III, 8).

risk, relative See *relative risk*.

role, physician/provider A set of normative expectations for the full-time professional activity of caring for the sick, involving the development of technical proficiency, affective neutrality, and objectivity and placing the welfare of the patient above that of the professional's personal interests (Parsons, 1951, 1975, in Salloway et al., II, 4).

role, sick See *patient role*; *sick role*.

safe sex Sexual behavior in which there is no chance of direct bloodstream access to infected blood, blood products, seminal fluid, vaginal fluid, or breast milk (Thomason & Campos, III, 8).

safer sex Sexual behavior that reduces the likelihood of exchange of bodily fluids (Thomason & Campos, III, 8).

secular trend Health behavioral changes in a community that are not attributable to health education or health promotion intervention (Glanz & Oldenburg, IV, 8).

selective survival Changes in the composition of a population due to the higher mortality rates at advancing age of individuals participating in risk behaviors (Prohaska & Clark, III, 2).

self-care A process whereby laypersons can function effectively on their own behalf in health promotion and prevention and in detecting and treating disease (Levin, 1976, in Gochman, I, Part IV); often used interchangeably with *self-management, self-regulation* (Di Iorio, II, 11). See *self health management*.

self-care agency An individual's capacity to gather information, make decisions, and perform skillfully the behaviors necessary to assume personal control in health promotion and maintenance as well as in the prevention and treatment of illness (e.g., Orem, 1985, in Blue & Brooks, IV, 5).

self-care autonomy Demonstrating the ability and skills necessary to self-manage a condition (Wysocki & Greco, II, 9).

self-care autonomy, appropriate Expecting a child to have the requisite ability and skills to manage a condition at a level appropriate to the child's maturity (Wysocki & Greco, II, 9).

self-care autonomy, constrained Expecting a child to have the requisite ability and skills to manage a condition at a level less than appropriate to the child's maturity (Wysocki & Greco, II, 9).

self-care autonomy, excessive Expecting a child to have the requisite ability and skills to manage a condition at a level greater than appropriate to the child's maturity (Wysocki, II, 9).

self-efficacy Belief or judgment about one's ability to execute some action successfully (Strecher et al., I, 4; Maddux & DuCharme, I, 7); confidence in one's ability to perform a particular behavior (Baranowski, I, 9). See *health belief model*; *perceived behavioral control*; *protection motivation theory*; *theory of reasoned action*.

self health management Undertaking of lay activities to promote health, to prevent illness, and to detect and treat illness when it occurs; includes a range of behaviors such as: health maintenance activities, illness prevention, symptom evaluation, self-treatment, and use of a variety of health resources such as lay network members as well as diverse health professionals (Segall, I, 14).

self-management, childhood diabetes Assumption of responsibility by a patient and the patient's family for monitoring, evaluating, and adjusting treatment; basic components include demographic factors, family functioning, psychological stress, and interactions with providers to acquire necessary skills (Wysocki & Greco, II, 9). See *self-regulation/self-regulatory skills*.

self-management, epilepsy Sum total of steps a person takes to control seizures and to control the effects of having a seizure disorder; common practices include taking medications at prescribed times, avoiding factors that trigger seizures, following safety precautions such as not driving when seizures are not under control, avoiding running out of medications, consulting with professionals about treatment or unexpected problems, and monitoring seizure frequency; often used interchangeably with *self-care, self-regulation* (Di Iorio, II, 11).

self-prediction What one states one will do in contrast to *behavioral intention*: what one predicts one will do (Maddux & DuCharme, I, 7). See *intention, behavioral*; *theory of reasoned action*.

self-regulation/self-regulatory skills   Ability to control or change one's health behavior, including goal setting, monitoring movement toward goals, exerting effort and skill to reach goals, and rewarding self for attaining goals (Baranowski, I, 9); used interchangeably with *self-care*, *self-management* (Di Iorio, II, 11); a conceptual framework designed to understand behavior change, particularly in relation to disease management; basic components include *self-efficacy*, *outcome expectancy*, monitoring feedback, role modeling, social support, and learning of necessary skills (Clark, II, 8).

sense of place   Personal and social meanings or particular significance that people attach to physical locations or settings, as distinct from the objective or physical space dimensions (Tuan, 1974, in Scarpaci & Kearns, II, 5; Gochman, IV, 20).

setting   The conventional "bricks and mortar" facilities in which health care takes place as well as the psychosocial implications of such places for provider–patient encounters (Scarpaci & Kearns, II, 5).

sex, safe   See *safe sex*.

sexism   In health care, a focus primarily on male health issues and on health roles for women that are subordinate to those of men (Elder, Humphreys, & Lakowski, 1988, in VanScoy, III, 7).

shared decision making model   A framework for physician–patient interaction in which the physician is obliged to present the patient with all available information without filtering it, and without giving advice, in order for the patient to be able to make the most informed decision about care (Wennberg, 1990, in Reed et al., IV, 2).

sick call   The processing of health complaints in correctional facilities, which requires that inmates sign up, have their requests reviewed and triaged, and then be seen by a provider; inmates have no choice of providers or of appointment time (Anno, III, 14).

sick role   A conceptual framework developed by Parsons (1951, in Segall, I, 14) for analyzing the behavior of a person who has been diagnosed as ill; basic components are the person's rights to be exempt from responsibility for the incapacity and from normal role and task obligations and the person's duties to seek professional care and to abide by professional advice and recover (Segall, I, 14).

sick role, alternative   Elaboration of the Parsonian *sick role* model, adding the person's rights to make decisions about health care and to be dependent on lay others for care and social support and the person's duties to maintain health and overcome illness and to engage in routine self-management; assumes that members of the person's social network are prepared to take on added responsibilities and to function as caregivers as needed (Segall, I, 14).

sickness   A departure from being healthy, often defined through a combination of symptoms experienced, not feeling "right" or "normal," and consequences such as restricted activity (Lau, I, 3); the social side of illness (Gochman, I, 1); the social construction of an episode of illness, the way illness is dealt with in society (Fabrega, I, 2); a form of deviance (Segall, I, 14); the contextualized definition of dysfunction, a process by which signs and symptoms are given socially recognizable meanings (Dressler & Oths, I, 17).

social action   An approach to community health promotion interventions involving advocacy or conflict strategy that entails mass mobilization of low-power components and use of political pressure (Rothman, 1979, in Schooler & Flora, IV, 15).

social cognitive theory   A general social psychological conceptual framework adapted to understand the acquisition or health behaviors; basic components are *outcome expectancy*, *self-efficacy*, skills, and social evaluation of and feedback on behavior (Baranowski, I, 9; Di Iorio, II, 11; Marcus et al., II, 18).

social epidemiology   See *psychosocial epidemiology*.

social learning theory   A conceptual framework for understanding the acquisition of health behaviors; basic components are observation, modeling, and reinforcement in interpersonal contexts (Tinsley, I, 11; Marcus et al., II, 18).

social marketing   Use of merchandising and advertising techniques to increase the effectiveness of health-related campaigns, e.g., for immunizations and family planning; basic components are lowering the price; responding to market demands, such as needs; emphasizing relative advantages of the service or product; making the service or product accessible to the population; and using a full range of mass media to promote the service or product (Buchanan, IV, 9).

social network   A broad conceptual framework for examining social ties and social support; includes dimensions of structure (e.g., number and density of linkages, interaction (e.g., nature and quality), and function (e.g., provision of information, resources, and emotional support). Not identical to *social support*; networks may be unsupportive (Ritter, 1988, in Gochman, I, Part IV).

social norms   Generally held beliefs about the appropriateness or desirability of some behavior.

social planning   A technical approach to community health promotion interventions using rational empirical processes of data accumulation, and persuasion involving experts (Rothman, 1979, in Schooler & Flora, IV, 15).

social structure   The organization or patterning of social ties; regularities in interpersonal linkages. *Parochialism/cosmpolitanism* has been a major typology of social structure relevant to health behavior research (Geertsen, I, 13).

social support   Aggregate of social ties involving interpersonal relationships that protect people from negative experiences, including both structural (e.g., living arrangements, participation in social activities) and functional (e.g., emotional support, encouraging expression of feelings, provision of advice) dimensions (e.g., Ritter, 1988, in Gochman, I, Part IV); a range of interpersonal exchanges that include not only the provision of physical, social, and emotional assistance, but also the subjective consequences of making individuals feel that they are the subject of enduring concern by others (Pilisuk & Parks, 1981, in Morisky & Cabrera, II, 14).

social support, directive   Assumption by others of responsibility for tasks or decisions in relation to *adherence* (Fisher et al., II, 10).

social support, nondirective   Participation by others in cooperating, sharing, and expressing understanding of feelings in relation to *adherence* without attempts to control or alter tasks or decisions (Fisher et al., II, 10).

social ties   Interpersonal linkages, including those with household members, relatives, and friends (Geertsen, I, 13).

sociology of medicine   See *medical sociology*.

specific etiology, doctrine of   An essentially mechanistic medical model that specified that for each illness there was a single, necessary, and sufficient causal agent or pathogen (Pasteur, 1873 [cited in Hamann, 1994], in Wiese & Gallagher, IV, 4).

stage models of adoption   See *transtheoretical model*.

stages of change models   See *transtheoretical model*.

stepped-care model   A conceptual framework for increasing smoking cessation that matches intensity of treatment to stages of change (Glasglow & Orleans, II, 19).

stereotyping   Physician's categorization of a patient as bad or undesirable, using the patient's behavior as a clue indicative of potential challenge to the physician's authority (Ben-Sira, II, 2).

support-mobilizing hypothesis   A conceptual framework for understanding caregiver behavior, based on the assumption that stress will motivate the caregiver to elicit support (Bass, Tausig, & Noelker, 1988/1989, in Wright, III, 13).

t'ai chi   An ancient Chinese system of exercise and meditation being introduced in selected religious communities as a health behavior intervention (Duckro, Magaletta, & Wolf, III, 15).

theory of planned behavior   See *theory of reasoned action*.

theory of reasoned action   A conceptual framework designed to predict intentions to engage in or change specified health behaviors (Maddux & DuCharme, I, 7); basic components are a person's attitudes toward a specified behavior and a person's perceptions of the social norms regarding the behavior. See *intention, behavioral*; *self-prediction*.

therapeutic landscape   See *landscape, therapeutic*.

threat appraisal   Evaluation of maladaptive responses (Rogers & Prentice-Dunn, I, 6). See *protection motivation theory*.

transtheoretical model   A conceptual framework for predicting behavior change that assumes a progression of stages from *precontemplation* of change through *contemplation*, *preparation*, *action*, maintenance, and *relapse*, with different intervention approaches appropriate for each stage (Prohaska & Di Clemente, 1992, in Gochman, I, Part II; Rimer et al., II, 15; Glasgow & Orleans, II, 19); incorporates behavioral intentions, *decisional balance theory*, *self-efficacy*, and individual processes of behavioral change (Marcus et al., II, 18).

utilitarianism   A conceptual framework applied to health issues that emphasizes the maximization of some desired state (Nilstun, IV, 11).

utilization framework   A refinement of the *health services utilization model* designed to predict type and purpose of health care use; basic components are societal determinants such as technology and social norms, health service system resources and organizations, and *predisposing*, *enabling*, and *need factors* (Andersen & Newman, 1973, in Aday & Awe, I, 8).

value-based learning   An approach to professional education that places values, ethics, and moral issues at the curricular core (Bruhn, IV, 1).

wellness   Realization of the optimum health potential of an individual, family, or community; achieved by enhancing physical, psychological, and sociological well-being through activities aimed at the promotion of health (Blue & Brooks, IV, 5).

window of vulnerability   A period in the family life cycle when the strength of the family's influence on health behaviors has the potential for diminishing (Lau, Quadrel, & Hartman, 1990, in Gochman, I, 10).

worksite program   One or more health promotion activities conducted in an occupational setting (Schooler & Flora, IV, 15).

Contents of Volumes I–IV

VOLUME II. PROVIDER DETERMINANTS

VOLUME III.   DEMOGRAPHY, DEVELOPMENT, AND DIVERSITY

Index to Volumes I–IV

In addition to the entries in this Index, the reader is encouraged to look at the Contents of each volume and the Contents of Volumes I–IV that appears at the end of each volume, as well as at the Glossary contained in each volume. Space limitations precluded listing *every* intervention or program, government document, or disease or condition identified in the chapters. Similarly, passages dealing *solely* with etiologies, morbidity, mortality, and demographic correlates of diseases with no relevance for health behavior were not indexed.

ISBN 0-306-45446-7

90000